OBSESSIVE-COMPULSIVE DISORDERS
Practical Management

OBSESSIVE-COMPULSIVE DISORDERS
Practical Management

Third Edition

Michael A. Jenike, M.D.
Director, Obsessive-Compulsive Disorders
Clinic and Research Unit
Massachusetts General Hospital
Professor of Psychiatry, Harvard Medical School,
Boston, Massachusetts

Lee Baer, Ph.D.
Director, Psychological Research
Obsessive-Compulsive Disorders Clinic and Research Unit
Massachusetts General Hospital
Associate Professor of Psychology
Department of Psychology, Harvard Medical School
Boston, Massachusetts

William E. Minichiello, Ed.D.
Director, Psychological Clinical Services, Behavior Therapist
Obsessive-Compulsive Disorders Clinic and Research Unit
Massachusetts General Hospital
Assistant Professor of Psychology, Department of Psychiatry
Harvard Medical School, Boston, Massachusetts

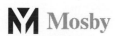

St. Louis Baltimore Boston Carlsbad Chicago Minneapolis New York Philadelphia Portland
London Milan Sydney Tokyo Toronto

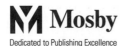

Mosby

Dedicated to Publishing Excellence

A Times Mirror
Company

Managing Editor: Laura DeYoung
Developmental Editor: Rebecca Gruliow
Production Manager: David Orzechowski
Production Editor: Anthony F. Trioli
Manufacturing Supervisor: William A. Winneberger, Jr.
Design Manager: Carolyn O'Brien
Cover Images: © Tony Stone Images

Third Edition
Copyright © 1998 by Mosby, Inc.

Previous editions copyrighted 1986 and 1990.

Printed in the United States of America
Composition by Barbara Crawford
Printing/binding by R.R. Donnelley & Sons, Co.

Mosby, Inc.
11830 Westline Industrial Drive
St. Louis, MO 63146

Library of Congress Cataloging-in-Publication Data
Obsessive-compulsive disorders : practical management / [edited by]
    Michael A. Jenike, Lee Baer, William E. Minichiello. -- 3rd ed.
        p.   cm.
    Includes biographical references and index.
    ISBN 0-8151-3840-7
    1. Obsessive-compulsive disorder.   2. Obsessive-compulsive
disorder--Treatment.   I. Jenike, Michael A.   II. Baer, Lee.
III. Minichiello, William E.
    [DNLM: 1. Obsessive-Compulsive Disorder--etiology.   2. Obsessive
-Compulsive Disorder--therapy.   WM 176 O146 1998]
RC533.028   1998
616.85'227--DC21   97-48499
                                                                                                          CIP

98 99 00 01 02 / 9 8 7 6 5 4 3 2 1

ABOUT THE EDITORS

Michael A. Jenike, M.D. is director of the Obsessive-Compulsive Disorders Clinic and Research Unit at Massachusetts General Hospital and professor of psychiatry at Harvard Medical School. He is associate chief of psychiatry in the Department of Psychiatry and director of the OCD Institute at McLean Hospital in Belmont, Massachusetts. From 1982 to 1987 he was director of the inpatient psychiatric service and co-director of the Geriatric Psychiatry Memory Disorders Clinic at Massachusetts General Hospital. He also is the chairman of the scientific advisory board of the National OC Foundation.

A psychiatrist with extensive experience in obsessive-compulsive disorder (OCD), Dr. Jenike has conducted a number of research studies on OCD and has published over 400 scientific and clinical papers. He is the author of three books, including *Handbook of Geriatric Psychopharmacology* and *Geriatric Psychiatry: A Clinical Approach*; and the editor of five other books, including *Obsessive-Compulsive Disorders: Practical Management*, and *Clinical Problems in Psychiatry*. He is the former editor of the psychiatry section of *Scientific American Medicine*, editor-in-chief of the *Journal of Geriatric Psychiatry and Neurology*, and a contributing editor to *Psychiatric Times*. He serves on the editorial boards of numerous journals and professional publications. He is a member of several professional societies, including the American Psychiatric Association, Alpha Omega Alpha, and Sigma Xi-the Scientific Research Society.

Dr. Jenike was a member of the DSM-IV committee on the obsessive-compulsive disorders. He has lectured nationally and internationally to physicians and mental health professionals on the topics of OCD, geriatric psychopharmacology, affective illness, and Alzheimer's disease; and has conducted numerous symposia on the drug treatment of psychiatric illness.

Lee Baer, Ph.D. is associate chief of psychology in the Department of Psychiatry at Massachusetts General Hospital and associate professor of psychology at Harvard Medical School. He is director of research at the Obsessive-Compulsive Disorders Clinic, and has extensive experience in the behavioral treatment of patients with OCD and other anxiety, tic, and mood disorders. Dr. Baer is director of the Harvard Telepsychiatry Project, which critically studies applications of telecommunication technologies to make psychiatric treatment more widely available, regardless of geographic barriers.

Dr. Baer has published more than one hundred scientific papers, books, and contributing chapters in the aforementioned areas. He has lectured internationally to mental health professionals and patients. He is the author of the widely acclaimed book *Getting Control*, which has now been published in four languages. He is a key behavior therapist at the OCD Institute at McLean Hospital in Belmont, Massachusetts.

Dr. Baer is on the editorial boards of many of the key scientific journals in psychiatry and is a member of the the scientific advisory board of the OCD Foundation. His professional affiliations include the American Psychological Association and the Association for the Advancement of Behavior Therapy.

William E. Minichiello, Ed.D. is an associate director of the Massachusetts General Hospital OCD Institute at McLean Hospital in Belmont, Massachusetts, and is an assistant professor of psychology at Harvard Medical School. He is on the staff of the Psychopharmacology and Behavior Therapy Units of the hospital.

A clinical psychologist and skilled clinician, Dr. Minichiello is actively engaged in the treatment of patients with severe OCD. He has had extensive experience applying the principles and techniques of behavior therapy to the treatment of patients with OCD, phobias, and psychophysiologic disorders. Dr. Minichiello also is an ordained priest with noncanonical status. His theologic training and pastoral experience have been particularly relevant and important in the management of those patients whose OCD has a religious dimension.

A member of the Association for the Advancement of Behavior Therapy, Dr. Minichiello maintains national accreditation as a member of the National Register of Health Service Providers in Psychology. He is a former member of the scientific advisory board of the National OC Foundation and is currently a member of the scientific advisory board of the OC Foundation of Greater Boston.

CONTRIBUTORS

John P. Alsobrook II, Ph.D.
Associate Research Scientist, Yale University Child Study Center, New Haven, Connecticut

Lee Baer, Ph.D.
Director, Psychological Research, Obsessive Compulsive Disorders Clinic and Research Unit, Massachusetts General Hospital, Charlestown, Massachusetts; Associate Professor of Psychology, Department of Psychiatry, Harvard Medical School, Boston, Massachusetts

Diane Baney, R.N., M.B.A.
Program Manager, Obsessive-Compulsive Disorders Institute, Massachusetts General Hospital, Charlestown, Massachusetts

Lewis R. Baxter, Jr., M.D.
Kathy Ireland Professor of Psychiatric Research, University of Alabama, Birmingham, Alabama

Maria Lynn Buttolph, M.D., Ph.D.
Instructor in Psychiatry, Harvard Medical School, Boston, Massachusetts

Sudeep Chakravorty, M.D.
Assistant Clinical Instructor, State University of New York at Buffalo; Chief Resident, State University of New York at Buffalo, Buffalo General Hospital, Buffalo, New York

Joseph W. Ciarrocchi, Ph.D.
Associate Professor and Director of Doctoral Clinical Education, Loyola College, Columbia, Maryland

Barbara J. Coffey, M.D.
Assistant Professor of Psychiatry, Harvard Medical School, Boston, Massachusetts; Director, Pediatric Psychopharmacology Clinic, McLean Hospital, Belmont, Massachusetts; Director, Tourette Syndrome Clinic, Massachusetts General Hospital, Charlestown, Massachusetts

Nicholas H. Dodman, B.V.M.S., M.R.C.V.S., D.A.C.V.B.
Professor, Tufts University Veterinary School, North Grafton, Massachusetts; Director, Animal Behavior Clinic, Grafton, Massachusetts

Darin Dougherty, M.D.
Instructor in Psychiatry, Harvard Medical School, Boston, Massachusetts; Department of Psychiatry, Massachusetts General Hospital, Charlestown, Massachusetts

Jane L. Eisen, M.D.
Assistant Professor, Department of Psychiatry and Human Behavior, Brown University; Butler Hospital, Providence, Rhode Island

Denise Egan, M.S.
Counselor Supervisor, Obsessive-
Compulsive Disorders Institute,
Massachusetts General Hospital,
Charlestown, Massachusetts

Steven Friedman, Ph.D.
Professor of Clinical Psychiatry, State
University of New York Health Science
Center at Brooklyn; Director, Phobia
and Anxiety Disorders Clinic,
Brooklyn, New York

Randy O. Frost, Ph.D.
Professor of Psychology, Smith College, Northampton, Massachusetts

**Daniel A. Geller, M.B.B.S.,
F.R.A.C.P.**
Instructor of Psychiatry, Harvard Med-
ical School, Boston, Massachusetts;
Director, Obsessive-Compulsive Disor-
ders Clinic; Co-Director, Tourette Syn-
drome Clinic; Assistant Director, Joint
Program in Pediatric Psychopharma-
cology, McLean Hospital, Belmont,
Massachusetts; Massachusetts General
Hospital, Charlestown, Massachusetts

Wayne K. Goodman, M.D.
Professor and Acting Chairman,
Department of Psychiatry, University
of Florida College of Medicine,
Gainesville, Florida

Marjorie Hatch, Ph.D.
Assistant Professor of Psychology,
Southern Methodist University, Dallas,
Texas

Amy D. Holland, M.Ed.
Marblehead, Massachusetts

Donald E. Jefferys, Ph.D.
Associate, Department of Psychiatry,
Austin Hospital, University of Melbourne; The Melbourne Clinic, Rich-
mond, Victoria, Australia

Michael A. Jenike, M.D.
Director, Obsessive-Compulsive Disor-
ders Clinic and Research Unit,
Massachusetts General Hospital,
Charlestown, Massachusetts;
Professor of Psychiatry, Harvard Med-
ical School, Boston, Massachusetts

Janice Jones, B.A.
Research Associate, Harvard Medical
School, Boston, Massachusetts;
Psychometrician, McLean Hospital,
Belmont, Massachusetts;
Massachusetts General Hospital,
Charlestown, Massachusetts

Nancy J. Keuthen, Ph.D.
Assistant Professor, Harvard Medical
School, Boston, Massachusetts;
Co-Director, Trichotillomania Clinic;
Staff Psychologist, Obsessive-
Compulsive Disorders Unit,
Massachusetts General Hospital,
Charlestown, Massachusetts

Peter Manzo, M.S.W.
Research Assistant, Obsessive-
Compulsive Disorders Clinic,
Massachusetts General Hospital,
Charlestown, Massachusetts

John S. March, M.D., M.P.H.
Director, Program in Child and Adolescent Anxiety Disorders, Duke University Medical Center, Durham, North
Carolina

William E. Minichiello, Ed.D.
Assistant Professor of Psychology, Department of Psychiatry, Harvard Medical School, Boston, Massachusetts; Director, Psychological Clinical Services; Behavior Therapist, Obsessive-Compulsive Disorders Clinic and Research Unit, Massachusetts General Hospital, Charlestown, Massachusetts

Richard L. O'Sullivan, M.D.
Assistant Professor of Psychiatry, Harvard Medical School, Boston, Massachusetts; Co-Director, Trichotillomania Clinic, Psychiatric Neuroscience Program, Massachusetts General Hospital, Charlestown, Massachusetts

Cheryl M. Paradis, Psy.D.
Clinical Associate Professor, State University of New York at Brooklyn, Health Science Center, Brooklyn, New York

Michele T. Pato, M.D.
Associate Professor, State University of New York at Buffalo; Director of Residency Training; Director of Ambulatory Services, Buffalo General Hospital, Buffalo, New York

David L. Pauls, Ph.D.
Associate Professor, Child Study Center, Yale University, New Haven, Connecticut

Kathleen E. Peets, B.A.
Boston, Massachusetts

Katharine A. Phillips, M.D.
Assistant Professor of Psychiatry and Human Behavior, Brown University School of Medicine; Chief, Outpatient Services; Director, Body Dysmorphic Disorder Program, Butler Hospital, Providence, Rhode Island

Lawrence H. Price, M.D.
Professor of Psychiatry, Brown University School of Medicine; Chief, Mood Disorders Program; Director of Research, Butler Hospital, Providence, Rhode Island

Steven A. Rasmussen, M.D.
Associate Professor, Brown University Medical Director, Butler Hospital, Providence, Rhode Island

Scott L. Rauch, M.D.
Associate Professor of Psychiatry, Harvard Medical School, Boston, Massachusetts; Director, Psychiatric Neuroimaging Research, Massachusetts General Hospital, Charlestown, Massachusetts

Josée Rhéaume, Ph.D.
Clinical Psychologist, University of Laval, Quebec, Canada

Johan Rosqvist, M.S.W.
Counselor, OCD Institute, MGH

Cary R. Savage, Ph.D.
Assistant Professor, Harvard Medical School, Boston, Massachusetts; Assistant in Psychology, Massachusetts General Hospital, Charlestown, Massachusetts

Stephanie Shapiro, B.A.
Research Assistant, Harvard Medical School, Boston, Massachusetts; Psychometrician, McLean Hospital, Belmont, Massachusetts; Massachusetts General Hospital, Charlestown, Massachusetts

Gail S. Steketee, Ph.D.
Professor and Associate Dean, School of Social Work, Boston University; Consultant, Center for Anxiety and Related Disorders, Boston, Massachusetts

Barbara L. Van Noppen, M.S.W., L.I.S.W.
Research Associate, Department of Psychiatry, Brown University; Senior Clinician, Obsessive-Compulsive Disorders Clinic, Butler Hospital; Private Practice, Providence, Rhode Island

Paul J. Whalen, Ph.D.
Instructor in Psychology, Harvard Medical School, Boston, Massachusetts; Department of Psychiatry, Massachusetts General Hospital, Charlestown, Massachusetts

Sabine Wilhem, Ph.D.
Clinical Fellow in Psychology (Psychiatry), Department of Psychiatry, Harvard Medical School, Boston, Massachusetts; Clinical Fellow in Psychology (Psychiatry), Massachusetts General Hospital, Charlestown, Massachusetts

B. Steven Willis, Ph.D.
Instructor in Psychiatry, Harvard Medical School, Boston, Massachusetts; Associate Director, Obsessive-Compulsive Disorders Institute, Massachusetts General Hospital, Charlestown, Massachusetts

To Julie, Lisa, Eric, Sara, Una, Andrew, Ian, Donna, and my patients,
with love and appreciation.

Michael A. Jenike

To Carole Ann, David, Emily, William, and Bernice, with love.

Lee Baer

To Marcia, Liz, Ann Marie, Aurelio, Connie, and all my patients, with
love and gratitude.

William E. Minichiello

FOREWORD TO THE FIRST EDITION

One of the first patients I treated when I was a psychiatric resident was a middle-aged gentleman with a compulsion to pull nails out of the walls. Until I met him, I had no idea of the number of random tacks, brads, bolts, screws, and pegs one could find on the vertical surfaces of a room. During one therapeutic hour he managed to strip my office of pictures, diplomas, and certificates in order to pluck out the supporting nail. While I was clearly able to see the association between his behavior and the expression of hostility and control, my insight did nothing to alter his actions. Nothing that I offered him in the way of treatment helped. None of the few available drugs in the late 1950s was effective, and ECT only served to confuse him. Eventually he left me for another therapist. Years later I learned he had found his way to Virginia and had been cured by behavior therapy. At that time I had only the scantiest acquaintance with this form of treatment, and it came as a surprise that a method as safe and simple as behavior modification could effect a change in so profound a disorder. Having witnessed the results of Dr. Minichiello's and Dr. Baer's work as described in this volume, I have developed substantial respect for their ability to mend behavior.

My experience with this patient is by no means atypical. Anyone who has labored to treat patients with obsessive-compulsive disorder (OCD) knows the awesome and unyielding power possessed by cleaning and checking rituals and obsessive thoughts. They often seem as fixed in the lives of these patients as a spinal reflex. It came as no surprise that psychosurgical lesions could sometimes extirpate these symptoms. Since they seemed as much a part of the patient's mental landscape as drumlins, one could expect to remove them only by excavation. The association between OCD and neurologic illness furthered the view that organic lesions caused this disorder.

While theories of Janet and Freud had served as models to explicate the mental mechanisms underlying these irrational rituals and thoughts, the failure of their application to bring about a cure caused even staunch advocates to view them skeptically. Despite the poor therapeutic results, the symptom complex of OCD continued to fascinate psychotherapists and scientists. We see enough of these traits in ourselves to suspect that they form the substrate for normalcy and civility as well as for disease. For example, most of us can measure our day by rituals. Like monks practicing canonical hours, we shave and drink coffee on arising, lunch with friends at noon, eat supper at 6:00 P.M., and go to bed after the 11:00 P.M. news. There are, of course, many variations and individual nuances built into this circadian framework. Rituals of living are fixed early in life and seldom change, despite major alterations in living circumstances. The English take tea at 4:00 P.M. whether living tranquilly in Surrey or fighting for their lives on the Somme.

While rituals can add stability and style to our human behavior, they must be adaptable over time, lest they undo us. Wearing a tie stems from the Croatian ritual custom of wrapping a thick cloth pad about the throat to reduce the cutting power of an enemy's sword. Louis XIV was so taken with the sartorial possibilities of this custom that he fashioned the cravat, inaugurating the age of neckwear. Some would, of course, question the utility of this adaptation.

This book, insofar as I know, is one of the most complete compendiums of OCD in the literature. Dr. Jenike and his colleagues offer a book that includes all of the current thinking on OCD. Since the symptoms of this condition are likely a part of other diagnostic entities in psychiatric classification, and since OCD in itself is being found in an increasing number of patients, this volume provides an immense service. It assembles the known current facts of this illness and puts them down in understandable prose that is both clear and unbiased. I recommend it to everyone involved in the practice of psychiatry. I predict it will become the standard text on this disorder for years to come. My only criticism may be remedied in the next edition. A chapter should be devoted to the quirky rituals that have become part of academic life. How many academics wear club ties on Thursdays, brown socks on Tuesdays, drive to work a certain way to ensure success before giving a lecture, or even make offerings to the heavens? I must admit that I carry a lucky piece and always wear the Massachusetts General Hospital tie when I meet with the trustees. Nothing wrong with that—as long as it works.

Thomas P. Hackett, M.D.
Eben S. Draper
Professor of Psychiatry
Harvard Medical School
Chief of Psychiatry (1976-1988)
Massachusetts General Hospital

PREFACE TO THE THIRD EDITION

In the first edition of our book, which was published in 1986, we attempted to include all the important thinking on OCD to that point, and we ended up with 11 chapters. Just 3 years later, in compiling the then current state of knowledge from the leading researchers in the field, the table of contents had more than doubled to 24 chapters. In addition to the steady growth in such areas as pharmacotherapy, behavior therapy, and epidemiology, which were covered in the first edition, several completely new areas that showed exceptional promise in OCD research and treatment were included in the second edition. Among these areas were neuroimaging studies in OCD, familial studies in OCD and Tourette's disorder, studies in childhood OCD, and new neurosurgical treatments for OCD.

Since the publication of the second edition of our book in 1990, further strides have been made in our understanding of obsessive-compulsive disorders. These advances are reflected by the vast increase of available information in this completely revised third edition. Although they were read by large numbers of patients and their families, the first two editions primarily were aimed at clinicians. In this edition, we attempted to make the book more accessible to the consumer while including the technical and clinical information required by professionals. Many patients will be able to understand material on the biology of OCD, whereas others will be more interested in the treatment aspects of this book. In addition to information on biology, genetics, and treatment, we have included material that should be helpful to consumers. For example, in the appendixes we included a section on OCD resources (e.g., physicians, support groups, Internet sites) for those who are interested in OCD. With the coming of age of the Internet, those who have computer access to this tremendously powerful media will be able to take advantage of unprecedented amounts of information. There now are OCD support groups on-line and in places where patients and families can ask questions of OCD experts.

This book begins with an overview of the illnesses of OCD, which includes its classic forms (Chapter 1) and its presentation at different times in the life cycle, such as in childhood (Chapter 3) or during pregnancy (Chapter 5). We review our current knowledge of the onset and course of OCD (Chapter 2) and its relationship to a variety of personality disorders (Chapter 4). Chapter 6 discusses rating scales for OCD.

We then discuss illnesses related to OCD, or so-called spectrum disorders, which are not classic OCD but are commonly encountered in OCD clinics and appear to be closely related, such as Tourette's disorder (Chapter 8), trichotillomania (Chapter 9), body dysmorphic disorder (Chapter 10), and others (Chapter 7).

The rapid growth of theories about the mechanisms and etiologies of OCD are then reviewed. Obsessive-compulsive disorder has progressed from relative obscurity to its current status as one of the most widely researched disorders in psychiatry. Chapters 11 and 12 review theories of the etiology and neurobiology of OCD. Promising technologies recently applied to OCD include neuroimagimg (Chapter 15), neuropsychological testing (Chapter 13), familial studies of OCD and Tourette's disorder (Chapter 14), and attempts to develop an animal model for OCD (Chapter 16).

The section on treatment includes detailed reviews of treatments proved to be at least partially effective for OCD, including behavior therapy (Chapters 17, 19, and 20), cognitive therapy (Chapter 18), medications (Chapter 22), and an often overlooked and controversial area, neurosurgical treatment (Chapter 26). These chapters provide detailed instructions for the clinician who treats patients with OCD. Specific clinical strategies and case vignettes are provided for behavior therapy (Chapter 20), medication discontinuation (Chapter 28), and psychotherapy (Chapter 27), along with a review of treatments for hoarding (Chapter 23) and scrupulosity (Chapter 24). New home-based and inpatient or residential treatments are discussed in Chapter 25, and group and family therapies are included in Chapter 21.

Chapter 29 specifically addresses the pertinent issues that relate to making treatment available to minority group members.

Step-by-step information on running an OCD clinic is included in Chapter 30.

The Appendixes contain helpful supplemental information, such as the history of the OCD Foundation and its pioneering work in establishing self-help treatment groups. Other appendixes contain copies of rating scales, helpful questionnaires that can be used in the evaluation of OCD patients in either research or clinical settings, a list of Internet sites, and a list of books helpful for OCD patients.

The chapters that follow provide an overview of the current state of knowledge of OCD written by experienced clinicians and researchers. The interdisciplinary nature of the research in this field is evident from the wide range of fields of expertise of the contributors, including psychiatry, psychology, neurology, veterinary medicine, neurosurgery, radiology, and social work. The success of this interdisciplinary approach has in a few short years moved us toward the goal we expressed in the first edition, to improve our treatments and to extend their effectiveness to a larger proportion of patients who suffer from OCD.

The authors thank the staff of our OCD clinic and newly formed OCD Institute, whose dedicated efforts are greatly appreciated. We thank Dr. Ned Cassem, chief of psychiatry at Massachusetts General Hospital, for maintaining an exciting and rigorous intellectual atmosphere within our department and for supporting our research, teaching, and clinical activities. We also thank Dr. Steven Willis, Diane Baney, Denise Egan, and Mary Dickie for their tireless efforts on behalf of our patients.

We have included the original foreword to the first edition of this book by Dr. Thomas Hackett, who has since passed away. We no longer hear his infectious laughter or his words of encouragement and wisdom, but fortunately his writings remain. We will never forget him or what he taught us. He remains our inspiration!

CONTENTS

Part I

The Clinical Picture

1

An Overview of Obsessive-Compulsive Disorder

Michael A. Jenike, M.D., Lee Baer, Ph.D., William E. Minichiello, Ed.D.

DEFINITIONS

Obsessive thoughts and compulsive urges or rituals are a part of everyday life. We return home to check that we locked a door, shut off a stove, or turned off our computer. We repetitively think about that stressful event next week. We refuse to eat with the fork that dropped on the floor, although we know the chance of contamination is remote. These events are part of the normal feedback and control loop between our thoughts and our actions. It is only when these obsessive thoughts become so frequent or intense, or these compulsive rituals become so extensive that they interfere with an individual's function that the diagnosis of obsessive-compulsive disorder (OCD) is made. Experts now know that part of the brain circuitry may be involved in OCD, producing the nagging concern that something is not right or that some action must be performed over and over. The brain seems to send itself an "error" message that the patient experiences as OCD.

Obsessive-compulsive disorder is categorized as an anxiety disorder (formerly called *obsessional neurosis*) because central factors seem to be anxiety and discomfort, which are usually increased by the obsessions (thoughts) and decreased by the compulsions or rituals (actions). Although patients with OCD frequently present with irrational or bizarre thoughts regarding their symptoms, they remain reality based in all other areas of their lives; therefore, OCD is not a psychotic disorder.

The currently accepted definition of OCD is given in the *Diagnostic and Statistical Manual of Mental Disorders* (DSM-IV).[1] To be diagnosed with OCD, a patient must have either obsessions or compulsions that are a significant source of distress or that interfere with the patient's social or role functioning.

Obsessions are defined as: "Recurrent, persistent ideas, thoughts, images, or impulses that are experienced, at least initially, as intrusive and senseless, e.g., a parent's having repeated impulses to kill a loved child, a religious person's having recurrent blasphemous thoughts." The person must attempt ". . . to ignore or suppress such thoughts or impulses or to neutralize them with some other thought or action." Finally "the person recognizes that the obsessions are the product of his or her own mind, not imposed from without (as in thought insertion)," and the content of the obsession must be unrelated to any other axis I disorder that may be present.

Compulsions are defined as: "Repetitive, purposeful, and intentional behaviors that are performed in response to an obsession, or according to certain rules or in a stereotyped fashion. The behavior is designed to neutralize or to prevent discomfort or some dreaded event or situation; however, either the activity is not connected in a realistic way with what it is designed to neutralize or prevent, or it is clearly excessive. The person recognizes that his or her behavior is excessive or unreasonable (this may not be true for young children; it may no longer be true for people whose obsessions have evolved into overvalued ideas)."[1]

In DSM-IV, it is now possible for patients to experience mental compulsions in which they repeat numbers or prayers or perform ritualistic thinking such as recalling a whole day's activities in minute detail. The basic principle is that obsessions generally produce anxiety, whereas compulsions are designed to at least temporarily alleviate or lessen anxiety. Thus if a patient mentally counts, prays, or recalls details when anxious or in response to an obsession, this action serves as an attempt to lessen anxiety and is termed a *compulsion*.

Additionally, obsessions or compulsions must cause the patient marked distress, be time consuming (e.g., involve more than 1 hour per day), or significantly interfere with the person's normal routine, occupational functioning, usual social activities, or relationships.[1]

Although DSM-III[2] required that obsession must not be the result of another mental disorder, such as Tourette's disorder, schizophrenia, major depression, or organic mental disorder, DSM-III-R and DSM-IV eliminate these exclusion criteria because it now is recognized that OCD can occur concomitantly with other disorders. This occurrence is seen most clearly when OCD predates the diagnosis of another psychiatric disorder, such as bipolar disorder[3] or major depression.

The syndrome of OCD is much more common than was previously believed. Traditional estimates of OCD in the general population were approximately 0.05%, although recent studies have suggested a significantly higher prevalence of between 2% and 3%. These issues are discussed in more detail in Chapter 2.

OCD can be severely incapacitating; depression is a frequent concomitant problem, and the symptoms can spread to interfere with the patient's social and occupational functioning, often involving the entire family. Rachman and Hodgson[4] have commented on the degree of impairment which can accompany OCD:

When the manifestations of obsessional and compulsive problems are described in print, it frequently is difficult for the reader to appreciate the seriousness of these problems. Without experience of people who have suffered from these difficulties, it is hard to imagine how a persistent compulsive urge to check the security of one's home before leaving for work each morning can grow into a problem of such magnitude as to distort and diminish the person's entire life. In the case of someone who is constantly troubled by intrusive, unacceptable thoughts, it is hard to imagine the amount of suffering involved, and how it can reach such proportions as to imprison the person and prevent him or her from carrying out any constructive work. Even more extreme, it is hard to imagine how a grossly exaggerated fear of dirt and disease can lead an entire family to move to a new house every six months and to avoid entire regions of the county. Of course, most people who suffer from obsessional-compulsive problems do not have them in this degree of severity, but it would be a mistake to underestimate the intensity and extent of the suffering involved.[4]

HISTORY

Obsessive-compulsive disorder has a long history; in the seventeenth century, obsessions and hand-washing rituals were immortalized by Shakespeare in the guilt-ridden character of Lady Macbeth. Even earlier, individuals with obsessive thoughts of a blasphemous or sexual nature were believed to be possessed by the devil. This view was consistent with beliefs of the time, and the logical treatment was designed to expel the demons from the unfortunate possessed soul. Exorcism was the treatment of choice, during which the person was subjected to torture in order to drive out the intruding entity. Such treatments were occasionally effective.

With time, the explanation of the cause of obsessions and compulsions moved from a religious to a medical view. Obsessions and compulsions were first described in psychiatric literature by Esquirol in 1838, and by the end of the nineteenth century, obsessions were generally regarded as manifestations of melancholy or depression.[4]

By the beginning of the twentieth century, the view of obsessive-compulsive neurosis had shifted toward a psychologic explanation. Janet[5] described the successful treatment of compulsive rituals with what would come to be known as *behavioral techniques* (see Chapters 17, 19, and 20). With Freud's publication in 1909 of the psychoanalysis of obsessional neurosis (the Rat Man), obsessive and compulsive actions were seen as the result of unconscious conflicts and of thoughts and actions being isolated from their emotional components.[6] As a result of this shift in theory, treatment of OCD turned away from the symptoms and toward the unconscious conflicts that were assumed to underlie the symptoms. Although this shift identified that actions can be motivated by factors of which the individual is unaware, it did little to improve the treatment outcome of OCD patients (see Chapter 27).

With the rise of behavior therapy in the 1950s, the learning theories useful in the conceptualization and treatment of phobic disorders were applied to OCD symptoms.[7] These theories are reviewed in Chapters 17, 19, and 20. Although learning theories did not encompass all OCD symptoms, they did lead to the development in the late 1960s and early 1970s of effective treatments for reducing compulsive rituals.

Today, OCD research has returned to a more medical view. For example, since the publication of the first edition of this book, research has accelerated in the areas of limbic system surgery (see Chapter 26); brain imaging (positron emission tomography, magnetic resonance imaging, and computed axial tomography; see Chapter 15); genetic studies (see Chapter 14); memory and other cognitive dysfunction (see Chapter 13); and Tourette's disorder (see Chapter 8). Theories of basal ganglia and frontal lobe dysfunction also have been proposed (see Chapters 12, 13, and 15). In addition, recent controlled studies have found that new pharmacologic agents yield impressive results in many OCD patients (see Chapter 22). Although there are experts who believe that affective illness is at the core of OCD symptoms, the viewpoint proposed by Rachman and Hodgson[4] appears to have gained wide support. In their view (1) biologic predisposition, (2) psychologic factors, (3) learning history, and (4) mood fluctuations can be crucial in the development and maintenance of OCD.

It is interesting to note that as the view of the causes of OCD changed over the centuries, the content of obsessions and rituals changed as well. Where once the predominant fear was contracting the dreaded plague, this fear then gave way to obsessions and rituals to ward off syphilis; more recently, fears of cancer have been predominant.[4] Now, fear of acquired immunodeficiency syndrome (AIDS) has become predominant in obsessions and rituals.

CLASSIFICATION OF OBSESSIVE-COMPULSIVE DISORDER SYMPTOMS

Obsessive-compulsive disorder is frequently viewed as a unitary concept, and a patient can meet DSM-IV criteria for diagnosis of OCD with obsessive thoughts (of any type), compulsive actions (of any type), or a combination of the two. In recent years, however, several specialized OCD clinics have been established, which accept sufficient numbers of patients to examine various subgroups of this disorder. As a result of this development, experts are now able to determine whether there are subgroups of OCD patients who respond to various treatments. In addition, if experts can clearly define the types of behaviors and subjective experiences of OCD patients, epidemiologic studies may be carried out to determine onset, prevalence, and course for the various subgroups.

Obsessive-compulsive complaints tend to fall into one of several major categories: (1) cleaning compulsions; (2) checking rituals; (3) obsessive thoughts alone; (4) obsessional slowness; and (5) mixed rituals. Hodgson and Rach-man[8] have developed a psychometric instrument (the Maudsley Obsessional-Compulsive Inventory) to delineate reliably the subclasses of rituals (see Chapter 6). They found that 53% of their patients showed checking rituals, 48% reported cleaning rituals, 52% had complaints of obsessional slowness, and 60% had doubting obsessions. The overlap in these categories illustrates that patients with OCD frequently have more than one type of complaint. Nonetheless, it is usually straightforward to categorize a patient's predominant complaint. For example, Rachman and Hodgson[4] found that patients could be separated into two categories—checkers and cleaners—based on the patients' questionnaire answers. On the other hand, obsessional slowness rarely is found as the major complaint.

The following case summaries illustrate the clinical presentations of patients with various subtypes of OCD.

Cleaning Compulsions

A 30-year-old man presented with fears of being contaminated by touching objects he considered dirty. He had to cover various "dirty objects" with paper towels before he was able to touch them. If, however, he did happen to touch his laundry, his bed, door handles in public restrooms, his shoes, the gas cap on his car, or other "dirty" objects, he experienced vague feelings of dirtiness and discomfort, and he engaged in extensive washing of his hands, along with any clothing he believed had come into contact with the "dirty" object. The patient kept one hand "clean" at all times and refused to place this hand in his trousers pocket or to use it to shake hands. As a result of these OCD symptoms and resultant avoidance behavior, the patient was unable to work full time, and his social life dwindled because he spent several hours each day engaged in cleaning.

Patients with cleaning rituals attempt to avoid contacting contaminated objects, and these patients usually engage in cleaning rituals only when they believe that they have touched a contaminated object. These patients, termed *cleaners*, are described by Rachman and Hodgson[4] as "phobic-compulsives," because their avoidance behavior resembles that of phobic patients.

Checking Rituals

A 50-year-old woman engaged in repetitive checking behaviors when she was not sure whether she had performed an action correctly. For example, she would plug and unplug electric appliances 20 times or more to be sure that she actually took the plug out of the socket. She would do the same with light switches, turning them on and off repeatedly to ensure that she in fact had turned them off. She stared at the address on envelopes for up to several minutes to ensure that she had actually seen her name on the envelope. She counted money over and over, and her arithmetic required so many recalculations that she totally avoided financial paperwork and could no longer work in her previous job as a bookkeeper. The patient was no longer able to read because she continually returned to sentences she had already read to be sure she had actually seen them.

Several patients with checking rituals similar to the above have remarked that "it just doesn't seem to register" that they have performed an action correctly; as a result, they have a terrible feeling that they did something wrong. These patients frequently ask others for reassurance and engage in less checking behavior if there is someone else present to share responsibility for their actions.[4] These patients repeatedly engage in checking behaviors to ensure that they (1) performed an action correctly; (2) did not harm someone in the process; or (3) did not create a hazard that might produce harm in the future. Unlike cleaners, these patients actively engage in their checking rituals to forestall catastrophes in the future. Rachman and Hodgson[4] have referred to these patients as engaging in active avoidance.

Obsessional Thoughts

Virtually all patients with cleaning or checking rituals also have frequent obsessive thoughts. However, there are some OCD patients whose primary problem is obsessive thoughts, with few or no behavioral rituals present. These obsessive thoughts are often of an aggressive, sexual, or religious nature. An example of a patient with obsessional thoughts but no associated rituals was a 30-year-old man who could no longer enter public places because of obsessive thoughts and impulses to shout obscenities or to accuse "unsavory" characters of having committed some illegal act. The patient's obsessions and impulses were so severe that he was no longer able to work, and he became increasingly housebound.

Other Types of Compulsions and Obsessions

Less common subgroups of OCD include patients who engage in rituals which involve placing objects in a certain order (ordering rituals), and patients with primary obsessional slowness, who become "stuck" for hours when performing a routine task and are unable to finish it. Some patients develop time-consuming grooming rituals, such as parting their hair exactly in the middle or cutting their sideburns to exactly the same length. We have seen young women who often spend hours at a time picking at small or imagined lesions on their face while looking in the mirror. Other disorders closely related to OCD are monosymptomatic hypochondriasis, dysmorphophobia, fear of AIDS and cancer, trichotillomania, and certain social phobias. Many of these disorders are covered in some detail in Chapters 7 through 10.

The categorization of OCD into various subgroups has begun to yield results in epidemiology and treatment outcome studies. For example, Rachman and Hodgson[4] have found that patients with checking rituals tend to have a slow onset of symptoms, and early social learning appears to play an important role in the development of the problem. On the other hand, patients with cleaning rituals tend to have sudden onset of their symptoms. Further, there is evidence of different ages of onset and gender ratios for various subtypes of OCD.[9,9a] Patients with checking versus cleaning rituals also appear to differ in their level of anxiety increase and decrease throughout obsessions and compulsions.

The relationship between OCD and other disorders, especially schizophrenia, has been confusing. Many patients are misdiagnosed and treated with ineffective methods which may have dangerous side effects (see Chapter 4). A subgroup of OCD patients suffer from concomitant schizotypal personality disorder. The presence of this personality disorder appears to be a poor prognostic indicator for treatment with medications, behavior therapy, or a combination of the two.[9–12]

Behavioral and psychopharmacologic treatments may proceed more smoothly and rapidly in patients with cleaning rituals than in those patients with checking rituals (see Chapter 17). For patients with obsessive thoughts without related ritualistic behavior, behavioral treatment is unpredictable at best. However, various antidepressant medications may help such patients (see Chapter 22), and newer cognitive approaches also offer promise (see Chapter 18).

TREATMENT OUTCOME

Traditionally, OCD has been considered to have one of the poorest prognoses of all psychiatric disorders. Several recent studies, however, indicate that the bleak outlook for OCD may have been seriously overstated. Three independent studies of the natural course of OCD (summarized by Black[13]) found that 24% to 33% of patients have a fluctuating course, in which symptoms are reduced greatly at times but never totally absent; another 11% to 14% of patients have a phasic course in which there are periods of complete remission. Thus, approximately 40% of OCD patients may be improved or asymptomatic at any point, even with no treatment. Likewise, summaries of treatment outcomes for OCD[13] indicate that 45% to 60% of patients are moderately to greatly improved following a variety of psychologic and somatic treatments.

With new developments in treatment, this outlook has improved further. For example, approximately 60% to 80% of OCD patients can expect moderate to marked improvement in compulsive rituals with brief behavioral (see Chapter 17) or pharmacologic (see Chapter 22) treatment.

Although OCD remains a difficult disorder to treat, several recent developments account for the improved prognosis: (1) the appearance of specialized clinics, which permit sufficient numbers of OCD patients to be studied; (2) the use of various effective medications in the treatment of OCD; (3) the use of behavioral treatments to reduce rituals; (4) the combination of behavior therapy and medication treatment in OCD patients, rather than two mutually exclusive treatments; (5) more formal studies of epidemiology, personality, and family history, rather than anecdotal suppositions about OCD; and (6) the recognition of modern psychosurgery as a possibly effective and safe last-resort treatment.

SUMMARY

Because of its complex nature, obsessive-compulsive disorder has attracted the attention of experts in various fields of medicine and psychology. It is, therefore, a field well suited for interdisciplinary treatment and research. Psychoanalysts have long been intrigued by the sexual and aggressive content of obsessive thoughts and the symbolism of rituals. Behaviorists have been interested in the way that most behavioral rituals precisely fit into an anxiety-reduction model of learning. Psychopharmacologists have noted that OCD is frequently accompanied by depression, and OCD symptoms can usually be reduced or eliminated with appropriate medications. Neurologists and neurosurgeons have noted that specific brain lesions can produce compulsive behaviors in humans, and conversely, that other surgical lesions can provide relief in some patients with intractable OCD. Finally, neuropsychologists have been interested in the possibility of memory or attention deficit in patients with obsessional thoughts and checking rituals. To date, no single viewpoint provides a comprehensive explanation of OCD. It is encouraging, however, that recent interdisciplinary approaches have yielded promising results with various subgroups of OCD patients.

Although much more research is needed to improve treatments and extend the effectiveness to a larger proportion of patients suffering from OCD, therapies now produce moderate to marked changes in the majority of patients within weeks or months. In addition, we now are aware of some of the factors that predict poor treatment response, permitting us to focus our research efforts in this direction. The following chapters present an overview of the current state of the art of this interdisciplinary approach to OCD, illustrating its benefits over reliance on a single theoretic system.

REFERENCES

1. American Psychiatric Association: *Diagnostic and statistical manual of mental disorders,* ed 4, Washington, 1994, American Psychiatric Association.
2. American Psychiatric Association: *Diagnostic and statistical manual of mental disorders,* ed 3, Washington, 1980, American Psychiatric Association.
3. Baer L, Minichiello WE, Jenike MA: Behavioral treatment in two cases of obsessive compulsive disorder with concomitant bipolar affective disorder, *Am J Psychiatry* 142:358–360, 1985.
4. Rachman S, Hodgson R: *Obsessions and compulsions,* Englewood Cliffs, 1980, Prentice Hall, p 203.
5. Marks IM: Review of behavioral psychotherapy, I: Obsessive compulsive disorders, *Am J Psychiatry* 138:584–592, 1981.
6. Freud S: *Three case histories,* New York, 1973, Macmillan. (Translated by P. Rieff; originally published in 1909.)

7. Wolpe J: *Psychotherapy by reciprocal inhibition*, Stanford, 1958, Stanford University Press.
8. Hodgson J, Rachman S: Obsessional compulsive complaints, *Behav Res Ther* 15:389–395, 1977.
9. Minichiello WE, Baer L, Jenike MA: Schizotypal personality disorder: a poor prognostic indicator for behavior therapy in the treatment of obsessive-compulsive disorder, *J Anx Disorders* 1:273–276, 1987.
9a. Minichiello WE, Baer L, Jenike MA, et al: Age of onset of major subtypes of obsessive-compulsive disorders, *J Anxiety Dis* 4:147–150, 1990.
10. Jenike MA, Baer L, Minichiello WE, et al: Concomitant obsessive-compulsive disorder and schizotypal personality disorder: A poor prognostic indicator, *Arch Gen Psychiatry* 43:296, 1986a.
11. Jenike MA, Baer L, Minichiello WE, et al: Concomitant obsessive-compulsive disorder and schizotypal personality disorder, *Am J Psychiatry* 143:530–533, 1986b.
12. Baer L, Jenike MA, Black DW, et al: Effect of axis II diagnoses on treatment outcome with clomipramine in 54 patients with obsessive compulsive disorder. *Arch Gen Psychiatry* 49:862–866, 1992.
13. Black A: The natural history of obsessional neurosis. In Beech HR, editor: *Obsessional states*, London, 1974, Methuen, pp 19–54.

2

The Epidemiology and Clinical Features of Obsessive-Compulsive Disorder

Steven A. Rasmussen, M.D., Jane L. Eisen, M.D.

Over the past 15 years, we have experienced a rapid growth in our understanding of the clinical features, pathophysiology, and treatment of obsessive-compulsive disorder (OCD). In the 1980s, both clinicians and researchers recognized that OCD was much more common than was previously believed, leading to ever-accelerating interest in this fascinating psychiatric condition. Epidemiologic studies in diverse cultures have confirmed earlier findings that 1% to 2% of the general population suffers from OCD at any given time.[1] Widespread media attention and a growing recognition of the disorder among health care professionals have led to the successful diagnosis and treatment of large numbers of obsessive-compulsive patients, who prior to the 1980s, would not have presented for treatment.

Much of the progress in the epidemiology of OCD over the past decade has centered on the surprisingly high prevalence rates for OCD initially reported in the National Epidemiologic Catchment Area Survey (ECA). Verification of the ECA prevalence figures has come from other studies using improved methodology[2,3] and from cross-cultural studies confirming that the unexpectedly high prevalence of OCD as a worldwide phenomenon.[4-6]

Knowledge of the disorder's clinical features also has expanded significantly in the past 10 years. Treatment centers specializing in OCD have succeeded in enrolling large cohorts of patients, allowing more sophisticated analysis of the disorder's heterogeneity, comorbidity and course of illness, and the relationship of these variables to treatment outcome. Prospective observational studies of OCD's longitudinal course have led to further insight into the clinical characteristics and prognosis of the illness. Improvements in methodology (e.g., the use of control groups, blind clinical assessments, structured interviews, reliable and valid diagnostic criteria, and better database management systems) have aided these analyses. Finally, significant progress has been made in identifying homogeneous subgroups of OCD patients, which should assist in unraveling the etiology of OCD and in the development of more specific and effective treatment strategies. This chapter reviews current knowledge of the epidemiology and clinical features of OCD. It focuses on the phenomenologic heterogeneity of OCD and its comorbidity with other axis I and axis II syndromes.

EPIDEMIOLOGY
Frequency in Psychiatric Populations

The incorrect impression that OCD was a relatively rare disorder arose from a series of retrospective chart review studies completed in the late 1950s and early 1960s, which examined the frequency of OCD probands in inpatient and outpatient psychiatric settings. OCD made up a small minority (1% to 4%) of the total patient pool. Such low figures reinforced the prevailing attitude at the time that OCD was a rare condition. This attitude was primarily shaped by epidemiologic study by Rudin, who estimated OCD prevalence to be 5 in 10,000 in the general population.[7] Some investigators believed that Rudin's figures were probably an underestimate, realizing that patients often did not seek treatment because of fear or shame. In a more recent study, Hantouche, et al[8] found that 9.2% of 4,364 psychiatric outpatients had a diagnosis of OCD, whereas 17% of these patients had obsessive-compulsive symptoms. These higher figures most likely represent a combination of increased recognition by clinicians and increasing numbers of patients seeking treatment.

Prevalence in the General Population

The National Epidemiologic Catchment Area Survey (ECA) was funded by the National Institute of Mental Health (NIMH) in the late 1970s to determine the lifetime and 6-month prevalence of axis I psychiatric disorders in the general population of the United States and to determine where patients sought treatment. One of the most striking findings of the study was that OCD was 50 to 100 times more common than was previously believed, with a 6-month point prevalence of 1.6%,[9] and a lifetime prevalence of 2.5%.[10] This finding suggested that OCD was the fourth most common psychiatric disorder, following the phobias, substance abuse, and major depression. The prevalence rate of OCD was double that for panic disorder or schizophrenia in this study.[1] In a Canadian epidemiologic study of 3,258 randomly selected residents of Edmonton, using similar methods and instruments, the Diagnostic Interview Schedule (DIS) confirmed the initial ECA findings. The 6-month point prevalence of OCD in that study was 1.6%,[11] and the lifetime prevalence was 3%.

Since the initial publication of the ECA data, studies using similar methodology have been completed in diverse cultures including Europe,[6] Taiwan,[4]

New Zealand, Korea, and Africa (Table 2-1).[18] Remarkably similar prevalence rates were reported across these countries. Recently, Tadai, et al[19] measured the prevalence of OCD in 424 Japanese students using the Maudsley Obsessional Inventory (MOI) and found that 1.7% met the *Diagnostic and Statistical Manual of Mental Disorders* (DSM-III-R) criteria for OCD.

The ECA study has been criticized because it used the DIS, which lacked validity for its diagnostic criteria, and because it was administered by lay interviewers. This may have led to the overestimation of the prevalence of some disorders, particularly phobias and OCD. These criticisms were supported by two follow-up studies of ECA subjects that used semistructured interviews conducted by psychiatrists,[12,13] both of which found significantly lower prevalence rates of OCD than were reported in the original ECA study. These studies have in turn been criticized because of the small number of subjects interviewed and the lack of objective rating instruments developed for OCD. Unfortunately, no follow-up study of the original ECA OCD subjects using obsessive-compulsive–specific scales was completed.

A carefully designed two-stage epidemiologic study of the prevalence of OCD in a population of high school students by Flament, et al[2] supported the ECA prevalence figures for OCD. Investigators screened 5,000 students with a modified Leyton Obsessional Inventory (LOI).[14] Students scoring above a predetermined cut-off score on the scale were interviewed by a psychiatrist specializing in childhood OCD. Fifteen (0.3%) of the total 5,000 students were diagnosed as meeting DSM-III-R criteria for OCD. The average age of the probands was 15.4 years, and the average age of onset of the disorder is approximately age 20. When an age correction is applied, the point prevalence estimate for the general population is 1%. In a similar two-stage study, Valleni-Basile, et al[15] screened 3,283 adolescents with a self-report screening questionnaire followed by the SADS for school-age children. The 1-year incidence rates of OCD and subclinical OCD were 0.7% and 8.4%. Douglass, et al[16] found that the 1-year prevalence rate of OCD in 930 18-year-olds as measured by the DIS was 4%.

In a similar epidemiologic study, Apter, et al[17] studied 861 16-year-old Israelis during preinduction military screening. Eight percent of the sample reported spending more than 1 hour daily on obsessions or compulsions. OCD and subclinical OCD cases differed significantly from non-OCD cases, but not from each other, in distress and mean number of symptoms.

Some studies have failed to support the ECA findings. The first epidemiologic prevalence study of psychiatric disorders completed in the United States found that none of the 500 probands interviewed suffered from clinically significant OCD.[20] Bebbington[21] reported in the Camberwell Epidemiologic Survey that none of 300 patients interviewed had clinically significant OCD, although several patients had subthreshold disorder. Unfortunately, no objective measures of obsessive-compulsive severity were used in either of these

Table 2-1 Epidemiologic Studies of Obsessive-Compulsive Disorder

Study	Patients (n)	Population	Diagnostic Instrument	Interview	Lifetime Prevalence (%)	Six-Month Prevalence (%)	One-Year Prevalence (%)
Robins (1982), et al	18,572	General	DIS	Lay	2.5	1.5	
Bland (1988), et al	3,258	General	DIS	Lay	3.0	1.6	
Anthony (1985), et al	810	General	PSE	Psychiatrist		1.0	
Melzer (1985), et al	360	General	DSM-III Cklst	Psychiatrist		0.8	
Weissman (1978), et al	511	General	SADS	Lay		0.0	
Henderson (1988), et al	497	General	ASI	Lay		2.8	
Haveral (1988), et al	11,000	General	DIS	Lay	0.7	0.4	
Wittchen (1992), et al	481	General	DIS	Lay	2.1	1.6	
Canino (1987), et al	513	General	DIS	Lay	2.5	1.8	
Lee (1990), et al	5,100	General	DIS	Lay	1.9	1.1	
Wells (1989), et al	1,498	General	DIS	Lay	2.2	1.1	
Chen (1993), et al	7,651	General	DIS	Lay	1.1		
Khanna (1995), et al	Unk.	General	Scan Y BOCS		0.6		
Degonda (1993), et al	2,220	General	SPIKE	Psychiatrist	1.0		
Hwu (1989), et al							
Tadai (1995), et al	424	Student	MOI	Self-Report		1.7	
Flament (1988), et al	5,000	Student	LOI/K-SADS	Psychiatrist		0.3	
Valleni (1995), et al	3,283	Student	LOI/K-SADS	Psychiatrist		0.7	
Douglass (1995), et al	930	Student	DIS	Lay			4.0
Apler (1996), et al	861	Student		Psychiatrist			8.0
Zoharetal (1992), et al	562	16–17 yrs old	Yale TS & OCD	Psychiatrist		3.6	

studies. Degonda, et al[22] investigated the longitudinal course of OCD and obsessive-compulsive symptoms over an 11-year period in a Swiss cohort. The prevalence of DSM-III OCD in the study was considerably less than 1%. When a lower diagnostic threshold, based on obsessive-compulsive symptoms and social impairment, was used, the weighted lifetime prevalence rate for OCD at 30 years of age was 5.5%.

One could ask, "Why did we underestimate the prevalence of OCD for so long?" Additional data from the ECA study suggested that as many as 60% of patients with anxiety disorders present to primary care physicians rather than mental health professionals.[23] We have found a significant number of obsessive-compulsive patients who have not yet sought psychiatric care in the practices of dermatologists, obstetrician/gynecologists, and internists.[24,25]

A study we completed several years ago illustrates how the disorder often presents in medical settings. We observed that several of our handwashers who had 10-year histories of contamination fears reported that they had sought medical treatment for their hands prior to seeking psychiatric help. We therefore interviewed 22 patients who had nonspecific functional dermatitis at a local dermatologic clinic with a diagnostic interview for OCD. Eight of the 22 (35%) met DSM-III-R criteria with an average Yale-Brown Obsessive-Compulsive Scale (Y-BOCS) score of 22—well within the clinical range. Even more telling was that none of the eight had told the dermatologist about their OCD.

Similarly, patients with somatic obsessions often present to primary medical settings. Patients who develop aggressive obsessions toward their newborn children often are diagnosed by obstetricians or pediatricians as depressed because they don't want to divulge the horrible thoughts. Dysmorphophobics often are found in plastic surgeons' offices. Recognition of obsessive-compulsive patients in primary care settings requires careful observation and listening skills. The availability of a reliable self-report inventory or screener that could be completed in physicians' offices would enhance the recognition of OCD in the general population. (See Chapter 6.)

Subthreshold Symptoms

An optimal threshold or diagnostic criterion that reliably distinguishes the clinical from the subthreshold syndrome of OCD has yet to be identified. After screening 861 16-year-old Israeli military recruits, Apter, et al[17] concluded that obsessive-compulsive phenomena appear to form a continuum with few symptoms and minimal severity at one end, and many symptoms and severe impairment at the other. Using Angst's longitudinal follow-up sample, Degonda, et al[22] found a weighted lifetime prevalence of 5.5% for obsessive-compulsive symptoms by 30 years of age.

Rachman, et al[26] reported that a high percentage of the normal population have some obsessions and compulsions. Most children also go through developmental stages characterized by obsessive-compulsive or superstitious behavior. The degree of interference and frequency of the obsessions and compulsions are what distinguish them from normal phenomena; specifically, the patient must have had 1 hour of obsessive-compulsive symptoms daily for a period of 6 months that interfere with social or occupational function. (This corresponds to a score of 16 or greater on the Y-BOCS.)

Determining where the clinical syndrome begins is significant for both pharmacologic trials and genetic studies. Multicenter studies of selective serotonin reuptake inhibitor (SSRI) drugs in OCD found greater placebo response in patients with lower Y-BOCS scores, prompting some investigators to suggest that patients with Y-BOCS scores below 20 (as opposed to the usual 16) should be excluded from controlled trials.[27] Family genetic studies have found increased risk for both subthreshold and clinical OCD in family members of OCD probands.[28] Any longitudinal change in diagnoses can have dramatic effects on linkage studies and may contribute to some of the problems in replication of linkage findings in other disorders.

DEMOGRAPHIC VARIABLES

The following demographic variables have been examined in both inpatient and outpatient populations: gender, marital status, fertility rate, social class, intelligence, parental attitude, occupational status, ordinal position, early parental loss, and cause of death. Significant variability exists between them because standardized diagnostic criteria for OCD were not in use prior to 1970, when most of these studies were completed.

Gender

Black[29] tabulated 11 studies of inpatients and outpatients with OCD and found a total of 651 men (48.6%) and 685 women (51.4%). Three hundred and two of 560 patients meeting DSM-III-R criteria for OCD in our own sample were women (53.8%). Adding our figures to those of two other studies collecting data on gender ratio since that review, we find 969 men and 1,071 women (53% women to 47% men). Hollingsworth, et al[30] found that 13 of 17 (76%) children and adolescents with OCD were male. A male predominance in children with OCD also was reported by Rapoport.[3] As noted in the following paragraphs, men also have a significantly earlier age of OCD onset, whereas women with OCD are more likely to be married and have children.[31]

Race

There is a lower than expected frequency of blacks with OCD presenting for treatment. In addition, black respondents to the ECA study reported significantly less lifetime OCD than white respondents.[1] However, the same phenomenon was found for nine other mental disorders. It appears that blacks are less likely to present for treatment of various psychiatric problems because of service delivery issues rather than true genetic differences. Epidemiologic studies of OCD in Korea[18] and Japan[19] found a similar prevalence in the general population compared with the United States, but it appears that an even greater percentage of these do not seek treatment with a physician or mental health professional.

Marital Status

Significantly more patients with OCD remain single compared with age-matched controls. Interestingly, the percentage of divorces among OCD sufferers is lower than expected, particularly given the stress that obsessive-compulsive symptoms place on spouses. It is generally believed that there is a significant degree of marital maladjustment in patients with OCD. However, Coryell[32] found no significant difference between the marital status of OCD patients compared with a matched group of unipolar depressives, suggesting that marital maladjustment may not be syndrome-specific.

Rachman and Hodgson[33] distinguished between "part-time" and "full-time" obsessive-compulsive patients. Full-timers are those patients who are preoccupied the majority of the day with their symptoms, whereas part-timers can voluntarily control their symptoms more easily and generally ritualize alone. Although severity of OCD correlates with marital maladjustment, personality factors and family function also are important predictors.

Religion

Freud was among the first to identify the relationship between religious practices and obsessive-compulsive symptoms.[34] There appears to be an overrepresentation of patients with religious symptoms who are raised in strict religious communities (e.g., Hasidic or fundamentalist Muslim).[35] Interestingly, we have found that a strict religious upbringing predicts the presence of religious, sexual, or aggressive obsessions.

Intelligence

Most early anecdotal studies concluded that OCD patients possess higher than average intelligence.[24,29,36,37] Three recent studies used the Wechsler Adult Intelligence Scale (WAIS)[32,38,39] and found a small nonsignificant difference in full-scale intelligence quotient (IQ) between OCD patients and a matched normal comparison group. A small but consistent discrepancy in verbal versus performance IQ scores in OCD patients as well as in neuropsychologic tests of frontal lobe function has been noted. These findings led Flor-Henry to hypothesize that there may be dominant frontal impairment in OCD.[38] Alternatively, compulsiveness and obsessional slowness during testing might interfere with performance of visuospatial tasks, accounting for the differences (This also may account for patients who undergo neurosurgery for relief of obsessive-compulsive symptoms showing increased IQ postoperatively.).

Birth Order

Three studies have investigated ordinal position in OCD. In the first, OCD patients showed no significant difference in size of sibship compared with a matched primary unipolar depressive sample.[32] In addition, ordinal position and frequency of parental loss before 15 years of age were not significantly different between the groups. Obsessive-compulsive patients were somewhat more likely to be first-born, although this difference did not reach statistical significance. In the second study, 21 of 40 patients (52%) with OCD were first-born or only children compared with 11 of 40 (27%) in the control groups—a highly significant difference.[40] A third study investigated the birth order of psychiatric inpatients with a wide variety of psychiatric diagnoses.[41] No significant difference in birth order was found between those patients with OCD and a control population. In a recent analysis of our sample, we found that 115 of 404 (34%) patients were first born. There was no significant relationship between ordinal status and clinical course.

CLINICAL FEATURES

Age of Onset

In our cohort, the mean age of onset of significant OCD symptoms was 20.9 ± 9.6 with males having a significantly earlier onset of illness, 19.5 ± 9.2 for men, 22.0 ± 9.8 for women ($p < 0.003$). Sixty-five percent developed OCD prior to 25 years of age, some as early as 2 years of age. Fewer than 15% of obsessionals develop the illness after 35 years of age (Figure 2-1) with a significant increase in prevalence at puberty. The majority of patients remember having minor obsessive-compulsive symptoms prior to the onset of full DSM-III-R OCD. Although men noticed minor obsessive-compulsive symptom onset earlier than women, the difference did not reach statistical significance. The majority of patients described a gradual onset of illness. In contrast, many patients with early prepubertal childhood onsets have an acute attack followed by an episodic course.[42] These patients frequently also suffer from comorbid tics and other movement disorders, including choreiform movements. Swedo, et al[43] studied 50 early-onset children suffering from what they have termed *pediatric autoimmune neuropsychiatric disorder* (PANDA). PANDAs are characterized by the following criteria: (1) the presence of OCD or a tic disorder; (2) prepubertal symptom onset; (3) episodic course of symptom severity; (4) dramatic exacerbation of symptoms following a group A β-hemolytic streptoccocal infection; and (5) association with neurologic abnormalities. These children had an average age of onset of 6.3 years for tics and 7.4 years for OCD symptoms.

Natural History and Course of Illness

Black[29] and Goodwin[44] reviewed 13 follow-up studies between 1936 and 1970, most of which were retrospective chart reviews. Relatively little is known about the temporal characteristics and patterns of the typical course of

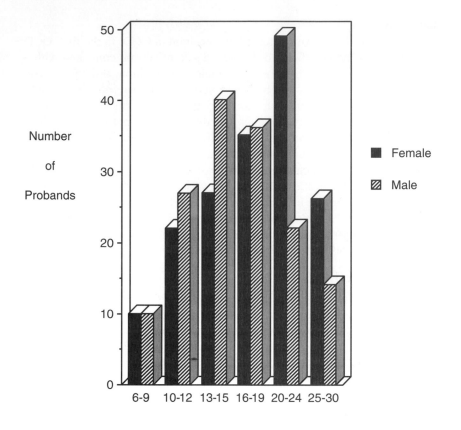

Fig. 2-1   Brown study: Age of onset in obsessive-compulsive disorder.

OCD, the switching of obsessive-compulsive symptoms over time (e.g., washing to checking), or of the patterns of comorbidity with other DSM-III-R disorders over time. Since 1970, several follow-up studies have measured the long-term efficacy of behavioral treatment for OCD (see Chapter 17). In contrast, most drug studies only have measured initial response with little or no long-term follow-up data. (A summary of follow-up studies from 1936 to 1983 is presented in Tables 2-2 and 2-3.)

The prevailing notion that OCD has a chronic deteriorating course has not been borne out by the evidence. In their review of follow-up studies, Goodwin, et al[44] found that the course of OCD could be divided into three categories: (1) unremitting and chronic; (2) phasic with periods of complete remission; and (3) episodic with incomplete remission that permitted normal social functioning.

Table 2-2 Outcome Studies of Behavioral Treatment in Obsessive-Compulsive Disorder

Author	Year	Diagnosis	Patients (n)	Mean Follow-Up	Treatment	Duration of Therapy	Asymptomatic (n)	Asymptomatic (%)	Improved (n)	Improved (%)	Unimproved (n)	Unimproved (%)
Rachman	1973	OCD Rituals	5	2 yr	ERP	?			3	66		
Boulougouris	1977	OCD Rituals	15	2.8 yr	ERP		9	60	6	40		
Emmelkamp, et al	1977	OCD Rituals	14	3.5 mo	ERP; Self-controlled; Therapist-controlled	10 sessions, 2 hr	Avg improvement 75% in both groups					
Foa, et al	1978	OCD Rituals	21	15 mo	ERP	10 sessions, 2 hr	14	66	4	20	3	14
Foa, et al	1980	OCD Rituals	15	11 mo	EI; ERP	10 sessions, 2 hr	Same outcome at 11 mo					
Steketee, et al	1982	OCD Rituals	51	1 yr	EI; ERP; EI/ERP; EI/ERP	Various	25	50	10	17	16	33
Mawson, et al	1982	OCD Rituals	40	2 yr	ERP and CMI (0–36 wk); ERP and placebo (0–36 wk)	15- or 30-min sessions	26	67	7	16	7	16
Emmelkamp, et al	1983	OCD Rituals	12	6 mo	ERP alone; ERP with spouse	10–45-min sessions	Improved 5 of 15 variables; Improved 13 of 15 variables					
Robertson, et al	1983	OCD Rituals and thoughts	3	2 yr	Systematic disruption; Cognitive restructuring	10–30 min; 1–2 hr	2	66	1	33		

CMI, clomipramine; EI, exposure in imagination; ERP, exposure with response prevention; OCD, obsessive-compulsive disorder.

Table 2-3 Retrospective Follow-Up Studies: 1936–1983

Author	Year	Diagnosis	Patients (n)	Mean Follow-Up	Treatment (n)	Much Improvement (%)	(n)	No Improvement (%)	(n)	Change (%)	Assessment
Lewis	1936	OCD	50	7.5	Mixed (16)	32	17	34	17	34	Therapist
Rudin	1953	OCD and mixed obsessional states	130	2–26	Mixed (16)	12	31	26	83	61	Self and therapist
Pollitt	1957	OCD	66	3.4	Mixed (16)	24	32	48	18	28	Self and therapist
Hastings	1957	OCD	23	6–12	Supportive (3) psychotherapy	13	9	40	11	47	Therapist
Ingram	1961	OCD and mixed obsessional states	46	5.9	Mixed (4)	9	14	30	28	61	Therapist
Grimshaw	1965	OCD	97	5.08	Electroshock (n = 31) Insight-oriented psychotherapy (n = 36) No psychotherapy (n = 14)	29	7	22	15	49	Self
Kringlen	1965	OCD and Phobia	85	16.6	Mixed (13)	15	38	44	34	41	Therapist
Lo	1967	OCD	87	3.9	Mixed (17)	20	43	50	27	30	Therapist
Coryell	1981	OCD	44	4.3	Mixed (10)	22	24	55	10	22	Research assistant

OCD, obsessive-compulsive disorder.

Although studies varied considerably regarding the percentage of patients in each category, the majority of patients in each study always fell into the last group, with approximately 10% of patients exhibiting a course marked by progressive deterioration. These figures are consistent with our own observational follow-up study (Table 2-4). Although previous descriptive studies found that 85% of patients have a chronic waxing and waning course, there were no previous studies to subdivide this waxing and waning into predictable patterns or subtypes.[45] More recent prospective studies using standardized criteria have shown that episodicity in this disorder (with clear periods of remission off medication) is uncommon. There is considerable variability in the periodicity, duration, and severity of OCD episodes. However, once present, obsessions and compulsions usually persist throughout a patient's life.

Over the past decade, there have been several prospective longitudinal studies of the course of OCD. Flament, et al[46] completed a 2-year follow-up study of 59 high school students identified as having OCD, subclinical OCD, or compulsive personality disorder. Of the 12 patients meeting criteria for OCD at baseline, only five met full criteria at follow-up. Four patients who had subclinical OCD at baseline later met full criteria for OCD at follow-up. Another 5-year prospective follow-up study of an obsessive-compulsive adolescent cohort by Leonard, et al[47] concluded that patterns of course were not easily predicted from baseline variables. Some patients who were suffering from subthreshold symptoms at baseline were severely ill at follow-up, and others who were classified as severely ill at baseline no longer suffered from clinical levels of symptoms at follow-up. Similarly, Valleni-Basile, et al[15] screened a community sample of 3,283 adolescents and found 1-year incidence rates of OCD and subthreshold OCD of 0.7% and 8.4%, respectively. Interestingly, transition probabilities were highest for moving from more severe to less severe categories. Seventeen percent of patients with OCD at baseline had OCD at follow-up, whereas only 1.5% of those with subclinical OCD had developed OCD that met syndromal criteria. In contrast, a Danish follow-up study of 23 adolescents presenting with OCD to a community clinic found that 12 of the subjects still had an OCD diagnosis at follow-up. One third of the subjects had an episodic course, and two thirds had a chronic course.[48]

The introduction of the SSRIs has led to a significant improvement in prognosis for patients suffering from OCD over the past decade. A follow-up study of 83 OCD patients[49] assessed 1 to 3 years after initial evaluation found that 64% had a greater than 50% decrease in Y-BOCS, and 33% had a greater than 75% decrease in Y-BOCS at follow-up. This study is at odds with two other prospective longitudinal observational studies that have recently been initiated at our site. Eisen, et al[50] examined 68 obsessive-compulsive outpatients evaluated at either the Brown or Yale Obsessive-Compulsive Clinics and followed them prospectively over a 2-year period. Of the 51 patients who entered the study meeting full criteria, 57% still met full criteria after 2 years. Survival analysis

Table 2-4   Prospective Follow-Up Studies of Obsessive-Compulsive Disorder

Author	Treatments	Patients (n)	Mean Follow-Up (yrs)	Remained in Episode (%)	Partial Remission (%)	Full Remission (%)	Comments
Children and adolescents							
Berg, et al (1989)		12	2	42	17[a]	8	17% had compulsive personality or traits
Leonard, et al (1993)	SSRIs, BT, psychotherapy, family therapy	54	3.4	43	46	11[b]	70% on medication at follow-up
Adults							
Orloff, et al (1994[c])	SSRIs, BT	85	2.1		31	33	
Eisen, et al (1995[b])	SSRIs, BT	51	2	57	31	12	
G. Steketee, et al (submitted for publication)	SSRIs, BT	107	0.5–5	47		22	Mainly outpatients

BT, behavior therapy; SSRIs, selective serotonin reuptake inhibitors.
[a] Subjects had subclinical OCD at follow-up (i.e., obsessions/compulsions present but not at full criteria).
[b] Three of the six subjects in remission (i.e., symptom free) were receiving medication.
[c] Course assessed by percentage change in Y-BOCS score only.

revealed a 47% probability of achieving at least partial remission during the 2-year study period. Another prospective study by Steketee, et al[51] examined 107 clinic patients with OCD followed up to 5 years after intake. The probability of partial remission for at least a 2-month period was 0.53 and for full remission (no longer meeting criteria), 0.22 at 5 years. Differences between these studies may be secondary to differences in the clinical populations or instruments used.

Quality of Life

There has been only one study to date of the impact of OCD on the quality of patients' lives: Koran, et al[52] studied 60 obsessive-compulsive outpatients and compared their quality of life reference scores with depressed or diabetic patients studied using the self-rated Medical Outcomes Study 36-Item-Short-Form Health Survey. Instrumental role performance and social functioning of OCD patients were worse than those of patients with diabetes and the general population. After adjustment for gender differences, quality of life ratings were similar for the patients with OCD and major depression.

Symptom Subtypes

The beginning clinician is often struck by the diversity of the clinical presentations of OCD. However, with sufficient experience with OCD patients, this initial impression is replaced by the realization that the number of types of obsessions and compulsions are remarkably limited and stereotypic. The basic types and frequencies of obsessive-compulsive symptoms are consistent across cultures and time.[19,53] Why a particular symptom type develops in a given individual remains unknown. The clinical descriptions of Freud,[54] Bleuler,[55] Janet,[56] Kraeplin,[57] and others are remarkably consistent with the clinical presentation of OCD seen today. Over the past 15 years, we have characterized the phenomenologic and clinical features of more than 1,000 obsessive-compulsive patients at Brown.[58] A summary of the obsessions and compulsions most commonly found is listed in Table 2-5. The most common obsessions involve contamination, pathologic doubt, aggressive and sexual thoughts, somatic concerns, and the need for symmetry and precision. The most common rituals are checking, cleaning, and counting compulsions. In the following paragraphs, we have attempted to convey the typical clinical presentation of the most common of the obsessive-compulsive symptoms.

Contamination Obsessions

Obsessive fear of contamination, coupled with handwashing, checking compulsions, and avoidance, is the most common phenomenologic presentation of OCD. Although handwashing is the most common compulsion seen in these patients, they will first try to avoid contaminated objects if given the opportunity. Of all obsessors, the fear structure is most closely linked to the phobias: (1) both are precipitated by specific external cues; (2) both are accompanied

Table 2-5   Obsessive-Compulsive Symptoms on Admission (n = 560)

Obsessions	(%)	Compulsions	(%)
Contamination	50	Checking	61
Pathologic doubt	42	Washing	50
Somatic	33	Counting	36
Need for symmetry	32	Need to ask or confess	34
Aggressive	31	Symmetry and precision	28
Sexual	24	Hoarding	18
Multiple obsessions	72	Multiple compulsions	58

Course of Illness (n = 560)

Age of Onset	Type	(%)	Precipitant	(%)
Men 19.6 ± 9.3	Continuous	85.0	Not present	71
Women 22.0 ± 9.8	Deteriorative	10.0	Present	29
Total 20.9 ± 9.6	Episodic	2.0		

by a high level of anxiety; and (3) for both, the coherence of their fear network is high. The most frequently identified contaminant is dirt or germs, but a wide variety of substances can serve as the contaminant (e.g., toxic chemicals, poisons, radiation, or heavy metals). Although these patients are usually obsessed with external cues or objects, some become morbidly preoccupied with cognitive rather than external cues. As is often the case in simple phobias, generalization from fear of a specific object to fear of a more abstract category of objects is frequently seen. Most report anxiety as the dominant effect, but the presence of disgust and shame also are commonly seen,[59] as are embarrassment and guilt. Unlike other phobic patients, contamination obsessive patients often report that they are more concerned that significant others might become ill because of them, rather than them becoming ill themselves. Contamination is "magically transmitted" from a dirty object to a clean object merely by coming into contact with it. Objects that have come into contact with the source of contamination, no matter how remote, are often viewed with as much trepidation or disgust as the original contaminant.

Checking Rituals

These patients are characterized by incessant worrisome thoughts that something bad will happen because they have failed to check something thoroughly or completely. This need for certainty is driven by the possibility that something terrible will happen that they will be responsible for (although they may recognize that the possibility is remote). They describe an internal conflict between a rational knowledge that the door is locked and an irrational urge that compels them to check anyway. If checking is postponed, there is a rise in anxiety that is difficult for most patients to tolerate.

The experience of pathologic doubt is part of many OCD symptoms, but is seen in its purest form in this subgroup of patients. If one asks these patients, "When are you satisfied that the door is *really* locked or the faucet is *really* off?" many say that if it was not for the fact that they would lose their job or family, they would check all day. One of several strategies is usually adopted to reduce the amount of time spent checking and permit limited functioning. The most common strategy is to limit the number of checks by counting, often involving a system of "good" numbers and "bad" numbers. Other patients describe the "click phenomena." One of our checkers told us: "I will be checking something over and over and the feeling that it is not totally shut is there, until suddenly, the feeling will no longer be there. It is like clicking a light switch off." Another is the use of physical force, often resulting in broken window handles, locks, and faucets. There is a sense of finality or completeness when this occurs. Janet felt that "incompleteness" underlies most obsessive and compulsive symptoms and tics.[56]

Checkers are usually perfectionists, possibly with overly meticulous or overly critical parents.[33] Although they usually fear something terrible will happen (e.g., a fire or their children being poisoned by medication left in the medicine cabinet), this is not always the case. Sometimes, these patients are plagued by constant doubts about nondangerous things (e.g., Is the refrigerator door totally shut? Is the car window totally shut?). Such patients report being truly incapable of cognitive and motor control over their behavior.

Sexual and Aggressive Obsessions

Some patients suffer from recurrent abhorrent thoughts that they have, or may have, committed an unacceptable sexual or aggressive thought or act toward others. Janet noted that the most objectionable thoughts or actions that the patient could imagine and that caused patients the most horror were the ones that invariably occurred.[56] For example, a very religious man in our clinic was compelled to link the word "damn" to "God" every time he saw, heard, or spoke the word "God." A 26-year-old mother was compelled to get rid of all the knives in her house because of a fear of stabbing her baby. A 30-year-old stewardess was obsessed with intrusive sexual thoughts and images of homosexuality and child molestation. A 42-year-old church secretary had intrusive sexual images of the Virgin Mary whenever she crossed the threshold of the church. Guilt and anxiety are the dominant affective symptoms. Patients may think they should be jailed for their thoughts (both to protect them from what they think they might do and because they feel they deserve to be punished).

The compulsion to ask or confess is also frequently present. Such patients repeatedly tell their therapist, spouse, or close friend a terrible thought or deed that they feel they have committed, as a way of seeking reassurance that they are really not capable of fulfilling these thoughts or deeds. Patients sometimes leave the therapist's office after having sought reassurance the whole hour, only to call back later to add an insignificant detail they earlier omitted. Distinguishing these patients from paraphiliacs and those patients with true homicidal impulses is not difficult in most cases. Most patients have had past histories that follow the typical course of OCD and have had other types of obsessions and compulsions during their course of illness. Obsessive-compulsive patients worry that they want to do these things they are obsessed with "What if I?" and "How do you know I?" and think they should be punished for even having the thought.

It is the patient's reaction to the thought or impulse, "Oh my God how could I think that?" that leads to the obsessive characteristic of the thought. Everyone experiences unacceptable sexual or aggressive thoughts, but most are able to quickly and usually preconsciously dismiss them. For obsessive-compulsive patients, the thought becomes labeled with intense negative affect and anxiety, and is therefore more likely to be conditionally linked to other neutral stimuli, stored, and subsequently replayed with increasing intrusiveness and frequency. Attempts to actively dismiss the thought without dissociation of affect often lead to increased preoccupation and anxiety.

Need for Symmetry and Precision

Here, the clinical picture is dominated by an obsession to have objects or events in a certain order or position, to do and undo certain motor actions in an exact fashion, or to have things exactly symmetrical or "evened up." In our experience, these patients can be divided into two groups: (1) those with primary obsessive slowness; and (2) those with primary magical thinking. Patients who suffer from primary obsessive slowness require an inordinate amount of time to complete even the simplest of tasks.[33] Unlike most obsessive-compulsive patients, those with obsessive slowness may not experience their symptoms as ego dystonic. Instead, these patients seem to have lost their goal directiveness in favor of completing a given subroutine perfectly. The basal ganglia control motor planning and therefore coordinate motor subroutines and what MacLean has termed the *master routine*.[60] It is, therefore, tempting to speculate that these patients suffer from some interference in fronto-limbic-basal ganglia function that interferes with their goal directedness, making them incapable of distinguishing the importance of subroutines versus overall goal-directed behavior (see Chapters 12 and 15). These patients often experience a subjective feeling as "discontent" or "tension" when things are not lined up "just so" or "perfectly," rather than fear or anxiety. It is the preoccupation many of us have with a picture hung crookedly, but magnified many times. In that sense, these patients can be seen as at the extreme end of the spectrum of compulsive personality, in which the need for every detail to be "perfect" or "just so" is extreme. Their description of rising tension followed by release after the act is more similar to the subjective sensory experience of Tourette's patients[56] than to the anxiety experienced by other obsessive-compulsive patients.

In contrast to patients with primary obsessive slowness, some patients' need for symmetry and precision is an attempt to magically ward off an imagined disaster. Such patients are usually beset with a bewildering variety of doing and undoing rituals, lucky and unlucky numbers, and counting rituals. They often are described as being superstitious during childhood, and the rituals are usually accompanied by severe anxiety.

Somatic Obsessions

The irrational, persistent fear of developing a serious life-threatening illness is seen in hypochondriasis, major depression with somatic features, panic disorder, and OCD. Somatic obsessions accompanied by checking compulsions are frequently seen in obsessive-compulsive patients at the time of evaluation.

Many of our patients with somatic obsessions are indistinguishable from hypochondriacs, except that they have multiple other obsessions and compulsions. Analysis of the multicenter clomipramine and fluvoxamine trials shows that patients with primary somatic obsessions respond to SSRIs similar to patients with other obsessive-compulsive symptoms. There is usually no difficulty in distinguishing these patients from those with somatization disorders. Patients with somatization disorders tend to complain about their symptoms, whereas somatic obsessive patients are highly anxious about an imagined disease they either fear they have or will develop. Somatic obsessions are most commonly linked to checking and the need for reassurance rituals. Unlike many OCD patients, those with somatic obsessions are primarily concerned with themselves dying rather than with being responsible for harm befalling others. Until recently, cancer, heart attacks, and venereal disease had been the most common fears in these patients. Patients with obsessions about AIDS are appearing in rapidly increasing numbers.

Hoarding

Approximately one fifth of the OCD patients in our clinic have some hoarding behaviors. Although the symptom is common, it rarely dominates the clinical presentation. The reason most hoarders come to treatment is complaints of family or friends or the fact that the person is unable to function because of the accumulation of material in the house or office. These patients often feel compelled to check possessions over and over to make certain nothing is missing, or to check the garbage to make certain that they have not inadvertently thrown away something valuable. The ego syntonic nature of such symptoms makes one question whether the syndrome should be seen as part of a compulsive personality instead of OCD. The checking rituals and anxiety attendant with the potential loss of valued possessions suggest, however, that these patients suffer from true OCD. Hoarders tend to be particularly resistant to behavioral and pharmacologic intervention, raising the specter that these patients may have a distinct pathophysiology.[60a]

Religious Obsessions

Approximately one in 10 patients in our clinic suffer from religious obsessions, such as fearing they have committed a mortal sin or whether they have followed the letter of the religious law or confessed completely. These patients tend to be overly serious and hypermoral and commonly suffer from the need to confess. Although suffering greatly from their obsessions, some see this as a religious suffering that God has asked them to endure. The frequency of religious obsessive-compulsive symptoms appear to be culturally bound: Areas of the world that have religions with strict moral codes have more OCD patients with religious obsessions.[35,53] The prevalence of religious symptoms in obsessive-compulsive patients, previously described in the literature on scrupulosity, appears to be on the decline in the United States, concurrent with the liberalization of church laws and procedures. This suggests that the content of an obsession is likely to be environmentally determined in at least some OCD cases. We agree with Greenberg,[35] who hypothesized that patients who develop obsessive-compulsive symptoms have a preexisting genotype, and that the development of religious obsessions and compulsions is dependent on that genotype.

Mental Rituals

Mental rituals were the third most common type of compulsion after hand-washing and checking in the DSM-IV field trial.[61] When faced with the choice of touching a contaminated object and washing their hands for 1 hour afterward versus avoiding the contaminated object, most patients would prefer to avoid. Similarly, most patients would prefer to avoid coming into contact with a situation that will provoke checking than to spend large amounts of time ritualizing. It is sometimes difficult to discern the difference between obsessions and preservative mental rituals that also can cause distress and anxiety. Mental rituals always are performed in the service of reducing anxiety associated with the obsessions. It is particularly important to take a careful inventory of mental rituals and avoidance patterns when the patient is engaged in exposure treatment. Mental rituals or avoidance often takes the place of overt motor behavior, and unless the therapist is alert to their development, the patient may extinguish his overt rituals with no significant improvement in outcome.

Obsessive-Compulsive Disorder with Poor Insight

There has been increasing interest in the role of insight in OCD over the past 5 years. Janet was the first to indicate that many obsessive-compulsive patients have psychotic features.[56] Eight percent of his sample had psychotic symptoms. Eisen and Rasmussen[62] found that 14% of 475 patients with DSM-III-R OCD also had psychotic symptoms.[62] Six percent of patients had lack of insight and high conviction about the reasonableness of the obsessions as their *only* psychotic symptom. Four percent had OCD and schizophrenia, and 2% had OCD and another delusional disorder. Probands with OCD and psychotic features were more likely to be men, single, and suffering from a chronic deteriorative course. As part of the DSM-IV field trial Foa, et al[61] reported that the majority of patients were uncertain about whether the obsessive-compulsive symptoms were unreasonable or excessive. (Four percent were "completely certain" that the feared consequence would occur if they did not perform the ritual.) More recently, Eisen, et al[63] have developed a scale with reliability and validity to measure the degree of insight or strength of conviction about a belief, The Brown Assessment of Beliefs Scale (BABS). They have found that, although 30% of obsessive-compulsive patients have limited insight into their obsessions, only 5% to 10% would be categorized as delusional compared with 70% of body dysmorphic patients who were considered delusional. Interestingly, Eisen, et al[64] found no correlation between the degree of insight in OCD as measured by the BABS and response to sertraline in a multicenter trial.

Comorbidity

In studying a disorder such as OCD, comorbidity with other axis I disorders is a serious obstacle for researchers wishing to obtain homogenous subgroups. This is particularly true of clinical neurobiologists and geneticists who are studying a discrete phenomenon that could have a very wide variation in nonhomogenous populations. The majority (57%) of 100 OCD patients presenting to our clinic had at least one other axis I DSM-III-R diagnosis. To further complicate matters, OCD is a chronic illness and an even higher percentage of our patients (77%) have had a lifetime history of another axis I disorder. Distinguishing primary from secondary diagnoses often can be difficult, if not impossible.

Studies examining the comorbidity of OCD with other psychiatric disorders can be divided into two groups: (1) those looking at the coexistence of other psychiatric disorders in a clinically defined population of obsessive-compulsive patients; and (2) those primarily focused on recording the frequency of obsessive-compulsive symptoms in other diagnostic groups. The coexistence of other anxiety states, depression, and psychotic symptoms with obsessive-compulsive symptoms was well documented in the early literature.[55-57] However, few systematic clinical psychopathologic studies had been completed before 1985 using standardized diagnostic criteria or reliable structured instruments.

The question of a relationship between OCD and schizophrenia has been of central interest. Some investigators have suggested that obsessions are a preliminary sign of schizophrenia, whereas other experts claim that obsessional symptoms are a defense against psychotic symptoms. Recent data suggest that the two disorders are distinct diagnostic entities that have no true relationship to one another. If OCD were closely related to schizophrenia, one would expect a significant percentage of OCD patients to develop schizophrenia; however, follow-up studies have found that few OCD probands go on to develop schizophrenia (i.e., 1.0% to 3.3%).[7,37,65] In a retrospective chart review of 850 inpatients with schizophrenia, Rosen[66] found that approximately 10% of patients exhibited prominent obsessive-compulsive symptoms. This finding was replicated by Fenton and McGlashan[67] who also found that 10% of schizophrenics in a Chestnut Lodge follow-up study exhibited prominent obsessive-compulsive symptoms. These "obsessive-compulsive schizophrenics" tended to have a more chronic course and a greater frequency of social or occupational impairment compared with a matched sample of schizophrenics without obsessive-compulsive features. A preliminary review of schizophrenic patients who were followed up in the Iowa 500 sample supports these data (Rasmussen & Tsuang, unpublished observation). Recently, Eisen, et al[68] interviewed 75 patients who met SADS (DSM-III-R) criteria for schizophrenia and found that 7.8% met DSM-III-R criteria for OCD. The average Y-BOCS score was 22.3% for those schizophrenics who also met DSM-III-R criteria for OCD.

The relation between obsessions, compulsions, and depression was the subject of several early studies.[36,69,70] These studies were primarily retrospective and failed to use diagnostic criteria or structured interviews, leaving many aspects of the association between depression and OCD unclear.

The phenomenologic and biologic evidence relating OCD to affective disorder has been reviewed by Insel, et al.[71] There is increasing evidence from biologic, genetic, and treatment efficacy studies that there is a shared vulnerability to the development of depressive illness and anxiety disorders.[72] It has been noted that obsessive-compulsive features are rarely, if ever, seen in mania. We have reported on a case of OCD in a bipolar patient whose obsessions and compulsions worsened in direct proportion to the severity of his depression and totally disappeared when he became manic.[73] Although preliminary evidence suggests that OCD is rarely seen in mania, no systematic data existed on the frequency of obsessive-compulsive symptoms in a bipolar population until recently. Chen, et al[75] found that 21% of patients with bipolar disorder, 12.2% of patients with unipolar depression, and 5.9% of patients with other disorders had OCD in the ECA sample. Kruger, et al[74] found that 35% of both bipolar and unipolar depressed patients suffered from an obsessive-compulsive syndrome. Many of these depressed patients suffer from obsessions which are at times difficult to differentiate from ruminations.

In our subsample of 250 patients who met DSM-III criteria for OCD, only 25% denied depression on admission.[45] Although the majority admitted to feelings of inadequacy and hopelessness, only one patient gave a history of euphoria. Over the course of their illness, most patients reported that depression developed *after* the OCD symptoms occurred, and these patients were, therefore, classified as having secondary depression. A minority (8%) of patients had concurrent onset of obsessive-compulsive symptoms with depressive episodes.

Kringlen[76] reported that more than 50% of 91 obsessional patients complained of phobic symptoms. Of Videbach's 104 depressed obsessionals, 42 (40%) reported phobic symptoms.[77] In contrast, Welner, et al[69] found associated phobias in only 7 (5%) of 150 patients with severe OCD. Additional evidence supporting covulnerability between OCD and other anxiety disorders is found in the high frequency of childhood phobias reported by obsessional patients. Lo[37] reported that 21 (35%) of his 59 obsessional patients had significant phobias during childhood. Videbach[77] observed this finding in 52 (50%) of 104 depressed ruminative patients. Similarly, Ingram[65] reported that 22 (25%) of 89 OCD patients had significant phobias in childhood. Over the past 5 years, there have been several studies that examined the comorbidity of OCD with other anxiety disorders. In a study of 60 panic disorder patients using the SADS-LA and personal interviews, Breier, et al[72] found that 17% suffered from DSM-III OCD. Subsequent studies by Mellman and Uhde[78] and Barlow, et al[79] have confirmed these initial findings of overlap between panic and OCD. Insel and colleagues[80] have indicated the important distinction between primary and secondary anxiety disorders; for example, it is often difficult to distinguish a primary social phobia with obsessive features from primary OCD that centered on completing a ritual in public. A high frequency of current and lifetime anxiety disorders suggests that OCD patients are vulnerable to many types of anxiety. The high prevalence of anxiety states in these patients may be the result of common developmental/temperamental traits in which phenotypic expression is secondary to shared genotypic and psychosocial factors. Of particular interest in this regard is the high lifetime prevalence of separation anxiety in this group of patients (12%)—a finding that also has been well documented in panic disorder.[81]

Table 2-6 summarizes common comorbid axis I disorders found in our OCD sample. Two thirds of patients had a lifetime history of a major depression, and one third of patients had major depression at the time of first evaluation. The majority (85%) have a mood disorder secondary to OCD, and 15% had a concurrent unipolar recurrent depression. There is also a significant overlap with the other axis I anxiety disorders, including panic disorder (with and without agoraphobia), social phobia, generalized anxiety disorder, and separation anxiety disorder. Other syndromes with greater comorbidity than one would expect from general population studies include eating disorders, Tourette's disorder, and schizophrenia. Comorbid axis I conditions can influence course of illness and affect choice and order of treatment.

Recently, attention has focused on patients with comorbid tics and OCD. Approximately 20% of patients with OCD have a lifetime history of multiple tics, and 5% to 10% of patients have a lifetime history of Tourette's disorder.[82] This subgroup has an earlier age of onset and family pedigrees that are loaded for both Tourette's disorder and OCD.[28] Miguel, et al[83] studied similarities and differences in the clinical symptoms of 15 OCD outpatients without tics

Table 2-6   Coexisting Axis I Diagnoses in Primary Obsessive-Compulsive Disorder (n = 100)

Diagnosis	Current	Lifetime	
	Semistructured (n = 100) (%)	Semistructured (n = 100) (%)	from Separation Anxiety Disorder (n = 60) (%)
Major depressive disorder	31	67	78
Simple phobia	7	22	28
Separation anxiety disorder	—	2	17
Social phobia	11	18	26
Eating disorder	8	17	8
Alcohol abuse (dependence)	8	14	16
Panic disorder	6	12	15
Tourette's disorder	5	7	6

and 12 adult Tourette's disorder patients without OCD. All OCD patients reported some cognitions preceding the compulsions whereas only 2 of 12 Tourette's disorder patients reported cognitions. In contrast, all Tourette's disorder patients reported sensory phenomena preceding repetitive behaviors, and no OCD patients reported such sensations.

There also has been interest in the overlap of OCD with eating disorders, particularly anorexia nervosa. Theil, et al[86] reported that 37% of 93 women who met criteria for anorexia or bulimia nervosa also met DSM-III-R criteria for OCD and had a score of 16 or higher on the Y-BOCS. Rastam, et al[87] also reported a high rate of OCD in 16-year-old girls diagnosed with anorexia nervosa.

Axis II conditions in OCD are covered extensively elsewhere in this volume.[88] The most commonly encountered diagnoses are dependent, avoidant, passive-aggressive, and compulsive. Schizotypal, paranoid, and borderline personalities are found less commonly in OCD but appear to be associated with poor outcome.[88] Compulsive personality is covered more fully here because of its relationship to the model that follows.

Compulsive Personality Disorder

Janet[56] viewed all obsessional patients as having a premorbid personality causally related to pathogenesis of the disorder. However, as early as 1936, Lewis[36] cautioned against acceptance of the connection between predisposing personality and emergence of obsessional illness. Despite the questions about the validity of current diagnostic criteria for compulsive personality, there is general agreement that obsessional traits also occur in many people who never become mentally ill, with conditions other than OCD. Several previous studies found a significant percentage of OCD patients who did not have premorbid compulsive personalities. In seven studies reviewed by Black,[29] marked obsessional traits were found in 31% of 254 obsessional patients, moderate traits in 40%, and no obsessional traits in 29%. All of these studies were completed prior to the introduction of DSM-III, so that comparisons among studies are difficult because of variations in methodology and sample selection. Studies completed after the introduction of DSM-III also have varied regarding the rates of comorbidity of compulsive personality with OCD. This variation is partly because of the arbitrary nature of how many of the criteria must be met to make the diagnosis and the fact that there are considerable variations between DSM-III and DSM-III-R. In spite of these problems, there is now ample evidence from recent studies supporting the discontinuity of obsessive-compulsive personality (OCP) and OCD. The majority of OCD patients do not suffer from compulsive personalities.[88] The classic distinction—rituals being ego syntonic in OCP as opposed to ego dystonic in OCD—is useful but not absolute. Some cleaners, hoarders, and those with the need for symmetry and precision or obsessive slowness, who strive for perfection or completeness, find their rituals ego syntonic until they begin to impair social and occupational function. Further empirical study is needed to determine if these patients should be classified as having OCP or subthreshold OCD. The relative validity of each of the criteria also needs further empirical validation.

Developmental Psychopathology

There has been little systematic study of the developmental antecedents of OCD since Janet. In his *Obsessions and Psychasthenia*, Janet[56] outlines how obsessions and compulsions are the most severe stage of an underlying state of psychasthenia (a syndrome consisting of feelings of incompleteness and imperfection). He hypothesized that, at one time, all patients with obsessions and compulsions passed through a psychasthenic stage. His clinical descriptions of the temperamental features of psychasthenics coincide remarkably well with current phenomenologic descriptions of the disorder. His description of the patient who "finds on the stairway, the word that needed to be said in the parlor" is a beautiful clinical description of the independent variable chosen by Kagan, et al[89] to measure behavioral inhibition (i.e., speech latency in a novel social situation). It is important to note that Janet includes four of five elements of DSM-III compulsive personality disorder in his description of the psychasthenic state: perfectionism, indecisiveness, restricted emotional expression, and indecisiveness, whereas the orderly and obstinate aspects of our current definition of compulsive personality derive from Freud. Previous studies have shown that many or most patients with OCD do not meet DSM-III-R criteria for compulsive personality disorder.[88] The European diagnostic schemata for anacastic personality are more directly related to Janet's original definition of psychasthenia and are consistent with the idea of an obsessive spectrum that ranges from normal obsessional behavior to obsessional personality to OCD.

We have conducted a retrospective study of 90 of our obsessive-compulsive probands using a semistructured format that was designed to elicit personality traits or temperamental factors commonly found in OCD (unpublished observations). We identified 9 factors that were commonly found in our adult obsessive-compulsive probands as children (Table 2-7 and Figure 2-2). These traits tended to be constant throughout development.

There is a significant overlap of these developmental antecedents of OCD with the behavioral inhibition syndrome in children that Kagan, et al[89] have described. Four developmental traits appear to be shared by adult OCD and panic probands: (1) separation anxiety; (2) resistance to change or novelty; (3) risk aversion; and (4) submissiveness. Four of the traits are more likely to be specific to OCD: (1) perfectionism; (2) ambivalence; (3) excessive devotion to work; and (4) hypermorality. The overlap of the developmental antecedents of panic disorder and OCD is consistent with Janet's original conception of the psychasthenic syndrome and adds credence to a shared genetic vulnerability among the anxiety disorders. It appears that some traits are more commonly seen in OCD symptoms (e.g., perfectionism with the need for symmetry and precision or incompleteness, and contamination fears with high levels of anxiety with abnormal risk assessment [Figure 2-2]). Further prospective study of the developmental antecedents of OCD should be an important area for future research.

The Relation of Heterogeneity and Comorbidity

We have become increasingly interested in developing a model of categorizing obsessive-compulsive patients based on what we see as the three core features of the disorder: (1) abnormal risk assessment; (2) pathologic doubt; and (3) incompleteness. These features cut across phenomenologic subtypes such as checking, cleaning, and the need for symmetry, although some symptom subtypes are more closely associated with one core feature than another.

Similar to phobics, obsessive-compulsive patients are continually worried that something will happen to them. If there is a one-in-a-million chance that the elevator cable will snap, the phobic is certain that it will snap on him or her. In the same way, many of our obsessive-compulsive patients' obsessions are

Table 2-7   Common Developmental Antecedents in Adult Obsessive-Compulsive Disorder Probands

Behavioral Inhibitions	Anacastic
Separation anxiety	Perfectionism
Resistance to change or novelty	Hypermorality
Risk aversion	Ambivalence
Submissiveness (compliance)	Excessive devotion to work
Sensitivity	

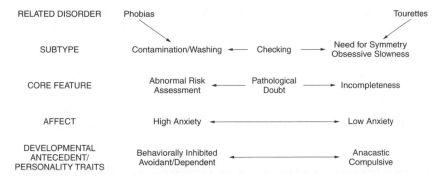

Fig. 2-2   Heterogeneity and comorbidity in obsessive-compulsive disorder.

dominated by the possibility of improbable events that most of us would not think twice about. Many checkers also suffer from "what if." "What if I didn't unplug the coffee machine and there's a fire?" Or, "What if I do pick up the knife?"

On the opposite side of the spectrum are obsessive-compulsive patients who experience little or no anxiety that something terrible will happen. Janet observed that many obsessive-compulsive patients were tormented by an inner sense of imperfection. Their actions were never completely achieved to satisfaction. Many of our patients describe an inner drive connected with a wish to have things perfect, absolutely certain, or completely under control. When they achieve this perfection, they describe a curious sensation that they can compare with no other feeling. Janet called it the *occasional brief appearance of sublime ecstasy*. This absolute feeling of certainty or perfection is rarely attained, and therefore, these patients experience a feeling of incompleteness.

The feeling of entering a door right through the middle, of having both shoelaces tied to exactly the same tension, of having one's hands perfectly clean, of saying one's prayers exactly right, or of having one's hair parted precisely down the middle are clinical examples. Most of us can relate to the feeling of wanting something "just so" or "perfect" and the feeling of accomplishment when we finally attain that, as well as the feelings of frustration and incompleteness when this doesn't happen. But for the obsessive patient, this feeling becomes attached to an action that would hold little significance for most of us, just as most of us don't think about the one-in-a-million chance of something going wrong. This feeling of incompleteness also is described by patients with Tourette's disorder and trichotillomania. Both describe a feeling of incompleteness with continued tension until they've pulled out an entire patch of hair or until they have completed a sequence of tics to their satisfaction. Both types of patients describe the impossibility of stopping in the middle of their compulsive actions, in spite of consequences. The core features appear to relate to both the clinical features of OCD and the relationship to comorbid disorders. Patients with abnormalities in risk assessment have high levels of anxiety associated with symptoms. In addition, these patients are more likely to have comorbid axis I panic GAD or social phobia, avoidant and dependent personality features, and a family history of an anxiety disorder. In contrast, patients with incompleteness are more likely to manifest low levels of anxiety, to have comorbid multiple tics or habit disorders such as trichotillomania or onychophagia, and to have compulsive personality features. Empirical validation of these subgroups may have important implications for diagnosis and treatment. There is already some evidence that patients with treatment-resistant OCD and tic spectrum disorder are particularly responsive to dopaminergic antagonists.[90] These patients also are more likely to exhibit incompleteness.

Baer [91] applied principal component analysis to 107 patients with OCD who completed the symptom checklist of the Y-BOCS and examined the correlations between the factor scores and the presence of comorbid tic or personality disorders. Three factors—symmetry/hoarding, contamination/cleaning, and pure obsessions—best explained the variance. Only the first factor was significantly related to OCPD or to a lifetime history of Tourette's disorder.

SUMMARY

Over the past 15 years, significant advances have been made that have revolutionized the way we conceptualize and treat OCD. Epidemiologic studies have confirmed that OCD is an underrecognized, common major psychiatric disorder with a lifetime prevalence of 2% to 3% in the general population and have been instrumental in focusing the attention of researchers, clinicians, and the media on this most interesting psychiatric disorder. Descriptions of the clinical features, course of illness, and comorbidity of the disorder have been in the literature since the turn of the century. However, the importance of using the clinical experience developed through years (working with OCD patients to develop and test new hypotheses about the etiology and treatment of OCD) is clear.

Future studies will benefit from the continuous refinement of our hypotheses on the heterogeneity and comorbidity of OCD and the search for homogeneous subtypes. The identification of an OCD/tic subtype has led to important new genetic and biologic studies and has been directly relevant to treatment. There is increasing evidence that patients with incompleteness may suffer from a different form of illness than patients with harm avoidance. Finally, the recent effort to clinically characterize pediatric autoimmune neuropsychiatric disorders and their relationship to genetic vulnerability to streptococcal infection offers a promising lead for further understanding of the pathophysiology of OCD. Increasing our understanding of the relationship between specific symptom patterns of OCD and the neurobiologic correlates over the next decade is a particularly exciting prospect for future research.

REFERENCES

1. Karno M, Goldin JM, Sorenson SB, Burnom A: The epidemiology of obsessive compulsive disorder in five U.S. communities, *Arch Gen Psychiatry* 45:1094–1099, 1988.
2. Flament M, Whitaker A, Rapoport J, et al: Obsessive compulsive disorder in adolescence in epidemiologic study, *J Am Acad Child Adolesc Psychiatry* 27(6):764–771, 1988.
3. Rapoport JL, editor: *Obsessive compulsive disorder in children and adolescents*, Washington, 1989, American Psychiatric Association.
4. Hwuh YE, Chang L: Prevalence of psychiatric disorders in Taiwan, *Acta Psychiatr Scand* 79:136, 1989.
5. Orly J, Wing JK: Psychiatric disorders in two African villages, *Arch Gen Psychiatry* 36:513, 1979.
6. Vaisaner E: Psychiatric disorders in Finland, *Acta Psychiatr Scand* 62(suppl 263):27, 1975.
7. Rudin E: Ein Beitrag zur Frage der Zwangskrankheit insebesondere ihrere hereditaren Beziehungen, *Arch Psychiatr Nervenkr* 191:14–54, 1953.
8. Hantouche EG, Bouhassira M, Lancrenon S, et al: Prevalence of obsessive compulsive disorders in a large French patient population in psychiatric consultation, *Encephale* 21(5):571–580, 1995.
9. Myers JK, Weissman MM, Tischler GL, et al: Six month prevalence of psychiatric disorders in three commitments, *Arch Gen Psychiatry* 41:949–958, 1984.
10. Robins LN, Helzer JE, Weissman MM, et al: Lifetime prevalence of specific psychiatric disorders in three sites, *Arch Gen Psychiatry* 41:958–967, 1984.
11. Bland RC, Newman SC, Orn H: Period prevalence of psychiatric disorders in Edmonton, *Acta Psychiatr Scand* 77(suppl 338):33–42, 1988.
12. Anthony JC, Folstein M, Romanoski AJ: Comparison of lay diagnostic interview schedule and a standardized psychiatric diagnosis. Experience in eastern Baltimore, *Arch Gen Psychiatry* 985:667–675, 1985.
13. Helzer JE, Robins LN, McEvoy LT: A comparison of clinical and diagnostic interview schedule diagnosis: Physician reexamination of lay interview cases in general population, *Arch Gen Psychiatry* 42:657–666, 1985.
14. Cooper J: The Leyton Obsessional Inventory, *Psychiatr Med* 1:48, 1970.
15. Valleni-Basile LA, Garrison CZ, Jackson KL, et al: Frequency of obsessive compulsive disorder in a community sample of young adolescents, *J Am Acad Child Adolesc Psychiatry* 34(2):782–791, 1995.
16. Douglass HM, Moffitt TE, Dar R, et al: Obsessive compulsive disorder in a birth cohort of 18 year olds: Prevalence and predictors, *J Am Acad Child Adolesc Psychiatry* 34(11):1424–1431, 1995.
17. Apter A, Fallon TJ, King RA, et al: Obsessive compulsive characteristics: From symptoms to syndrome, *J Am Acad Child Adolesc Psychiatry* 35(7):907–912, 1996.
18. Weissman MM, Bland RC, Canino GJ, et al: The cross national epidemiology of obsessive compulsive disorder, *J Clin Psychiatry* (suppl 55):5–10, 1994.
19. Tadai T, Nakamura M, Okazaki S, et al: The prevalence of obsessive compulsive disorder in Japan: A study of students using the Maudsley Obsessional-Compulsive Inventory and DSM-III-R, *Psychiatr Clin Neurosci* 49(1):39–41, 1995.

20. Weissman MM, Myers JK, Harding PS: Psychiatric disorders in a U.S. urban community, *Am J Psychiatry* 135:459, 1978.
21. Bebbington P: Personal communication.
22. Degonda M, Wyss M, Angst J: The Zurich study. XVIII. Obsessive compulsive disorders and syndromes in the general population, *Eur Arch Psychiatr Clin Neurosci* 243(1):16–22, 1993.
23. Shapiro S, Skinner EA, Kessler LG, et al: Utilization of health and mental health services, *Arch Gen Psychiatry* 41:971–978, 1984.
24. Rasmussen SA: Obsessive compulsive disorder in dermatologic practice, *J Am Acad Dermatol* 13:965, 1986.
25. Rasmussen S, Tsuang MT: Epidemiology of obsessive compulsive disorder: A review, *J Clin Psychiatry* 45:450–457, 1984.
26. Rachman S, DeSilva P: Abnormal and normal obsessions, *Behav Res Ther* 16: 233–248, 1978.
27. Greist JH, Jefferson JW, Kobak KA, et al: Efficacy and tolerability of serotonin transport inhibitors in obsessive compulsive disorder, *Arch Gen Psychiatry* 52:53–60, 1995.
28. Pauls DL, Alsobrook JP, Goodman W, et al: A family study of obsessive compulsive disorder, *Am J Psychiatry* 152(1):76–84, 1995.
29. Black A: The natural history of obsessional neurosis. In Beech HR, editor: *Obsessional states*, London, 1974, Methuen, pp 1–23.
30. Hollingsworth C, Tanguay P, Grossman L, et al: Long-term outcome of obsessive compulsive disorder in childhood, *J Am Acad Child Psychiatry* 9:134–144, 1980.
31. Castle DJ, Deale A, Marks IM: Gender differences in obsessive compulsive disorder, *Aust N Z J Psychiatry* 29(1):114–117, 1995.
32. Coryell W: Obsessive compulsive disorder and primary unipolar depression: Comparisons of background, family history, course and mortality, *J Nerv Ment Dis* 169:220–224, 1981.
33. Rachman S, Hodgson RL: *Obsessions and compulsions*, Englewood Cliffs, 1980, Prentice-Hall.
34. Freud S: Obsessive actions and religious practices. In *The standard edition of the complete psychological works of Sigmund Freud*, vol IX, London, 1952, Hogarth, pp 115–129.
35. Greenberg D, Chir B: Are religious compulsions religious or compulsive: A phenomenological study, *Am J Psychother* 38:524, 1984.
36. Lewis AJ: Problems of obsessional illness, *Proc R Soc Med* 29:325–336, 1936.
37. Lo WH: A followup study of obsessional neurotics in Hong Kong Chinese, *Br J Psychiatry* 113:823–832, 1967.
38. Flor-Henry P, Yeudall LT, Kiles ZJ, et al: Neuropsychological and power spectral EEG investigations of the obsessive compulsive syndrome, *Biol Psychiatry* 14:119–130, 1979.
39. Insel TR, Donnelly EG, Lalaken NL, et al: Neurological and neuropsychological studies of patients with obsessive-compulsive disorder, *Biol Psychiatry* 18:741–751, 1983a.
40. Kayton L, Borge GF: Birth order and obsessive compulsive character, *Arch Gen Psychiatry* 17:751–754, 1967.

41. Tsuang MT: Birth order and maternal age of psychiatric inpatients, *Br J Psychiatry* 112:1131–1141, 1966.
42. Swedo SE, Leonard HL: Childhood movement disorders and obsessive compulsive disorder, *J Clin Psychiatry* (suppl 55)32–37, 1994.
43. Swedo SE, Leonard HL, Garvey M, et al: Pediatric autoimmune neuropsychiatric disorders associated with streptococcal infections (PANDAs: A clinical description of the first fifty cases), *Am J Psychiatry* 155(2):264–271, 1998.
44. Goodwin DW, Guze SB, Robins E: Followup studies in obsessional neurosis, *Arch Gen Psychiatry* 20:182–187, 1969.
45. Rasmussen SA, Tsuang MT: DSM-III obsessive compulsive disorder: Clinical characteristics and family history, *Am J Psychiatry* 143:317–322, 1986.
46. Flament MF, Koby E, Rapoport JL, et al: Childhood obsessive compulsive disorder: A prospective follow-up study, *J Child Psychol Psychiatry* 31:363–380, 1990.
47. Leonard HL, Swedo SE, Lenane MC, et al: A two to seven year follow-up study of 54 obsessive compulsive children and adolescents, *Arch Gen Psychiatry* 50:429–439, 1993.
48. Thomsen PH: Obsessive compulsive disorder in children and adolescents in Denmark, *Acta Psychiatr Scand* 88(3):212–217, 1993.
49. Orloff LM, Battle MA, Baer L, et al: Long term follow-up of 85 patients with obsessive compulsive disorder, *Am J Psychiatry* 51:441–442, 1994.
50. Eisen JL, Rasmussen SA, Goodman W, et al: A two year prospective followup study of OCD, submitted for publication.
51. Steketee G, Eisen JL, Rasmussen SA, et al: A five year followup study of obsessive compulsive disorder, submitted for publication.
52. Koran LM, Thienemann ML, Davenport R: Quality of life for patients with obsessive compulsive disorder, *Am J Psychiatry* 153(6):783–788, 1996.
53. Okasha A, Kamel M, Hassan AH: Preliminary psychiatric observations in Egypt, *Am J Psychiatry* 114:949, 1968.
54. Freud S: *The complete psychological works of Sigmund Freud*, vols 1–24, London, 1983, Hogarth Press. Translated by J Strachey.
55. Bleuler E: *Lehrbuch der Psychiatrie,* ed 2, Berlin, 1920, Springer-Verlag.
56. Janet P: *Les obsessions et al psychasthenie*, ed 2, Paris, 1904, Bailliere.
57. Kraeplin E: *Lectures on clinical psychiatry*, New York, 1913, William Wood.
58. Rasmussen SA, Eisen JL: Clinical and epidemiologic findings of significance to neuropharmacologic trials in OCD, *Psychopharmacol Bull* 24(3):466–470, 1988.
59. Straus EW: On obsession: A clinical and methodological study, *Nerv Ment Dis Mon* 73:1, 1948.
60. MacLean PD: Brain evolution relating to family, play, and the separation call, *Arch Gen Psychiatry* 42:405, 1985.
60a. Marsland, Rasmussen: unpublished data.
61. Foa EB, Kozak MJ, Goodman W, et al: DSM-IV field trial: Obsessive compulsive disorder, *Am J Psychiatry* 152:90–96, 1995.
62. Eisen JL, Rasmussen SA: Obsessive compulsive disorder with psychotic features, *J Clin Psychiatry* 54:373–379, 1993.
63. Eisen JL, Phillips K, Rasmussen SA, et al: The Brown Assessment of Beliefs Scale (BABS): Reliability and validity, *Am J Psychiatry* 155(1):102–108, 1998.

64. Eisen JL, Rasmussen SA, Goodman WK, et al: Does insight predict response to SSRIs in OCD? *Am J Psychiatry,* submitted for publication.
65. Ingram E: Obsessional illness in mental hospital patients, *J Ment Sci* 107:382–402, 1961.
66. Rosen I: The clinical significance of obsessions in schizophrenia, *J Ment Sci* 103:773–785, 1957.
67. Fenton WS, McGlashan TH: The prognostic significance of obsessive compulsive symptoms in schizophrenia, *Am J Psychiatry* 143:437–441, 1986.
68. Eisen JL, Beer D, Pato MT, et al: Obsessive compulsive disorder in patients with schizophrenia or schizoaffective disorder, *Am J Psychiatry* 154(2):271–273, 1997.
69. Welner A, Reich T, Robins E, et al: Obsessive compulsive neurosis: Record, follow-up, and family studies. I. Inpatient record study, *Comp Psychiatry* 17:527–539, 1976.
70. Gittleson NL: Depression in the obsessional neurotic, *Br J Psychiatry* 112:883–887, 1966.
71. Insel 1983.
72. Breier A, Charney DS, Heninger GR: Agoraphobia and panic disorder: Development, diagnostic stability and course of illness, *Arch Gen Psychiatry* 43:1029–1036, 1986.
73. Gordon A, Rasmussen SA: Mood related obsessive compulsive symptoms in a patient with bipolar affective disorder, *J Clin Psychiatry* 49:27–28, 1988.
74. Kruger, Cooke RG, Hasey GM, et al: Comorbidity of obsessive compulsive disorder in bipolar disorder, *J Affect Disord* 34(2):117–120, 1995.
75. Chen YW, Dilsaver C: Comorbidity for obsessive compulsive disorder in bipolar and unipolar disorders, *Psychiatr Res* 59(1):57–64, 1995.
76. Kringlen E: Obsessional neurotics: A long term followup, *Br J Psychiatry* 111:709–722, 1965.
77. Videbach T: The psychopathology of anacastic endogenous depression, *Acta Psychiatr Scand* 52:336–373, 1975.
78. Mellman TA, Uhde TW: Obsessive compulsive symptoms in panic disorder, *Am J Psychiatry* 144:1573–1576, 1986.
79. Barlow DH: *Anxiety and its disorders*, New York, 1988, Guilford Press.
80. Insel TR: Obsessive compulsive disorder—Five clinical questions and a suggested approach, *Comp Psychiatry* 23(3):241–251, 1982.
81. Lipsitz JD, Martin LY, Mannuzza S, et al: Childhood separation anxiety disorder in patients with adult anxiety disorders, *Am J Psychiatry* 151(6):927–929, 1994.
82. Leckman JF, Walker DE, Goodman WK, et al: "Just right" perceptions associated with compulsive behavior in Tourette's syndrome, *Am J Psychiatry* 151(5): 675–680, 1994.
83. Miguel EC, Coffey BJ, Baer L, et al: Phenomenology of intentional repetitive behaviors in obsessive compulsive disorder and Tourette's disorder, *J Clin Psychiatry* 56(6):246–255, 1995.
84. Pitman RK, Green RC, Jenike MA, et al: Clinical comparison of Tourette's disorder and obsessive compulsive disorder, *Am J Psychiatry* 144:1166–1171, 1987.
85. Holzer JC, Goodman WK, McDougle CJ, et al: Obsessive compulsive disorder with and without a chronic tic disorder, *Br J Psychiatry* 164:469–473, 1994.
86. Theil A, Broocks A, Ohlmeier M, et al: Obsessive compulsive disorder among

patients with anorexia nervosa and bulimia nervosa, *Am J Psychiatry* 152(1): 72–75, 1995.

87. Rastam M, Gillberg IC, Gillberg C: Anorexia nervosa 6 years after onset: Part II. Comorbid psychiatric problems, *Comp Psychiatry* 36(1):70–76, 1995.

88. Baer L, Jenike MA: Personality disorders in obsessive-compulsive disorder. In Jenike MA, Baer L, Minichiello WE, editors: *Obsessive-compulsive disorders: theory and management,* ed 3, St. Louis, Mosby (in press).

89. Kagan J, Reznick JS, Snidman N: The physiology and psychology of behavioral inhibition in children, *Child Dev* 58:459, 1987.

90. McDougle CJ, Goodman WK, Leckman JF, et al: Haloperidol addition in fluvoxamine refractory obsessive compulsive disorder. A double blind placebo controlled study in patients with and without tics, *Arch Gen Psychiatry* 51(4):302–308, 1994.

91. Baer L: Factor analysis of symptom subtypes of obsessive compulsive disorder and their relation to personality and tic disorders, *J Clin Psychiatry* (suppl 55): 18–23, 1994.

3

Juvenile Obsessive-Compulsive Disorder

Daniel A. Geller, M.B.B.S., F.R.A.C.P.

Obsessive-compulsive disorder (OCD) can affect children, adolescents, and adults.[1-10] Early indications of the existence of OCD in juveniles came from occasional case reports of children who were afflicted with the disorder[11] and from observations that a substantial proportion of adult OCD sufferers had onset of the disorder during childhood.[12] Later reports of adults with OCD confirmed that approximately one third of these patients had a childhood onset.[13,14] Further case reports of children and adolescents with OCD appeared between the 1940s and 1970s (Berman, n = 6; Despert, n = 68; Judd, n = 5; Adams, n = 49).[15-18] Although early theories regarding the etiology (and by corollary, treatment) of obsessional and compulsive behavior in children were based on psychodynamic formulations,[19-23] early clinical observations found mostly normal premorbid function without evidence of sexual trauma or of abnormal bowel training[17] in these children. Although the varied methodologies and changing diagnostic criteria of OCD make critical assessment of these earlier reports difficult, the reports do illustrate that OCD in children and adolescents has long been recognized.

EPIDEMIOLOGY

In the northeastern United States, Flament, et al[1] reported a lifetime prevalence rate of 1.9% in a survey of more than 5,000 high school students. The Leyton Obsessional Inventory (LOI)[24] was used as a screening tool, and structured clinical interviews were used to confirm diagnoses. It is noteworthy that few of the clinical cases identified in this study had been diagnosed correctly, and the study challenged the notion that the presence of OCD was relatively rare in juveniles. Rather, this study suggested that the diagnosis was often unrecognized. This initial study was subsequently confirmed by several American and international reports.[23,25] Valleni-Basile,[25] in a two-stage epidemiologic study in the southeastern United States, reported a lifetime prevalence rate of juvenile OCD of 3% and a 1-year incidence of 0.7%. Similarly, international studies have reported prevalence rates of 2.3% of OCD in juveniles in Israel,[26] 3.9% in New Zealand,[27] and 4.1% in Denmark.[28] All six epidemiologic studies were conducted on adolescent populations and most used school surveys to obtain samples. They also reported an equal gender ratio and high levels of lifetime comorbidity with rates of other psychiatric disorders ranging from 75% to 84%.[1,27] In addition, obsessive-compulsive phenomena and subclinical OCD appear to be quite common in juveniles and may be on a continuum with OCD.[26] Thus, OCD affecting children and adolescents appears to be at least as prevalent as the adult-onset disorder.[1,8,25,29–31]

PATHOPHYSIOLOGY AND NEUROBIOLOGY

It is likely that OCD is a heterogeneous disorder. Although the etiologies remain unknown, evidence for a neurobiologic basis for OCD is derived from multiple sources. The efficacy and specificity of serotonergic antidepressants[32–34] in the treatment of OCD, and the evidence of abnormalities in serotonin binding capacity[35] and decreases in platelet serotonin concentration[36] during clomipramine treatment in pediatric OCD subjects contribute to the hypothesis derived from adult studies that central serotonin pathways are implicated in the pathophysiology of the disorder. Neuroimaging, including functional neuroimaging, studies[37–39] have also implicated the basal ganglia, caudate nucleus, and frontal cortex in the genesis of obsessive-compulsive symptoms, but replication of these findings is needed in pediatric subjects.

Clinical and family studies provide strong evidence for a genetic etiology in some patients with OCD. The available studies of juveniles with OCD report the disorder as highly familial in children and adolescents. OCD and subclinical obsessive-compulsive symptoms were found in 18% to 30% of first-degree relatives.[40,41] Lenane, et al[41] found that fathers of pediatric OCD patients were more likely to be affected with OCD than mothers and that father-son pairs were the most common familial pattern. Pauls, et al[40] also found a higher risk for tic disorders (Tourette's disorder and chronic tics) in first-degree relatives of OCD juveniles and a significantly increased risk for both OCD and tics in the relatives of patients with early-onset OCD compared with relatives of later-onset OCD patients. Leonard, et al[42] found an earlier age at onset of OCD in subjects with comorbid OCD and Tourette's disorder. These reports also support the notion that the hypothesized link between OCD and Tourette's disorder occurs in juvenile-onset OCD patients. Clinical studies suggest that the familiality of OCD is increased in patients with childhood-onset disorder[4,40,41,43,44] compared with adult-onset OCD patients. In the National Institute of Mental Health (NIMH) series,[4] the Riddle, et al[44] series, and the Geller, et al[45] series, the vast majority of OCD patients with a positive family history of the disorder were subjects 12 years of age and younger. Together, these findings indicate that there could be an inverse relationship between age of onset and genetic loading of OCD. Because younger age of onset is associated with a positive family history, and a family history of psychiatric disorder has been reported to be an adverse prognostic factor in juvenile OCD patients,[46] childhood-onset OCD may herald a more complicated course in affected patients.

Three clinical studies noted the presence of adverse neurologic and perinatal events in childhood OCD patients.[44,47,48] These events included cerebral hemorrhage in one,[48] traumatic head injury in two,[47] and unspecified "perinatal difficulties" in 9 of 21 patients in Riddle, et al.[49] However, it is difficult to say whether these neurologic events represent the same pathophysiologic mechanisms as those reported in the adult-onset OCD literature. In another study, Rapoport[3] found abnormal neurologic examinations in 44 of 54 juvenile OCD patients (18 had choreiform movements) clustering among the younger subjects; however, no comparison group was studied. In a review of adverse birth events from a national birth registry, Thomsen[50] found that although 20% of 61 juvenile OCD patients were placed in the "organic" class, this rate was not different than that of non-OCD psychiatric controls. In contrast, Douglass et al[27] longitudinally followed a consecutive birth cohort from Dunedin, New Zealand. They reported no significant differences in recorded adverse perinatal events in subjects who had developed OCD by 18 years of age compared with psychologically healthy patients and psychiatric controls. Thus, clinical and epidemiologic samples may differ in the presence or absence of abnormal neurologic findings. The association between childhood movement disorders that are presumed to have a neurologic basis, such as Sydenham's chorea, and pediatric OCD has been reviewed by Swedo and Leonard,[51] who speculate that basal ganglia disturbance is associated with OCD symptoms.

As noted in Chapter 2, recent investigations have focused on the possibility that autoimmune disturbance may produce obsessive-compulsive and tic behavior in some children infected with group A β-hemolytic streptococcus through autoantibodies reacting with neuronal tissue.[52–55] An observed association between juvenile OCD and Sydenham's chorea,[56] which was presumed to be caused by autoimmune pathophysiology affecting the basal ganglia following streptococcal infection, led to the search for non-Sydenham's–mediated, streptococcal-induced OCD. Although these putative "pediatric autoimmune neuropsychiatric disorders associated with streptococcal infections" (or "PANDAS") probably account for only a subset of juvenile OCD patients, they have nonetheless generated great interest both as possible models for the development of neuropsychiatric symptoms and as implications that antibiotic treatment of upper respiratory streptococcal infections may impact OCD and Tourette's disorder severity. Measurement of antistreptolysin O titers (ASOT) or anti-DNAse B antibodies provides indirect evidence for such a process because direct assay of antineuronal antibodies is largely experimental at present.

Further evidence for etiologic heterogeneity of OCD derives from neuro-endocrine studies in adults and children.[57–61] These studies suggest that some forms of OCD may be mediated by increased levels of oxytocin. Hamburger[62] described height and weight deficits in juveniles with OCD when compared with age- and gender-matched normal and psychiatric controls and a flattened growth curve, suggesting subtle neuroendocrine dysfunction. Further, Kreusi, et al[63] found increased cerebrospinal fluid levels of somatostatin in OCD children compared with matched disruptive behavior disordered subjects. These findings provide direct and indirect evidence of a role for somatostatin in the pathophysiology of juvenile OCD in some subjects. Other neuroendocrine studies of cerebrospinal fluid levels of corticotrophin-releasing hormone, somatostatin, vasopressin, and oxytocin and monoamine metabolites before[61] and after treatment[58] are also consistent with a role for these neuropeptides in the pathophysiology of OCD in some children.

CLINICAL FEATURES
Phenomenology and Diagnosis

Rituals and superstitions that occur as part of normal childhood development[64] are distinct from clinical obsessions and compulsions;[65] the latter provoke anxiety, impair function, and have a later onset. Although insistence on routines and rituals is common in preschool-age children, this behavior usually fades in early school-age children. In later childhood, formalized games, hobbies, and collections are common and promote social interaction. Leonard, et al[65] compared early childhood rituals and superstitions in a clinical sample of OCD children with those of normal controls. They found that, although parents of OCD children gave a history of more childhood rituals, when rituals resembling OCD behaviors were excluded, these patients did not differ significantly from controls. Further study is needed to determine if this finding indicates an insidious subclinical onset of the disorder or a behavioral marker for later OCD.

The clinical phenotype and diagnostic criteria for OCD are similar in children and in adults.[66] The decision to de-emphasize insight as a DSM-IV[66] diagnostic requirement for OCD (which followed DSM-IV OCD field trial recommendations[67]) may be especially relevant to children and adolescents with the disorder. One of the few studies addressing this issue reported that 30% of OCD children have poor or little insight regarding their disorder,[45] and Allsop[47] found that poor insight was evident in more than 50% of his sample. It is unknown if the limited insight in some OCD children reflects immature cognitive development of the child or specific developmental differences.

Although diagnostic criteria for OCD are well operationalized for juvenile patients, the diagnosis may sometimes be missed because of (1) children's limited ability to articulate their obsessions; and (2) failure of mental health professionals to inquire about obsessive-compulsive symptoms (particularly when more prominent psychopathologic features are present). For example, our group recently reviewed pediatric OCD literature and found that the mean time between onset of OCD and presentation was 2.5 years.[45]

Although the majority of children exhibit both multiple obsessions and compulsions (mean number over lifetime was 4.0 and 4.8, respectively, in one study[68]), compulsions with no accompanying obsessions were significantly more common in children than in adolescents.[68] Neither gender nor age of onset was significantly related to the type, number, or severity of OCD symptoms.[68]

Prior to the development of the Yale-Brown Obsessive Compulsive Scale (Y-BOCS),[69] there was no available standardized method to record or quantify symptomatology. However, the most commonly reported obsessions in children and adolescents with OCD in these studies concerned contamination, sex, the body, magic, and scruples. Washing, repeating, checking, ordering, and touching were the most common compulsions. Frequently, children's obsessions center on fear of a catastrophic family event (e.g., the death of a parent). Mental rituals such as praying, chanting, and counting are also common and patients should be asked specifically about them.

Although OCD symptoms tend to wax and wane, they persist in the majority of pediatric patients and frequently change over time (i.e., the presenting symptom constellation is often not maintained).[70] Often, parents have been noted to be intimately involved in their child's rituals, especially in the child's reassurance seeking, which is a form of vicarious checking. Specific psychosocial events associated with the onset of OCD were described in several reports, which suggest that these events may be precipitants in 38% to 54% of juvenile OCD cases.[17,47,70–72]

Age of Onset

Perhaps the clearest difference between juvenile and adult OCD is age of onset. Studies have shown a *bimodal* distribution of age of onset, with one peak in childhood and a second in early adulthood. In contrast to adult OCD studies that reported mean age of onset at 21 years,[6,8,40,73–75] studies of pediatric OCD have consistently found a prepubertal age of onset.[4,28,44,45,68,72,76] The mean age of onset in these studies ranged from 7.5 to 12.5 years of age, and the age at assessment ranged from 12 to 15.2 years of age.

Gender Representation

In contrast to adult OCD patients who demonstrate either equal gender representation or a slight preponderance in women,[7,8] pediatric clinical OCD patients show a male-to-female ratio of approximately 3:2.[4,17,45,68,72] Two reports found that boys had an earlier age of onset than girls.[4,68]

Comorbidity

Studies of juvenile OCD have indicated that comorbidity is the rule, whereas OCD as an only diagnosis is the exception; thus, at least two thirds of juveniles with OCD will have one or more additional axis I diagnoses (including both internalizing and externalizing disorders). Aside from the high rates of comorbidity with tic, mood, and anxiety disorders seen in OCD adults (Figure 3-1),[77,78] juvenile OCD also is frequently characterized by high rates of (1) comorbid disruptive behavior disorders (i.e., attention deficit hyperactivity disorder and oppositional defiant disorder); (2) specific developmental disorders; and (3) enuresis. Comorbid conditions appear in a chronologic sequence with attention deficit hyperactivity disorder, specific developmental and other anxiety disorders, and Tourette's disorder often identifiable years before the OCD symptoms.[45] Our group recently used structured diagnostic interview methodology[45] and found rates of psychiatric comorbidity in more than 90% of juveniles presenting to a specialized OCD clinic, including a rate of 50% for disruptive behavior disorders.[45] Although these types of comorbid psychiatric problems in juvenile OCD patients are partly distinct from adult OCD, it is not known whether they represent unique developmental hallmarks of juvenile-onset OCD, because studies of OCD adults do not screen subjects for some of these disorders.

The comorbidity of Tourette's disorder plus OCD has long been recognized. This overlap appears to be bidirectional and has been shown to affect approximately one third of patients with each disorder.[42,79–81] Although rates of Tourette's disorder of 0.03% to 0.4% have been reported in selected community samples,[82–84] much higher rates of chronic tic disorders have been reported in juvenile clinical samples.[42,45] For example, Leonard, et al[42] found Tourette's disorder in 15% and chronic tics in 31% of children and adolescents within 2 to 7 years following treatment for OCD, although patients with Tourette's disorder were initially excluded. Our group recently reviewed the pediatric OCD literature and found Tourette's disorder or chronic tics were reported in 21% of juvenile OCD patients across eleven studies.[45] Similarly, family studies of probands with Tourette's disorder[80,85–87] support evidence for a genetic relationship between these two disorders (see Chapter 14). Although Tourette's disorder and OCD are believed to result from common underlying etiologic risk factors, the reason some patients express only one or both of these disorders remains unknown. Nevertheless, the presence of the comorbid type of Tourette's disorder and OCD may herald a more serious phenotype than that of either disorder alone. For example, Leonard, et al[5] reported that the presence of tic disorder and OCD was associated with poorer treatment outcome, compared with children without comorbid tics.

Cognitive, Neuropsychologic, and School Function

A number of studies report neuropsychologic deficits in patients with juvenile OCD.[27,88] Rapoport[89] found significantly lower scores on performance subtests of the Wechsler Intelligence Scale for Children-Revised (WISC-R)[90]

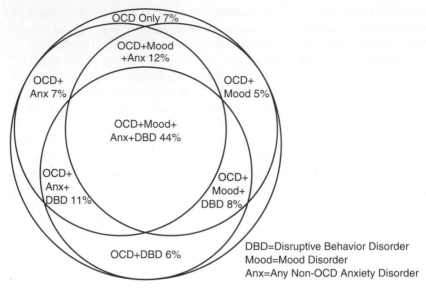

Fig. 3-1 Comorbidity of juvenile obsessive-compulsive disorder (n = 217). (Courtesy of McLean Hospital Pediatric OCD Clinic and Massachusetts General Hospital Psycho-Pharmacological Clinic.)

in adolescent OCD patients compared with normal controls. The NIMH subjects also performed less well in several neuropsychologic tests deemed sensitive to frontal and/or caudate lesions at baseline and at posttreatment follow-up.[91,92] Behar, et al[91] also found significantly increased mean ventricular-brain ratios in these 16 adolescents with OCD compared with control subjects. In the 34 pediatric OCD subjects of an epidemiologic survey by Douglass,[27] neither IQ assessed using the WISC-R nor a battery of neuropsychologic test results differed from the psychiatric or normal controls.

Many authors[47,48,68,71,72] note school avoidance, school refusal, and academic difficulties in juvenile OCD subjects. In one report,[45] 48% of patients had received remedial help, 40% were placed in a special class, and 7% had repeated a grade. Other researchers[4,43,68] have reported rates of specific developmental disorders in their pediatric OCD patients, ranging from 23% to 27%. Although the causes of impaired school performance are probably multidetermined, the learning disabilities often predate the OCD. A relative academic decline is therefore not uncommon in juveniles with OCD and is a sign of more serious decompensation.

OBSESSIVE-COMPULSIVE SPECTRUM DISORDERS

Trichotillomania, compulsive nail biting and skin picking, body dysmorphic disorder, anorexia nervosa, and bulimia nervosa occur in pediatric patients and share some characteristics, but some important differences, with OCD. In fact, the comorbidity between these disorders is not very common. For example, trichotillomania is concurrent with OCD in approximately 10% to 15% of cases.[93,94] The "habit" or impulse-control disorders, such as trichotillomania and onychophagia, may not share treatment responsivity with OCD, although little data exist on drug treatment of these disorders in the pediatric population. Our group often has found that the serotonergic antidepressants have minimal impact on these behaviors in juvenile patients, although comorbid psychopathology, especially depression, is common and medications may be otherwise helpful. Behavioral treatments are often the treatment of choice for these patients. Somatic obsessions and dysmorphophobia (i.e., body dysmorphic disorder) occur in juvenile OCD patients and may represent the only symptom. These characteristics are more common in adolescents than in prepubertal children and may present as a preoccupation and dissatisfaction with hairstyle, leading to grooming behaviors. Antiobsessional agents are the first-choice treatment in these patients, even in the absence of insight. Young patients with anorexia nervosa and bulimia nervosa require a comprehensive treatment approach that ideally involves pediatric or adolescent medical supervision, behavioral management, family therapy, and often psychopharmacologic treatment and an alliance between mental health and medical personnel, which is usually best achieved in specialized programs for eating disorders.

ASSESSMENT

Once the categorical diagnosis of OCD is made, the clinician can use a number of dimensional scales to rate the severity and treatment responsiveness of symptoms in juvenile patients. Global assessment of severity (GAS)[95] scales and clinical global impairment (CGI)[96] scales permit an overall quantitative assessment of the impact of symptoms. A more detailed quantifiable instrument is the Children's Yale-Brown Obsessive Compulsive Scale (CY-BOCS),[97] a clinician-rated, 10-item scale, in which each item is rated on a five-point scale from 0 ("no symptoms") to 4 ("extreme symptoms") and a total range from 0 to 40, with subtotals for obsessions (items 1 through 5) and compulsions (items 6 through 10). Ratings for the amount of time consumed by obsessions or compulsions, degree of life interference, degree of internal distress, and resistance to and control over symptoms are recorded and totaled. Further questions probe for the amount of insight, avoidance, indecisiveness, sense of overvalued responsibility, and pervasive slowness, although these items do not contribute to the total score. The CY-BOCS includes a symptom checklist of more than 60 examples of obsessions and compulsions organized into several larger categories according to their thematic content (e.g., contamination, aggressive, sexual, hoarding, somatic, religious obsessions or magical thoughts and rituals, washing, checking, repeating, counting, ordering). The parent version, the Y-BOCS,[69] has proved both a reliable and valid measure of OCD symptomatology in adults and a measure responsive to changes with treatment. Preliminary data[98,99] also indicate good interrater reliability, internal consistency, and convergent validity of the child version. One potential problem with this instrument relates to obsessional avoidance of a feared stimulus. If a child has a great degree of passive avoidance, for example, of touching household items or other family members, then the impairment caused by this restriction may not be reflected in the total CY-BOCS score. Treatment responsivity also has been shown with the CY-BOCS in open and controlled studies,[100–102] and it is the current gold standard for assessment of juvenile OCD.

The original Leyton Obsessional Inventory (LOI),[24,103] a 69-item self-report questionnaire for obsessional adults, was adapted by Berg[104] for use with children and adolescents and then further adapted into a 20-item survey form (LOI-Child Version)[105] used in a two-stage epidemiologic study assessing the prevalence of OCD in a community sample of adolescents. The 20-item Leyton demonstrated high internal reliability,[105] high sensitivity but low specificity and predictive value,[1] and appeared useful primarily as a screening tool for current obsessive-compulsive symptomatology. Because it is a self-report instrument, use of the LOI may be limited in those younger subjects with poor insight.

TREATMENT
Pharmacotherapy

Treatment studies (Table 3-1), including a total of 376 juvenile OCD patients, all found that serotonergic medications were effective in both the short-term and medium-term treatment of children and adolescents with OCD. Although most studies were acute-treatment trials lasting no longer than 10 weeks, all longer-term studies found efficacy maintained over time.[34,43,101] Prospective controlled trials with both placebo[32,101,106] and nonserotonergic drugs[33,34] also indicated specificity of response for the serotonergic antidepressants. Four studies evaluated clomipramine, five evaluated fluoxetine, and two evaluated fluvoxamine (Table 3-1), with reported response rates ranging from 50% to 75% and amount of symptom abatement ranging from 25% to 57%. Our group[43] has found that both preadolescent and adolescent OCD patients respond equally well to fluoxetine over a treatment period averaging 19 months.

These studies document that the need for aggressive dosing in pediatric OCD is shared with the adult disorder. For example, clomipramine at 3 to 5 mg/kg/day was used in the NIMH cohort.[32–34] In a retrospective series of children and adolescents treated for OCD with fluoxetine, doses averaged 1.0 mg/kg/day or 35 mg/day in children (12 years of age or younger) and 64 mg/day in adolescents (older than 12 years of age).[43] Dosing for sertraline and fluvoxamine is somewhat higher at 1 to 3 mg/kg/day. Industry-sponsored trials of both sertraline and fluvoxamine used doses of 50 to 200 mg/day in

Table 3-1   Pharmacologic Treatment Studies in Pediatric Obsessive-Compulsive Disorder

Author/Year	Design of Study	Results
Flament, et al, 1985	10-week randomized, double-blind, placebo-controlled, cross-over trial of clomipramine	75% showed at least moderate improvement Response independent of depressive symptoms
Leonard, et al, 1989	10-week randomized, double-blind, placebo-controlled, cross-over trial of clomipramine versus desipramine	Clomipramine superior to desipramine 64% relapsed when switched from clomipramine to desipramine Little placebo response
Liebowitz, et al, 1990	Open trial of fluoxetine in adolescents	50% or more improved clinically
Riddle, et al, 1990	Open trial of fluoxetine	50% response rate
Como and Kurlan, 1991	Open trial of fluoxetine in adolescents	54%–85% response rate
Leonard, et al, 1991	8-month double-blind desipramine substitution during clomipramine maintenance treatment	89% relapsed on desipramine, compared with 18% on clomipramine Younger age predicted increased risk for relapse
DeVeaugh-Geiss, 1992	Multicenter 8-week randomized, double-blind, placebo-controlled, parallel trial, with 1-year open-label extension phase of clomipramine	Obsessive-compulsive symptoms decreased 37% in treated group, compared with 8% in placebo group 60% were very much improved Response was maintained over 1-year extension
Riddle, et al, 1992	20-week randomized, double-blind, placebo-controlled, cross-over trial of fluoxetine	Significant differences between groups in improving global obsessive-compulsive disorder scores, but not in CY-BOCS scores
Apter, et al, 1994	8-month open-label, variable-dose trial of fluvoxamine in adolescents	29% decrease in obsessive-compulsive symptoms
Geller, et al, 1995	Retrospective review of fluoxetine treatment in clinical series of juveniles	75% moderate/marked improvement Effect size 47%
Riddle, et al, 1996	10-week randomized, double-blind, placebo-controlled, parallel trial of fluvoxamine	Children and adolescents responded equally well Significant difference between fluvoxamine and placebo in obsessive-compulsive symptoms Well tolerated

children. Although the use of paroxetine in pediatric OCD is now being systematically studied (by SmithKline Beecham Pharmaceuticals), clear guidelines for dosing in this age group (younger than 16 years of age) are not yet available. However, doses of paroxetine 10 to 60 mg/day (0.5 to 1.0 mg/kg/day) appear to be equivalent to the other SSRI dose ranges noted previously.

Placebo response in the studies in Table 3-1 ranged from 10%[32,101] to 27%.[106] The recently completed industry-sponsored controlled trial of fluvoxamine in 120 juvenile patients[102] showed similar efficacy but a higher placebo response rate than other studies. This study represents the largest controlled pharmacologic trial to date in pediatric OCD. Although no predictors of response were statistically significant, Leonard, et al[34] found that discontinuation of serotonergic medication at a younger age predicted later relapse. Serum levels did not correlate with clinical response.

In the most comprehensive study to date of the use of clomipramine in juvenile OCD,[101] adverse effects were common and included anticholinergic symptoms (e.g., dry mouth), 63%; tremor, 33%; dizziness, 41%; and sedation, 46%, making the drug difficult for some patients to tolerate even in the context of a robust clinical response. Adverse effects are also common, although generally better tolerated in juveniles treated with the SSRIs. For example, reported adverse effects of fluoxetine treatment included insomnia, 16%; somnolence, 11%; weight change and appetite disturbance, 8%; dry mouth and headache, 5%; and myoclonus, increased tics, bruising, and nervousness, 3%.[43] One of the most common adverse effects found with the use of fluoxetine and other SSRIs (as well as clomipramine) is behavioral activation/agitation,[107] which may occur in up to 25% of treated patients[43] and may be severe enough to warrant a diagnosis of organically induced mania or hypomania. Whether children with this adverse effect are predisposed to the development of bipolar disorder, which is then unmasked by the SSRI, remains unknown.

To date, controlled trials of augmentation in treatment-resistant adult OCD have shown only haloperidol[108] (inpatients with a chronic tic disorder or possibly psychotic symptoms) and clonazepam[109] to be helpful. One study suggests that clonazepam also may be a useful adjunct in the treatment of pediatric cases.[56] Although the addition of neuroleptics has not been systematically studied in children, such a trial may be indicated in those patients with comorbid Tourette's disorder or psychotic symptoms.

A more common and perhaps safer combined pharmacotherapeutic approach for the OCD juvenile with a chronic tic disorder or attention deficit hyperactivity disorder is clomipramine plus an SSRI. Although attention to blood levels is mandatory because of hepatic inhibition of clomipramine metabolism by SSRIs and consequent increased blood levels, this combination may be extremely useful in certain patients. In addition, because the secondary amine tricyclic antidepressants recently have proved useful in both tic disorders and attention deficit hyperactivity disorder,[110-114] the noradrenergic tricyclic metabolite of clomipramine (desmethylclomipramine) may have a unique role in the treatment of these comorbid patients.

The use of clomipramine mandates a thoughtful evaluation of the pediatric patient's general medical condition—cardiac status in particular. Baseline evaluation should include a systems review and questions about personal or family history of heart disease. If in doubt, a general pediatric examination including auscultation of the heart and measurement of pulse and blood pressure is indicated. A history of nonfebrile seizures should also be noted but is not an absolute contraindication to clomipramine. A baseline (i.e., pretreatment) electrocardiogram should be requested. Indices of interest are heart rate and rhythm, and cardiac electrocardiographic cycle intervals such as PR, QRS, and QTc. Because all tricyclics are type 1 antiarrhythmic agents, they may slow electrical conduction in the heart. Although statistically significant changes in conduction intervals and heart rate may occur, these changes are rarely of clinical significance. However, in view of the current debate in pediatric psychopharmacology circles regarding the safety of desipramine, the prudent practitioner will evaluate and document these cardiac parameters. These issues have been reviewed by Biederman,[115] and Food and Drug Administration guidelines regarding unacceptable electrocardiographic indices for not using, or not increasing, clomipramine are: (1) PR interval greater than 200 ms; (2) QRS interval greater than 30% increased over baseline or greater than 120 ms; (3) blood pressure greater than 140 systolic or 90 diastolic; and (4) heart rate greater than 130 bpm at rest.[116,117] Finally, a prolonged QTc (corrected QT interval $\geq$ 450 ms) is associated with increased risk of ventricular tachycardias and is a relative contraindication for clomipramine use (or further increase). Despite these concerns, clomipramine remains an important drug in the armamentarium of antiobsessional medications.

Behavioral Treatment

Although many anecdotal reports (27 case reports) of some form of behavioral therapy[118] suggest the usefulness of behavioral treatments in juvenile OCD, the very limited scientific information on this subject does not permit a straightforward comparison with this treatment modality in adult OCD. Four behavioral treatment reports,[119–122] which included a total of 60 patients, reported some improvement in OCD symptoms. However, none of these studies were controlled and most included medicated patients. For example, a report by de Haan[121] of 22 OCD children indicated a 75% to 95% improvement in 16 cases at follow-up using outpatient behavioral techniques. March, et al,[122] using a manualized cognitive behavior treatment protocol, found that 9 of 15 adolescent outpatients had a 50% or greater improvement on the CY-BOCS[97] and that medication could be discontinued in six cases. Benefits were maintained at follow-up periods of up to 18 months. Several reports, however, remarked that the presence of disruptive or oppositional behavior made successful implementation of behavioral treatments more difficult.[47,48,122]

Despite the limited evidence demonstrating efficacy in well-designed scientific studies, strong empirical support exists for the use of cognitive behavioral treatment in juveniles OCD, and it may be the treatment of choice for some patients (e.g., very young patients or those with serious adverse reactions to medications). The younger the patient, the more parental involvement is needed for the successful implementation of behavioral treatment. Some experts routinely advocate a trial of behavioral therapy before beginning medication, but this decision is a clinical one based on many factors, including patient and family attitudes toward drugs, the cognitive capacity, insight, and motivation of the young patient, the intactness of the family, and the presence of comorbid psychiatric conditions. Most often, the greatest benefit will derive from combined pharmacologic and behavioral approaches because drug treatment rarely removes all symptoms yet may increase tolerance to behavioral techniques.

Other Treatments

Although scientific evidence for the usefulness of individual or family therapy is very limited, most clinicians experienced in the treatment of OCD agree that some individuals and their families benefit greatly from these interventions. Family interactions, parental perceptions, self-concept, and identity formation of the juvenile patient may be altered by the presence of OCD and associated morbidity. Such issues can be best addressed by a more traditional psychotherapeutic approach, although these issues may not directly impact obsessive-compulsive behaviors.

On the other hand, little support currently exists for intensive psychoanalytic psychotherapy of OCD symptoms per se in pediatric patients. Finally, because social impairment is frequently perceived as more severe than academic impairment[68] and social withdrawal and isolation are common, group therapy or patient-sponsored support groups can be very helpful for some juvenile OCD sufferers. Local and state affiliates of the National Obsessive-Compulsive Foundation sometimes facilitate groups for teenagers.

OUTCOME AND PROGNOSIS

Eight studies describing 208 subjects (mean, 26; range, 14 to 54 subjects) with a mean follow-up of 7 years (range, 2 to 22 years) all report chronicity of symptoms in outcome and long-term follow-up studies of children and adolescents with OCD. Four of these studies were retrospective; one[123] was a 2-year follow-up of a community sample of adolescents with OCD, who were identified during an epidemiologic survey; seven studies were of clinical samples. Combined, 50% of subjects still met diagnostic criteria for OCD at follow-up (range, 23% to 70%). Seven studies that examined treatment outcome indicated that improvement of OCD symptoms was maintained over time. For example, Leonard, et al[46] found at 2- to 7-year follow-up, only 19% of patients were rated as unchanged or worse. However, 70% of patients were still taking psychoactive medication, 43% continued to meet time and impairment criteria for a full diagnosis, and only 6% were considered to be in true remission.

Less rigorous data are available for psychosocial treatments. Authors of these studies all reported improvement in their subjects. Four reports[124–127] stress a poor social outcome (including those compared with psychiatric controls[127]) associated with juvenile OCD, with isolation and failure of patients to achieve developmentally appropriate psychosocial milestones. Some studies reported that poor outcome was associated with (1) poor response to initial treatment;[46] (2) presence of family psychiatric illness;[46,125] and (3) a lifetime history of tics.[46] Leonard, et al[42] found that despite efforts to exclude subjects with Tourette's disorder, 8 boys out of 54 pediatric OCD subjects had Tourette's disorder at follow-up, and these patients had an earlier age of OCD onset than the rest.

SUMMARY

The available literature indicates that OCD affecting juveniles has a prevalence of 2% to 3%. Although normal developmental rituals can usually be distinguished easily from clinical OCD, pediatric patients frequently demonstrate poor insight into the nature of their obsessions, which, along with their limited verbal expression, may make the diagnosis more difficult. Although the diagnostic criteria and clinical phenotype of OCD are similar between children and adults, rituals involving family members are more common in younger patients. Multiple obsessions and compulsions tend to wax and wane over time yet remain chronic.

Evidence from pathophysiologic and neuroanatomic studies suggests that OCD may be a heterogeneous disorder. Although the etiology of OCD is still unknown, genetic factors are strongly implicated because the disorder is highly familial and a juvenile onset of the disorder appears to be associated with an increased risk for familial transmission. Recent interest has focused on a possible autoimmune etiology, involving antineuronal antibodies in a subset of child OCD cases associated with tic disorders. A unique preadolescent peak of age at onset in juveniles provides evidence that OCD is a disorder with a bimodal incidence. The juvenile form is male preponderant and is frequently comorbid with a distinct pattern of comorbidity, including attention deficit hyperactivity disorder and developmental disorders, as well as tic, mood, and anxiety disorders. It is important for clinicians to appreciate the full scope of comorbidity when considering their treatment approach. Serotonergic antidepressants are effective in two thirds to three quarters of juvenile OCD patients but usually approximately 25% to 50% of symptoms are abated. Aggressive dosing is needed for some patients. Other treatments, including cognitive behavioral therapy, have not been well studied, but cumulative anecdotal evidence and experience suggest that these treatments are a valuable option for many children and adolescents and may even be the first-choice treatment for some.

In conclusion, there appear to be important similarities and differences between juvenile and adult OCD. The literature provides some evidence for considering age of onset as an important variable in the expression of OCD across the patient's life cycle.

REFERENCES

1. Flament M, Whitaker A, Rapoport J, et al: Obsessive compulsive disorder in adolescence: an epidemiological study, *J Am Acad Child Adolesc Psychiatry* 27: 764–771, 1988.
2. Flament M, Whitaker A, Rapoport J, et al: An epidemiological study of obsessive-compulsive disorder in adolescence. In Rapoport J, editor: *Obsessive-compulsive disorder in children and adolescents*, Washington, 1989, American Psychiatric Press.
3. Rapoport JL: *Obsessive-compulsive disorder in children and adolescents*, Washington, 1989, American Psychiatric Press.
4. Swedo S, Rapoport J, Leonard H, et al: Obsessive-compulsive disorder in children and adolescents: clinical phenomenology of 70 consecutive cases, *Arch Gen Psychiatry* 46:335–341, 1989.
5. Leonard HL, Lenane MC, Swedo SE: Obsessive-compulsive disorder, *Psych Clin North Am* 2:655–666, 1993.
6. Rasmussen SA, Eisen JL: The epidemiology and differential diagnosis of obsessive compulsive disorder, *J Clin Psychiatry* 53:4–10, 1992.
7. Rasmussen S, Eisen J: The epidemiology and clinical features of obsessive compulsive disorder, *Psychiatr Clin North Am* 15:743–758, 1992.
8. Karno M, Golding J, Sorenson S, et al: The epidemiology of obsessive-compulsive disorder in five U.S. communities, *Arch Gen Psychiatry* 45:1094–1099, 1988.
9. Weissman M, Bland R, Canino G, et al: The cross national epidemiology of obsessive compulsive disorder, *Am J Psychiatry* 55:5–10, 1994.
10. Jenike MA, Baer L, Minichiello WE: *Obsessive-compulsive disorders: Theory and management*, Littleton, Colo, 1990, Mosby.
11. Janet P: *Les obsessions et la psychasthenie*, Paris, 1903, Felix Alcan.
12. Pitres A, Regis E: *Les obsessions et les impulsions*, Paris, 1902, Doin.
13. Black A: The natural history of obsessional neurosis. In Beech H, editor: *Obsessional states*, London, 1974, Methuen.
14. Rachman SJ, Hodgson RJ: *Obsessions and compulsions*, Englewood Cliffs, NJ, 1980, Prentice Hall.
15. Berman L: The obsessive-compulsive neurosis in children, *J Nerv Ment Dis* 95:26–39, 1942.
16. Despert JL: Differential diagnosis between obsessive compulsive neurosis and schizophrenia in children. In Hoch P, Zubin J, editors: *Psychopathology in children*, New York, 1955, Grune & Stratton.
17. Judd L: Obsessive-compulsive neurosis in children, *Arch Gen Psychiatry* 12: 136–144, 1965.
18. Adams P: *Obsessive children,* New York, 1973, Brunner Mazel.
19. Freud S: The predisposition to obsessional neurosis. In Riviere J, editor: *Sigmund Freud: Collected Papers,* vol 2, New York, 1913, Basic Books.

20. Freud S: Neurosis and psychosis. In Strachey J, editor: *Standard edition of the complete psychological works of Sigmund Freud, Volume XIX (1923–1925): The ego and the id and other works,* London, 1924, Hogarth Press.
21. Freud A: *The ego and the mechanisms of defence,* New York, 1966, International Universities.
22. Klein M: *The psycho-analysis of children,* London, 1932, Hogarth Press.
23. Kanner L: *Child psychiatry,* Springfield, Ill, 1957, Charles C Thomas.
24. Murray RM, Cooper JE, Smith A: The Leyton Obsessional Inventory: An analysis of the responses of 73 obsessional patients, *Psychol Med* 9:305–311, 1979.
25. Valleni-Basile L, Garrison C, Jackson K, et al: Frequency of obsessive-compulsive disorder in a community sample of young adolescents, *J Am Acad Child Adolesc Psychiatry* 33:782–791, 1994.
26. Apter A, Fallon Jr, TJ, King RA, et al: Obsessive-compulsive characteristics: from symptoms to syndrome, *J Am Acad Child Adolesc Psychiatry* 35:907–912, 1996.
27. Douglass HM, Moffitt TE, Dar R, et al: Obsessive-compulsive disorder in a birth cohort of 18-year-olds: prevalence and predictors, *J Am Acad Child Adolesc Psychiatry* 34:1424–1431, 1995.
28. Thomsen P: Obsessive-compulsive disorder in children and adolescents: self-reported obsessive-compulsive behaviour in pupils in Denmark, *Acta Psychiatr Scand* 88:212–217, 1993.
29. Degonda M, Wyss M, Angst J: The Zurich Study: XVIII. Obsessive-compulsive disorders and syndromes in the general population, *Eur Arch Psychiatry Clin Neurosci* 243:16–22, 1993.
30. Kolada JL, Bland RC, Newman SC: Obsessive-compulsive disorder, *Acta Psychiatr Scand Suppl* 376:24–35, 1994.
31. Rasmussen S, Tsuang M: The epidemiology of obsessive compulsive disorder, *J Clin Psychiatry* 45:450–457, 1984.
32. Flament MF, Rapoport JL, Berg CJ, et al: Clomipramine treatment of childhood obsessive-compulsive disorder: A double blind controlled study, *Arch Gen Psychiatry* 42:977–983, 1985.
33. Leonard H, Swedo S, Rapoport J, et al: Treatment of obsessive-compulsive disorder with clomipramine and desipramine in children and adolescents, *Arch Gen Psychiatry* 46:1088–1092, 1989.
34. Leonard HL, Swedo SE, Lenane MC, et al: A double-blind desipramine substitution during long-term clomipramine treatment in children and adolescents with obsessive-compulsive disorder, *Arch Gen Psychiatry* 48:922–927, 1991.
35. Sallee FR, Richman H, Beach K, et al: Platelet serotonin transporter in children and adolescents with obsessive-compulsive disorder or Tourette's syndrome, *J Am Acad Child Adolesc Psychiatry* 35:1647–1656, 1996.
36. Flament MF, Rapoport JL, Murphy DL, et al: Biochemical changes during clomipramine treatment of childhood obsessive-compulsive disorder, *Arch Gen Psychiatry* 44:219–225, 1987.
37. Rauch SL, Jenike MA, Alpert NM, et al: Regional cerebral blood flow measured during symptom provocation in obsessive-compulsive disorder using oxygen 15-labeled carbon dioxide and positron emission tomography, *Arch Gen Psychiatry* 51:62–70, 1994.

38. Swedo SE, Schapiro MB, Grady CL: Cerebral glucose metabolism in childhood-onset obsessive-compulsive disorder, *Arch Gen Psychiatry* 46:518–523, 1989.

39. Luxenberg J, Swedo S, Flament M, et al: Neuroanatomical abnormalities in obsessive-compulsive disorder detected with quantitative X-ray computed tomography, *Am J Psychiatry* 45:1089–1093, 1988.

40. Pauls D, Alsobrook J II, Goodman W, et al: A family study of obsessive-compulsive disorder, *Am J Psychiatry* 152:76–84, 1995.

41. Lenane M, Swedo S, Leonard H, et al: Psychiatric disorders in first degree relatives of children and adolescents with obsessive compulsive disorder, *J Am Acad Child Adolesc Psychiatry* 29:407–412, 1990.

42. Leonard HL, Lenane MC, Swedo SE, et al: Tics and Tourette's disorder: A 2- to 7-year follow-up of 54 obsessive-compulsive children, *Am J Psychiatry* 149:1244–1251, 1992.

43. Geller D, Biederman J, Reed E, et al: Similarities in response to fluoxetine in the treatment of children and adolescents with obsessive-compulsive disorder, *J Am Acad Child Adolesc Psychiatry* 34:36–44, 1995.

44. Riddle M, Scahill L, King R, et al: Obsessive compulsive disorder in children and adolescents: phenomenology and family history, *J Am Acad Child Adolesc Psychiatry* 29:766–772, 1990.

45. Geller D, Biederman J, Griffin S, et al: Comorbidity of juvenile obsessive-compulsive disorder with disruptive behavior disorders, *J Am Acad Child Adolesc Psychiatry* 35:1637–1646, 1996.

46. Leonard H, Swedo S, Lenane M, et al: A 2- to 7-year follow-up study of 54 obsessive-compulsive children and adolescents, *Arch Gen Psychiatry* 50:429–439, 1993.

47. Allsopp M, Verduyn C: Adolescents with obsessive-compulsive disorder: a case note review of consecutive patients referred to a provincial regional adolescent psychiatry unit, *J Adolesc* 13:157–169, 1990.

48. Apter A, Tyano S: Obsessive compulsive disorders in adolescence, *J Adolesc* 11:183–194, 1988.

49. Riddle MA, Hardin MT, King R, et al: Fluoxetine treatment of children and adolescents with Tourette's and obsessive compulsive disorders: preliminary clinical experience, *J Am Acad Child Adolesc Psychiatry* 29:45–48, 1990.

50. Thomsen PH, Mikkelsen HU: Children and adolescents with obsessive-compulsive disorder: the demographic and diagnostic characteristics of 61 Danish patients, *Acta Psychiatr Scand* 83:262–266, 1991.

51. Swedo S, Leonard H: Childhood movement disorders and obsessive compulsive disorder, *J Clin Psychiatry* 55:32–37, 1994.

52. Swedo S, Kiessling L: Speculations on antineuronal antibody-mediated neuropsychiatric disorders of childhood, *Pediatrics* 93:323–326, 1994.

53. Allen A, Leonard H, Swedo S: Case study: a new infection-triggered, autoimmune subtype of pediatric OCD and Tourette's syndrome, *J Am Acad Child Adolesc Psychiatry* 34:307–311, 1995.

54. Giedd JN, Rapoport JL, Leonard HL, et al: Case study: acute basal ganglia enlargement and obsessive-compulsive symptoms in an adolescent boy, *J Am Acad Child Adolesc Psychiatry* 35:913–915, 1996.

55. Tucker DM, Leckman JF, Scahill L, et al: A putative poststreptococcal case of

OCD with chronic tic disorder, not otherwise specified, *J Am Acad Child Adolesc Psychiatry* 35:1684–1691, 1996.

56. Leonard HL, Topol D, Bukstein O, et al: Clonazepam as an augmenting agent in the treatment of childhood-onset obsessive-compulsive disorder, *J Am Acad Child Adolesc Psychiatry* 33:792–794, 1994.

57. Leckman J, Goodman W, North W, et al: Elevated cerebrospinal fluid levels of oxytocin in obsessive-compulsive disorder: comparison with Tourette's syndrome and healthy controls, *Arch Gen Psychiatry* 51:782–793, 1994.

58. Altemus M, Swedo S, Leonard H, et al: Changes in cerebrospinal fluid neuro-chemistry during treatment of obsessive-compulsive disorder with clomipramine, *Arch Gen Psychiatry* 51:794–803, 1994.

59. Leckman JF, Goodman WK, North WG, et al: The role of central oxytocin in obsessive compulsive disorder and related normal behavior, *Psychoneuroendocrinology* 19:723–749, 1994.

60. Epperson CN, McDougle CJ, Price LH: Intranasal oxytocin in obsessive-compulsive disorder, *Biol Psychiatry* 40:547–549, 1996.

61. Swedo SE, Leonard HL, Kruesi MJ, et al: Cerebrospinal fluid neurochemistry in children and adolescents with obsessive-compulsive disorder, *Arch Gen Psychiatry* 49:29 36, 1992.

62. Hamburger S, Swedo S, Whitaker A, et al: Growth rate in adolescents with obsessive-compulsive disorder, *Am J Psychiatry* 146:652–655, 1989.

63. Kruesi MJ, Swedo S, Leonard H, et al: CSF somatostatin in childhood psychiatric disorders: a preliminary investigation, *Psychiatry Res* 33:277–284, 1990.

64. Gesell A, Amatruda CS: *Developmental diagnosis: normal and abnormal child development*, New York, 1941, Hoeber.

65. Leonard HL, Goldberger EL, Rapoport JL, et al: Childhood rituals: normal development or obsessive-compulsive symptoms, *J Am Acad Child Adolesc Psychiatry* 29:17–23, 1990.

66. American Psychiatric Association: *Diagnostic and statistical manual of mental disorders*, ed 4, Washington, 1994, American Psychiatric Press.

67. Foa EB, Kozak MJ: DSM-IV field trial: obsessive-compulsive disorder, *Am J Psychiatry* 152:90–96, 1995.

68. Hanna GL: Demographic and clinical features of obsessive-compulsive disorder in children and adolescents, *J Am Acad Child Adolesc Psychiatry* 34:19–27, 1995.

69. Goodman WK, Price LH, Rasmussen SA, et al: Yale-Brown Obsessive Compulsive Scale (Y-BOCS): Part II. Validity, *Arch Gen Psychiatry* 46:1012–1016, 1989.

70. Rettew DC, Swedo SE, Leonard HL, et al: Obsessions and compulsions across time in 79 children and adolescents with obsessive-compulsive disorder, *J Am Acad Child Adolesc Psychiatry* 31:1050–1056, 1992.

71. Honjo S, Hirano C, Murase S, et al: Obsessive-compulsive symptoms in childhood and adolescents, *Acta Psychiatr Scand* 80:83–91, 1989.

72. Toro J, Cervera M, Osejo E, Salamero M: Obsessive-compulsive disorder in childhood and adolescence: a clinical study, *J Child Psychol Psychiatry* 33:1025–1037, 1992.

73. Burke KC, Burke JD Jr, Regier DA, et al: Age at onset of selected mental disorders in five community populations, *Arch Gen Psychiatry* 47:511–518, 1990.

74. Minichiello WE, Baer L, Jenike MA, et al: Age of onset of major subtypes of obsessive-compulsive disorder, *J Anx Dis* 4:147–150, 1990.

75. Thyer BA, Parrish RT, Curtis GC, et al: Ages of onset of DSM-III anxiety disorders, *Compr Psychiatry* 26:113–122, 1985.
76. Last CG, Strauss CC: Obsessive-compulsive disorder in childhood, *J Anx Dis* 3:295–302, 1989.
77. Pigott TA, L'Heureux F, Dubbert B, et al: Obsessive-compulsive disorder: comorbid conditions, *J Clin Psychiatry* 55:15–27, 1994.
78. Rasmussen SA, Eisen JL: The epidemiology and differential diagnosis of obsessive compulsive disorder, *J Clin Psychiatry* 55:5–14, 1994.
79. Grad LR, Pelcovitz D, Olson M, et al: Obsessive-compulsive symptomatology in children with Tourette's syndrome, *J Am Acad Child Adolesc Psychiatry* 26:69–73, 1987.
80. Pauls DL, Leckman JF: The inheritance of Gilles de la Tourette's syndrome and associated behaviors: Evidence for autosomal dominant transmission, *N Engl J Med* 315:993–997, 1986.
81. Pauls D: Continuity and discontinuity between obsessive compulsive disorder and Gilles de la Tourette's syndrome with the adult phenotypes, Scientific Proceedings of the American Academy of Child and Adolescent Psychiatry, New Orleans, 1995.
82. Caine ED, McBride MC, Chiverton P, et al: Tourette's syndrome in Monroe County school children, *Neurology* 38:472–475, 1988.
83. Burd L, Kerbeshian J, Fisher W, et al: Anticonvulsant medications: an iatrogenic cause of tic disorders, *Can J Psychiatry* 31:419–423, 1986.
84. Comings DE, Himes JA, Comings BG: An epidemiologic study of Tourette's syndrome in a single school district, *J Clin Psychiatry* 51:463–469, 1990.
85. Pitman R, Green R, Jenike M, et al: Clinical comparison of Tourette's disorder and obsessive-compulsive disorder, *Am J Psychiatry* 144:1166–1171, 1987.
86. Robertson M: Familial Tourette's syndrome in a large British pedigree: associated psychopathology, severity, and potential for linkage analysis, *Br J Psychiatry* 156:515–521, 1990.
87. Pauls DL, Raymond CL, Stevenson JM, et al: A family study of Gilles de la Tourette syndrome, *Am J Hum Genet* 48:154–163, 1991.
88. Keller B: Cognitive assessment of obsessive-compulsive children. In Rapoport J, editor: *Obsessive-compulsive disorder in children and adolescents,* Washington, 1989, American Psychiatric Press.
89. Rapoport J: The biology of obsessions and compulsions, *Sci Am* 83–89, 1989.
90. Wechsler D: *Manual for the Wechsler Intelligence Scale for Children—Revised,* New York, 1974, Psychological Corporation.
91. Behar D, Rapoport J, Berg C, et al: Computerized tomography and neuropsychological test measures in adolescents with obsessive compulsive disorder, *Am J Psychiatry* 141:363–369, 1984.
92. Cox C, Fedio P, Rapoport J: Neuropsychological testing of obsessive-compulsive adolescents. In Rapoport J, editor: *Obsessive-compulsive disorder in children and adolescents,* Washington, 1989, American Psychiatric Press.
93. Leonard HL, Swedo SE, Rapoport JL, et al: Tourette syndrome and obsessive-compulsive disorder [review], *Adv Neurol* 58:83–93, 1992.
94. King RA, Scahill L, Vitulano LA, et al: Childhood trichotillomania: clinical phenomenology, comorbidity, and family genetics, *J Am Acad Child Adolesc Psychiatry* 34:1451–1459, 1995.

95. Patterson DA, Lee MS: Field trial of the Global Assessment of Functioning Scale, modified, *Am J Psychiatry* 152:1386–1388, 1995.

96. National Institute of Mental Health: CGI (Clinical Global Impression) Scale— NIMH, *Psychopharmacol Bull* 21:839–844, 1985.

97. Goodman WK, Rasmussen SA, Price LH: *Children's Yale-Brown Obsessive Compulsive Scale (CY-BOCS),* New Haven, Conn, 1986, Yale University Press.

98. Riddle MA, Scahill L, Smith J, et al: *Children's Yale-Brown Obsessive Compulsive Scale (CY-BOCS),* Scientific Proceedings, 48th Annual Meeting of the Society of Biological Psychiatry, 1993.

99. Scahill L, Riddle M, McSwiggin-Hardin M, et al: Children's Yale-Brown Obsessive Compulsive Scale: reliability and validity, *J Am Acad Child Adolesc Psychiatry* 36:844–852, 1997.

100. AuBuchon PG, Malatesta VJ: Obsessive compulsive patients with comorbid personality disorder: associated problems and response to a comprehensive behavior therapy, *J Clin Psychiatry* 55:448–453, 1994.

101. DeVeaugh-Geiss J, Moroz G, Biederman J, et al: Clomipramine hydrochloride in childhood and adolescent obsessive-compulsive disorder: a multicenter trial, *J Am Acad Child Adolesc Psychiatry* 31:45–49, 1992.

102. Riddle M, Claghorn J, Gaffney G, et al: Fluvoxamine for OCD in children and adolescents: a controlled trial. Presented at Scientific Proceedings of the Annual Meeting of the American Academy of Child and Adolescent Psychiatry, 1996.

103. Cooper J: The Leyton Obsessional Inventory, *Psychol Med* 1:48–64, 1970.

104. Berg CJ, Rapoport JL, Flament M: The Leyton Obsessional Inventory—child version, *J Am Acad Child Adolesc Psychiatry* 25:84–91, 1986.

105. Berg CZ, Whitaker A, Davies M, et al: The survey form of the Leyton Obsessional Inventory—child version, *J Am Acad Child Adolesc Psychiatry* 27:759–763, 1988.

106. Riddle M, Scahill L, King R, et al: Double-blind, crossover trial of fluoxetine and placebo in children and adolescents with obsessive-compulsive disorder, *J Am Acad Child Adolesc Psychiatry* 31:1062–1069, 1992.

107. King RA, Riddle MA, Chappell PB, et al: Emergence of self-destructive phenomena in children and adolescents during fluoxetine treatment, *J Am Acad Child Adolesc Psychiatry* 30:179–186, 1991.

108. McDougle CJ, Goodman WK, Price LH: Dopamine antagonists in tic-related and psychotic spectrum obsessive compulsive disorder, *J Clin Psychiatry* 55:24–31, 1994.

109. Hewlett WA: The use of benzodiazepines in obsessive compulsive disorder and Tourette's syndrome, *Psychiat Ann* 23:309–316, 1993.

110. Singer HS, Brown J, Quaskey S, et al: The treatment of attention-deficit hyperactivity disorder in Tourette's syndrome: a double-blind placebo-controlled study with clonidine and desipramine, *Pediatrics* 95:74–81, 1995.

111. Singer HS, Walkup JT: Tourette syndrome and other tic disorders: Diagnosis, pathophysiology, and treatment [review], *Medicine* 70:15–32, 1991.

112. Spencer T, Biederman J, Wilens T, et al: Nortriptyline treatment of children with attention-deficit hyperactivity disorder and tic disorder or Tourette's syndrome, *J Am Acad Child Adolesc Psychiatry* 32:205–210, 1993.

113. Spencer T, Biederman J, Wilens T, Faraone S: Is attention-deficit hyperactivity

disorder in adults a valid disorder? *Harv Rev Psychiatry* March/April:326–335, 1994.

114. Spencer T, Biederman J, Kerman K, et al: Desipramine treatment of children with attention deficit hyperactivity disorder and tic disorder or Tourette's syndrome, *J Am Acad Child Adolesc Psychiatry* 32:354–360, 1993.

115. Biederman J: Sudden death in children treated with a tricyclic antidepressant: a commentary, *J Am Acad Child Adolesc Psychiatry* 30:495–497, 1991.

116. Puig-Antich J, Perel JM, Lupatkin W, et al: Plasma levels of imipramine (IMI) and desmethylimipramine (DMI) and clinical response in prepubertal major depressive disorder, *J Am Acad Child Psychiatry* 18:616–627, 1979.

117. Puig-Antich J, Perel JM, Lupatkin W, et al: Imipramine in prepubertal major depressive disorders, *Arch Gen Psychiatry* 44:81–89, 1987.

118. March JS: Cognitive-behavioral psychotherapy for children and adolescents with OCD: a review and recommendations for treatment, *J Am Acad Child Adolesc Psychiatry* 34:7–18, 1995.

119. Bolton D, Collins S, Steinberg D: The treatment of obsessive-compulsive disorder in adolescence: a report of fifteen cases, *Br J Psychiatry* 142:456–464, 1983.

120. Apter A, Bernhout E, Tyano S: Severe obsessive compulsive disorder in adolescence: a report of eight cases, *J Adolesc* 7:349–358, 1984.

121. de Haan E, Hoogduin C: The treatment of children with obsessive-compulsive disorder, *Acta Paedopsychiatrica* 55:93–97, 1992.

122. March JS, Mulle K, Herbel B: Behavioral psychotherapy for children and adolescents with obsessive-compulsive disorder: an open trial of a new protocol-driven treatment package, *J Am Acad Child Adolesc Psychiatry* 33:333–341, 1994.

123. Berg CZ, Rapoport JL, Whitaker A, et al: Childhood obsessive compulsive disorder: a two-year prospective follow-up of a community sample, *J Am Acad Child Adolesc Psychiatry* 28:528–533, 1989.

124. Hollingsworth C, Tanguay E, Grossman L, et al: Long-term outcome of obsessive-compulsive disorder in childhood, *J Am Acad Child Adolesc Psychiatry* 19:134–144, 1980.

125. Allsopp M, Verduyn C: A follow-up of adolescents with obsessive-compulsive disorder, *Br J Psychiatry* 154:829–834, 1988.

126. Flament M, Koby E, Rapoport J, et al: Childhood obsessive-compulsive disorder: A prospective follow-up study, *J Child Psychol Psychiatry* 31:363–380, 1990.

127. Thomsen PH: Obsessive-compulsive disorder in children and adolescents: a 6–22 year follow-up study of social outcome, *Eur Child Adolesc Psychiatry* 4:112–122, 1995.

4

Personality Disorders in Obsessive-Compulsive Disorder

Lee Baer, Ph.D., Michael A. Jenike, M.D.

Psychology and psychiatry have differed historically in their conception of personality assessment: whereas psychology has focused on personality characteristics that can be measured along a dimension, including both normal and abnormal traits, psychiatry has focused on categorical personality disorders that fit into the axis II diagnostic categories most recently enumerated in *Diagnostic and Statistical Manual of Mental Disorders* (DSM-IV).[1] The current state-of-the-art of personality assessment in psychology was recently summarized by McCrae and Costa[2] of the National Institute of Aging:

> Many psychologists are now convinced that the best representation of trait structure is provided by the five-factor model (FFM). According to the FFM, most personality traits can be described in terms of five basic dimensions, called Neuroticism versus Emotional Stability (N); Extroversion or Surgency (E); Openness to Experience or Intellect, Imagination, or Culture (O); Agreeableness versus Antagonism (A); and Conscientiousness or Will to Achieve (C). (McCrae & Costa, 1997, p. 509).

These authors then went on to provide evidence that these five personality traits may be universal across human cultures by demonstrating almost identical factor analysis results confirming these five traits in large populations of individuals from the United States, Germany, Portugal, Israel, China, Korea, and Japan,[2] using the Revised NEO Personality Inventory these authors had developed earlier.[3]

The current state-of-the-art of personality disorder research in psychiatry was recently reviewed in detail by a number of experts in the area as part of the DSM-IV field trial process (with the chapter focusing on Obsessive-Compulsive Personality Disorder [OCPD] contributed by Pfohl[4]). Today, diagnoses of Axis II personality disorders are made most reliably with the aid of a structured interview, such as the structured clinical interview for diagnosis (SCID-II) or the structured interview for the diagnosis of personality disorders revised (SIDP-R). One difficulty in studying personality disorders is that criteria have changed over time, as have cutpoints used to define "caseness." This raises problems in the assessment of the prevalence of given axis II disorders and in the determination of their predictive validity in treatment studies. To illustrate this, Table 4-1 shows the changing criteria of obsessive-compulsive personality disorder between DSM-II and the current DSM-IV.

As the footnote to Table 4-1 illustrates, DSM-II criteria were closer to the obsessional personality or anal-erotic character described by Freud.[5] More recent conceptions of OCPD, however, have been suggested to be "a much more pathological entity than the classical obsessive-compulsive character"[6] (similarly, "borderline character structure," as used in the psychoanalytic literature, is a much less illness-oriented construct than the DSM diagnosis of "borderline personality disorder").

Prior to the publication of DSM-III in 1980,[7] there were no clear criteria for the diagnosis of obsessive-compulsive personality disorder (even the disorder's name has changed over the years, with the word "obsessive" absent in DSM-III and added in DSM-III-R[8] and DSM-IV[1]). Only three criteria have been present continuously since the publication of DSM-III: "perfectionism," "excessive devotion to work," and "stubbornness or being interpersonally controlling." All other criteria either have been dropped or added over time (the rationale for changes between DSM-III-R and DSM-IV is given by Pfohl[4]). There has been no mention of the inability to discard worthless objects prior to DSM-III-R; this fact is particularly important for obsessive-compulsive disorder (OCD) research because hoarding is believed to be a symptom of OCD, although its responsiveness to current treatment is unclear. Finally, over the years, the percentage of criteria required to make the diagnosis of OCPD has changed, making it progressively easier for a patient to be diagnosed with this disorder and influencing prevalence estimates in patients with OCD (generally increasing the estimates). Researchers sometimes comment on the number of personality traits for which an individual qualifies (i.e., the individual criteria of OCPD, as shown for DSM-IV in Table 4-2), although the reliability of individual traits has been little studied.

The only reliable epidemiologic study of OCPD to date was performed by Nestadt et al[9] in conjunction with the Epidemiologic Catchment Area survey conducted in the Baltimore area. These researchers observed patients diagnosed with *either* compulsive personality disorder or compulsive personality traits. Researchers estimated a prevalence of 1.7% in a general population, with white, married, and employed men most often receiving the diagnosis. These authors concluded that compulsive personality has a dimensional rather than a categorical character, and that the condition imparts a vulnerability for development of anxiety disorders.[9]

Despite methodologic problems, interest has continued in personality assessment in OCD for at least two reasons: (1) the clinical question of whether

Table 4-1   Changes Over Time in DSM Criteria for Obsessive-Compulsive Personality Disorder*

Criteria	DSM-III	DSM-III-R	DSM-IV
Perfectionism	+	+	+
Excessive devotion to work	+	+	+
Stubbornness, interpersonally controlling	+	+	+
Restricted expression of affection	+	+	
Indecisiveness	+	+	
Preoccupation with details		+	+
Overconscientiousness regarding ethics		+	+
Lack of generosity		+	+
Inability to discard worthless objects		+	+
Number of criteria required for diagnosis	4 of 5 (80%)	5 of 9 (56%)	4 of 8 (50%)

* DSM-II criteria (1968) stated: "characterized by excessive concern with conformity and adherence to standards of conscience. Consequently individuals in this group may be rigid, over-inhibited, over-conscientious, over-dutiful, and unable to relax easily."
(From American Psychiatric Association: *Diagnostic and statistical manual of mental disorders*, ed 2, Washington, 1968, American Psychiatric Association; with permission.)

certain personality disorders may be helpful in predicting poorer outcome to both behavioral and drug treatments for OCD and (2) a theoretical question as to whether OCPD or traits are closely linked to OCD and can lead to OCD (as was stated in DSM-II).[10] In the traditional psychoanalytic explanation of obsessional disorders, obsessional personality has been described as a predisposing feature of obsessional neurosis, with the two conditions existing side by side along a continuum.[11] On this continuum (which is believed to result from conflicts over bowel training), individuals with obsessional personality (characterized by orderliness, parsimoniousness, and obstinacy[5]) differ from those individuals with obsessive-compulsive symptoms (obsessions and compulsions) only in that they are asymptomatic.[5] In fact, DSM-II[10] cautioned that obsessive-compulsive personality "may lead to an obsessive-compulsive neurosis, from which it must be distinguished." The current state of the literature regarding each of these issues is described in the following paragraphs.

PREDICTING OBSESSIVE-COMPULSIVE DISORDER TREATMENT OUTCOME FROM PERSONALITY

Despite anecdotal clinical impressions of a connection, until recently there was little experimental literature demonstrating a negative effect of personality disorder diagnosis on drug or behavioral treatment outcome.

Nonstandardized Assessment

In a study of 316 patients, Tyrer, et al[12] provided evidence that presence of a personality disorder can predict a poor response to phenelzine in affective

Table 4-2   DSM-IV Criteria for Obsessive-Compulsive Personality Disorder

A pervasive pattern of preoccupation with orderliness, perfectionism, and mental and interpersonal control, at the expense of flexibility, openness, and efficiency, beginning by early adulthood and present in a variety of contexts, as indicated by four (or more) of the following:

1. Preoccupation with details, rules, lists, order, organization, or schedules to the extent that the major point of the activity is lost
2. Perfectionism that interferes with task completion (e.g., is unable to complete a project because his or her own overly strict standards are not met)
3. Excessive devotion to work and productivity to the exclusion of leisure activities and friendships (not accounted for by obvious economic necessity)
4. Overconscientiousness, scrupulousness, and inflexibility about matters of morality, ethics, or values (not accounted for by cultural or religious identification)
5. Inability to discard worn-out or worthless objects, even when they have no sentimental value
6. Reluctance to delegate tasks or to work with others unless they submit to exactly his or her way of doing things
7. Adoption of a miserly spending style toward both self and others; money is viewed as something to be hoarded for future catastrophes
8. Rigidity and stubbornness

(From American Psychiatric Association: *Diagnostic and statistical manual of mental disorders*, ed 4, Washington, 1994, American Psychiatric Association; with permission.)

disorder. Despite the important clinical and theoretic implications of such a finding, few studies have assessed the impact of personality disorders on treatment outcome in OCD. Our group has reported that in a retrospective chart review study, the presence of schizotypal personality was a negative predictor for outcome with both drug[13] and behavioral[14] treatments.

Schizotypal personality disorder, which along with schizoid and paranoid personality disorders form Cluster A of DSM-III personality disorders, has been reported to be genetically related to schizophrenia.[15, 16] In a retrospective study of 43 consecutive OCD patients, Jenike et al[13] reported that a subgroup of 14 (33%) treatment-resistant patients were found by chart review to meet DSM-III criteria for schizotypal personality disorder, with negative implications for treatment outcome. As described in the following paragraphs regarding MMPI findings, many of these patients had been previously misdiagnosed as schizophrenic and had not benefited from neuroleptic treatment.

Standardized Assessment

As part of a multicenter trial of clomipramine for OCD, the SIDP was used to assess the effect of DSM-III personality disorders on outcome in a controlled trial of clomipramine, which to date has been the most-studied drug treatment for OCD.[17] This study involved 54 patients, seen at six sites, who were in the clomipramine treatment group of the double-blind trial. Because the 60 subjects in the placebo group did not significantly improve in the trial, their data were excluded from the present study. As part of the study protocol, patients were assessed with the Structured Interview for DSM-III Personality Disorders,[18] which has established reliability and validity. Raters in all sites were trained by one of two experts with this scale.[19] The major outcome measures were the clinician-administered Yale-Brown Obsessive-Compulsive Scale (Y-BOCS), two clinician-rated subjective improvement measures—the National Institute of Mental Health (NIMH) Global Improvement Scale and Clinician Rated Assessment Scale—and the Patient-Rated Assessment Scale which is a patient-rated subjective scale. All four measures have been widely used in controlled drug trials in OCD patients. Because of unequal sample sizes among the various personality disorders, the primary data analyses were multiple linear regressions for the two main outcome measures: Y-BOCS and NIMH Global Scale. For these regressions, the dependent variable was the final score on each outcome scale, with the baseline score on the same scale forced first into the equation as a covariate. Other independent variables of interest were then entered into the equation,[20] and we examined the partial correlation of each of the predictor variables (Table 4-3).

We found that presence of any personality disorder was unrelated to improvement on any OCD outcome measure in these patients treated with clomipramine. However, the number of personality disorders present was consistently related to poorer outcome, as was the presence of a DSM-III Cluster A personality diagnosis. Among the individual personality disorders, schizotypal personality disorder was found to be negatively related to outcome on all dependent variables; this finding was consistent with our earlier findings summarized in the previous paragraphs. Avoidant personality disorder also was related negatively to outcome on several dependent variables, as were borderline and paranoid personality disorders.

Later, Fals-Stewart and Lucente[21] gave the Millon Clinical Multiaxial Inventory personality scale to 137 OCD patients seeking outpatient behavioral treatment, and Y-BOCS scores were assessed at baseline, at posttreatment, and at 6-month follow-up. They found that patients with either no personality difficulties or with dependent personality traits had the best outcomes. On the other hand, those patients whose personality problems included difficulties with interpersonal interactions were most likely to refuse behavior therapy, and among those patients who did agree to undergo behavior therapy, no reduction in OCD symptoms was found at either posttreatment or follow-up. Those patients with histrionic or borderline traits at baseline had OCD reductions at posttreatment, but they did not maintain these treatment gains at follow-up.[21]

Most recently, AuBuchon and Malatesta[22] compared consecutively 26 OCD patients with a comorbid DSM-III-R personality disorder (by 100% agreement

Table 4-3 Personality Disorders and Outcome with Clomipramine: Partial Correlations with Week 12 Outcome Variables (with Baseline Score Partialed Out)

Personality Disorder	Patients n (%)	Total = 54 Y-BOCS	NIMH
Paranoid	4 (7)	0.23	0.41[†]
Schizoid	1 (2)	0.01	0.08
Schizotypal	5 (8)	0.36[†]	0.44[‡]
Histrionic	5 (8)	0.00	0.06
Narcissistic	0 (0)	—	—
Antisocial	0 (0)	—	—
Borderline	6 (10)	0.34*	0.38[†]
Avoidant	15 (25)	0.35[†]	0.24
Dependent	14 (23)	0.08	0.08
Compulsive	10 (17)	0.11	0.21
Passive-aggressive	9 (15)	0.20	0.26
Mixed	5 (8)	0.09	0.07
Any personality disorder	38 (63)	0.17	0.16
Any Cluster A personality disorder		0.31*	0.49[‡]
Any Cluster B personality disorder		0.25	0.33*
Any Cluster C personality disorder		0.10	0.08

* $p < 0.05$
[†] $p < 0.01$
[‡] $p < 0.001$
(From Baer L, et al: Effect of axis II diagnoses on treatment outcome with clomipramine in 55 patients with obsessive-compulsive disorder, *Arch Gen Psychiatry* 49:862–866, 1992.)

of their psychiatrist and consulting psychologist) to five consecutive OCD patients without a personality disorder who underwent "comprehensive behavior therapy" for OCD. Researchers found that those patients with comorbid personality disorders had greater symptomatic and psychosocial impairment before treatment, responded less well to behavior therapy (although still "moderately" better), were rated as more difficult to treat, required more psychiatric hospitalizations during treatment, and were more likely to terminate behavior therapy prematurely. The authors reported that when patients were treated with comprehensive behavior therapy that focused on other clinical problems besides the OCD, those patients with comorbid personality disorders "had an enhanced response to treatment."[22]

Balancing these studies, which all found that presence of personality disorders negatively influenced treatment of OCD with both drugs and behavior therapy, is a study by Steketee,[23] which administered the Personality Diagnostic Questionnaire (PDQ) to the relatives of 26 OCD patients and found that presence of various personality disorders in the relatives was unrelated to the patients' outcome with behavior therapy. This study differed from the others in assessing personality traits of relatives rather than of OCD sufferers themselves.

RELATION OF OBSESSIVE-COMPULSIVE PERSONALITY TRAITS TO OBSESSIVE-COMPULSIVE DISORDER
Nonstandardized Assessment

Rorschach Inkblot Test

One traditional approach to personality assessment has been the use of projective psychologic tests to assess the primary issues and defenses of patients with OCD. Coursey[24] administered the Rorschach inkblot test to 15 patients with OCD and found that, although it is rare to have any explicit hostility on the Rorschach, OCD patients had explicitly aggressive responses on 60% of the protocols. When mild or symbolically hostile responses were included, this number increased to 80%. Coursey noted that these typical responses contrasted markedly with the socially timid, inhibited, and fearful demeanor and behavior of these patients. Although oral-dependent Rorschach responses such as mouth, food, touching, and oral-aggressive responses are uncommon in adults, two thirds of the OCD patients gave mouth and food responses and more than one third gave touching and holding responses. In addition, one third of the patients gave unusual genital and anal content in more than 10% of their responses.

These Rorschach responses suggested that to control and neutralize the hostile impulses that had erupted into consciousness, approximately 50% of these OCD patients used classical defenses such as undoing and denial; these defense mechanisms were usually seen across responses, balancing the impulse with its opposite. For instance, one patient first saw "piercing mean eyes peering at me through the dark," then, "some type of face smiling, a cartoon figure." Interestingly, 20% of the subjects demonstrated denial that failed, that is, first denying any response, then revealing a sexual or hostile one. Approximately two thirds of these patients controlled their affect through cold, factual language, mostly through the choice of emotionally flat, neutral words.

Coursey[24] concluded that obsessive-compulsive patients are marked by the extent to which primitive material has invaded their consciousness and the neutralizing strategies these patients have developed to handle these impulses. Unlike other neurotic patients, in whom primitive drives never fully reach consciousness except in symbolic or symptomatic forms, and unlike psychotics, in whom primary process is conscious and defenses have completely failed, most of the OCD patients represented a third possibility: primitive impulse material is conscious and the defenses, other than repression and denial, have not failed. Instead, the defenses that succeed are those that neutralize and contain the primary process material. Thus, the central characteristics of most of these patients include this highly charged impasse, a deadlock between the failure of repression and denial, and the success of the aforementioned neutralizing strategies and other containing defenses such as preoccupation with detail. Coursey felt that his Rorschach data confirmed the observations of Freud and others and that hostile and sadistic impulses are a central component of this disorder. They are also in accord with a descriptive study by Rachman and DeSilva[25] of the obsessions of patients and normals, which found that 70% of the obsessions in their patients focused on violence and physical aggression, 17% on deviant sexual impulses, another 9% on being out of control, and only 4% on neutral phrases. The descriptive Rorschach material presented by Coursey also suggests that repression and denial are not effective in preventing primary process material from becoming conscious. In contradiction to some Freudian theories, there is no evidence from this study that there are "even more horrible" unconscious underlying impulses. Coursey concluded that this finding is strong evidence that the psychotherapeutic process may better focus on what is present than on what might be underlying. This process would entail working with the secondary features of the disorder—the anxiety, rituals, and obsessions. In addition, this process would be important to help patients deal with and accept the heightened impulses they experience.

Clinical Judgment of Personality Traits

In an early report, Ingram[5] studied 31 OCD inpatients using subjective descriptions by patients, clinicians, and relatives regarding the patients' premorbid personality. Ten patients (32%) had "marked obsessional traits," and four patients (13%) had no obsessional traits. This study concluded that obsessional personality and obsessional illness are intimately connected. It is likely that in this study the number of patients without premorbid traits was underestimated because patients with early-onset OCD were eliminated from analysis.

Slade[26] reviewed a number of psychometric studies of obsessive patients and reached a different conclusion: "The evidence presented seems to support fairly strongly the distinction between obsessional personality traits and obsessional neurosis."

A more recent review of the literature concluded that obsessive-compulsive personality can be statistically differentiated through factor analysis from obsessive-compulsive symptoms as distinct phenomena, with obsessive-compulsive symptoms positively related to measures of neuroticism, whereas obsessive-compulsive personality was not.[27] Pollack[27,28] concluded that, although obsessive-compulsive personality has been reported to occur premorbidly, it is neither a necessary nor sufficient condition for the development of OCD.

Standardized Assessment

The early studies reviewed previously provided hypotheses of heuristic value regarding personality structure in OCD; however, the conclusions are limited by the questionable reliability of clinical interview and projective tests.

More recently, standardized psychometric instruments have been used to provide more reliable assessment of personality in OCD. These instruments have been of two types: (1) self-report scales for personality traits, such as the Minnesota Multiphasic Personality Inventory (MMPI), Personality Diagnostic Question-naire (PDQ), and Tridimensional Personality Questionnaire (TPQ) described in the following paragraphs; and (2) structured interviews keyed to DSM-III crite-ria for personality diagnoses, such as the Structured Interview for the Diagnosis of Personality Disorders (SIDP), also described in the following paragraphs.

Minnesota Multiphasic Personality Inventory

In patients referred to our OCD clinic, we noted on several occasions that the results of the MMPI had been used to corroborate a misdiagnosis of schiz-ophrenia in patients who had never been psychotic but clearly met DSM-III criteria for OCD. A computerized literature search revealed only one unpub-lished doctoral dissertation on the relationship of the MMPI to OCD.[29] Because the differential diagnosis between OCD and formal thought disorder is crucial in terms of treatment, we administered the MMPI to 32 consecutive patients referred to our OCD clinic who met DSM-III criteria for OCD.[30] Of the 32 subjects (16 men and 16 women), five displayed no compulsive behav-ior despite the presence of obsessive thoughts. Each subject's medical records were examined for previous diagnoses, indicating that 12 of the 32 patients had previously been diagnosed as schizophrenic. Seven patients—one of whom had also been previously diagnosed as schizophrenic—satisfied DSM-III cri-teria for major depression, but in all seven cases the obsessive-compulsive symptoms predated the depressive symptoms by at least 3 months.

Subjects' K-corrected T-scores were examined for the three MMPI validity scales (L,F,K) and the 10 clinical scales: hypochondriasis (scale 1); depression (scale 2); hysteria (scale 3); psychopathic deviance (scale 4); masculinity-femininity (scale 5); paranoia (scale 6); psychasthenia (scale 7); schizophrenia (scale 8); mania (scale 9); and social introversion (scale 10). Separate mean pro-files were obtained for both men and women, and for each gender, those patients with previous diagnoses of schizophrenia were compared with those patients without such previous diagnoses. Validity of the profiles was determined by the criteria commonly used and described by Graham.[31]

For both men and women, the mean MMPI profile was characterized by elevations on scales 2, 7, and 8, with 4 the next highest scale (Table 4-4). This pattern was found both for patients with a prior schizophrenic diagnosis and for those patients without such a diagnosis. Although the shape of the profile was essentially the same for the two subgroups, those subjects with a prior diagnosis of schizophrenia displayed higher elevations on a number of scales, including F, 6, 7, and 8 for men, and F, 4, and 6 for women. Small sample size provided inadequate statistical power for tests comparing the mean scores of the subgroups.[30]

Table 4-4 Mean MMPI T-Scores for 32 Patients with Obsessive-Compulsive Disorder

MMPI scale		Previously Diagnosed Schizophrenic		Not Previously Diagnosed Schizophrenic	
		Men (n = 8)	Women (n = 4)	Men (n = 8)	Women (n = 12)
—	L	47	48	49	50
—	F	68	69	61	61
—	K	52	48	53	53
1	Hypochondriasis	68	54	62	60
2	Depression	89	79	85	79
3	Hysteria	68	61	73	67
4	Psychopathic deviance	78	79	76	69
5	Masculinity-Femininity	69	53	68	52
6	Paranoia	77	73	64	63
7	Psychasthenia	94	77	84	77
8	Schizophrenia	95	74	76	73
9	Mania	61	62	55	54
10	Social introversion	59	58	55	57

(From Carey RJ, et al: MMPI correlates of obsessive-compulsive disorder, *J Clin Psychiatry* 47: 371–372, 1986; with permission.)

The results of this study are consistent with those reported by Doppelt,[29] and these results support the hypothesis that individuals meeting criteria for OCD typically produce MMPI profiles with primary elevations on scales 2 (depression), 7 (psychasthenia), 8 (schizophrenia), and 4 (psychopathic deviance). Elevation on scale 8 reflects "odd thinking," which can be produced by OCD patients' reports of obsessions or superstitious fears; it need not reflect classical "schizophrenic thinking." Elevation on scale 4 may reflect OCD patients' fears of "losing control" in socially unacceptable ways, such as shoplifting or causing an accident.

Our results suggest that the MMPIs of those OCD patients who have been previously diagnosed as schizophrenic may be characterized by somewhat higher elevations on a number of scales while yielding the same basic profile pattern as those produced by OCD patients with more benign previous diagnoses. These preliminary results suggest that the MMPI may be useful in making the important distinction between OCD and more insidious formal thought disorders. The parallels between the pretreatment MMPI results of Doppelt's sample and those of Carey et al[30] provide tentative support for the delineation of a "classic" OCD profile, considerably different from those profiles typically produced by schizophrenics.

On the other hand, Schotte, et al[32] attempted to use the MMPI to differentiate psychiatric inpatients with and without OCPD as diagnosed by the SCID-II structured interview. They found that neither ROC analysis nor other methods showed good diagnostic performance of MMPI for detecting DSM-III-R OCPD. Unlike our findings in an OCD population, these researchers found that the OCPD group had a mean MMPI profile of 2-6-1 (depression-paranoia-hypochondriasis) with a tendency for a lowered scale 4 (psychopathic deviance), compared with non–OCPDs. However, this study differed in that it examined the axis II diagnosis of OCPD rather than the axis I diagnosis of OCD.

Dimensional Personality Assessment

A modified method of dimensional assessment of personality (as described previously) was proposed by Cloninger[33] as an alternate method to the standard categorical personality disorder approach as used in DSM. In Cloninger's typology, three dimensions of personality are defined in terms of "novelty seeking," "harm avoidance," and "reward dependence." These dimensions are assessed by means of a self-report scale—the Tridimensional Personality Questionnaire (TPQ)—and underlying genetic and neuroanatomic bases for these dimensions have also been proposed.[33]

Pfohl et al[32] applied this dimensional concept of personality to OCD and tested the prediction that the traits of "low novelty seeking" and "high harm avoidance" would be prevalent in OCD patients. These researchers used the TPQ to compare OCD patients to nonpsychiatric controls and found significant differences in the predicted direction on these two dimensions, although they did not find evidence for the neurotransmitter mechanisms underlying this theory.

On the other hand, Richter et al[35] administered the TPQ to 32 OCD patients and found that *only* the Harm Avoidance score was significantly different from that of normal controls.

Joffee et al[36] administered a computer-scored Millon Clinical Multiaxial Inventory to 23 OCD patients and found that 19 (83%) met criteria for a personality disorder, with only one patient (4%) meeting criteria for compulsive personality disorder and four (17%) patients meeting criteria for schizotypal personality disorder. Avoidant (44%), passive-aggressive (44%), and dependent (35%) personality disorders were most common. It is possible that this instrument may have overestimated sample prevalences of personality disorders, because in the same report 20 of 23 (87%) patients with a lifetime diagnosis of major depressive disorder also met criteria for at least one personality disorder.

Structured DSM Interviews

In a study of 44 OCD outpatients, Rasmussen and Tsuang[37] reported that 29 (66%) manifested an axis II diagnosis, with 55% of patients meeting criteria for compulsive, 9% of patients for histrionic, 7% of patients for schizoid, 5%

of patients for dependents, and 0% for schizotypal personality disorder. Diagnosis was based on a broad, semistructured interview which included symptom checklists from DSM-III axis II criteria.

Steketee[23] administered the Personality Diagnostic Questionnaire (PDQ), a self-report instrument, to relatives of 26 OCD patients and found that only one patient (4%) met criteria for compulsive personality disorder, and nine patients (35%) met criteria for schizotypal personality disorder. Dependent (39%), histrionic (31%), and avoidant (27%) personality disorders were also frequently diagnosed. Black et al[38] also administered the PDQ to 21 OCD patients and 42 age- and gender-matched normal controls. These authors found that 52% of the OCD patients had DSM-III Cluster B (dramatic) personality diagnoses or traits compared with 7% for the controls—a statistically significant difference. The two groups did not differ in prevalence of Cluster A (eccentric) or Cluster C (anxious) diagnoses or traits. Dependent, histrionic, and borderline personality disorders (all 24%) were most frequent. No OCD patient was diagnosed with compulsive personality disorder, and three (14%) were diagnosed with schizotypal personality disorder.

The SIDP is a structured interview designed specifically to diagnose all DSM-III personality disorders,[18] and it has been used in several recent studies assessing personality in OCD patients. It consists of 160 questions, which are asked by a trained interviewer, and requires 60 to 90 minutes to complete.[18] This instrument has been demonstrated to have adequate interrater reliability for presence of any personality disorder (kappa = 0.71 for simultaneous interviews with two raters, and kappa = 0.66 for separate interviews in a test-retest format). Kappa coefficients (based on simultaneous interviews) for specific personality disorders ranged from 0.30 for compulsive to 0.90 for dependent.[39] The reliability of the scale is improved when supplemented with a 20- to 45-minute interview of a relative or close friend after interview of the subject.[40] Comparison of SIDP diagnoses to scores on the MMPI and the Marke-Nyman Temperament Scale has provided evidence for the ability of the SIDP to discriminate between presence and absence of a personality disorder, as well as among the three DSM-III personality disorder clusters.[18]

A patient is diagnosed with an axis II personality disorder if the requisite number of criteria specified in DSM-III is met. To qualify for the diagnosis of mixed personality disorder, the subject must have missed the requisite number of criteria by one for two or more personality disorders, and must not have met full criteria for any other personality disorder.[18] The diagnosis of passive-aggressive personality disorder is rarely made on the SIDP because the presence of any other personality disorder disallowed this diagnosis in DSM-III (changed in DSM-III-R and DSM-IV).

There is poor reliability of axis II diagnoses made by experienced clinicians based on a clinical interview, and according to the developers of the SIDP, this reliability provides "an unacceptable standard for comparison with the SIDP."[18] Specifically, the kappa for presence of a personality disorder has been reported to be between 0.41[41] and 0.56[42] for experienced clinicians; both reliabilities are lower than the kappa of 0.66 reported for the SIDP administered in separate interviews.[18] Thus, despite improvements, there remains no accepted "gold standard" for personality diagnosis to date.

We evaluated 96 consecutive DSM-III OCD patients in our clinic with the SIDP evaluation and found that 50 (52%) received one or more axis II personality disorder diagnoses.[43] If mixed personality disorder is excluded, 35 patients (36%) met full criteria for one or more of the personality disorders. Mixed personality disorder (personality disorder not otherwise specified in DSM-III-R) was most frequently diagnosed (15%), followed in frequency by dependent (12%), histrionic (9%), compulsive (6%), and schizotypal, paranoid, and avoidant personality disorders with equal frequencies (5% each). No patients received a diagnosis of antisocial, narcissistic, or passive-aggressive personality disorders. The majority of diagnoses were within Cluster C (patients described in DSM-III as "anxious or fearful"). Presence of a personality disorder was not gender-related. Twenty five of the 46 men (54%), and 25 of the 50 women (50%) received an axis II diagnosis ($X^2(1) = 0.2$, n.s.).

As noted previously, dependent, histrionic, and compulsive personality disorders were most commonly found.[43] Similarly, Mavissakalian and Hamann[44] found dependent, avoidant, and histrionic personality disorders to be most common in a sample of 60 agoraphobic patients. Thus dependent and histrionic personality disorders may be relatively common in a variety of anxiety disorders, although in neither sample was the frequency greater than 15% for any of these personality disorders.

As noted previously, we found that compulsive personality disorder was diagnosed in six patients (6%), all with age of onset of OCD prior to 20 years of age. These results replicate two earlier studies[23,36] in finding that compulsive personality disorder is less frequent in OCD than was once believed. The prevalence of compulsive personality disorder of from 4% to 6% in OCD outpatients in these studies indicates that compulsive personality disorder, as defined by DSM-III, is not a necessary condition for the development of OCD, and in fact, is not the most common personality disorder in OCD. When patients with significant compulsive features were combined with this personality disorder diagnosis (i.e., including the mixed personality disorder with compulsive features), our sample prevalence increased to only 14%. These conclusions are limited to the DSM-III diagnosis of compulsive personality disorder, rather than the traditional psychodynamic concept of obsessional personality. However, changes in the diagnostic criteria in DSM-III-R moved the diagnostic entity of OCPD somewhat closer to the traditional concept;[6] as a result, prevalence of this personality disorder in OCD became somewhat higher when we applied DSM-III-R criteria, approaching 25%.[43]

Mavissakalian, et al[45,46] administered the PDQ to 43 OCD sufferers. The most frequent diagnoses were avoidant, histrionic, dependent, and schizotypal. Looking at individual traits regardless of diagnostic categories and avoidant and dependent personality disorder characteristics, OCD patients had strong passive-aggressive and compulsive tendencies, and substantial histrionic, paranoid, and schizotypal traits. The more personality traits, the more symptomatic the patients were with OCD. The strongest predictor of personality disorder presence was depression (measured by Beck Depression Inventory). Presence of a personality disorder was not predicted by social background, OCD symptoms, or age of OCD onset.

In a review of this literature, Pfohl,[4] as part of the DSM-IV Taskforce Project, recently concluded:

> In summary, available studies suggest that the majority of patients with OCD do not meet criteria for OCPD. Among patients with OCD who do have a PD, several other PDs may be just as common or more common than OCPD. The relationship between OCPD and other Axis I disorders is even less clear. (Pfohl, 1996, p. 783.)

CHANGES IN OBSESSIVE-COMPULSIVE PERSONALITY DISORDER OVER TIME

The fact that OCPD traits (but not OCPD) are common in OCD may simply represent confounding of axis II traits by axis I symptoms. For example, in the previous revision of this textbook, Swedo and associates[47] advanced the hypothesis that some children may develop compulsive personality traits as an adaptive mechanism to handle OCD. This hypothesis is in accord with our finding that of 96 adult patients with OCD, the presence of mixed personality disorder was more likely with longer duration of OCD; this finding suggests that patients who do not have premorbid personality disorders may develop significant personality traits (especially avoidant, compulsive, and dependent), which may be related to behavioral and lifestyle changes secondary to OCD.[43]

Supporting Swedo, et al's[45] hypothesis, Thomsen and Mikkelsen[48] compared 47 adults who had earlier had a hospital admission for childhood OCD to 49 adult controls with no psychiatric history. As adults, the number of personality disorders diagnosed by SCID-II did not significantly differ between the groups. However, adults who *still had* OCD as adults had significantly more OCPD than those who no longer had OCD.

Mavissakalian et al[45] reported 27 OCD subjects who completed the PDQ pretreatment and 12 weeks of treatment with clomipramine. These authors reported reduction on several personality variables, including number of personality diagnoses assigned, distribution of traits, and number of items endorsed in each disorder category. Significantly, they found that improvement in personality functioning was greater among responders than among either nonresponders or partial responders to clomipramine.[45]

In our Massachusetts General Hospital OCD clinic, Ricciardi et al[49] studied 17 patients with OCD and concomitant personality disorder who were treated pharmacologically and behaviorally and reassessed for presence of DSM-III-R personality disorder after 4 months. Ten of 12 patients who responded to treatment no longer met criteria for a personality disorder, but of five patients who were unresponsive to treatment, four patients continued to meet criteria for personality disorder (Table 4-5). Because none of these patients had Cluster A personality disorders at baseline, we cannot yet conclude whether these personality disorders also change with successful treatment, although we have evidence that treatment is less likely to be successful in this group.

These studies imply that perhaps the diagnosis of current OCPD made in the presence of current OCD provides little useful information. These findings also indicate the "fuzzy" distinction between axis I and axis II symptoms and the response of each of these symptom groups to drug and behavioral treatments. Because the question of symptom overlap across axes I and II between OCD and OCPD has been a subject of interest to us, we conducted factor analyses of DSM-III-R OCD symptoms and OCPD symptoms (diagnosed by SIDP-R) and then examined their overlap.[50] We found that in OCPD, a first factor accounted for 28.7% of the variance in the nine criteria and included items often seen in patients with OCD: (1) "preoccupation with details;" (2) "inability to throw things away (i.e., hoarding);" (3) "indecision;" and (4) "perfectionism" (the other criterion that loaded on this factor was restricted expression of affection). A smaller second factor accounted for 21.2% of the variance, and the criteria were: (1) "overconscientiousness;" (2) "devotion to work;" (3) "insistence that others comply;" and (4) "lack of generosity" (loaded 0.35 or more on this second factor). Only the first factor was related to our factor-analysis OCD symptoms, particularly symmetry, hoarding, repeating, ordering, and counting symptoms.[50] We hypothesized that the first OCPD factor reflected OCD–type symptoms, whereas the second factor reflected interpersonal personality traits possibly secondary to the OCD–type symptoms.

TREATMENT FOR OBSESSIVE-COMPULSIVE DISORDER SUFFERERS WITH PERSONALITY DISORDERS

If, as research summarized previously indicates, individuals with OCD and one or more comorbid personality disorders are less responsive to standard drug and behavioral treatments, what can be done to help them? Although research in this important clinical area is sparse, two recent reports offer hope and may help guide future research.

McKay and Neziroglu[51] reported an OCD patient with comorbid schizotypal personality disorder who underwent social skills treatment and at 6-month follow-up, had considerable OCD symptom reduction (although OCD, anxiety, and depressive symptoms remained). This coincides with the study cited previously, indicating that when treated with comprehensive behavior

Table 4-5   Changes in DSM-III-R Personality Disorders in Responders and Nonresponders to Fluoxetine and/or Behavior Therapy

Responders to Treatment*	
Personality Disorder Pretreatment	**Personality Disorder Posttreatment**
1. Avoidant, dependent	—
2. Mixed	—
3. Avoidant	—
4. Obsessive-compulsive	—
5. Obsessive-compulsive	—
6. Obsessive-compulsive	—
7. Avoidant	—
8. Obsessive-compulsive	Dependent
9. Obsessive-compulsive, avoidant, dependent	Obsessive-compulsive
10. Avoidant	—
11. Mixed	—
12. Avoidant	—

Nonresponders to Treatment*	
Personality Disorder Pretreatment	**Personality Disorder Posttreatment**
1. [†]Obsessive-compulsive	—
2. Mixed	Self-defeating
3. Obsessive-compulsive	Obsessive-compulsive
4. Self-defeating	Self-defeating
5. Mixed	Mixed

* Responders, Y-BOCS decreased by 25% or more; Nonresponders, Y-BOCS decreased by less than 25%.
[†] Y-BOCS decreased by 24%.
(From Ricciardi, et al: Changes in axis II diagnoses following treatment of obsessive-compulsive disorder, *Am J Psychiatry* 149:829–831, 1992; with permission.)

therapy that focused on other clinical problems *besides* the OCD, those patients with comorbid personality disorders "had an enhanced response to treatment."[22]

Steinert, et al[52] reported a treatment-resistant 27-year-old woman with OCD and borderline personality disorder who responded to clozapine after having failed previous trials with paroxetine, clomipramine, various classical and atypical neuroleptics, and psychotherapy.

REFERENCES

1. American Psychiatric Association: *Diagnostic and statistical manual of mental disorders*, ed 4, Washington, 1994, American Psychiatric Association.
2. McCrae RR, Costa PT Jr: Personality trait structure as a human universal, *Am Psychol* 52:509–516, 1997.

3. Costa PT Jr, McRae RR: *Revised NEO Personality Inventory (NEO-PI-R) and NEO Five-Factor Inventory (NEO-FFI) professional manual*, Odessa, 1992, Psychological Assessment Resources.
4. Pfohl B: Obsessive-compulsive personality disorder. In Widiger TA, Frances AJ, Pincus HA, Ross R, First MB, Davis WW, editors: *DSM-IV sourcebook*, Washington, 1996, American Psychiatric Association, pp 777–788.
5. Ingram IM: The obsessional personality and obsessional illness, *Am J Psychiatry* 117:1016–1019, 1961.
6. Goldstein WN: Obsessive-compulsive behavior, DSM-III and a psychodynamic classification of psychopathology, *Am J Psychother* 39:346–359, 1985.
7. American Psychiatric Association: *Diagnostic and statistical manual of mental disorders*, ed 3, Washington, 1980, American Psychiatric Association.
8. American Psychiatric Association: *Diagnostic and statistical manual of mental disorders*, ed 3, revised, Washington, 1987, American Psychiatric Association.
9. Nestadt G, Romanski AJ, Brown CH, et al: DSM-III compulsive personality disorder: An epidemiological survey, *Psychol Med* 21:461–471, 1991.
10. American Psychiatric Association: *Diagnostic and statistical manual of mental disorders*, ed 2, Washington, 1968, American Psychiatric Association.
11. Salzman L: *Obsessional personality*, New York, 1968, Science House.
12. Tyrer P, Casey P, Gall J: Relationship between neurosis and personality, *Br J Psychiatry* 142:404–408, 1983.
13. Jenike MA, Baer L, Minichiello WE, et al: Concomitant obsessive-compulsive disorder and schizotypal personality disorder, *Am J Psychiatry* 143:530–532, 1986.
14. Minichiello WE, Baer L, Jenike MA: Schizotypal personality disorder: A poor prognostic indicator for behavior therapy in the treatment of obsessive-compulsive disorder, *J Anx Dis* 1:273–276, 1987.
15. Kendler KS, Masterson CC, Ungaro R, et al: A family history study of schizophrenia-related personality disorders, *Am J Psychiatry* 141:424–427, 1984.
16. Kendler KS, Masterson CC, Davis KL: Psychiatric illness in first-degree relatives of patients with paranoid psychosis, schizophrenia and medical illness, *Br J Psychiatry* 147:524–531, 1985.
17. Baer L, Jenike MA, Black DW, et al: Effect of axis II diagnoses on treatment outcome with clomipramine in 54 patients with obsessive compulsive disorder, *Arch Gen Psychiatry* 49:862–866, 1992.
18. Stangl D, Pfohl B, Zimmerman M, et al: A structured interview for the DSM-III personality disorders, *Arch Gen Psychiatry* 42:591–596, 1985.
19. Pfohl B: Personal communication, 1989.
20. Cohen J, Cohen P: *Applied multiple regression/correlation analysis for the behavioral sciences*, Hillsdale, 1975, Lawrence Erlbaum Associates.
21. Fals-Stewart W, Lucente S: An MCMI cluster typology of obsessive-compulsives: a measure of personality characteristics and its relationship to treatment participation, compliance and outcome in behavior therapy, *J Psychiatr Res* 27:139–254, 1993.
22. AuBuchon PG, Malatesta VJ: Obsessive compulsive patients with comorbid personality disorder: Associated problems and response to a comprehensive behavior therapy, *J Clin Psychiatry* 55:448–453, 1994.
23. Steketee G: Personality traits and diagnoses in obsessive-compulsive disorder.

Paper presented at the annual meeting of The Association for the Advancement of Behavior Therapy, November 1988.

24. Coursey RD: The dynamics of obsessive-compulsive disorder. In Insel TR, editor: *New findings in OCD,* Washington, DC, 1984, American Psychiatric Press, pp 104–121.

25. Rachman S, DeSilva P: Abnormal and normal obsessions, *Behav Res Ther* 16: 233–248, 1978.

26. Slade PD: Psychometric studies of obsessional illness and obsessional personality. In Beech HR, editor: *Obsessional states*, London, 1974, Methuen.

27. Pollack JM: Obsessive-compulsive personality: A review. *Psychol Bull* 2:225–241, 1979.

28. Pollack J: Relationship of obsessive-compulsive personality to obsessive-compulsive disorder: A review of the literature, *J Psychology* 121:137–148, 1987.

29. Doppelt HG: A topological investigation of the MMPI scores of clients with an obsessive-compulsive disorder and the relationship of their MMPI scores to behavioral treatment outcome, *Dissertation Abstracts International*, Ann Arbor, 1983, University Microfilms No. DA8311133.

30. Carey RJ, Baer L, Jenike MA, et al: MMPI correlates of obsessive-compulsive disorder, *J Clin Psychiatry* 47:371–372, 1986.

31. Graham JR: *The MMPI: A practical guide*, New York, 1977, Oxford University Press.

32. Schotte C, De Doncker D, Maes M, et al: Low MMPI diagnostic performance for the DSM-III-R obsessive-compulsive personality disorder, *Psychol Rep* 69:795–800, 1991.

33. Cloninger CR: A systematic method for clinical description and classification of personality variants: A proposal, *Arch Gen Psychiatry* 44:573–588, 1987.

34. Pfohl B, Black D, Noyes R, et al: Harm avoidance and serotonin in obsessive-compulsive disorder: A test of the Tridimensional Personality Questionnaire by association with diagnosis and platelet imipramine binding. Paper presented at the annual meeting of The American Psychiatric Association, San Francisco, May 1989.

35. Richter MA, Summerfeldt LJ, Joffe T, Swinson RP: The Tridimensional Personality Questionnaire in obsessive-compulsive disorder, *Psychiatr Res* 65:185–188, 1996.

36. Joffee RT, Swinson RP, Regan JJ: Personality features of obsessive-compulsive disorder, *Am J Psychiatry* 145:1127–1129, 1988.

37. Rasmussen SA, Tsuang MT: Clinical characteristics and family history in DSM-III obsessive-compulsive disorder, *Am J Psychiatry* 143:317–322, 1986.

38. Black DW, Yates WR, Noyes R, et al: DSM-III personality disorder in obsessive-compulsive study volunteers: A controlled study, *J Personality Dis* 3:58–62, 1989.

39. Pfohl B, Coryell W, Zimmerman M, et al: DSM-III personality disorders: Diagnostic overlap and internal consistency of individual DSM-III criteria, *Comp Psychiatry* 27:21–34, 1986.

40. Zimmerman M, Pfohl B, Stangl D, et al: Assessment of DSM-III personality disorders: The importance of using an informant, *J Clin Psychiatry* 47:261–263, 1986.

41. Mellsop G, Varghese F, Joshua S, et al: The reliability of Axis II of DSM-III, *Am J Psychiatry* 139:1360–1361, 1982.

42. Spitzer RL, Forman JBW, Nee J: DSM-III field trials: I. Initial interrater diagnostic reliability, *Am J Psychiatry* 136:815–817, 1979.

43. Baer L, Jenike MA, Ricciardi JN, et al: Standardized assessment of personality disorders in obsessive-compulsive disorder, *Arch Gen Psychiatry* 47:826–832, 1990.
44. Mavissakalian M, Hamann MS: DSM-III personality disorder in agoraphobia, *Compr Psychiatry* 27:471–479, 1986.
45. Mavissakalian M, Hamann MS, Jones B: Correlates of DSM-III personality disorder in obsessive-compulsive disorder, *Compr Psychiatry* 31:481–489, 1990.
46. Mavissakalian M, Hamann MS, Jones B: DSM-III personality disorders in obsessive-compulsive disorder: Changes with treatment, *Compr Psychiatry* 31:432–437, 1990a.
47. Swedo SE, Leonard HL, Rapoport JL: Childhood-onset obsessive-compulsive disorder. In Jenike MA, Baer L, Minichiello WE, editors: *Obsessive-compulsive disorders: Theory and management*, ed 2, Chicago, 1990, Mosby–Year Book, pp 28–38.
48. Thomsen PH, Mikkelsen HU: Development of personality disorders in children and adolescents with obsessive-compulsive disorder. A 6- to 22-year follow-up study, *Acta Psychiatr Scand* 87:456–462, 1993.
49. Ricciardi JN, Baer L, Fischer S, et al: Changes in axis II diagnoses following treatment of obsessive-compulsive disorder, *Am J Psychiatry* 149:829–831, 1992.
50. Baer L. Factor analysis of symptom subtypes of obsessive compulsive disorder and their relation to personality and tic disorders, *J Clin Psychiatry* 55(suppl 3):18–23, 1994.
51. McKay D, Neziroglu F: Social skills training in a case of obsessive-compulsive disorder with schizotypal personality disorder, *J Behav Ther Exp Psychiatry* 27: 189–194, 1996.
52. Steinert T, Schmidt-Michel PO, Kaschka WP: Considerable improvement in a case of obsessive-compulsive disorder in an emotionally unstable personality disorder, borderline type under treatment with clozapine, *Pharmacopsychiatry* 29:111–114, 1996.

5

Obsessive-Compulsive Disorder Symptoms and Medication Treatment in Pregnancy

Maria Lynn Buttolph, M.D., Ph.D., Kathleen E. Peets, B.A., Amy D. Holland, M.Ed.

This chapter reviews the literature bearing on two important questions: (1) what is the relation between obsessive-compulsive disorder (OCD) symptom onset or worsening and pregnancy or childbirth; and (2) what is the effect on the fetus or newborn of OCD medications taken by pregnant or breastfeeding women?

OBSESSIVE-COMPULSIVE DISORDER SYMPTOM ONSET OR WORSENING IN PREGNANCY

Findings in the earliest reports, prior to the *Diagnostic and Statistical Manual of Mental Disorders* (DSM) diagnoses, were mixed: Pollitt[1] found pregnancy and childbirth to be precipitating factors in 10 (11%) of 93 obsessional patients, whereas Ingram[2] found pregnancy to be the most common precipitating event, occurring in 15 (17%) of 89 OCD patients, and Lo[3] reported pregnancy and delivery to be precipitants in 3 (5%) of 56 OCD patients. However, all these percentages are misleadingly low because these studies include both women and men.

More recently, a follow-up study of 82 patients who were treated for a postpartum illness found that only 1% had an obsessional state with depression, and no patients had an obsessional state alone.[4] Brandt and MacKenzie[5] described one patient in whom OCD worsened during pregnancy, and proposed several possible explanations for the worsening of symptoms: (1) the biologic and psychosocial demands of pregnancy; (2) decreases in psychotropic medication used during pregnancy; (3) the nature of the obsession (fear of harming the fetus); and (4) development of concurrent depression.

Several case reports have shown onset of OCD during pregnancy and describe symptoms of obsessive thoughts—primarily fears about harming the fetus or neonate.[6-8] Significantly, several of our clinic patients have reported significant improvements in their obsessions as their children become older and more independent. Keuthen, et al[9] recently reported a relation between worsening of trichotillomania symptoms during pregnancy and menstruation.

In 1989, to examine the relationship between OCD and pregnancy or childbirth, we developed a questionnaire (Box 5-1) and mailed it with a self-addressed stamped envelope to the 180 consecutively evaluated OCD patients in our database as of December 1988.[10] Sixty (33%) questionnaires were returned, from 39 women and 21 men. Of the men respondents, only one (5%) stated that the birth of his two children worsened his OCD symptoms. Of the 39 women respondents, 27 (69%) related onset or worsening of OCD to pregnancy or childbirth. Triggering events appeared to be infertility, miscarriage, pregnancy, birth and care of first child, and birth and care of subsequent child. Case reports are presented to illustrate the clinical presentation of these patients, along with their response to behavior therapy, medication, or both. Table 5-1 presents the frequency and percentage of women in whom OCD was triggered or worsened by the events of each category.

Case 1: Onset of Obsessive-Compulsive Disorder in Pregnancy

A 31-year-old woman reported onset of OCD during the ninth month of her first pregnancy. She began to have excessive fears of asbestos and rat poison; as her obsessions worsened, washing rituals also increased. She used antiseptic solution to wash doorknobs and washed her clothes repeatedly. If she thought that her husband had touched something that was contaminated, she demanded that he shower. She did not go to the supermarket because she feared the aisle that contained rat poison. She did not receive any treatment.

During her second pregnancy, her symptoms became more severe. She thought that she was bringing traces of rat poison into her house on her shoes, which then spread to every room. She feared the whole house was contaminated, and cleaned it repeatedly. In addition, she had to change her child's clothes several times a day. During her pregnancy, she was referred for behavior therapy, and the compulsive behaviors decreased significantly.

After the birth of her second child she was given fluoxetine 20 mg/day, which was slowly increased to 80 mg/day because her obsessions with rat poison were not helped by behavior therapy. These fears were causing her to obsessively wash herself and her children.

Prior to medication treatment, her Yale-Brown Obsessive-Compulsive Scale (Y-BOCS) score was 17 (a score of 16 or higher usually indicates clinically significant OCD) and her Beck Depression Inventory was 13. Three months after beginning fluoxetine, she felt very much improved; the Y-BOCS decreased to

Box 5-1 Obsessive-Compulsive Disorder Questionnaire

As part of our continuing research on obsessive-compulsive disorder through the Massachusetts General Hospital OCD Clinic and Research Unit, we would like you to fill out the following questionnaire and return it in the enclosed self-addressed envelope. Thank you very much for your time and help.

Birthdate _____

Age when your OCD symptoms became problematic _____

We would like to know if any of the following events either triggered the onset of your OCD symptoms or significantly worsened them. Please place a T on the line to the left of the number for triggered the onset of OCD symptoms and a W for worsening them. You may write on the back if more space is needed.

_____ 1. Accident or head injury (please explain) _____

_____ 2. School-related event (i.e., college; please explain) _____

_____ 3. Job-related event (please explain)_____

_____ 4. Death of close friend or family member (please explain) _____

_____ 5. Illness (please explain) _____

_____ 6. Birth of a child
      a. _____ First child
      b. _____ Second child
      c. _____ Subsequent child

IF YES: Did you have any problems with cleaning the child?_____
_____

Did you have any problems feeding the child?_____
_____

Did you have difficulties putting the child to bed?_____
_____

FOR WOMEN:
_____ 7. Pregnancy (please explain) _____

For those of you who answered yes to either question 6 or 7, we would like to contact you for further information regarding the effect of pregnancy and childbirth on OCD. If you would be willing to be contacted, please put your name and phone number in the space below. This is optional and will only be done with your permission; however, it will be extremely helpful to have as much information about these areas as we can.

Anyone who responded to the questionnaire who would be willing to be contacted for further information, please put your name and phone number in the space below.

Table 5-1   Percentage of Women (n = 27) Reporting a Relationship Between Obsessive-Compulsive Disorder and Pregnancy or Childbirth

Category	Targeted Obsessive-Compulsive Disorder		Worsened Obsessive-Compulsive Disorder		Category Total	
	Number	%	Number	%	Number	%
Infertility	2	7.5	0		2	7.5
Miscarriage	0		2	7.5	2	7.5
Pregnancy	6	22	3	11	9	33
Birth and care						
First child	6	22	4	15	10	37
Subsequent child	2	7.5	2	7.5	4	15
Total, n	16	59	11	41	27	100

9 and the Beck Depression Inventory to 1. She was able to let her children go out and play without making them bathe when they returned. In addition, she allowed other children to come into her house, and she went to the supermarket three to four times per week and walked past the rat poison each time.

Case 2: Worsening of Obsessive-Compulsive Disorder During Pregnancy

A 35-year-old woman had severe OCD symptoms. She reported onset of OCD when she was in the sixth grade, when she began to fear broken glass. This progressed to the fear that she may have caused an accident, and ultimately led to her avoidance of driving for the previous 4 years. Her symptoms worsened during pregnancy, when she was obsessed with contamination and feared that harm would come to the fetus. Her compulsions included checking the stove to prevent fire and checking doors and windows to make sure they were locked. She also washed her hands approximately 100 times per day because of fear that she would contaminate the baby with germs. After her baby was born, she washed the baby's hands and any objects the baby came in contact with and spent hours sterilizing the baby's bottles. She frequently called the poison control hotline to find out if she had inadvertently poisoned her child; she has avoided using many cleaning products since the birth of her child.

On initial evaluation, her Y-BOCS score was 35, her Beck Depression Inventory was 29, and her Maudsley Obsessive Compulsive Inventory was 19. Her child was 4 months old, and she was afraid of having a second child.

The recommended treatment for this patient was a trial of fluoxetine 20 mg/day, with the dosage slowly increased to a maximum dose of 80 mg/day, along with behavior therapy. After 3 months, she was much improved and handwashing was decreased from 100 to 30 times per day. In addition, she decreased the time spent sterilizing bottles from 3 hours to half an hour. She also decreased the time spent cleaning her kitchen from 3 hours to half an hour per day, and stated that she was using this extra time to enjoy her child. She was allowing her child to chew on a pacifier. At 3-month follow-up, her Y-BOCS score was 27, and the Beck Depression Inventory was 8. At 4-month follow-up, the patient continued to take fluoxetine 80 mg/day and remained in behavior therapy; Y-BOCS was 20 and Beck Depression Inventory 5.

Case 3: Onset of Obsessive-Compulsive Disorder in Postpartum Period

A 42-year-old woman reported that her OCD symptoms began immediately after the birth of her first child, while she was still in the hospital and learning from nurses how to care for her infant. She was instructed that she needed to scrub and use sterile techniques, such as using a fingernail brush and antiseptic to clean her hands before touching her child. She was also instructed not to touch the telephone, the bed rail, or any of her personal items before touching her baby. When she was leaving the hospital with her 3-day-old infant, she instructed her husband to wash his hands before touching the baby. She was concerned that he had been driving and that the steering wheel was covered with germs. However, he refused to wash his hands, and this upset her. After returning home, she read literature recommending handwashing prior to nursing and cautioning that hospitals were often full of germs. This led her to wash her slippers and other clothes she had brought to the hospital. When her child was 2 weeks old, she visited the pediatrician, and believed that the office door handle was contaminated. She became upset when anyone touched the baby. In addition, she could not buy any new clothes because she believed that her breast milk would become contaminated by trying them on.

Over the following 2 years her obsessions changed to fears of contamination by urine from the baby's diapers, which was accompanied by an increase in her washing rituals. This fear of urine contamination persisted for the next 11 years, and eventually led to her total inability to touch her daughter, then 13 years of age. The patient totally isolated herself, did not allow anyone to come into her home, lost her job, and was divorced.

At the time of evaluation at our clinic, the patient had tried several medications, including fluvoxamine and clomipramine, with no improvement of symptoms. On initial evaluation, her Y-BOCS score was 31 and the Beck Depression Inventory 26. Fluoxetine 20 mg/day was begun, and slowly increased to a dose of 80 mg/day; she was also given clonazepam 0.5 mg twice a day, because of the anxiety that accompanied the symptoms. Over the next 3 months, her Y-BOCS score decreased to 21, and her Beck Depression Inventory decreased to 0. After 10 months of medication and behavior therapy, the Y-BOCS score decreased further to 10, and the Beck remained at 0. The symptoms had decreased to the extent that the patient was able to return to teaching children without being disabled by her previous obsessions about urine and contamination.

Case 4: Worsening of Symptoms in Postpartum Period

A 34-year-old mother of twins came to our clinic because her OCD symptoms were worsening with the care of her 9-month-old infants. She reported the onset of OCD at age 18 years, when she saw an occult movie and became obsessed with anything associated with it. She had almost constant obsessions and reported that she performed rituals to keep the devils away.

For the first 2 months after the birth of her twins, she noticed that her symptoms decreased significantly when she was breastfeeding. However, when the children were 3 months old, her symptoms worsened and she began to fear being responsible for harm coming to her children. She also became obsessed with symmetry, exactness, superstitious fears, and lucky and unlucky numbers.

Her compulsions included excessive showers, repetition of routine activities, ordering and rearranging, and superstitious behaviors. She was unable to dress her children in red or black because those colors increased her rituals. In addition, she could not dress them in clothing that had an apostrophe on its label, such as Oshkosh B'Gosh; she stated that the apostrophe was the symbol of possessiveness, which was associated with the devil and the occult. She also described difficulty feeding her children at certain unlucky times of the day. Although she was aware that her obsessions and compulsions were not rational, she felt unable to control them.

On initial examination, her Y-BOCS score was 31 and her Beck Depression Inventory 19, indicating severe OCD with mild depression.

Recommendations were made for her to begin a trial of fluoxetine therapy and to consider behavior therapy after beginning the medication. Follow-up data are not yet available.

Case 5: Onset of Symptoms Related to Infertility

A 25-year-old woman stated that her OCD symptoms began when she was trying to conceive and she became concerned that chemicals in her environment were preventing her from becoming pregnant. She became pregnant 4 years later, and began to avoid cleaning fluids, insecticides, and animals, because she feared that her unborn child would be harmed. She became very anxious when doing laundry and feared that touching the dirty laundry would cause a birth defect in her baby. She engaged in compulsive handwashing and bathing rituals to protect her unborn child.

She reported that her mother had compulsions to check the stove and light switches, and her grandmother liked things to be symmetrical and in order. However, neither had been treated for OCD.

When evaluated at our clinic, the patient's Y-BOCS score was 29 and her Beck Depression Inventory score was 24, indicating severe OCD and moderate depression.

Because the patient was pregnant and did not want to take medication, she was referred for behavior therapy. One month after beginning behavior therapy, her Y-BOCS score decreased to 14 and at 2 months, it decreased to 5.

In our 1989 study described previously,[10] both patients who reported that miscarriage worsened their OCD symptoms had severe obsessions. One patient worried that her obsessions about harming others had actually caused her miscarriage. The second patient's obsession was that she had venereal disease, which caused her to miscarry; this patient also believed that her obsessions about harming others might have caused her miscarriage.

The most striking finding of our survey was that 69% of the women who answered the questionnaire described a relationship between the onset or worsening of OCD symptoms and some aspect of pregnancy, birth, or care of their children. Because OCD is now recognized as a relatively common psychiatric disorder,[11] with mean age of onset in the childbearing years,[12] it is difficult to determine retrospectively whether pregnancy and childbirth are causative in development of OCD.

If future research identifies these events as causative factors in developing OCD, there are several possible explanations for this finding. First, the biologic and psychosocial demands of pregnancy may increase tension and anxiety in the pregnant woman with OCD. Studies have reported exacerbation of OCD during environmental stress[3] or increased tension.[13]

Stern and Cobb[14] reported that the most common underlying theme in OCD is the fear of harming oneself or others. All cases included in Table 5-1 had obsessive fears of harming themselves or others. It was striking that all 11 patients who reported worsening of symptoms developed fear of harming the fetus or child. Pregnant women and patients caring for small children cannot avoid situations that provoke their symptoms, which may contribute to the increased severity of the disorder.

Similarly, in a pilot study of 27 consecutive women presenting for treatment for postpartum major depression, Wisner[15] found that 12 (44%) endorsed aggressive obsessions on the Y-BOCS symptom checklist (and six checking compulsions), and that 9 of the 12 reported obsessions about harming their babies. This result, if replicated, would be very important, because Dr. Wisner asked women explicitly about the presence of various obsessive thoughts of an embarrassing nature, which may explain the higher prevalence of aggressive obsessions in this series.

The observation that many women relate their OCD symptoms to pregnancy or childbirth is an interesting finding without an adequate biochemical explanation. There is no unified hypothesis linking the serotonin system with hormonal changes in pregnancy and birth. Future research into the cause of OCD may offer new insights into possible relationships. Recently, Leckman and associates[16] reported an association between elevated oxytocin levels and OCD symptoms.

There have been several hypotheses to explain the association between elevated oxytocin levels and OCD symptoms, including high gonadal steroid secretion during pregnancy.[17] Neziroglu, et al[18] agreed that the gonadal-steroid subsystem may be involved in some form of obsessive-compulsive disorder. Williams and Koran[19] found premenstrual and postpartum exacerbation of OCD symptoms in some women and also suggested that changes in gonadal hormones may be involved. In addition, it has been our clinical experience that patients report a worsening of their obsessive-compulsive symptoms premenstrually, and Keuthen, et al[9] from our group have noted premenstrual worsening of trichotillomania symptoms. It would be helpful to explore this hypothesized correlation between levels of gonadal steroids and OCD onset and symptoms by documenting concurrently steroid levels with symptom severity.

EFFECTS OF PHARMACOTHERAPY FOR OBSESSIVE-COMPULSIVE DISORDER

Pregnancy

Fluoxetine, clomipramine, and fluvoxamine are among the most commonly prescribed medications for OCD. Because of a lack of relevant research on other medications, we limited our focus to the effects of these three medications.

The majority of the research on the effects of psychotropic medications during pregnancy has investigated fluoxetine, one of the most frequently used medications for depression. Although it is often prescribed for OCD, most studies examine the effects of fluoxetine in pregnant patients treated for depression.[20,21]

The largest prospective study to date included 228 women taking fluoxetine and 254 who were medication-free. No significant difference in the rate of spontaneous pregnancy loss or major structural anomalies was reported between women who used fluoxetine during pregnancy and women in a control group.[22] However, infants of mothers in the fluoxetine group had significantly more minor anomalies (three or more) than the control infants. Also measured was the difference in the effect of fluoxetine exposure in the first trimester versus the third trimester. Results indicated a greater risk for perinatal complications with third-trimester exposure. Criticism of the study[23,24] indicated the lack of a relevant control group. However, as the authors explained in their response to this criticism,[25] setting up a well-matched control group of severely depressed pregnant women is unlikely. An earlier study by Goldstein[24] found no apparent significant complications in pregnancy outcome with third-trimester fluoxetine exposure. Similarly, no increased risk of major malformations was found in another earlier study by Pastuszak, et al,[26] which examined first-trimester fluoxetine exposure.

To date, only one study has addressed the critical issue of the long-term effects of psychotropic medication exposure during pregnancy. Nulman et al[27] examined the preschool-age children of 80 women who had taken a tricyclic antidepressant (55 had been treated with fluoxetine) and compared them with 84 children whose mothers were not exposed to such medications during pregnancy. This study concluded that exposure to either tricyclic antidepressants or fluoxetine during pregnancy did not have a long-term impact on global IQ, language, or behavioral development.

Case reports on the use of clomipramine during pregnancy have shown a significant impact on the neonate. One infant born a few days after the mother abruptly discontinued the medication suffered apparent withdrawal symptoms minutes after birth.[28] Other infants, whose mothers remained on clomipramine throughout their pregnancy, also suffered withdrawal symptoms shortly after birth.[29,30] After their literature review, Goldberg and Nissim[31] did not recommend clomipramine during pregnancy because of the risk of neonatal seizures. If it is necessary, however, for a patient to remain on clomipramine during pregnancy, a gradual tapering off of the medication prior to delivery may be helpful in minimizing the risk of seizures.[32]

Fluvoxamine has not been specifically studied for its impact on pregnancy. The research available suggests that fluvoxamine is generally safer for use than tricyclic antidepressants.[33] In a personal communication, Wagner[34] reported that, in data collected by Solvay Pharmaceuticals as of 1993, 63 women were maintained on fluvoxamine during their pregnancy. Of this group, there were eight therapeutic abortions and eight spontaneous abortions. In addition, there was one report of a congenital cardiac anomaly resulting in the infant's death during surgery. It is the company's recommendation that fluvoxamine be used during pregnancy only if there is a potential benefit to outweigh the risk to the fetus. Another report[35] on a group of British patients exposed to fluvoxamine during pregnancy showed low numbers of spontaneous abortions or gross anomalies.

Breastfeeding

The decision to breastfeed may be complicated in OCD patients who need medication treatment. The importance of this issue is underscored from the results of our earlier survey. Twenty-two percent of the women reported new-onset OCD after the birth of their child, and another fifteen percent reported worsening of their symptoms.[10] There is an obvious need to consider both the use of psychotropic drugs during breastfeeding and the effects of the concentrations in breast milk.

A few reviews have summarized these effects.[31,36,37] Goldberg and Nissim[31] begin their review of research on psychotropic drugs and lactation with the observation that "all psychotropic drugs . . . are secreted into milk," although at varying concentrations. The decision to take psychotropic medication during pregnancy or when nursing is a difficult one that requires a careful analysis of the risks and benefits to both the mother and the infant. When medication is needed, Goldberg and Nissim[31] strongly recommend close monitoring of the drug levels in both the infants and the mothers' breast milk.

One recent study[38] measured serum clomipramine and its metabolites in four breastfeeding mother-infant pairs. The mothers showed a wide range of serum concentrations, whereas the infants' levels were either nondetectable or below quantifiable limit. Previous studies of women taking tricyclics who breastfed their infants have also failed to detect harmful levels of the drug in the infants.[39,40]

Similar findings were obtained in studies of the effect of sertraline and its metabolite, norsertraline, on breastfed infants.[41,42] Although the patients in both studies were suffering from postpartum depression rather than OCD, sertraline is among the medications often used in the treatment of OCD. Mammen and colleagues[41] measured sertraline and norsertraline plasma concentrations in three mother-infant pairs and found one or both present at very low levels, but with no adverse effects on the infants. In the Epperson[42] study, four infant-mother pairs were studied and the whole-blood serotonin levels measured before and after sertraline therapy. Platelet serotonin transport was suppressed in 90% of the mothers; however, there was little or no effect in the infants. An earlier case report[43] found levels of sertraline in breast milk to be variable over a 24-hour period, but again found no detectable levels of sertraline in the infant serum. A metabolite of sertraline, desmethylsertraline, was detected in six infant serum samples, although the concentration was below the detection limit of most commercial laboratories.[44]

Nulman and Koran[45] studied the safety of fluoxetine by measuring both the amount of the drug and its active metabolite, norfluoxetine, in the breast milk of 10 women. They also evaluated the short-term adverse effects on the 11 infants who were nursed by women undergoing treatment with fluoxetine. None of the 11 infants were reported to have any short-term adverse effects, and the researchers concluded that less than 10% of the adult therapeutic dose of fluoxetine is passed on to an infant through breast milk. On the other hand, a previous case study[46] suggested the possibility of a relationship between colic and fluoxetine hydrochloride passed to a 6-week-old infant through maternal breast milk. This possible connection highlights the need for further research on short- and long-term effects, as well as for careful consideration of each individual situation before any medication is prescribed for nursing mothers.

One case report of a woman with OCD[47] quantified the level of paroxetine in her breast milk. Measurement of the concentration of paroxetine in a milk sample was taken 4 hours after a dose intake of 20 mg. No adverse effects were noted in the infant during breastfeeding.

Thus far, there has been only one report measuring the level of fluvoxamine in breast milk,[48] which suggested a minimal risk of significant levels being passed to infants.

SUMMARY

It is generally considered that in severely ill women, the benefits of pharmacotherapy outweigh the risks to the fetus or infant. It is also agreed, however, that considerably more research is necessary to determine potential risks and benefits of OCD treatment medications.

Given that the mean age of the onset of OCD is in the childbearing years[12,49] and the efficacy of medication treatment for OCD, a need for comprehensive research to determine the effects of drug therapy during pregnancy and breastfeeding remains. As more data are collected on both the short- and long-term effects of medication treatment during pregnancy and lactation, a more informed decision can be made. Behavior therapy is an effective treatment for OCD[50] (see Chapters 17, 19, and 20) and should be the first-choice treatment for pregnant or nursing OCD sufferers.

REFERENCES

1. Pollitt J: Natural history of obsessional states, *Br Med J* 1:194–198, 1975.
2. Ingram IM: Obsessional illness in mental hospital patients, *J Ment Sci* 107: 382–402, 1961.
3. Lo WH: A follow-up study of obsessional neurotics in Hong Kong Chinese, *Br J Psychiatry* 113:823–832, 1967.
4. Davidson J, Robertston E: A follow-up study of post-partum illness (1946–1978), *Acta Psychiatr Scand* 71:451–457, 1985.
5. Brandt KR, MacKenzie TB: Obsessive-compulsive disorder exacerbated during pregnancy: a case report, *Int J Psychiatry Med* 17:361–366, 1987.
6. Sichel DA, Cohen LS, Rosenbaum JF, et al: Postpartum onset of obsessive-compulsive disorder, *Psychosomatics* 34:277–279, 1993.
7. Sichel DA, Cohen LS, Dimmock JA, et al: Postpartum obsessive compulsive disorder: a case series, *J Clin Psychiatry* 54:156–159, 1993.
8. Iancu I, Lepkifker E, Dannon P, Kotler M: Obsessive-compulsive disorder limited to pregnancy, *Psychother Psychosom* 64:109–112, 1995.
9. Keuthen NJ, O'Sullivan RL, Hayday CF, et al: The relationship of menstrual cycle and pregnancy to compulsive hairpulling, *Psychother Psychosom* 66:33–37, 1997.
10. Buttolph ML, Holland AD: Obsessive compulsive disorders in pregnancy and childbirth. In Jenike MA, Baer L, Minichiello WE (editors): *Obsessive-compulsive disorders: theory and treatment*, ed 2, Chicago, 1990, Mosby.
11. Robins LV, Helzer JE, Weissman MM, et al: Lifetime prevalence of specific psychiatric disorders in three sites, *Arch Gen Psychiatry* 41:949–958, 1984.
12. Minichiello WE, Baer L, Jenike MA, et al: Age of onset of major subtypes of obsessive-compulsive disorder, *J Anx Dis* 4:147–150, 1990.
13. Pollitt J: Obsessional states, *Br Med J* 9:133–140, 1975.
14. Stern RS, Cobb JP: Phenomenology of obsessive-compulsive neurosis, *Br J Psychiatry* 132:233–239, 1978.
15. Wisner KL: personal communication, November 5, 1996.

16. Leckman JF, Goodman WK, North WG, et al: Elevated levels of CSF oxytocin in obsessive-compulsive disorder, *Arch Gen Psychiatry* 51:782–792, 1994.
17. Stein DJ, Hollander E, Simeon D, et al: Pregnancy and obsessive-compulsive disorder, *Am J Psychiatry* 150:1131–1132, 1993 (letter).
18. Neziroglu FA, Yaryura-Tobias JA, Anemone R: *Am J Psychiatry* 150:1132, 1993 (letter).
19. Williams KE, Koran LM: Obsessive-compulsive disorder in pregnancy, the puerperium, and the premenstruum, *J Clin Psychiatry* 58:330–334, 1997.
20. Altshuler LL, Szuba MP: Course of psychiatric disorders in pregnancy: dilemmas in pharmacologic management, *Neurol Clin* 12:613–635, 1994.
21. Spencer MJ: Fluoxetine hydrochloride (Prozac) toxicity in a neonate, *Pediatrics* 92:721–722, 1993.
22. Chambers CD, Johnson KA, Dick LM, et al: Birth outcomes in pregnant women taking fluoxetine, *N Engl J Med* 335:1010–1015, 1996.
23. Cohen LS, Rosenbaum JF: Birth outcomes in pregnant women taking fluoxetine, *N Engl J Med* 236:872, 1997 (letter).
24. Goldstein DJ, Sundell KL, Corbin LA: *N Engl J Med* 236:872–873, 1997 (Letter to the Editor).
25. Jones KL, Johnson KA, Chambers CD: Birth outcomes in pregnant women taking fluoxetine, *N Engl J Med* 236:873, 1997 (letter).
26. Pastuszak A, Schick-Boschetto B, Zuber C, et al: Pregnancy outcome following first-trimester exposure to fluvoxamine (Prozac), *JAMA* 269:2246–2248, 1993.
27. Nulman I, Rovet J, Stewart DE, et al: Neurodevelopment of children exposed in utero to antidepressant drugs, *N Engl J Med* 336:258–262, 1997.
28. Bromiker R, Kaplan M: Apparent intrauterine fetal withdrawal from clomipramine hydrochloride, *JAMA* 272:1722–1723, 1994.
29. Østergaard GZ, Pedersen SE: Neonatal effects of maternal clomipramine treatment, *Pediatrics* 69:233–234, 1982.
30. Cowe L, Lloyd DJ: Neonatal convulsions caused by withdrawal from maternal clomipramine, *Br Med J* 284:1837–1838, 1982.
31. Goldberg HL, Nissim R: Psychotropic drugs in pregnancy and lactation, *Int J Psychiatry Med* 24:129–147, 1994.
32. Calabrese JR, Gulledge AD: Psychotropics during pregnancy and lactation: a review, *Psychotropics* 26:413–426, 1985.
33. Palmer KJ, Benfield P: Fluvoxamine: an overview of its pharmacological properties and review of its therapeutic potential in non-depressive disorders, *CNS Drugs* 1:57–87, 1994.
34. Wagner B: Solvay Pharmaceuticals, personal communication, October 2, 1997.
35. Edwards JG, Inman WHW, Wilton L, et al: Prescription-event monitoring of 10,401 patients treated with fluvoxamine, *Br J Psychiatry* 164:387–395, 1994.
36. Buist A, Normann TR, Dennerstein L: Breast feeding and the use of psychotropic medication: a review, *J Affect Disord* 19:197–206, 1990.
37. Wisner KL, Perel JM, Findling RL: Antidepressant treatment during breast feeding, *Am J Psychiatry* 153:1132–1137, 1996.
38. Wisner KL, Perel JM, Foglia JP: Serum clomipramine and metabolite levels in four nursing mother-infant pairs. *J Clin Psychiatry* 56:17–20, 1995.

39. Schimmell MS, Katz EZ, Shaag Y, et al: Toxic neonatal effects following maternal clomipramine therapy, *J Toxicol Clin Toxicol* 29:479–484, 1991.
40. Wisner KL, Perel JM: Serum nortriptyline levels in nursing mothers and their infants, *Am J Psychiatry* 148:1234–1236, 1991.
41. Mammen OK, Perel JM, Rudolph G, et al: Sertraline and norsertraline levels in three breastfed infants, *J Clin Psychiatry* 58:100–103, 1997.
42. Epperson CN, Anderson GM, McDougle CJ: Sertraline and breast feeding, *N Engl J Med* 336:1189–1190, 1997.
43. Altshuler LL, Burt VK, McMullen M: Breast feeding and sertraline: a 24-hour analysis, *J Clin Psychiatry* 56:243–245, 1995.
44. Stowe ZN, Owens MJ, Landry JC, et al: Sertraline and desmethylsertraline in human breast milk and nursing infants, *Am J Psychiatry* 154:1255–1260, 1997.
45. Nulman I, Koran G: The safety of fluoxetine during pregnancy and lactation, *Teratology* 53:304–308, 1996.
46. Lester BM, Cucca J, Andreozzi L, et al: Possible association between fluoxetine hydrochloride and colic in an infant, *J Am Acad Child Adolesc Psychiatry* 32:1253–1255, 1993.
47. Spigset O, Carleborg L, Norstrom A, et al: Paroxetine level in breast milk, *J Clin Psychiatry* 57:39, 1996.
48. Wright S, Dawling S, Ashford JJ: Excretion of fluvoxamine in breast milk, *J Clin Pharmacol* 31:209, 1991.
49. Leckman JF, Grice DE, Boardman J, et al: Symptoms of obsessive-compulsive disorder, *Am J Psychiatry* 154:911–917, 1997.
50. March JS, Frances A, Carpenter D, et al: The expert consensus guideline series: treatment of obsessive-compulsive disorder, *J Clin Psychiatry* 58:25, 1997.

6

Rating Scales for Obsessive-Compulsive Disorder

Wayne K. Goodman, M.D., Lawrence H. Price, M.D.

Reliable and valid symptom measures are essential to investigations of obsessive-compulsive disorder (OCD). Use of rating scales may also enhance the quality of clinical care by refining the evaluation and documentation of a patient's state. The recognition that OCD is common, coupled with the need to evaluate new and more effective treatments, has highlighted the importance of outcome measures that are specific and sensitive to change in severity of obsessive-compulsive symptoms. Until recently, accurate assessment of treatment response in patients with OCD was handicapped by the limitations of many of the existing rating instruments. These shortcomings included lack of specificity for obsessive-compulsive symptoms, confusion of trait with state measures, examination of only certain types of obsessions and compulsions, and inadequate analysis of scale psychometric properties. The absence of a generally accepted scale for OCD also made it difficult to compare results across different studies.

Since its introduction a decade ago, the Yale-Brown Obsessive-Compulsive Scale (Y-BOCS) has gained acceptance as the standard outcome measure in clinical studies of OCD in the United States and elsewhere and is described in detail in this chapter. The construction and psychometric properties of other widely used observer- and self-rated scales for OCD are also described. (For readers interested in additional coverage of this subject, see reviews by Taylor[1] and Feske and Chambless.[2])

PSYCHOMETRIC TERMINOLOGY

Adequate appraisal of any rating instrument must include an evaluation of its psychometric properties. A detailed discussion of approaches to scale development and psychometric analysis can be found elsewhere;[3] however, for the purposes of this chapter it may be helpful to define key psychometric terms. To begin with, reliability and validity must be distinguished. The *reliability* of a scale refers to the consistency with which it performs its measurements; *validity* refers to how well the scale actually measures what it is designed to measure. The reliability of a scale provides an index of the contribution of measurement error in the obtained scores. Demonstration of adequate reliability is a necessary, but not sufficient, condition for establishing the adequacy of a scale's psychometric performance; evidence of both reliability and validity is required to assess how well a scale is fulfilling its intended function. Although sensitivity to change is not viewed traditionally as an aspect of scale validity, information about the capacity of a scale to detect treatment-induced changes in symptom severity is highly relevant to outcome studies. (As noted later in this chapter, adequate data regarding reliability, validity, and sensitivity to treatment effects are not available for some of the scales currently in use for OCD.)

A number of different types of reliability have been described. Interrater reliability is a measure of the degree of agreement among different raters for the same subject. It can be assessed by calculating the agreement of scores obtained by different raters for the same subject during a single interview. Internal consistency measures the interim homogeneity of the scale. This factor is influenced both by the uniformity of the behavioral domain that is being sampled and by how well the items of the scale sample the content of that domain.[3] Test-retest reliability evaluates the concordance of scores obtained for the same subject on repeat administrations of a scale under similar test conditions. Test-retest reliability is more germane to scales that assess trait variables (e.g., characteristics of obsessive-compulsive personality) than to those scales that measure state variables (e.g., severity of obsessive-compulsive symptoms).[4]

Content, construct, and criterion-related validity are three generally accepted categories of validity.[3] "Face validity" is a nonstatistical term used to describe the "appearance" of the scale as valid; that is, the scale contains items that appear pertinent to the phenomenon being measured. Conversely, content validity involves statistical examination of scale content to determine if this content does, in fact, adequately represent the domain being measured, irrespective of item appearance. Construct validity refers to how well a scale measures the theoretic construct it is designed to assess. Techniques used to evaluate construct validity include comparing scores from other measures of the same (convergent) or different (divergent) constructs. Criterion-related validity measures the correlation between scale scores and independent criteria that are known to relate directly to the phenomenon under study. The criterion-related validity of OCD scales has not been carefully examined, in part because objective evaluation of covert obsessive-compulsive symptoms (e.g., silent checking) is problematic.[5]

OBSERVER-RATED SCALES

The Yale-Brown Obsessive-Compulsive Scale

Construction of the Yale-Brown Obsessive-Compulsive Scale

The Y-BOCS was designed to provide a specific measure of the severity of OCD symptoms that would not be influenced by the type or number of obsessions or compulsions present.[4] This scale was originally intended for use as an outcome measure in drug trials for patients already diagnosed as meeting criteria for OCD. The core portion of the Y-BOCS is a clinician-rated, 10-item scale, with each item rated on a four-point scale from 0 (no symptoms) to 4 (extreme symptoms) (total range, 0 to 40), with separate subtotals for severity of obsessions (sum of items 1 through 5) and compulsions (sum of items 6 through 10) (see Appendices 8 and 12). Obsessions and compulsions are assessed in an analogous fashion with regard to how much they occupy the patient's time, interfere with functioning, cause subjective distress, are resisted by the patient, and can actually be controlled by the patient. Information about symptom severity is elicited from a semistructured interview, which includes detailed criteria for scoring these items (see Appendix 8).

"Resistance," as it is defined in the Y-BOCS, differs from the use of this term in both the Leyton Obsession Inventory (LOI)[6] and the National Institute of Mental Health Global Obsessive-Compulsive Scale (NIMH Global OC). In the Y-BOCS, resistance is defined as the amount of effort spent by the patient to oppose obsessions or compulsions by means other than avoidance or performance of compulsions. It is assumed that a lower score (greater resistance) on the resistance items is a manifestation of health. In contrast, on the LOI and the NIMH Global OC, resistance is equated with the "internal struggle" of the patient against distressing symptoms. The resistance item on the LOI combines measures of distress and insight to evaluate the diagnostic significance of symptoms rather than the severity of symptoms. As used in the LOI, higher resistance scores reflect greater distress from the symptoms and hence a higher ranking for the clinical significance of the corresponding symptom score.

The balanced weighting of obsessions and compulsions conforms with the criteria of DSM-IV, which allows either obsessions or compulsions to be present alone. This design was also intended to facilitate comparisons between the severity of obsessions and compulsions. One application of this feature is to enable the rate and magnitude of treatment response of obsessions and compulsions to be analyzed separately.

The original full version of the Y-BOCS contained 19 items: items 1 through 10 corresponding to the core features of OCD (described previously); items 11 through 16, the investigational component of the Y-BOCS; and items 17 (global severity), 18 (global improvement), and 19 (reliability). The investigational items (11 through 16) assess insight, avoidance, indecisiveness, pathologic responsibility, pathologic slowness, and pathologic doubting, respectively. Ratings on these six items are not included in the computation of the total Y-BOCS score, because it is unclear whether they measure the core features of OCD and because of insufficient psychometric data. Items 17 and 18 were adapted from the Clinical Global Impressions (CGI) scale[7] to provide overall measures of severity (CGI-OCS) and improvement (CGI-OCI) in obsessive-compulsive symptoms, respectively. Both are rated on a seven-point scale. In some trials, two additional items have been added to the Y-BOCS: one (1b) to complement item number 1 (time occupied by obsessions) and the other (6b) to complement item number 6 (time occupied by compulsions). Item 1b is the "obsession-free interval" and item 6b is the "compulsion-free interval." These items were added because during the course of clinical improvement some patients with OCD reported lengthening of their symptom-free interval before they reported shortening of the total hours occupied by their obsessive-compulsive symptoms. To date, data reviewed are inconclusive as to the advantages of including these two items. The remainder of this discussion will be confined mainly to the first 10 standard items of the Y-BOCS.

Administration of the Yale-Brown Obsessive-Compulsive Scale

The first step in administering the Y-BOCS is to provide the patient with easy-to-understand definitions of obsessions and compulsions. Most patients can be educated about what these terms mean and how to distinguish between them. In some cases, depending on the level of education and psychologic sophistication of the patient, other words may be substituted. For example, with children, it is often necessary to simplify technical language and use the Children's Yale-Brown Obsessive Compulsive Scale (CY-BOCS) in such cases.[8] The interviewer is asked to read aloud the definitions of obsessions and compulsions and to illustrate with some common examples. Although this is important to do on the first rating interview, it is generally not necessary in subsequent rating sessions. As long as it can be established that the patient understands the meaning of these terms, it is usually sufficient to remind patients that obsessions are their thoughts and that compulsions are the behaviors that they feel driven to perform (with the reminder that compulsions are not always observable behaviors, but may also be thoughts, such as silent checking and silent recitation of nonsense prayers).

The next task of the rater is to help the patient enumerate his or her current obsessions and compulsions by generating a list of target symptoms. In treatment studies, it is crucial to conduct a comprehensive screening of all obsessions and compulsions present. The recognition of previously unidentified obsessive-compulsive symptoms during the course of treatment creates a dilemma for the rater because scoring them may falsely suggest that the severity of the patient's symptoms worsened or that new symptoms developed. By the same token, it is also useful to identify and be aware of past symptoms because they might reemerge later. The Y-BOCS Symptom Checklist, which includes more than 50 examples of obsessions and compulsions, is intended as an adjunct to facilitate symptom identification (see Appendix 12). For the convenience of ascertainment, these symptoms are organized into 15 larger categories according to their thematic content (e.g., aggression or contamination) or behavioral expression (e.g., checking or washing). The Checklist is not designed to be scored as an inventory nor is it usually necessary to readminister it during the course of a treatment study. Greist and others have adapted the checklist for computerized self-administration.[9]

In some cases, it can be difficult to decide whether a patient has both obsessions and compulsions or compulsions alone. For example, if a patient describes that hours are wasted aligning or symmetrically arranging objects in the immediate environment, the patient has a compulsion; but does this constitute also an obsession? One can infer that this "obsession" is a need for symmetry, but is this merely a construct invented by the clinician to explain the patient's senseless behaviors? At present, there is no unequivocal answer to this issue. If the patient describes rearranging pencils on a desk in an effort to suppress horrific images of the patient's parents in a car crash, the behavior clearly seems driven by ideation (obsessions). But if the patient performs these actions just because it "feels right," perhaps it is a pure compulsion.

The next step is to list specific descriptions of the patient's obsessive-compulsive symptoms on the Y-BOCS Target Symptom List (see Appendix 12). The target symptoms represent the types of obsessions and compulsions that will be assessed in sequential ratings. Together they constitute a symptom profile for the patient that can be reviewed at the beginning of each rating session. There are no set rules as to how to list the target symptoms. The rater must rely on his or her clinical judgment in considering whether the list accurately represents the symptoms of the patient. In any case, it should be readily comprehensible to a substitute rater. All current obsessive-compulsive symptoms should be concisely recorded on the Target List, but those symptoms that will be the primary focus of the ratings should be clearly indicated. The patient may have several different target obsessions and compulsions, each of greater or lesser severity; however, the final severity ratings are based on the combined effect of the individual target symptoms. For example, a patient whose major problem involves contamination by urine may also be overly concerned with arrangement and order. However, if the patient reports that the need for order is not distressing and does not cause significant interference, then this particular obsession will contribute minimally to the patient's overall rating.

The rater must ascertain whether reported behaviors are bona fide symptoms of OCD and not symptoms of another disorder, such as simple phobia or a paraphilia. The differential diagnosis between certain complex motor tics and compulsions (e.g., touching objects) may be difficult. In such cases, it is particularly important to provide explicit descriptions of the target symptoms and to be consistent in subsequent ratings. Separate assessment of tic severity with a tic rating instrument may be necessary in such cases. Some of the items listed on the checklist, such as trichotillomania, are currently classified in the *Diagnostic and Statistical Manual of Mental Disorders* (DSM-IV) as symptoms of an impulse control disorder, but it is not known whether the Y-BOCS is suitable for use in disorders other than DSM-IV–defined OCD. When using the Y-BOCS to rate severity of symptoms not strictly classified under OCD (e.g., trichotillomania) in a patient who otherwise meets criteria for OCD, it has been our practice to administer the Y-BOCS twice: once for conventional obsessive-compulsive symptoms, and a second time for putative OCD–related phenomena. In this fashion, separate Y-BOCS scores are generated for severity of OCD and severity of other symptoms in which the relationship to OCD is still unsettled. A special version of the Y-BOCS has been developed by Stanley, et al[10] for assessment of trichotillomania.

The Target List also provides a space for "avoidance," because many patients deal with their obsessive fears through avoidance of things or situations that trigger them. In the course of successful treatment, some patients may avoid these trigger factors less; however, this action may lead to increased exposure to anxiogenic stimuli and thus to more compulsive behavior. On the 10-item Y-BOCS, this occurrence may be reflected as increased severity of OCD unless the rater is careful to include assessment of avoidance on the interference items 2 and 7. Investigational item 12 separately assesses degree of avoidance, but this item is not included in the total Y-BOCS score. Woody et al[11] have suggested modifying the Y-BOCS by adding this avoidance item to the total score, but this addition is not standard practice.

Once the Target List is completed (including avoidance behaviors), the interviewer is instructed to assess the Y-BOCS items in the listed order and use the questions provided for each item. However, the interviewer is free to ask additional questions for purposes of clarification; if the patient volunteers information at any time during the interview, that information also can be considered. Additional information supplied by outside observers may be included in a determination of the ratings, provided such information is deemed essential to adequate assessment, and reliable week-to-week reporting can be ensured. For example, the use of the patient's parents as informants is often necessary when assessing children, as discussed later. The interviewer is asked to rate the average occurrence of each item's characteristics during the prior week up until and including the interview. The final score for each item reflects the composite rating of all of the patient's obsessions or compulsions.

For a new patient, the administration of the Y-BOCS takes approximately 30 to 45 minutes, because completion of the Y-BOCS Checklist and Target Symptom List is required. Subsequent administrations of the Y-BOCS to the same patient usually take from 10 to 20 minutes.

Psychometric Properties of the Yale-Brown Obsessive-Compulsive Scale

Studies of the psychometric properties of the Y-BOCS suggest that it is a highly reliable instrument for measuring the severity of illness in patients with OCD with a range of severity and types of obsessive-compulsive symptoms.[4] In a study involving four raters and 40 patients with OCD at various stages of treatment, interrater reliability and internal consistency of the Y-BOCS were excellent (intraclass correlation r = 0.98 and Cronbach's alpha coefficient = 0.89, respectively). Excellent interrater reliability was also obtained in studies by other investigators.[11,12] Test-retest reliability of the Y-BOCS was good when readministered within 2 weeks.[11,13,14]

The absence of a "gold standard" at the time the Y-BOCS was being introduced in 1986 made it difficult to establish construct validity. Nevertheless, the Y-BOCS is considered both a valid measure of severity in OCD, and the yardstick against which all new instruments are measured. In an early study, convergent and discriminant validity were examined in 81 patients with OCD and total Y-BOCS baseline score was significantly correlated with two independent measures of OCD (the CGI-OCS and NIMH Global OC), but not with a third (the MOCI).[5] Examination of discriminant validity found weak correlations between total Y-BOCS score and ratings of depression and anxiety in these patients, only for patients with low depression scores. Other investigators[11,13,15] have found good convergent validity for the Y-BOCS but also found that its discriminant validity is less satisfactory, as reflected in high correlations with measures of depression or anxiety.[11,15] The shortcoming is not unique to the Y-BOCS[2] and may be inherent to the measurement of OCD, in which more severe obsessive-compulsive symptoms are often accompanied by more severe symptoms of anxiety and depression. To control the effects of mood treatment, Richter, et al[15] have recommended always including a measure of depression in studies of OCD.

Numerous drug treatment studies in OCD have found the Y-BOCS to be a sensitive measure of changes in symptom severity. The Y-BOCS was sensitive to drug-induced changes in obsessive-compulsive symptoms in double-blind, placebo-controlled trials of fluvoxamine,[16,17] clomipramine,[18] fluoxetine,[19] sertraline,[20] and paroxetine[21] in patients with OCD. The Y-BOCS is a specific and sensitive measure of change because OCD response (as measured by global ratings of OCD) was significantly correlated with improvement on the Y-BOCS, but not with changes in depression or anxiety ratings.[5] Multicenter drug trials have found the Y-BOCS to be stable in untreated conditions. For example, after 10 weeks of treatment in the clomipramine multicenter trials, Y-BOCS scores in the placebo-treated group showed a mean decrease of only 4% from baseline; in contrast, Y-BOCS scores in the clomipramine-treated group showed a mean reduction of 40% from baseline.[18]

Together, these data indicate that the Y-BOCS is a reliable and valid instrument for assessing severity of obsessive-compulsive symptoms in patients with OCD. It does not appear useful in discriminating severity of OCD from severity of depression or anxiety in OCD patients with prominent secondary depression. The Y-BOCS provides a sensitive and specific measure of changes in symptom severity and is well suited to drug treatment studies. The usefulness of the Y-BOCS as an outcome measure in behavioral treatment studies has also been substantiated.[22,23] In contrast to inventories such as the LOI and MOCI, the total Y-BOCS score is not determined by the number or particular types of obsessive-compulsive symptoms present. This feature of the Y-BOCS facilitates comparisons of illness severity in patients with different types of obsessions and compulsions. Thus, the Y-BOCS emphasizes the functional impact, not content, of symptoms, while preserving information about content in the Checklist and Target List. This process orientation of the Y-BOCS has been adopted as a central feature of scales developed for the assessment of eating disorders,[24] pathologic gambling, alcoholism,[25] trichotillomania,[10] body dysmorphic disorder,[26] and hypochondriasis.[27]

Although the Y-BOCS was not intended as a diagnostic instrument, it can be a useful adjunct to diagnosis. For example, the Schedule for Tourette's and Other Behavioral Syndromes (STOBS) developed by Pauls, et al[28] contains an adaptation of the Y-BOCS for use in a structured diagnostic interview.

There are now at least 15 foreign-language translations of the Y-BOCS, including Spanish,[29] Portuguese, Italian, French,[30] Greek, Dutch, Danish, Turkish,[31] Japanese,[32] Hebrew, Slovak, Swedish, German,[33] Mandarin, and three Indian dialects (i.e., Hindi, Kannada, and Tamil). Published psychometric data are available for the versions in Spanish,[29] German,[33] Japanese,[32] French,[30] and Turkish.[31] The availability of these translations has facilitated cross-national studies of OCD.

The Comprehensive Psychopathologic Rating Scale– Obsessive-Compulsive Disorder Subscale

The Comprehensive Psychopathologic Rating Scale (CPRS) is a clinician-rated scale based on a semistructured clinical interview.[34] It was designed to measure change in the severity of psychiatric signs and symptoms. The CPRS contains 65 items, each rated on a four-point scale, covering a broad range of psychopathology. The eight-item OCD subscale of the CPRS was derived from a parent scale by selecting the highest ranked items endorsed by 24 patients with OCD who were administered the full-scale CPRS. These eight items were "rituals," "inner tension," "compulsive thoughts," "concentration difficulties," "worrying over trifles," "sadness," "lassitude," and "indecision." Four of these items were also included in a similarly derived depression subscale of the CPRS. Insel and colleagues[35] later dropped three items (sadness, inner tension, and worrying over trifles) from the original OCD subscale to form a five-item CPRS-OCD subscale, but two items of this version still overlap with the depression subscale.

Interrater reliability for the total score of the eight-item CPRS-OCD subscale is high (r = 0.87).[36] However, other formal studies of the reliability the CPRS-OCD subscale, such as tests of internal consistency, are lacking. Likewise, the CPRS-OCD subscale has not been formally validated. Inspection of the scale items raises concerns about the content validity of the scale, because it contains items that are not specific to OCD, including some items commonly associated with depression (e.g., sadness). Despite these psychometric shortcomings, the CPRS-OCD subscale has demonstrated sensitivity to change in several drug treatment studies of OCD.[35-37] Nevertheless, because the specificity of this instrument for OCD is not sufficiently supported, changes in CPRS-OCD subscale scores may also reflect changes in another condition, such as depression.

The National Institute of Mental Health Global Obsessive-Compulsive Scale

The National Institute of Mental Health (NIMH) has introduced several different rating instruments for OCD.[35,38] Of these, an overall measure of obsessive-compulsive symptom severity, the NIMH Global Obsessive-Compulsive Scale (NIMH Global OC), has had the most widespread use. The NIMH Global OC has been employed as a secondary outcome measure in several multicenter drug trials in patients with OCD.[18] The NIMH Global OC is a single-item, Likert-type, clinician-rated measure with 15 gradations of severity ranging from 1 (minimal) to 15 (very severe). Anchor points are provided for 5 of the 15 possible scores. Scores above 6 reflect clinically significant obsessive-compulsive behavior.

Formal psychometric data on the NIMH Global OC are incomplete, but the available evidence supports the convergent validity and sensitivity to change of this instrument. Interrater reliability has been reported to be high for other NIMH–developed OCD rating scales,[35] but these data have not been reported for the NIMH Global OC. Data from several multicenter drug trials on OCD found that, in general, scores on the NIMH Global OC are convergent with those on the Y-BOCS. These studies have also shown that the NIMH Global OC is sensitive to drug-induced symptom changes. The specificity of the NIMH Global OC for detecting changes in obsessive-compulsive symptoms (e.g., as opposed to depressive symptoms) is supported by pharmacologic challenge studies.[39] The NIMH Global OC is easy to administer and well suited to treatment studies of OCD in which an overall measure of obsessive-compulsive symptoms is desired, in addition to the Y-BOCS. It cannot, however, be relied on as a "stand-alone" measure of OCD, because it contains no instructions for ascertaining only OCD–specific symptoms.

SELF-RATED SCALES

Maudsley Obsessional-Compulsive Inventory

The Maudsley Obsessional-Compulsive Inventory (MOCI) is a 30-item dichotomous (true-false), self-rated questionnaire that was developed to investigate the different types of obsessive-compulsive complaints in patients with observable rituals (see Appendix 7).[40] The MOCI was derived from a larger set of 65 items after it was determined that these 30 items differentiated a group of obsessional patients from a control group of nonobsessional neurotic patients.[40] The MOCI was not intended as a diagnostic instrument, but rather as a research tool in the typology of obsessional patients who were already diagnosed (although the authors suggested that it might be used for other clinical research purposes, such as measuring treatment outcome).

Principal components analysis of the MOCI in 100 adult obsessional patients identified four orthogonal components, which together accounted for 43% of the total variance.[40] These components were labelled as "checking," "cleaning," "slowness," or "doubting." Separate ratings can be obtained for these four factors or all endorsements can be summed to arrive at a total obsessionality score (range = 0 to 30). Compared with several items about checking and cleaning compulsions, a variety of other obsessive-compulsive symptoms are insufficiently represented on the MOCI (e.g., aggressive obsession and hoarding).[5] Because the item selection of the MOCI is biased toward patients with checking or cleaning behaviors, patients with these types of symptoms (e.g., contamination-related behaviors) may score disproportionately higher on the MOCI than patients who are monosymptomatic (e.g., scrupulosity only), but who otherwise have equally severe illness.[5] This is a general limitation of using symptom inventories to compare patients' symptom severity using different symptom profiles. (The LOI addresses this problem by including item scores which assess the degree of distress and interference, thus providing supplemental measures of clinical severity.)

The internal consistency and test-retest reliability of the MOCI are satisfactory,[40] and convergent validity of retrospective clinician ratings with the cleaning and checking subscales and the total scale score of the MOCI yielded acceptable correlations.[40] In 30 obsessional patients, the total MOCI score correlated significantly with the LOI ($r = 0.60$). Although there is some evidence that the MOCI is sensitive to changes in OCD symptom severity,[40] in two trials of fluvoxamine, clinically significant, drug-induced improvement was reflected in statistically significant, but small, decreases in MOCI scores from baseline.[16,41] The dichotomous structure of the MOCI may contribute to its low sensitivity to change. Some of the items on the MOCI seem to overlap with obsessive-compulsive personality traits (e.g., following a very strict routine when doing ordinary things). Hence, in some cases the MOCI may measure personality characteristics that are relatively resistant to drug treatment.

One group of investigators has modified the true-false MOCI to include a graded response (four-point scale). Preliminary studies of this 20-item version suggest that it may be sensitive to change, but clear superiority to the original scale has yet to be demonstrated.[42]

In summary, the MOCI is short, easy to administer, and its reliability and validity are relatively well established. On the other hand, MOCI does not adequately cover the range of obsessive-compulsive symptoms seen in clinical practice, and it is relatively insensitive to drug-induced changes in obsessive-compulsive symptoms.

Leyton Obsessional Inventory

Up until the introduction of the Y-BOCS in 1986, the most widely used self-rating scale was the Leyton Obsessional Inventory (LOI)[6] and its variants.[43–45] The LOI is a 69-question inventory designed to assess obsessional symptoms and traits. It was first devised to provide an independent measure of child-rearing attitudes in a group of "house-proud" mothers and to diagnose obsessional symptoms and obsessional personality traits. Cooper[6] suggested, however, that it might also have broader clinical applications, such as monitoring change in obsessional symptoms during treatment. The original form of the LOI used a card-sorting ("postbox") procedure that required close supervision. Paper-and-pencil forms of the LOI have since been developed to facilitate scale administration,[43] but the postbox form has remained the most widely used. Several authors have introduced modified and shortened versions of the LOI,[44] including a version for children.[46]

Although the LOI addresses a wide range of obsessive-compulsive symptoms, coverage of obsessions involving aggression, violence, and other unacceptable ideation (e.g., blasphemous thoughts) is less adequate. In addition to "yes or no" responses to each item, scores are obtained for feelings of "resistance" and the degree of "interference" with other activities. These items (range, 0 to 3) were constructed to help differentiate patients with OCD from healthy subjects and subjects with obsessional traits. That is, higher scores on the resistance items indicate more intense subjective distress from obsessional symptoms, which in turn is assumed to reflect greater likelihood of having OCD (e.g., a score of 3 on the resistance item corresponds to the response, "This upsets me a great deal, and I try very hard to stop it").

Findings from studies of the reliability and validity of the LOI are incomplete and inconsistent. Reliability data are very limited, although Cooper[6] suggested that test-retest reliability of the LOI in depressed patients was encouraging. In one study, scores on the LOI successfully distinguished obsessional patients from healthy subjects.[6] In contrast, other studies have failed to support the convergent and discriminant validity of the LOI.[47,48] In several small studies, the LOI has been a useful measure of drug-induced changes in severity of obsessive-compulsive symptoms,[49–51] but most larger drug trials raise serious questions about the sensitivity of the instrument to detect change in symptom severity.[35,36] For example, in two different studies, clomipramine treatment was associated with significant reductions in severity of OCD on several other outcome measures, whereas scores on the LOI failed to reflect clinical improvement.[35,36]

In summary, the LOI has enjoyed extensive use and is more comprehensive than preceding inventories. The inclusion of items that estimate distress and interference may enable it to be used as a screening device in specialized situations. The postbox form is time consuming and cumbersome to administer,[44] but conventional self-report versions are available. Good agreement has been reported between these two forms of the LOI, although most of these reliability data were obtained in healthy subjects.[43] The most serious shortcomings of the LOI concern its reliability, validity, and sensitivity to change. Overall, these disadvantages of the LOI typically outweigh its advantages, especially an outcome measure in drug-treatment studies of patients with OCD.

Padua Inventory

The original 60-item Padua Inventory (PI) was devised by Sanavio[52] to measure degree of distress from obsessive-compulsive symptoms. Unfortunately, most publications on the properties and use of the PI have been based on non-clinical samples.[53] The 41-item revised PI (PI-R), on the other hand, has been studied in patients with OCD.[54] Each item is rated on a five-point scale from 0 (not at all) to 4 (very much), so that the total scale range is 0 to 164. Scores on the 41-item PI-R are subdivided into five subscales that were derived from factor analysis: (1) "impulses"; (2) "washing"; (3) "checking"; (4) "rumination"; and (5) "precision."[54] Internal consistency, interrater reliability, and test-retest reliability of the PI and PI-R have been reported to be satisfactory. In a study of patients with OCD, the PI-R was sensitive to clinical improvement from both medication and cognitive-behavior therapy.[55] The main drawbacks of the PI and its variants concern content and convergent/discriminant validity.[2] For example, some items on the PI do not clearly differentiate obsessions from worries.[56] To address this weakness, Burns, et al[57] created a 39-item version of the PI, omitting items that seemed to measure both worries and obsessions. When tested in a nonclinical population, this 39-item PI performed better with respect to this aspect. Despite this improvement, some other items of the PI do not seem specific to OCD and may reflect symptoms of depression or other anxiety disorders. Although scores on the PI and the PI-R show good agreement with other self-report measures of OCD, correlations with clinician-administered scales, including the Y-BOCS, are weak.[2]

Self-Report Yale-Brown Obsessive-Compulsive Disorder Scale

The Symptom Checklist of the Y-BOCS has been modified for use as a self-administered screening device for community-based populations as the

Screening Test for Obsessive-compulsive Problems (STOP) and for clinical settings as the Florida Obsessive-Compulsive Inventory (FOCI). Both the STOP and FOCI are intended for use as screening instruments and not as severity measures. A diagnosis of OCD should not be based on the results of these tests alone, but must be confirmed by clinical interview. The STOP consists of 12 dichotomous (true-false) questions that are divided into two parts. Part I (questions 1–6) determines whether the subject has been experiencing obsessive-compulsive symptoms during the past month. If any of the questions from Part I is answered "yes," the subject is instructed to complete Part II, which elicits information on the clinical significance of the obsessive-compulsive symptoms. Preliminary data on the psychometric propertics of the STOP are available from studies in patients with OCD,[58] from college students in introductory psychology classes,[59] and from respondents to an advertisement in a local newspaper (Ward, et al, unpublished data, 1997). Results from these studies are encouraging, but the sensitivity and specificity of the STOP have yet to be studied. The FOCI, like the STOP, consists of two parts: Part I, a true-false inventory and Part II, questions pertaining to the severity and clinical sig nificance of items endorsed in Part I. In contrast to the STOP, Part I of the FOCI contains additional examples of obsessive-compulsive symptoms (i.e., 20 versus 6 items) and Part II consists of five questions with graded, not dichotomous, response choices. Accordingly, the STOP takes less time to administer and is easier to use; on the other hand, the more-detailed FOCI has the potential for being more sensitive and specific. At present, however, even less psychometric information is available on the FOCI than on the STOP. In an anxiety disorders clinic, high concordance was observed between scores on Part II of the FOCI and the clinician-administered Y-BOCS (Ward, et al, unpublished data, 1997). A study of the psychometric properties of the FOCI in a primary care setting is currently under way. Additional work is required to establish the optimal cutoffs on the STOP and FOCI.

Computer-administered versions of the Y-BOCS have been developed to be used as severity and outcome measures. An interactive computer-assisted Y-BOCS test is available for use at a computer terminal in the clinician's office[9] or at a touch-tone telephone in the subject's home.[60] Excellent agreement has been found between computer- and clinician-administered Y-BOCS scores among patients with a diagnosis of OCD.[9,60] In one study,[9] the computer version of the Y-BOCS was administered in a counterbalanced fashion with the clinician-administered version to three cohorts: (1) patients with OCD; (2) patients with other anxiety disorders; and (3) healthy subjects. Convergent validity was excellent in the OCD group and good in the anxiety disorders group. Healthy controls scored themselves higher (more symptomatic) than did clinicians. These data suggest that computer-derived Y-BOCS scores may be less accurate outside of an established OCD sample. As long as satisfactory agreement is shown between the computer and clinician during the initial assessment, follow-up evaluations by computer Y-BOCS may offer a cost-effective alternative to live interviews in monitoring outcome.

Steketee, et al[61] compared a self-report, paper-and-pencil form of the Y-BOCS (originally developed by Baer[62]) with the clinician-administered Y-BOCS in several different clinical and nonclinical samples. The psychometric performance of the self-report version was comparable with that of the usual interview format. Within the nonclinical group, there were few differences between the scales in frequency of items endorsed on the Symptom Checklist. Within the clinical sample, however, OCD patients tended to endorse more symptoms on the self-report version. The self-report version demonstrated good convergent validity with the clinician-administered Y-BOCS, and it discriminated well between OCD and non–OCD patients.[61]

Compulsive Activity Checklist

The Compulsive Activity Checklist (CAC) has been widely used outside the United States for more than 20 years. The original 62-item CAC developed by Hallam was intended as a clinician interview of daily interference from overt rituals.[47] The CAC does not assess mental rituals. Several different self- and clinician-administered versions are available. One of the more popular versions of the CAC has 37 items,[63] each about a different compulsive symptom, rated on a four-point (0–3) scale regarding duration, repetition, and avoidance (total score range, 0–111). Neither distress nor interference with social relationships is evaluated. Recent versions of the CAC have shown good internal consistency.[64–67] Results for interrater and test-retest reliability have been more variable. The psychometric properties of the CAC and the clinician-administered, 10-item Y-BOCS were compared in a trial of behavior therapy in OCD.[22] The CAC and the Y-BOCS were significantly correlated both at baseline and at end of treatment. The Y-BOCS was superior to the CAC with respect to measuring OCD–related disability. We agree with the conclusion of Feske and Chambless[2] that there is little reason to recommend the CAC over the MOCI.

Assessment of Children

Assessment of obsessive-compulsive symptoms in children and adolescents has been reviewed in detail elsewhere (see Chapter 3).[68] A 44-item version of the LOI has been adapted for use in children,[46] with the scale extensively modified to shorten administration time and to better conform with the symptom profile of children. Because it is a postbox form of the scale, this version requires close supervision by the examiner. Psychometric studies of the LOI for children and adolescents found good test-retest reliability, discriminant validity, and sensitivity to drug-induced changes.[46,69] However, convergent validity with several other measures of OCD could not be demonstrated before treatment.[46] Although the latter validity studies are discouraging, this version of the LOI has the advantage of being carefully tailored to younger patients.

The CY-BOCS is a modification of the Y-BOCS for use in children.[8] It is identical to the Y-BOCS except for substitution of simpler language (e.g., obsessions are referred to as "thoughts" and compulsions as "habits"). Types of obsessive-compulsive symptoms more frequently found in children (e.g., bedtime rituals) have also been added to the CY-BOCS Symptom Checklist. Scahill, et al[70] studied the psychometric performance of the CY-BOCS in 65 children (8 to 17 years of age) with OCD. Reliability was satisfactory, as reflected in high internal consistency and good to excellent interrater agreement for the CY-BOCS total score and subscales for obsessions and compulsions. The CY-BOCS had high convergent and discriminant validity. The CY-BOCS total score showed a significantly higher correlation with a self-report measure of obsessive-compulsive symptoms ($r = 0.62$ for the LOI) as compared with the Children's Depression Inventory ($r = 0.34$) and the Children's Manifest Anxiety Scale ($r = 0.37$). Sensitivity of the CY-BOCS to drug-induced changes in symptom severity was found in several multicenter clinical trials in children and adolescents with OCD.[71,72]

Pharmacologic Challenge Studies

A number of investigators have applied the pharmacologic challenge strategy to the evaluation of the neurobiology of OCD.[39] In brief, this paradigm involves measuring the behavioral and neurochemical changes in response to the acute administration of a pharmacologic agent with predictable behavioral effects or well-characterized neurochemical properties. One of the problems associated with assessment of obsessive-compulsive symptoms in this setting is the short time period over which behavioral measurements must be made.[39] Unlike mood state, severity of OCD cannot be adequately assessed at a single time point. At any given moment, depressed patients can describe how depressed they feel, but OCD patients cannot readily describe how obsessive-compulsive they are. In fact, a major measure of OCD severity is the amount of time occupied by the symptoms. In our experience, a 1-hour interval is the shortest time over which obsessive-compulsive symptoms can be validly rated, because the anchor points of the Y-BOCS do not allow for reliable evaluation of a time period shorter than 24 hours.

In pharmacologic challenge studies, we have adopted the following approach: on the morning of the challenge study, the standard clinician-rated, 10-item Y-BOCS is completed. The period of assessment ranges from 1 week to a minimum of 1 hour, depending on the design of the study (e.g., frequency between repeat test days). An abbreviated and modified version of the Y-BOCS has been adapted for use during the challenge test day. The Yale-Brown Obsessive-Compulsive Challenge Scale (Y-BOCCS) is a 10-item analog scale, each item scored by a vertical mark on a 100-mm horizontal line, with greatest symptom severity corresponding to the extreme right of the line.[39] The total score of the Y-BOCCS equals the sum of the 10 items (to the nearest mm) divided by 10 (maximal score equals $1000 \div 10$, or 100).

The item composition of the Y-BOCCS is similar to that of the Y-BOCS. However, the resistance and interference items (which, in general, are not germane to the challenge setting) have been omitted and items that rate indecisiveness, pathologic responsibility (labelled as "guilt"), and insight (labelled as "conviction") have been added. Analogous clinician- and self-rated versions of the Y-BOCCS are intended for evaluation of symptoms over the 1 hour prior to the time of scale administration. The patient and clinician are instructed to refer to the obsessive-compulsive symptoms on the Target Symptom List generated during initial administration of the standard Y-BOCS. Formal psychometric studies of the Y-BOCCS have not been conducted. In addition to the Y-BOCCS, we administer a modified version of the CGI Scale global improvement item[7] to assess global change in obsessive-compulsive symptoms since the time the challenge agent was administered. Careful observation and documentation of the patient's behavior by trained research personnel are essential.

SUMMARY

The clinician-administered Y-BOCS has become the standard for both measuring symptom severity and monitoring treatment outcome in patients with OCD. It is sensitive to changes induced by either drugs or behavior therapy. Unlike some of the symptom inventories, such as the LOI, scores on the Y-BOCS are not usually influenced by the type or number of obsessions and compulsions present. Some rating scales have been adapted for use in children with OCD and for the assessment of change in obsessive-compulsive behavior following a pharmacologic challenge. The children's version of the Y-BOCS (or CY-BOCS) has demonstrated reliability, validity, and sensitivity to change.

Some currently available patient-rated instruments (e.g., the MOCI) suffer from serious shortcomings, including insensitivity to change and less relevance for patients with monosymptomatic syndromes (e.g., hoarding alone). To remedy the inadequacies of earlier self-report instruments, several self-report measures of OCD have been introduced in recent years, including the PI and variants of the Y-BOCS (i.e., the FOCI, STOP, and computerized formats). The PI, FOCI, and STOP show promise as screening instruments for detecting OCD in various clinical and nonclinical populations. However, there is insufficient evidence to support a diagnosis of OCD on the basis of these scale scores alone—the findings must be verified by a structured or expert clinical interview. Some versions of the PI and the computer-administered Y-BOCS are being used to monitor clinical change in OCD. Excellent convergent validity has been shown between computer-derived and clinician-administered Y-BOCS scores in established cases of OCD.

Several groups, including our own, have elected to use change scores on the 10-item Y-BOCS and a global measure of OCD such as the NIMH Global OC or modified CGI as the principal outcome variables in drug trials in patients with OCD. Most clinical trials have noted a 25% decrease in Y-BOCS scores from baseline as indicative of clinically significant improvement. A 35% reduction in the Y-BOCS has been used as a more stringent definition of responder status in some studies.

ACKNOWLEDGEMENTS

The authors wish to acknowledge Donna Epting and Candy Hill for their assistance with the preparation of this manuscript. This study was supported in part by a research grant from the National Institute of Mental Health, #MH45802.

REFERENCES

1. Taylor S: Assessment of obsessions and compulsions: reliability, validity, and sensitivity to treatment effects, *Clin Psychology Rev* 15:261–296, 1995.
2. Feske U, Chambless DL: A review of assessment measures for obsessive-compulsive disorder. In Goodman WK, Ruderfer M, Maser J, editors: *Treatment challenges in obsessive compulsive disorder*, Mahwah, NJ, 1997, Lawrence Earlbaum Associates.
3. Anastasi A: *Psychological testing*, ed 6, New York, 1988, Macmillan Publishing.
4. Goodman WK, Price LH, Rasmussen SA, et al: The Yale-Brown Obsessive Compulsive Scale (Y-BOCS). Part 1: Development, use and reliability, *Arch Gen Psychiatry* 46:1006–1011, 1989.
5. Goodman WK, Price LH, Rasmussen SA, et al: The Yale-Brown Obsessive-Compulsive Scale (Y-BOCS). Part II: Validity, *Arch Gen Psychiatry* 46:1012–1016, 1989.
6. Cooper J: The Leyton Obsessional Inventory, *Psychol Med* 1:48–64, 1970.
7. Guy W: *ECDEU Assessment manual for psychopharmacology*, Washington, 1976, United States Department of Health, Education and Welfare, publication number 76–338.
8. Goodman WK, Rasmussen SA, Price LH, et al: *Children's Yale-Brown Obsessive-Compulsive Scale* (CY-BOCS), ed 1, Departments of Psychiatry of Yale and Brown Universities, and Child Psychiatry Branch, 1986, National Institute of Mental Health.
9. Rosenfeld R, Dar R, Anderson D, et al: A computer-administered version of the Yale-Brown Obsessive-Compulsive Scale, *Psychol Assess* 4:329–332, 1992.
10. Stanley MA, Prather RC, Wagner AL, et al: Can the Yale-Brown Obsessive-Compulsive Scale be used to assess trichotillomania? A preliminary report, *Behav Res Ther* 31:171–177, 1993.
11. Woody SR, Steketee G, Chambless DL: Reliability and validity of the Yale-Brown Obsessive-Compulsive Scale, *Behav Res Ther* 33:597–605, 1995.
12. Jenike MA, Hyman S, Baer L, et al: A controlled trial of fluvoxamine in obsessive-compulsive disorder—implications for a serotonergic theory, *Am J Psychiatry* 147:1209–1215, 1990.
13. Kim SW, Dysken MW, Katz R: The Yale-Brown Obsessive-Compulsive Scale: A reliability and validity study, *Psychiatry Res* 34:99–106, 1990.

14. Kim SW, Dysken MW, Kuskowski M, et al: The Yale-Brown Obsessive-Compulsive Scale (Y-BOCS) and the NIMH Global Obsessive-Compulsive Scale (NIMH-GOCS): a reliability and validity study, *Int J Meth Psychiatric Res* 3: 37–44, 1993.

15. Richter MA, Cox BJ, Direnfeld DM: A comparison of three assessment instruments for obsessive-compulsive symptoms, *J Behav Ther Exp Psychiatry* 25:143–147, 1994.

16. Goodman WK, Price LH, Rasmussen SA, et al: Efficacy of fluvoxamine in obsessive-compulsive disorder: a double-blind comparison with placebo, *Arch Gen Psychiatry* 46:36–44, 1989.

17. Rasmussen SA, Goodman WK, Greist JH, et al: Fluvoxamine in the treatment of obsessive-compulsive disorder: a multi-center double-blind placebo-controlled study in outpatients, *Am J Psychiatry* in press.

18. Clomipramine Collaborative Study Group: Clomipramine in the treatment of patients with obsessive-compulsive disorder, *Arch Gen Psychiatry* 48:730–738, 1991.

19. Tollefson GD, Rampey AH Jr, Potvin JH, et al: A multicenter investigation of fixed-dose fluoxetine in the treatment of obsessive-compulsive disorder, *Arch Gen Psychiatry* 51:559–567, 1994.

20. Greist J, Chouinard G, DuBoff E, et al: Double-blind parallel comparison of three dosages of sertraline and placebo in outpatients with obsessive-compulsive disorder, *Arch Gen Psychiatry* 52:289–295, 1995.

21. Wheadon DE, Bushnell WD, Steiner M: A fixed dose comparison of 20, 40 or 60 mg paroxetine to placebo in the treatment of obsessive-compulsive disorder, Abstract, ACNP Meeting, Hawaii, 1993.

22. Nakagawa A, Marks IM, Takei N, et al: Comparisons among the Yale-Brown Obsessive-Compulsive Scale, Compulsion Checklist, and other measures of obsessive-compulsive disorder, *Br J Psychiatry* 169:108–112, 1996.

23. Fals-Stewart W, Marks AP, Schafer J: A comparison of behavioral group and individual behavior therapy in treating obsessive-compulsive disorder, *J Nerv Mental Dis* 181:189–193, 1993.

24. Mazure CM, Halmi KA, Sunday SR, et al: Yale-Brown-Cornell Eating Disorder Scale: development, use, reliability, and validity, *J Psychiatr Res* 28:425–445, 1994.

25. Anton RF, Moak DH, Latham PK: The obsessive compulsive drinking scale: a new method of assessing outcome in alcoholism treatment studies, *Arch Gen Psychiatry* 53:225–231, 1996.

26. Phillips KA, Hollander E, Rasmussen SA, et al: A severity rating scale for body dysmorphic disorder: development, reliability, and validity of a modified version of the Yale-Brown Obsessive Compulsive Scale, *Psychopharmacol Bull* 33(1): 17–22, 1997.

27. VanBalkom AKLM, et al: *Hypochondriasis—Y-BOCS assessment tool,* 1997.

28. Pauls DL, Hurst CR: *Schedule for Tourette and other behavioral syndromes,* Department of Psychiatry, Yale University, April 1987.

29. Nicolini H, Herrera K, Paez F, et al: Traducción al espanol y confiabilidad de la Escala Yale-Brown para et Trastomo Obsesivo-Compulsivo, *Salud Mental* 19:13–16, 1996.

30. Bouvard M, Sauteraud A, Notel, et al: Cottraux étude de validation et analyse

factorielle de la version Francaise de l'echelle d'obsession compulsion de Yale-Brown, *Therapie Comportementale et Cognitive* 2:18–22, 1992.

31. Tek C, Ulug B, Gursoy RB, et al: Yale-Brown Obsessive Compulsive Scale and United States National Institute of Mental Health Global Obsessive Compulsive Scale in Turkish: Reliability and validity, *Acta Psychiatr Scand* 91:410–413, 1995.

32. Nakajima T, Nakamura M, Taga C, et al: Reliability and validity of the Japanese version of the Yale-Brown Obsessive-Compulsive Scale, *Psychiatry Clin Neurosci* 49:121–126, 1995.

33. Hand l, Büttner-Westphal: Die Yale-Brown Obsessive Compulsive Scale (Y-BOCS): Ein halbstrukturietes interview zur beurteilung des schweregrades von denk—und haniungszdngen, *Verhaltenstherapie* 1:223–225, 1991.

34. Asberg M, Montgomery SA, Peris C, et al: A comprehensive psychopathological rating scale, *Acta Psychiatr Scand* (suppl)271:5–9, 1978.

35. Insel TR, Murphy DL, Cohen RM, et al: Obsessive-compulsive disorder: a double-blind trial of clomipramine and clorgyline, *Arch Gen Psychiatry* 40:605–612, 1983.

36. Thorn P, Asberc M, Cronholm B, et al: Clomipramine treatment of obsessive-compulsive disorder. I: A controlled clinical trial, *Arch Gen Psychiatry* 37:1281–1285, 1980.

37. Montgomery SA: Clomipramine in obsessional neurosis: a placebo controlled trial, *Pharm Med* 1:189–192, 1980.

38. Rapoport J, Elkins R, Mikkelsen E: Clinical controlled trial of chlorimipamine in adolescents with obsessive compulsive disorder, *Psychopharmacol Bull* 16:61–63, 1980.

39. Goodman WK, Price LH, Woods SW, et al: Pharmacological challenges in obsessive compulsive disorder. In Zohar J, Insel TR, Rasmussen SA, editors: *The psychobiology of obsessive compulsive disorder*, New York, 1991, Springer Publishing.

40. Hodgson RJ, Rachman S: Obsessional-compulsive complaints, *Behav Res Ther* 15:389–395, 1977.

41. Perse TL, Greist JH, Jefferson JW, et al: Fluvoxamine treatment of obsessive-compulsive disorder, *Am J Psychiatry* 144:1543–1548, 1987.

42. Dominguez RA, Jacobson AF, de la Gandara J, et al: Drug response assessed by modified Maudsley Obsessive-Compulsive Inventory, *Psychopharmacol Bull* 25:215–218, 1989.

43. Snowdon J: A comparison of written and postbox forms of the Leyton Obsessional Inventory, *Psychol Med* 10:165–170, 1980.

44. Allen JJ, Tune GS: The Lynfield Obsessional/Compulsive Questionnaires, *Scott Med J* 20:21–24, 1975.

45. Evans DR, Kazarian SS: Development of a reaction inventory to measure obsessive compulsive behaviors, Research Bulletin no. 315, 1974, Department of Psychology, University of Western Ontario.

46. Berg CJ, Rapoport JL, Flament M: The Leyton Obsessional Inventory—child version, *Psychopharmacol Bull* 21:1057–1059, 1985.

47. Philpott R: Recent advances in the behavioural measurement of obsessional illness. Difficulties common to these and other instruments, *Scott Med J* 20:33–40, 1975.

48. Clark DA, Bolton D: An investigation of two self report measures of obsessional

phenomena in obsessive-compulsive adolescents: research note, *J Child Psychol Psychiatr* 26:429–437, 1985.

49. Allen JJ, Rack PH: Changes in obsessive/compulsive patients as measured by the Leyton Inventory before and after treatment with clomipramine, *Scott Med J* 20:41–44, 1975.

50. Ananth J, Solyom L, Bryntwick S, et al: Chlorimipramine therapy for obsessive compulsive neurosis, *Am J Psychiatry* 136:700–701, 1979.

51. Prasad A: A double blind study of imipramine versus zimelidine in treatment of obsessive compulsive neurosis, *Pharmacopsychiatry* 17:61–72, 1984.

52. Sanavio E: Obsessions and compulsions: The Padua Inventory, *Behav Res Ther* 26:167–177, 1988.

53. Stemberger LG, Bums GL: Obsessions and compulsions: psychometric properties of the Padua Inventory with an American college population, *Behav Res Ther* 28:314–345, 1990.

54. van Oppen P, Hoekstra RJ, Emmelkamp PMG: The structure of obsessive compulsive symptoms, *Behav Res Ther* 33:15–23, 1995.

55. van Oppen P, Emmelkamp PMG, van Balkom AJLM, et al: The sensitivity to change of measures for obsessive-compulsive disorder, *J Anxiety Dis* 9:241–248, 1995.

56. Freeston MH, Ladouceur R, Rheume J, et al: Self-report of obsessions and worry, *Behav Res Ther* 32:29–36, 1994.

57. Bums LG, Keortge SG, Formea GM, et al: Revision of the Padua Inventory of obsessive compulsive disorder symptoms: Distinctions between worry, obsessions, and compulsions, *Behav Res Ther* 34:163–173, 1996.

58. Goodman WK: Introduction of a new OCD screening test. Presented at The 14th National Conference of the Anxiety Disorders Association of America, Santa Monica, California, March 17–20, 1994.

59. Morris NM, Blashfield RK, Rankupalli B, et al: Subclinical obsessive compulsive disorder in college students, *Depression-Anxiety* XX 1997.

60. Baer L, Brown-Bcasley MW, Sorce J, et al: Computer-assisted telephone administration of a structured interview for obsessive-compulsive disorder, *Am J Psychiatry* 150:1737–1738, 1993.

61. Steketee G, Frost R, Bogart K: The Yale-Brown Obsessive-Compulsive Scale: Interview versus self-report, *Behav Res Ther* 34:675–684, 1996.

62. Baer L: *Getting control: Overcoming your obsessions*, Boston, 1991, Little, Brown.

63. Marks IM, Connolly J, Philpott R: *Nursing in behavioral psychotherapy*, London, 1977, Royal College of Nursing.

64. Cottraux J, Bouvard M, Defayolle M, et al: Validity and factorial structure study of the Compulsive Activity Checklist, *Behav Ther* 19:45–53, 1988.

65. Frost RO, Steketee GS, Krause MS, et al: The relationship of the Yale-Brown Obsessive Compulsive Scale (Y-BOCS) to other measures of obsessive compulsive symptoms in a nonclinical population, *J Person Assess* 65:158–168, 1995.

66. Steketee G, Freund B: Compulsive Activity Checklist (CAC): further psychometric analyses and revision, *Behav Psychother* 21:13–25, 1993.

67. Stemberger LG, Bums GL: Compulsive Activity Checklist and the Maudsley Obsessional-Compulsive Inventory: psychometric properties of two measures of obsessive-compulsive disorder, *Behav Ther* 21:117–127, 1990.

68. Berg CZ: Behavioral assessment techniques for childhood obsessive compulsive disorder. In Rapoport JL, editor: *Obsessive compulsive disorder in children and adolescents*, New York, 1989, American Psychiatric Association.
69. Flament MF, Rapoport JL, Berg CA, et al: Clomipramine treatment of childhood obsessive compulsive disorder, *Arch Gen Psychiatry* 42:977–983, 1985.
70. Scahill L, Riddle NM, McSwiggin-Hardin M, et al: Children's Yale-Brown Obsessive-Compulsive Scales: reliability and validity, *Am J Child Adolesc Psychiatry* 36(6):844–852, 1997.
71. DeVeaugh-Geiss J, Moroz G, Biedeman J, et al: Clomipramine in child and adolescent obsessive-compulsive disorder: a multicenter trial, *J Am Acad Child Adolesc Psychiatry* 31:45–49, 1992.
72. Riddle MA, Scahill L, King RA, et al: Double-blind, crossover trial of fluoxetine and placebo in children and adolescents with obsessive-compulsive disorder, *J Am Acad Child Adolesc Psychiatry* 31:1062–1069, 1992.

Part II

**Illnesses Related to Obsessive-Compulsive Disorder:
Spectrum Disorders**

7

Illnesses Related to Obsessive-Compulsive Disorder: Introduction

Michael A. Jenike, M.D., Sabine Wilhelm, Ph.D.

A number of psychiatric illnesses resemble obsessive-compulsive disorder (OCD), including alcoholism, drug abuse, and compulsive sex, gambling, and eating; in each of these disorders, the patient feels compelled to perform some self-destructive act. By definition, however, these are not included under the category of OCD because patients do not necessarily resist the "compulsions," nor do they generally recognize the senselessness of their actions. In addition, patients derive some pleasure from carrying out these activities.

Many disorders can present with comorbid obsessive-compulsive symptoms; these include Tourette's disorder (see Chapter 8), schizophrenia, major depressive disorders, and organic mental disorders. Obsessions and compulsions are presumably secondary to the primary illness in these disorders. There are also a few syndromes in which symptoms are so similar to OCD that diagnostic distinctions are not always clear; in many cases treatment approaches similar to those employed in the treatment of OCD have been successful. These syndromes include trichotillomania (listed under Impulse Control Disorders Not Elsewhere Classified in *The Diagnosis and Statistical Manual of Mental Disorders* [DSM-IV]), monosymptomatic hypochondriasis, body dysmorphic disorder, globus hystericus, bowel obsessions, urinary obsessions, and compulsive skin picking. In addition, many patients with eating disorders, besides being obsessed with food, have concomitant obsessive-compulsive rituals such as repetitive handwashing. One group of researchers theorized that some patients who mutilate themselves may do so primarily to relieve anxiety and thus might be considered as having OCD.

In DSM-IV,[1] a number of related disorders are classified as impulse control disorders—these include kleptomania (compulsive stealing), pathologic gambling, pyromania (compulsive fire setting), and trichotillomania (compulsive hair pulling). Perhaps compulsive shopping and severe nail biting should also be included in this category.

Because patients with these related disorders are frequently referred to OCD clinics, and the treatments are often similar to those used for OCD, their clinical and therapeutic similarities to more classical OCD patients will be reviewed in this section. There are good reference text books that cover each of these disorders. Tourette's disorder, body dysmorphic disorder, and trichotillomania will be covered in their own chapters in this section in detail, because these represent the major diagnostic categories of related disorders. A few of the other common related disorders will be briefly reviewed in this chapter.

COMPULSIVE SKIN PICKING (NEUROTIC EXCORIATIONS)
Clinical Picture

Neurotic excoriations are lesions produced by patients as a result of repetitive skin picking.[2,3] Usually the behavior takes the form of an extensive cleaning ritual,[4] and the patients intend to remove small irregularities on the skin (e.g., blemishes, mosquito bites, dry skin). In more severe cases, the habit is uncontrollable and may turn into an urge to dig deep into the skin. Unlike patients with dermatitis artefacta, those with neurotic excoriations usually admit the self-inflicted nature of their lesions.[2] Skin picking can also occur secondary to delusions of parasitosis, but these patients have a psychotic character and therefore differ from those with typical presentations of neurotic excoriations.

We have seen approximately 40 patients over the past few years suffering from neurotic excoriations and many engage in picking for several hours per day. Patients frequently require dermatologic interventions for their skin wounds and infections. Some of our patients reported medical hospitalizations and surgical revisions for wounds that did not heal because they were not able to stop picking. Recently, a patient was described who picked a hole through the skin and neck muscles and nearly lacerated her carotid artery. In this case, the skin picking had an almost fatal outcome.[5] The lesions are typically in areas of the body that the patients can easily reach, such as face, upper and lower extremities, and upper back.[6] They are usually a few millimeters in diameter and crusted, weeping, or scarred.[6,7] The excoriations are produced with fingernails or small instruments such as tweezers or pins. Picking occurs most frequently in the evening or at night.[8,9]

Visual inspection and touching of the skin often precedes picking. Patients describe an uncontrollable urge to pick blemishes, and they report a temporary feeling of relief when blemishes are removed. However, this is soon replaced by a sense of disgust, depression, or anxiety.[10] Stressful circumstances usually increase picking behaviors. Some patients describe being in an almost trance-like state when picking at lesions. Patients often report that they try to resist the urge, but they usually find it difficult to control. A few of the patients we saw in our clinic looked somewhat disfigured because of scarring that resulted from skin picking, and most patients had mild acne. Patients were generally very embarrassed about their behavior and camouflaged the resulting lesions with make-up or clothing. Skin picking typically does not occur in the presence of other people, but interestingly, occasional patients reported picking at other people's skin.

Several studies described patients suffering from neurotic excoriations as "perfectionistic or having obsessive-compulsive traits, depressive symptoms, anxiety, hysteria, hypochondriasis" (for a review see Gutpa, et al[11]). However, the lack of modern diagnostic criteria limits the value of these studies. Skin picking has many similarities with OCD, because it is ego dystonic, repetitive, ritualistic, and temporarily relieves tension.[3,12,13] The compulsive and self-destructive quality of the behavior also resembles nail biting and trichotillomania. In a recent study, Phillips and Taub[10] showed that skin picking may be a symptom of body dysmorphic disorder. It can also occur in Tourette's disorder,[1] stereotypic movement disorder[1] or Prader-Willi syndrome.[14,15]

Demographics and Course

No data are available on the rate of occurrence of neurotic excoriations in the general population, but the incidence is estimated to be 2% among dermatology patients.[16] Prevalence is higher in women than in men[8,17] and the mean age of onset is in the range of 30 to 40 years; however, some researchers reported a peak in the range of 20 to 29 years of age.[6]

The intensity of compulsive skin picking seems to fluctuate, and the mean duration of symptoms is reported to be 5 years[18] with many patients having symptoms for 10 to 12 years.[8]

Treatment

Although dermatologic treatment may help to improve the skin condition, the treatment for neurotic excoriations is primarily psychiatric. Several case reports describe that these patients benefit from treatment with serotonin reuptake inhibitors.[3,12,13] In our anecdotal experience, the patients responded well to the use of serotonin reuptake inhibitor medications and/or with behavior therapy. Sometimes, symptoms have been completely eliminated with these approaches.

The following are two cases of patients suffering from compulsive skin picking who responded well to cognitive-behavior therapy:

Case 1

A 22-year-old woman had been picking at blemishes on her face and back for approximately 3 hours per day since she was 16 years of age. On inspection, she had mild acne and her skin was somewhat scarred as a result of the picking. She had constant and severe urges to pick at her skin and reported having no control over the picking. She frequently avoided leaving the house or going to work because she was embarrassed about the redness or scabs that resulted from the picking. She was often late for work because she could not stop picking at her skin, or because it took her so long to apply make-up to cover up the damaged skin. When she started to abuse alcohol and to cut her skin with a knife to stop the urge to pick, her parents became so worried that they encouraged her to seek treatment in our clinic. At the time of her intake evaluation, she met criteria for major depression, obsessive-compulsive personality disorder, and had some mild obsessions and compulsions focusing on symmetry and exactness. She had been treated with a trial of supportive psychotherapy (1 year) and fluvoxamine (200 mg/day for 10 weeks), which did not relieve her symptoms. She refused to take any further medication and requested cognitive-behavior therapy. The cognitive aspect of the treatment focused on changing distorted and unrealistic perfectionistic beliefs and the behavioral aspect focused on helping her to engage in activities that were incompatible with skin picking. Moreover, she learned to identify and regulate intense negative emotions that triggered the picking. After 14 sessions of cognitive-behavior therapy, her symptoms were very much improved. After 3 months of treatment, she still occasionally picked at her skin, but it did not interfere with social or occupational functioning.

Case 2

A 39-year-old woman had been picking at the skin on her feet to relieve tension for approximately 1 to 3 hours per day. The skin picking had originally been triggered by cracked heels or dehydrated skin. By the time she sought treatment she had been picking her skin for approximately 3 months and she mostly picked at healthy skin. The picking usually resulted in bleeding, extensive pain and difficulty walking. She was so embarrassed about the skin picking that she avoided all social and work settings. She described severe anxiety if the skin picking was interrupted and the urge that she always needed to carry out the behavior until she had a small pile of skin. Her history was remarkable for depression, alcohol abuse, and subclinical contamination fears. She had been treated with fluoxetine 60 mg/day for 10 weeks which did not relieve her symptoms. She began weekly cognitive behavioral therapy, focusing on cognitive restructuring and emotion regulation skills. The skin picking was very much improved after just nine sessions and improvement was maintained at 6 months' follow-up.

PATHOLOGIC GAMBLING

The DSM-IV criteria for pathologic gambling require that the patient have at least five of the following: (1) a frequent preoccupation with gambling; (2) a need to increase the size of bets to achieve the desired excitement; (3) repeated unsuccessful efforts to control, cut back, or stop gambling; (4) restlessness or irritability when attempting to cut down or stop gambling; (5) a tendency to gamble as a way of escaping from problems or of relieving a dysphoric mood; (6) a tendency to return another day to get even after losing money gambling; (7) a tendency to lie to family members, therapist, or others to conceal the extent of involvement with gambling; (8) committed illegal acts such as forgery, fraud, theft, or embezzlement to finance gambling; (9) jeopardized or lost a significant relationship, job, or educational or career opportunity because of gambling; and (10) a tendency to relie on others to provide money to relieve a desperate financial situation caused by gambling. In addition, the gambling behavior is not better accounted for by a manic episode.

Generally, the gambling urges and activity increase during periods of stress. Gamblers usually feel that money is both the cause of and the solution to their problems.[19] As gambling increases, patients usually are forced to lie to obtain money and to continue gambling; antisocial activities are not uncommon.

The disorder usually begins in adolescence in men and later in life in women and estimates of prevalence range from 1% to 3% of the adult population.[1]

Pyles[19] has suggested that personality disorders are extremely common in gamblers and that more than 50% of the disorders are of the narcissistic type,[20] although gambling also occurs among patients with borderline personality disorder, schizophrenia, sociopathy, cyclothymia, and manic-depressive disorder. There seems to be a high incidence of individuals with a history of attention deficit disorder, and affective disorders occur in up to three quarters of the patients.[21] It has been suggested that compulsive gambling may represent a self-medicating attempt to regulate affects.[19] Almost half of the patients have problems controlling alcohol intake.[21]

By the time the gambler presents for help, he or she often has a debt of between $55,000 and $92,000.[19] Pyles[19] reports that the therapist's initial dilemma is how to work with a patient who denies any problem except lack of money and who constantly lies and manipulates. Most treatment programs handle these patients as if they suffer from a serious character disorder. Inpatient and outpatient[22] programs are available, and Gamblers Anonymous is growing nationally. Unfortunately, medications have not been very helpful in decreasing the craving for gambling,[19] but there are no reports of attempts in gamblers to use the potent serotonergic reuptake inhibitors that have been successfully used in patients with frank OCD. Current approaches involve development of a repayment plan, therapy including the spouse and family members, group therapy with peer pressure, daily meetings with Gamblers Anonymous, and the possible use of medication.

MONOSYMPTOMATIC HYPOCHONDRIASIS/BODY DYSMORPHIC DISORDER

Patients manifesting circumscribed delusional beliefs that their body parts are distorted (body dysmorphic disorder [BDD]) or that they emit foul body odors (olfactory reference syndrome) suffer from a syndrome that has been called monosymptomatic hypochondriasis.[23–25] Another frequent manifestation of this disorder is delusions of parasitic infestation. Some define monosymptomatic hypochondriac patients as delusional and body dysmorphic patients as having an overvalued idea;[26] others feel that, at best, these distinctions are difficult to make.[25,25a] Although monosymptomatic hypochondriasis is frequently classified as a psychosis in the European literature,[26] the patient's single delusion may be the only evidence of a thought disorder.

Dysmorphophobia or body dysmorphic disorder, in which patients describe preoccupation with a minor bodily defect or imagined defect that they believe is conspicuous to others, is classified in the DSM-IV[1] as a somatoform disorder and is covered in detail in Chapter 10. Many of these patients initially consult surgeons, dermatologists, or internists,[27] seeking help for what they believe is a medical condition (e.g., extremely large nose, face is large, huge veins on leg, etc.). These symptoms have increasingly been treated with medication; Riding and Munro[28] report that the antipsychotic drug, pimozide (Orap), is effective. However, more benign drugs are often helpful.[29]

The following is a case of a patient suffering from one manifestation of monosymptomatic hypochondriasis—the olfactory reference syndrome—who responded to a tricyclic antidepressant[25]:

Case 1

A 31-year-old homosexual man complained of an "anal odor" of 1 year's duration that had begun after his lover of 7 years left him to enter the seminary. The results of multiple medical evaluations, including a complete gastrointestinal workup, were normal. He left his job because of embarrassment, wore several pairs of underwear, showered at least three times a day, and checked his anal area for seepage several times a day. He had no other evidence of a thought disorder, and an electroencephalogram after sleep deprivation was normal. He also had no history of drug or alcohol abuse and no family history of depression and did not meet criteria for depression. He did, however, meet criteria for OCD on the basis of his rituals associated with the odor.

Trials of insight-oriented psychotherapy (for 28 months) and amitriptyline (150 mg/day for 8 weeks); alprazolam (0.5 mg three times a day for 3 weeks); haloperidol (5 mg twice a day for 2 weeks); and tranylcypromine (60 mg/day for 8 weeks) did not alleviate his symptoms, and he refused further medication. After 2 years of continued disability, he finally agreed to take imipramine, which was increased to 250 mg/day producing a blood level of 165 ng/ml (imipramine plus desipramine). After 3 weeks of treatment, symptoms were reduced, his ritualized behavior ceased, and he began seeing friends again. Improvement continued after 6 months of treatment with imipramine. He occasionally detected an anal odor when stressed, but it no longer affected his daily behavior.

The patient described here had a circumscribed fixed "delusion" in the context of a clear sensorium with otherwise logical and rational thought processes. Many such patients do not meet criteria for depression when they come for treatment, although they often do develop some neurovegetative signs after several months of symptoms. They experience a single hypochondriac delusion, which is distinct from the remainder of their personality. The "obsessions" occurred in a clear consciousness and were not secondary to depressive illness, schizophrenia, organic brain disorder, or histrionic personality disorder. Also, the symptoms fluctuated over time but never vanished spontaneously.

Munro and Chmara,[24] who reviewed the characteristics of this disorder in a series of 50 patients, noted that these patients often had previous personality and interpersonal difficulties and that a specific precipitating factor was reported in approximately one third of the patients. Although the delusions (obsessions) are encapsulated, the patients' distress is widespread and their lives are profoundly disrupted by their illness. Typically, these patients are rational in all other areas but are profoundly illogical with respect to the delusions and obsessions accompanying them.

Some authors have considered body dysmorphic disorder as an ominous symptom—even part of a schizophrenic prodrome. As mentioned earlier, many patients present initially to general physicians or plastic surgeons because of their conviction that their perceived disfigurements are real. Connolly and Gipson[27] followed 187 rhinoplasty patients for a mean of 15 years, none of whom were believed to be psychologically disturbed when first seen. Of the 187 patients, 86 received rhinoplasty for aesthetic reasons and 101 for deformity caused by injury or disease. At follow-up, of the 86 subjects who had the operation for aesthetic reasons alone, 32 (37%) were "severely neurotic" and six (7%) were diagnosed as schizophrenic. Of the 101 who had the operation because of deformity, nine (9%) were "severely neurotic" and only one (1%) was psychotic. These differences were highly significant. The authors concluded that many of those patients who had the operation for aesthetic reasons suffered from BDD, and these were the patients who later exhibited severe psychopathology.

GLOBUS HYSTERICUS (CHOKING PHOBIA)

Patients with the globus hystericus syndrome are obsessed with a fear that they are intermittently choking and unable to breathe. This is a frequently misdiagnosed syndrome. If untreated, these patients may become profoundly disabled or may develop life-threatening weight loss requiring aggressive medical care. The prevalence of this syndrome is poorly described in the literature, but our experience would indicate that its occurrence is not rare. These patients are difficult to treat, and a computerized literature search revealed little management information. Successful treatment of outpatients with behavior therapy was described in only one paper.[30] The following three cases respond to antidepressant medication[31]:

Case 1

A 66-year-old woman had been treated for anxiety over 4 years with occasional diazepam. Her father's recent death precipitated a depressive episode and a previously mild sensation of throat tightness had become so severe that she had difficulty eating and drinking for fear that she would choke; she was admitted to an inpatient psychiatric service. Her history was remarkable for panic attacks and somatization disorders dating back to 16 years of age. Her fear of choking, however, had occurred within the year prior to hospitalization. Her mood and symptoms of throat tightness improved over the next week when she was taking imipramine, 50 mg three times a day, and she was discharged after 3 weeks. After 6 months of feeling well, the imipramine was discontinued and her depression remained in remission, but the choking sensation worsened and again became so severe that she was constantly preoccupied. She was hospitalized and again begun on imipramine, which was gradually increased to 250 mg/day. Over the next 2 weeks, her symptoms gradually improved.

At 1-year follow-up on imipramine 250 mg/day, she remained markedly improved and was able to function adequately as a housewife.

Case 2

A 40-year-old woman was admitted to an inpatient psychiatric service with complaints of anorexia. She refused to eat because of a fear that she would not be able to breathe when swallowing food. Several months prior to admission, she had a panic attack when eating, which caused her to hyperventilate and fear that she might choke. Since then she had been unable to eat solids, with a resultant 26-pound weight loss (74 pounds on admission). She had a 20-year history of agoraphobia as well as fears about swallowing and choking. In the past, she had refused all medications except diazepam because she feared they would cause her mouth to become dry. She denied a family history of formal psychiatric illness, except for her father who was an alcoholic.

On admission to the psychiatric unit, she looked extremely cachectic with disheveled hair and clothes and complained of feeling hopeless and depressed. There was no evidence of psychosis. She had difficulty falling asleep, had early morning awakening, and suffered from loss of energy and inability to concentrate. She felt hungry but could not eat for fear of choking.

Physical examination was unremarkable except for cachexia and tachycardia and laboratory data revealed ketones in her urine. Because of the patient's degree of dehydration and continued inability to eat, a feeding tube was placed. On the sixth hospital day, she began a trial of phenelzine, which was gradually increased to 60 mg and then reduced to 45 mg/day because of signs and symptoms of orthostatic hypotension. After three days of phenelzine, she was noted to be taking foods by mouth and was less depressed. On the thirteenth hospital day, the feeding tube was removed and she ate at least 1500 calories/day with a resultant weight gain to 102 pounds over the following month. At 1-year follow-up, she remained on phenelzine, 15 mg three times daily, with no recurrence of her swallowing difficulties with a stable weight of approximately 100 pounds.

Case 3

A 78-year-old woman with moderately advanced Alzheimer's disease spontaneously developed the fear that she would choke if she tried to swallow and complained vigorously of episodic difficulty in breathing. She had no previous history of depression or a family history of psychiatric illness. Her son reported one episode many years earlier when the patient choked on a piece of meat but reported no subsequent fears of swallowing until the present. Her symptoms became so frightening to her that her son brought her into the emergency service where she underwent a complete physical and otolaryngologic examination, in which no abnormalities were found. Complete blood count and electrolytes were normal. Because of the extent of the woman's distress, she received radiologic evaluation, including cervical films and a barium swallow; again, no pathology was found.

Despite continued reassurance, her fears persisted. Refusing to eat, she lost 30 pounds over the next 2 months. When she began to have difficulty swallowing liquids and required constant supervision and reassurance, she was admitted to an inpatient psychiatric service. After failing to improve with the administration of neuroleptics and benzodiazepines, although the patient did not have any characteristics of a major depression, she was begun on a trial of tranylcypromine because of our previous success with antidepressants in patients with similar symptoms. Tranylcypromine was slowly increased to 30 mg/day and the patient became asymptomatic within 7 days, resumed eating, and was back to her normal weight within a month. After 4 weeks, she developed symptoms of orthostatic hypotension and medication was discontinued. She remained symptom-free and received no medication at 4-month follow-up.

Case 4

A 20-year-old hairdresser choked on a piece of meat and immediately developed a severe fear of choking. Although she was hungry, she refused to eat anything but soups, yogurt, and pudding, and thus, rapidly lost weight. By the time she came for treatment, she had not eaten any "dry" food for more than 2 weeks. She had a history of panic disorder and histrionic personality style. After four sessions of cognitive-behavioral therapy, which mainly focused on encouraging the patient to gradually eat more difficult (i.e., dry) food, she resumed eating normally. She was symptom-free at 3 months' follow-up.

There is controversy about the etiology and the appropriate diagnostic criteria for the globus hystericus syndrome. Clearly, the patients do not all meet

DSM-IV criteria for conversion disorder. The similarities to OCD are quite striking. Defined as a lump in the throat or the globus sensation without true dysphagia, globus hystericus is sometimes described as a manifestation of a physiologic disorder[32,33] or as a psychosomatic illness.[30,34] Lehtinen and Puhakka[35] defined two populations with globus hystericus: one group with abnormal esophageal physiology, the other without abnormal physical findings. In those patients without demonstrated physiologic abnormalities, psychiatric disturbances, particularly of an obsessive or hysterical personality style, were common. Additionally, depressive features were found in 11 of 20 patients studied.

As noted earlier, patients with related disorders such as monosymptomatic hypochondriasis[24] and body dysmorphic disorder[36-38] have been reported to respond to antidepressants. These reports, in fact, prompted the authors to begin antidepressant therapy in these patients. In Cases 1 and 2 in the previous paragraphs, an antidepressant trial was also indicated for clinical depression and the globus symptoms remitted with the depression. In Case 1, however, the globus sensation returned when the antidepressant was stopped, although the depressive symptoms remained in remission. In Case 3, depression was not clinically apparent, but again the symptoms remitted with antidepressant medication. In each of these patients, the primary reason for hospitalization was the presence of the globus symptoms. The psychologic basis of these symptoms and their relation to depression and OCD require further study.

All patients with severe manifestations of this syndrome should receive a thorough physical and otolaryngologic examination, as well as radiographic and psychiatric evaluation. Based on the cases presented here, when no somatic abnormalities are found, a trial of antidepressants (including MAOI) is recommended even in the absence of clinical depression.

BOWEL OBSESSIONS

Over the past decade we have seen many patients with a primary symptom of overwhelming fear of losing bowel control and having a bowel movement in public.[39] Many had become progressively more disabled by their fears, and all planned their lives around bowel movements. These patients spent more than 1 hour on the toilet, straining to get rid of every bit of feces before going out of the house, and located toilets wherever they went to be prepared for an "emergency." Most of these patients had almost total resolution of symptoms after tricyclic antidepressant therapy, although the majority did not meet criteria for major depression. A few representative case reports follow[39]:

Case 1

A 24-year-old executive spent up to 2 hours a day straining to have a bowel movement before going out and planned his whole life around going to the bathroom. He limited all his activities because he feared becoming incontinent. His symptoms were particularly prominent when he was anxious or in unfamiliar surroundings.

Although the patient had always been concerned about regular bowel movements, his disabling symptoms did not begin until he was 21 years of age. He denied having symptoms of depression, psychosis, panic attacks, or other psychopathology. His mother was fearful, occasionally depressed, and obsessive, and his sister often spent up to 1 hour clearing her bowels. A distant aunt with an unknown diagnosis died in a state hospital. The patient's father was an alcoholic.

Imipramine was prescribed and the dose was increased to 150 mg/day within a week; within 10 days, he had no obsessive fears about bowels, stopped bathroom rituals, started dating again, and reported feeling normal. Three months later, his symptoms returned when he decreased the dose to 50 mg/day, but these symptoms remitted when the dose was increased to 100 mg/day.

Case 2

A 56-year-old manager reported "increasing anxiety about my diarrhea." She noted severe anticipatory anxiety about diarrhea and persistently searched for bathrooms in case she could not control her bowels. She restricted her work activities and often called in ill if major meetings were planned. She spent $180 a month for parking because she feared becoming incontinent on the subway.

The patient's symptoms began without a precipitating event when she was approximately 50 years of age and gradually worsened. She denied having diarrhea and stated that her bowel movements were, in fact, quite normal. She denied having symptoms of depression, thought disorder, panic attacks, or other psychopathology but admitted to mild checking behaviors, particularly checking the stove and doors. Her family was without psychopathology, but her mother had similar bowel concerns and spent excessive time in the bathroom.

The patient began taking imipramine at a dose that was increased to 100 mg/day within 1 week. Within 1 month, she was symptom-free and had resumed her previous level of activity. She resisted attempts to taper her medication and continued to do well at 15-month follow-up.

Case 3

A 34-year-old executive had an overwhelming fear that he would not be able to get to a bathroom and would defecate in his pants. Whenever he became anxious, he felt the urge to defecate. On two occasions over the previous 15 years, he was slightly incontinent of feces.

The patient reported that his symptoms began in the seventh grade when he left school permanently because a teacher told him he could not go to the

bathroom and he feared that he might defecate in his pants. He denied performing compulsive rituals or having psychotic thoughts or depressive symptoms but
described himself as anxious and as occasionally having classic panic attacks.
One brother had milder bowel concerns. His sister and father were "nervous"
individuals, and his father died of alcohol-related difficulties.

Doxepin was prescribed and the dose was increased to 150 mg/day within 3
days. Within 2 weeks, his bowel obsessions had largely disappeared, and he discontinued his lengthy bathroom sessions and search for toilets. His panic attacks
ceased when his dose of doxepin was increased to 200 mg at bedtime. Because
of secondary agoraphobia and extreme shyness, he was referred for behavior
therapy, which consisted of assertiveness training and exposure. His symptoms
remained in remission at a 48-month follow-up; he completed high school equiv-
alency examinations and finished three years of college with an A– average.

Case 4

A 57-year-old mother who came to be evaluated for agoraphobia and anxiety
had first developed symptoms 20 years earlier when she felt an overwhelming urge to defecate when shopping. From then on, she feared losing bowel
control, particularly in stores. She was unable to leave home without going to
the bathroom first. She developed panic attacks a few years before coming to our
clinic and avoided situations in which these attacks might occur. She appeared
anxious but denied having depressive symptoms.

When her symptoms began, the patient had undergone a barium enema and
psychiatric evaluation and was told that it was all in her head. She had been treated unsuccessfully with Lomotil and chlordiazepoxide. She denied having any
prior psychiatric symptoms or family history of psychiatric disorder, except for
her 31-year-old daughter who suffered from agoraphobia with panic attacks.

She became free of agoraphobic, bowel-obsessive, and panic symptoms after
taking 50 to 75 mg at bedtime of imipramine for 2 weeks at blood levels of 126
and 169 μg/l, respectively. At the same time that she began taking imipramine,
she was also seen for behavior treatment, which consisted of relaxation, thought
stopping, cognitive restructuring, and *in vivo* exposure (i.e., taking increasingly
longer walks and entering stores either accompanied by the therapist or alone).
At the latest follow-up, she had been seen for 21 sessions of behavior therapy
and remained free of bowel obsessions.

As noted throughout this book, patients with OCD are commonly separated
into subgroups on the basis of symptom clusters. A number of features suggest
that the patients described previously may represent another distinct subgroup.
First, these patients have remarkably similar symptoms, including obsessive fear
of having a bowel movement in public and spending long periods in the bathroom trying to completely rid themselves of feces. In addition, most of the

patients spent considerable time searching for bathrooms in case of an "emergency." A second feature is the relative absence of other compulsive rituals or obsessive thoughts not related to bowel movements.

The patient in Case 2 experienced very mild checking behavior. A third feature in those patients that have been carefully studied is the presence of psychopathology in the family. Although each of these patients functioned at an extremely high level, most had relatives with severe psychiatric illnesses. In addition, the patients in Case 1 and Case 3 had siblings with bowel obsessions, and the patient in Case 2 had a mother who may have had a similar disorder.

After these case reports appeared in the psychiatric literature[39] and were picked up by the Associated Press, we had hundreds of calls and letters from patients who suffered from this syndrome; this response led us to believe that the disorder may be very prevalent. The most remarkable feature of this syndrome is its response to medication.

In some respects, this syndrome is similar to social phobia in that the individual fears that he or she may act out in a way that will be humiliating or embarrassing. The observation that these patients did not exhibit symptoms when at home with no plans to go out strengthens this similarity. Despite the considerable disability of such phobias, there are almost no data on pharmacologic treatment. A few double-blind studies found phenelzine beneficial in subjects with both agoraphobia and social phobia,[40–44] but none reported response among subjects with social phobia alone. Because agoraphobic patients have been shown to benefit from treatment with monoamine oxidase inhibitors (MAOIs), one cannot be sure that subjects with social phobia and without agoraphobia would benefit from MAOI therapy. Liebowitz, et al[44] reported that 11 patients meeting DSM-III criteria for social phobia showed at least moderate improvement with phenelzine.

Whatever the mechanism of pharmacologic response or the relationship to other psychopathology, it is clinically important that similar patients receive trials of antidepressants for this extremely disabling syndrome.

URINARY OBSESSIONS

Urinary obsessions may represent a similar, but less common, variant of the above syndrome. Epstein and Jenike[45] reported two patients who presented with debilitating fear of urinary incontinence and excessive preoccupation with their urinary tracts to such an extent that there was major interference with work and social functioning. Both patients had similar symptoms, which included: fear of urinary incontinence, urinary frequency without organic etiology, temporary relief of distress by bladder evacuation, and extreme efforts to be near a bathroom. Neither patient had other symptoms of OCD such as washing or checking rituals. Since bowel obsessions were responsive to antidepressant medication,[39] we gave imipramine to one patient who had almost complete resolution of symptoms. The other patient left treatment prior to such a trial.[45]

Case 1

A 25-year-old student reported 5 months of "feeling like I have to urinate every time I'm stressed." He feared that he would become incontinent when in classes, cars, or subways. After these bladder concerns began, he experienced bladder pressure, nausea, tachycardia, weakness, and sweaty palms, which were completely relieved by urination. Occurring seven to nine times daily, these symptoms were so debilitating that he quit school and avoided public transportation.

The patient's symptoms began at 24 years of age with a gradually increasing need to leave classes to urinate; he was never incontinent. Symptoms became so intense that he sought urologic consultation; examination, urine culture, and intravenous pyelogram were reportedly normal. He denied bedwetting as a child, substance abuse or caffeine use, medication use, and symptoms of depression or thought disorder. His family was without psychopathology.

Imipramine was prescribed and increased to 100 mg at bedtime over 2 weeks. Within 5 days of starting medication, tachycardia and sweatiness resolved, and within 6 weeks, urinary obsessions were largely relieved. At 6-month follow-up he did not mention urinary symptoms and wanted to reduce his medication. Two months later, he discontinued imipramine and remained symptom-free. He plans to take imipramine in the future should his symptoms recur.

Case 2

A 37-year-old clerk presented with concerns that he had to urinate an average of 10 times a day and at worst every half-hour. Although never incontinent, he persistently feared that he would lose urine in public. He planned his life around bathrooms to the extent that it interfered with work and social activities. When urinating, he spent at least 5 minutes straining to rid himself of every drop of urine.

The patient's symptoms began at 16 years of age and he received 1 year of psychotherapy but no further psychiatric treatment, despite persistent symptoms until 29 years of age when he was diagnosed as having compulsive and borderline personality disorders and again treated with psychotherapy and low doses of thioridazine. Because of increasing depressive symptoms and suicidal ideation, he was admitted to an inpatient psychiatric unit and treated with thiothixene and chlorpromazine. Over the subsequent 2 weeks, he became less preoccupied. On physical examination, he was noted to have a midsystolic click.

At the time of presentation to our clinic, at 36 years of age, the patient denied substance abuse; symptoms of depression, panic, and anxiety; and had no evidence of a thought disorder. He denied family psychopathology, except for his father who had engaged in some checking of doors and windows. He was given an 8-week trial of buspirone, up to 60 mg/day, without positive effect. Diazepam, 8 mg/day, relieved some anxiety, but urinary symptoms persisted. He was given a prescription for fluoxetine but stopped treatment prior to taking it.

The patient in Case 1 had marked alleviation of urinary symptoms with imipramine, whereas the Case 2 patient had no relief with buspirone and refused antidepressant medication. In a recent open trial, buspirone was ineffective for patients with typical OCD.[46]

In Case 1, the symptoms included autonomic features suggestive of panic disorder; his cognitions, however, were not typical of these patients, and autonomic symptoms occurred only subsequent to the predominant fear of incontinence. Both patients had symptoms that were characteristic of agoraphobia. The patient in Case 2 did not have a panic disorder, but was found to have a midsystolic click, which is often reported in this disorder.[47,48] Mellman and Uhde,[49] in evaluating panic disorder patients for the presence of OCD, highlighted the difficulty in distinguishing panic-phobic from obsessive-compulsive symptoms in some patients. However, our patients clearly presented with urinary obsessions as their most disabling symptom, and the Case 2 patient had no panic symptoms. Neither patient had evidence of a social phobia and both were able to urinate comfortably in public facilities.

When more than 300 psychiatrists were queried at a recent conference, more than 50% had treated at least one similar patient, often successfully with antidepressant medication. As with bowel obsessions, this disorder may not be rare.

These patients may constitute a small subgroup of OCD patients comparable with patients who wash, check, or only have obsessional thoughts. Urinary obsessions might be a manifestation of OCD, and these patients may respond to the same treatments. Antidepressant medications have been shown to be useful for a number of anxiety disorders,[50] including panic disorder or agoraphobia with panic attacks,[51] classical OCD,[51a] posttraumatic stress disorder,[52] and social phobia.[44] It is possible that urinary and bowel obsessions could be added to this list. We must first understand the underlying pathophysiology to determine whether or not these disorders are related in some fundamental way to OCD. Until definitive answers are available, when patients with urinary obsessions present to clinicians, antidepressant medications should be considered, even when clinical depression is not present.

COMPULSIVE WATER DRINKING

Compulsive water drinking, or psychogenic polydipsia, is characterized by excessive intake of water. According to some reports, most patients with this disorder have serious psychiatric disturbances, often requiring chronic institutionalization, and the majority are women.[52] One author,[53] however, reported that up to 80% are "neurotic, middle-aged females." The disorder has been diagnosed in patients as early as 3 years of age.[54,55]

Thirst represents a normal physiologic response to a true water deficit; in pathologic thirst, a patient is thirsty despite the fact that the body is well hydrated or even overhydrated. Medical etiologies of pathologic thirst include primary polydipsia caused by continued irritation of thirst neurons (e.g., trauma, inflammation, tumor), high plasma renin levels, and direct stimulation of the thirst centers by hypokalemia or hypercalcemia.

Barlow and de Wardener[56] wrote the classic paper on this disorder and outlined features such as hysteria, delusional hypochondriasis, and depression. The presenting complaints usually are increased thirst and polyuria and bizarre reasons are usually offered for such behavior;[52] for example, the water will wash away worms or poisons. Water intakes of as much as 43 liters/day have been recorded.[56]

Cronin[52] reported in his series that 7 of 11 patients justified their drinking behavior as an attempt to rid themselves of hiccups. His patients differed from earlier samples in that they were not institutionalized, and only three patients were diagnosed as schizophrenic. Ten of the patients had a history of alcoholism, although it was a current problem in only four patients.

There is very little information on the treatment of these patients. One group[55] recommended water restriction to stabilize metabolic abnormalities and subsequent treatment of any underlying psychologic disorder. Another group[57] describes the successful behavioral treatment of a mentally retarded autistic woman. Interventions included rewarding water refusal with edible reinforcements and reductions in activity demands, whereas water drinking was followed by activity demands.

In summary, there are little more than anecdotal case reports about patients with this apparently uncommon disorder. No reports have been identified that give psychologic profiles of these patients, and there is no evidence that they are likely to have other symptoms that are more typical of OCD. Reports of concomitant psychopathology are conflicting; it is said on one hand that the disorder appears almost always in psychotic patients and on the other that the majority of the patients are neurotic women. There is no helpful literature addressing the psychologic treatment of these patients, although a few good reviews address management of the metabolic and physiologic disturbances.[52,55]

EATING DISORDERS

Eating disorders can be viewed as a form of obsessive-compulsive behavior centered around a morbid preoccupation or obsession with food and thinness. Many of the patients with severe anorexia nervosa, however, who are admitted to our inpatient service manifest symptoms of frank OCD apart from eating habits. The majority of these patients spend much of their time in ritualistic behaviors such as handwashing, arranging and rearranging, and checking.

Common aspects of anorexia nervosa and what had been called obsessive-compulsive neurosis have been pointed out by Schultze.[58] In his view, patients with OCD and many patients with anorexia nervosa develop their illness on the background of a premorbid anancastic personality. In his view, the pre-illness personality, in combination with problems typically present in adolescence, leads to the onset of the anorexia nervosa syndrome. Other authors[59,60] did not, in fact, regard anorexia nervosa as a separate clinical entity but rather as a subtype of OCD; these authors, however, also emphasize the hypothesized importance of the premorbid anacastic personality and problems of adolescence in development of the syndrome. Several others have commented on the occurrence of obsessive-compulsive symptoms in patients with anorexia nervosa.[61–64] There is a report of identical female twins, one of whom developed OCD and the other anorexia nervosa, both at 13 years of age.[64] Baba[65] theorized that there are subgroups of anorexia nervosa with schizoid, infantile, hysterical, and obsessive-compulsive features.

Hecht, et al[64] compared clinical characteristics and psychologic data from nine female anorexia nervosa patients, who had obsessive-compulsive symptoms during the course of their illness, with similar data from 16 anorexic patients without obsessive-compulsive features. Those patients with obsessive-compulsive symptoms showed higher scores in general psychiatric symptoms and in anorexic behavior. Deficiencies in social adjustment were pronounced. As in our experience, the combination of marked obsessive-compulsive and anorexic behaviors seems to coincide with more severe disturbances and chronicity. The data from this study suggest that there is a strong relationship between anorexia nervosa and OCD. To our knowledge, there are no data on the differential effects of medication in those anorexic patients with and without obsessive-compulsive symptoms.

COMPULSIVE SELF-MUTILATION

Primeau and Fontaine[66] have reported that self-destructive behavior and OCD share some striking characteristics, and that the most frequently reported driving force behind self-mutilation is relief of tension[67,68] in a similar manner to the performance of a compulsive ritual. They presented the case reports of two patients who had OCD features with unusual self-destructive behavior as the principal way to relieve tension and they proposed that such patients may form a new subgroup of OCD.

Case 1

A 29-year-old machinist had a compulsion to push his eyes in. This compulsion led to major injuries in both eyes and he required several operations for complications such as detachment of the retina, thrombosis, and related conditions. He was constantly obsessed with his eyes and said that pushing his eyes in gave him a feeling of relief. After not responding to a number of antidepressants and benzodiazepines, he was treated with 200 mg/day of clomipramine and his behaviors decreased markedly within 6 weeks. He remained somewhat obsessed but had no rituals and no longer needed repetitive eye surgery. When he stopped taking clomipramine, the symptoms returned and amitriptyline did not relieve them. Restarting clomipramine again had the same beneficial effect.

Case 2

A 20-year-old single woman presented with trichotillomania, horrific temptations (e.g., she might hurt her mother), insomnia, and anxiety. She also responded to clomipramine when other medications had failed. It was unclear from the report how this patient was different from other patients with trichotillomania.

Case 3

Hollander and associates[69] reported a 44-year-old male patient, whose primary problem centered around compulsive urges to harm himself, accompanied by anxiety. He had a history of inserting various objects into his mouth and down his throat, and had strong urges to slam a door on his finger. Hypothesizing that he had OCD, they entered him into a trial, examining the effect of pharmacologic challenges designed to evaluate the clinical effect of serotonergic agonists and antagonists. Following a 2-week, drug-free period, the patient underwent randomized, double-blind pharmacologic challenges with 0.5% mg/kg of m-chlorophenylpiperzine (m-CPP) and placebo. M-CPP, a selective 5-HT (serotonin) agonist, had previously been shown to provoke exacerbation of obsessions and compulsions in OCD patients but not controls.[70,71] Following the placebo challenge, there was no change in obsessions or self-mutilation urges; however, following the oral m-CPP challenge, the patient developed a new and strong compulsion to kick a speaker that was hanging on the wall so that it would fall on his foot and cause him pain. This compulsion began at 60 minutes, peaked at 90 minutes, and subsided by 210 minutes following the challenge, closely paralleling the time course of the plasma m-CPP metabolite. As part of this trial, the patient received a 15-week trial of placebo medication and he was blindly rated as a nonresponder. He could not tolerate clomipramine because of anorgasmia and severe anticholinergic effects; the drug was discontinued after 10 weeks of a fairly low dose. Eight weeks following the start of an open trial of fluoxetine at 80 mg/day, he reported a considerable decrease in compulsive, self-damaging urges, such as the desire to put his finger in a door crack and this improvement continued for 8 months of follow-up treatment.

We must first understand the basic mechanisms of these disorders before making the determination of whether or not patients who perform such self-damaging acts suffer from the same pathophysiologic disorder as patients with typical OCD. Until then, it is clinically important to give such patients a trial of pharmacologic agents (see Chapter 22) in light of the often dramatic improvements reported by these authors.

SUMMARY

Disorders that may present with obsessive-compulsive symptoms include major depression, schizophrenia, Tourette's disorder, and organic mental disorders. In addition, many self-destructive habits have elements in common with OCD, including trichotillomania, drug abuse, alcoholism, some self-mutilation, and compulsive eating, sex, and gambling. These are generally not considered to fall under the category of OCD in DSM-IV terminology, and a number of these related disorders are classified as impulse control disorders—these include kleptomania (compulsive stealing), pathologic gambling, pyromania (compulsive fire setting), and trichotillomania (compulsive hair pulling). Compulsive shopping and severe nail biting may also fall into such a category.

Other syndromes have been described that are so similar to OCD that diagnostic overlap and confusion are common. These include monosymptomatic hypochondriasis, including body dysmorphic disorder and the olfactory reference syndrome; globus hystericus; and bowel and urinary obsessions. Many of these patients are referred to psychiatrists, and their symptoms may be remarkably responsive to antidepressant agents, even in the absence of signs of clinical depression. There are few controlled studies, but a trial of antidepressant-antiobsessional medication should be attempted in any patient presenting with these disorders. Behavior therapy also may play a role in the treatment of many of these disorders.

REFERENCES

1. American Psychiatric Association: *Diagnostic and statistical manual of mental disorders*, ed 4, Washington, 1994, American Psychiatric Association Press.
2. Gutpa MA, Gutpa AK, Haberman HF: The self-inflicted dermatoses: a critical review, *Gen Hosp Psychiatry* 9:45–52, 1987.
3. Stein DJ, Hutt CS, Spitz JL, et al: Compulsive skin picking and obsessive-compulsive disorder, *Psychosomatics* 34:177–181, 1993.
4. Van Moffaert M: Psychodermatology: an overview, *Psychother Psychosom* 58: 125–136, 1992.
5. O'Sullivan RL, Philips KA, Keuthen NJ, et al: Near fatal skin picking from delusional body dysmorphic disorder responsive to fluvoxamine. Manuscript submitted for publication, 1997.
6. Obermayer ME: *Psychocutaneous medicine*, Springfield, Ill, 1955, Charles C Thomas.
7. Griesemer RD, Nadelson T: Emotional aspects of cutaneous disease. In Fitzpatrick TB, Eisen AZ, Wolff K, et al, editors: *Dermatology in general medicine*, ed 2, New York, 1979, McGraw-Hill.
8. Freunsgaard K: Neurotic excretions: a controlled psychiatric examination, *Acta Psychiatr Scand* (suppl) 312:1–52, 1984.
9. Zaidens SH: Self-induced dermatoses, *Skin* 3:135, 1964.
10. Phillips KA, Taub SL: Skin picking as a symptom of body dysmorphic disorder, *Psychopharmacol Bull* 31(2):279–288, 1995.

11. Gutpa MA, Gutpa AK, Haberman HF: Neurotic excoriations: a review and some new perspectives, *Compr Psychiatry* 27:381–386, 1986.
12. Gutpa MA, Gutpa AK: Fluoxetine is an effective treatment for neurotic excoriations: case report, *Cutis* 51:386–387, 1993.
13. Stout RJ: Fluoxetine for the treatment of compulsive skin picking, *Am J Psychiatry* 147:370, 1990 (letter).
14. Hellings JA, Warnock JK: Self-injurious behavior and serotonin in Prader-Willi syndrome, *Psychopharmacol Bull* 30(2):245–250, 1994.
15. Warnock JK, Kestenbaum T: Pharmacologic treatment of severe skin-picking behaviors in Prader-Willi syndrome, *Arch Dermatol* 128:1623–1625, 1992.
16. Griesemer RD: Emotionally triggered disease in a dermatologic practice, *Psychiatr Ann* 8:407–412, 1978.
17. Fisher BK, Pearce KI: Neurotic excoriations: a personality evaluation, *Cutis* 14:251–254, 1974.
18. Seitz PFD: Dynamically oriented brief psychotherapy: psychocutaneous excoriation syndromes, *Psychosom Med* 15:200–213, 1953.
19. Pyles R: Therapeutic challenges in the treatment of pathological gambling, *The Psychiatric Times* 6:23–25, 1989.
20. Barlow ED, de Wardener HE: Compulsive water drinking, *Q J Med* 28:235–258, 1979.
21. Taber J, McCormick R, Russow A, et al: Follow-up of pathological gamblers after treatment, *Am J Psychiatry* 144:757–761, 1987.
22. Miller W: Individual outpatient treatment of pathological gambling, *J Gamb Behav* 2:108–120, 1986.
23. Bishop ER: Monosymptomatic hypochondriasis, *Psychosomatics* 21:731–747, 1980.
24. Munro A, Chmara J: Monosymptomatic hypochondriacal psychosis: a diagnostic checklist based on 50 cases of the disorder, *Can J Psychiatry* 27:374–376, 1982.
25. Brotman AW, Jenike MA: Monosymptomatic hypochondriasis treated with tricyclic antidepressants, *Am J Psychiatry* 141:1608–1609, 1984.
25a. Brotman AW, Jenike MA: Dysmorphophobia and monosymptomatic hypochondriasis, *Am J Psychiatry* 142:917–918, 1986.
26. Thomas CS: Dysmorphophobia and monosymptomatic hypochondriasis, *Am J Psychiatry* 142:1121, 1985.
27. Connolly FH, Gipson M: Dysmorphophobia—a long-term study, *Br J Psychiatry* 132:568–570, 1978.
28. Riding J, Munro A: Pimozide in the treatment of monosymptomatic hypochondriacal psychosis, *Acta Psychiatr Scand* 52:23–30, 1975.
29. Deleted in proofs.
30. Solyom L, Sookman D: Fear of choking and its treatment, *Can J Psychiatry* 25:30–34, 1980.
31. Brown SR, Schwartz JM, Summergrad P, et al: Globus hystericus syndrome responsive to antidepressants, *Am J Psychiatry* 143:917–918, 1986.
32. Flores TC, Cross FS, Jones RD: Abnormal esophageal manometry in globus hystericus, *Ann Otol Rhinol Laryngol* 90:383–386, 1981.
33. Ardran GM: Feeling of a lump in the throat: thoughts of a radiologist, *J R Soc Med* 75:242–244, 1982.

34. Barber HO: Psychosomatic disorders of ear, nose, and throat, *Postgrad Med* 5:156–159, 1970.
35. Lehtinen V, Puhakka H: A psychosomatic approach to the globus hystericus syndrome, *Acta Psychiatr Scand* 53:21–28, 1976.
36. Jenike MA: Dysmorphophobia, *Br J Psychiatry* 3:326, 1985.
37. Jenike MA: A case report of successful treatment of dysmorphophobia with tranylcypromine, *Am J Psychiatry* 141:1463–1464, 1984.
38. Phillips KA: *The broken mirror*, New York, 1996, Oxford University Press.
39. Jenike MA, Vitagliano HL, Rabinowitz J, et al: Bowel obsessions responsive to tricyclic antidepressants in four patients, *Am J Psychiatry* 144:1347–1348, 1987.
40. Tyrer P, Candy J, Kelly D: A study of the clinical effects of phenelzine and placebo in the treatment of phobic anxiety, *Psychopharmacologia* 32:237–254, 1973.
41. Solyom L, Heseltine GFD, McClure DJ, et al: Behavior therapy vs drug therapy in the treatment of phobic neurosis, *Can Psychiatr Assoc J* 18:25–31, 1973.
42. Solyom C, Solyom L, LaPierre Y, et al: Phenelzine and exposure in the treatment of phobias, *Biol Psychiatry* 16:239–247, 1981.
43. Mountjoy CO, Roth M, Garside RF, et al: A clinical trial of phenelzine in anxiety depressive and phobic neuroses, *Br J Psychiatry* 131:486–492, 1977.
44. Liebowitz MR, Fyer AJ, Gorman JM, et al: Phenelzine in social phobia, *J Clin Psychopharmacol* 6:93–98, 1986.
45. Epstein S, Jenike MA: Disabling urinary obsessions: an uncommon variant of obsessive-compulsive disorder, *Psychosomatics* 31:450–452, 1990.
46. Jenike MA, Baer L: Buspirone in obsessive-compulsive disorder: an open trial, *Am J Psychiatry* 145:1285–1286, 1988.
47. Dager SR, Comess KA, Dunner DL: Differentiation of anxious patients by two dimensional echocardiographic evaluation of the mitral valve, *Am J Psychiatry* 1143:533–536, 1986.
48. Liberthson R, Sheehan DV, King ME, et al: The prevalence of mitral valve prolapse in patients with panic disorder, *Am J Psychiatry* 143:511–515, 1986.
49. Mellman TA, Uhde TW: Obsessive-compulsive symptoms in panic disorder, *Am J Psychiatry* 144:1573–1576, 1987.
50. Liebowitz MR: The efficacy of antidepressants in DSM-III anxiety disorders. In Grinspoon L, editor: *Psychiatry update: The American Psychiatric Association annual review*, vol 3, Washington, 1984, American Psychiatric Press.
51. Golger S, Grunhaus L, Birmacher B, et al: Treatment of spontaneous panic attacks with clomipramine, *Am J Psychiatry* 138:1215–1217, 1981.
51a. Jenike MA: Health care reform for Americans with severe mental illnesses: Report of the National Advisory Mental Health Council: Obsessive-compulsive disorder: Efficacy of specific treatments as assessed by controlled trials, *Psychopharmacol Bull* 29:487–499, 1993.
52. Cronin RE: Psychogenic polydipsia with hyponatremia: report of eleven cases, *Am J Kidney Dis* 11:410–426, 1987.
52. Hogben GL, Cornfield RB: Treatment of traumatic war neurosis with phenelzine, *Arch Gen Psychiatry* 38:440–445, 1981.
53. Chinn TA: Compulsive water drinking, *J Nerv Ment Dis* 158:78, 1974.
54. Kohn B, Normal ME, Feldman H, et al: Hysterical polydipsia (compulsive water drinking) in children, *Am J Dis Child* 130:210, 1976.

55. Walls LL, Supinski CR, Cotton WK, et al: Compulsive water drinking: a review with report on an additional case, *J Fam Pract* 5:531–533, 1977.
56. Hariprasad MK, Eisinger RP, Nadler IM: Hyponatremia in psychogenic polydipsia, *Arch Intern Med* 140:1639–1642, 1980.
57. McNally RJ, Calamari JE, Hansen PM, Kaliher C: Behavioral treatment of psychogenic polydipsia, *J Behav Ther Exp Psychiatry* 19:57–61, 1988.
58. Schultze G: *Anorexia nervosa,* Bern, 1980, Huber Verlag.
59. DuBois F: Compulsion neurosis with cachexia, *Am J Psychiatry* 106:107, 1949.
60. Palmer HD, Jones MS: Anorexia nervosa as a manifestation of compulsion neurosis: a study of psychogenic factors, *Arch Neurol Psychiatry* 41:856, 1939.
61. Rahman L, Richardson HB, Ripley HS: Anorexia nervosa with psychiatric observations, *Psychosom Med* 1:3, 1939.
62. Cantwell D, Sturzenberger S, Borroughs J, et al: Anorexia nervosa: an affective disorder? *Arch Gen Psychiatry* 34:1087–1093, 1977.
63. Dally P: *Anorexia nervosa,* London, 1969, William Heinemann.
64. Hecht AM, Fichter M, Postpischil P: Obsessive-compulsive neurosis and anorexia nervosa, *Int J Eating Dis* 2:69–77, 1983.
65. Baba K: Anorexia nervosa: A einige Beobachtungen zur Psychogenese und Psychotherapie, *J Psychosom Med Psychoanal* 22:267–277, 1976.
66. Primeau F, Fontaine R: Obsessive disorder with self-mutilation: a subgroup responsive to pharmacotherapy, *Can J Psychiatry* 32:699–700, 1987.
67. Gardner AR, Gardner AJ: Self-mutilation: obsessionality and narcissism, *Br J Psychiatry* 127:127–132, 1975.
68. Carroll J, Schaffer C, et al: Family experiences of self-mutilating patients, *Am J Psychiatry* 137:852–853, 1980.
69. Hollander E, Papp L, Campeas R, et al: More on self mutilation and obsessive compulsive disorder, *Can J Psychiatry* 33:675, 1988.
70. Hollander E, Fay M, Cohen B, et al: Serotonergic and noradrenergic function in obsessive compulsive disorder, *Am J Psychiatry* 145:1015–1017, 1988.
71. Zohar J, Mueller I, Insel TR, et al: Serotonergic responsivity in obsessive compulsive disorder: comparison of patients and healthy controls, *Arch Gen Psychiatry* 44:946–951, 1987.

8

Tourette's Disorder and Obsessive-Compulsive Disorder: Clinical Similarities and Differences

Barbara J. Coffey, M.D., Janice Jones, B.A., Stephanie Shapiro, B.A.

Tourette's disorder (TD), formerly known as Tourette's syndrome, is a childhood-onset neuropsychiatric disorder characterized by multiple motor and vocal tics. It was originally described by a French physician, Jean Marie Itard, in 1825 and named for Gilles de la Tourette who wrote the first clinical paper on tic disorders in 1885.[1] The early twentieth century view of TD was characterized by single case reports and psychoanalytic theory about the etiology of the disorder—then seen as an expression of unconscious sexual and aggressive conflict. Frau Emmy Von N. in Freud's *Case Studies of Hysteria*, with facial tics and nervousness, most likely had Tourette's disorder, although this was not diagnosed.[2]

Beginning in the 1960s, the work of Drs. Arthur and Elaine Shapiro brought scientific methodology to the understanding of TD. Haloperidol and other neuroleptics then became the cornerstone of treatment over the next decades.

The phenomenologic orientation of the *Diagnostic and Statistical Manual of Mental Disorders* (DSM-III)[3] and DSM-III-R[4] resulted in systematic description and classification of tic disorders, including TD.[5] The past decade has brought scientific advances in the understanding of the etiology, genetics, epidemiology, and clinical phenomenology and relationship between TD and obsessive-compulsive disorder (OCD). Treatment studies now have been conducted on a variety of alternatives to traditional neuroleptics including α-adrenergic agonists, tricyclic antidepressants, stimulants, benzodiazepines, and the newer atypical neuroleptics.[6-16]

Clinical literature has documented an overlap between TD and OCD: OCD is overrepresented in TD patients and TD is overrepresented in OCD patients.

For example, a recent study of 134 TD patients found that 23% met full criteria for OCD and 46% met criteria for the subthreshold form.[17] Conversely, lifetime occurrence of tics in patients with OCD has been reported to be approximately 7% to 20% in children.[18]

Studies examining clinical correlates of TD and OCD also have documented that both disorders share many characteristics.[19,20] Specifically, both disorders have a juvenile or young-adult onset; a chronic waxing and waning course; a familial occurrence; involuntary, intrusive repetitive behaviors; aggressive, sexual, or scatologic themes in the content of thoughts and behaviors; exacerbation of symptoms by stress or anxiety; and overlapping neuroanatomic sites of dysfunction in the basal ganglia and related structures such as the cortico-striatothalamocortical tracts and frontal lobes.[21–23]

This chapter reviews the relationship and overlap between TD and OCD, including classification, clinical phenomenology, epidemiology, etiology, clinical assessment, and treatment.

CLASSIFICATION

Tics are sudden, repetitive, "involuntary," stereotyped movements or vocalizations involving one or a group of muscles. Most patients can voluntarily suppress their tics for limited periods of time. Tics can be characterized by their anatomic location, number, frequency, duration, and complexity.[24] Simple motor tics (involving a single muscle) include eye blinking, nose twitching, and shoulder shrugging; complex motor tics (involving multiple muscle groups and considered more "purposeful") include touching objects or self, squatting, and jumping. Simple vocal tics (single sounds) include throat clearing, coughing, and sniffing/grunting; complex vocal tics include syllables, words, or phrases such as echolalia (repeating others' words), palilalia (repeating own words), and coprolalia (swearing).

Tic disorders can be classified as transient (lasting at least 4 weeks, but less than 12 months) or chronic (either motor or vocal tics or both, lasting more than 1 year). As many as 15% of all children may develop transient tics during childhood; chronic tics are less common and frequently coexist with other psychiatric disorders. The boundary between complex motor tics and compulsions is not always clear, because both involve repetitive behaviors performed in a stereotyped manner. Table 8-1 lists DSM-IV classification criteria for tic disorders.[25]

TOURETTE'S DISORDER AND OBSESSIVE-COMPULSIVE DISORDER: CLINICAL RELATIONSHIP
Clinical Course

The clinical course of TD usually includes onset of eye blinking, facial, or head/neck tics at approximately 6 or 7 years of age, followed by a rostral-caudal progression of motor tics over several years; vocal tics typically begin at 8 or

Table 8-1   Tic Disorder Classification

Transient Tic Disorder

A. Single or multiple motor and/or vocal tics (i.e., sudden, rapid, recurrent, nonrhythmic, stereotyped motor movements or vocalizations).
B. The tics occur many times a day, nearly every day for at least 4 weeks, for no longer than 12 consecutive months.
C. The disturbance causes marked distress or significant impairment in social, occupational, or other important areas of functioning.
D. The onset is before 18 years of age.
E. The disturbance is not the result of direct physiologic effects of a substance (i.e., stimulants) or a general medical condition (e.g., Huntington's disease or postviral encephalitis).
F. Criteria have never been met for Tourette's, chronic motor, or vocal tic disorder.

Chronic Motor or Vocal Tic Disorder

A. Single or multiple motor or vocal tics (i.e., sudden, rapid, recurrent, nonrhythmic stereotyped motor movements or vocalizations), but not both, present at some time during the illness.
B. The tics occur many times a day, nearly every day, or intermittently throughout a period of more than 1 year, and during this period there was never a tic-free period of more than 3 consecutive months.
C. The disturbance causes marked distress or significant impairment in social, occupational, or other important areas of functioning.
D. The onset is before 18 years of age.
E. The disturbance is not the result of direct physiologic effects of a substance (i.e., stimulants) or a general medical condition (e.g., Huntington's disease or postviral encephalitis).
F. Criteria have never been met for Tourette's disorder.

Tourette's Disorder

A. Both multiple motor and one or more vocal tics have been present at some time during the illness, although not necessarily concurrently.
B. The tics occur many times a day (usually in bouts), nearly every day or intermittently throughout a period of more than 1 year, and during this period there was never a tic-free period of more than 3 consecutive months.
C. The disturbance causes marked distress or significant impairment in social, occupational, or other important areas of functioning.
D. The onset is before 18 years of age.
E. The disturbance is not the result of direct physiologic effects of a substance (i.e., stimulants) or a general medical condition (e.g., Huntington's disease or postviral encephalitis).

9 years of age and obsessive-compulsive symptoms and complex tics later at 11 or 12 years of age. As many as 50% of patients may present initially with signs of motoric hyperactivity and inattention in early childhood prior to the onset of tics.[26]

Tics and obsessive-compulsive symptoms typically persist for a lifetime. Tics tend to stabilize over time, and some patients report lengthy periods in which symptoms diminish or remit altogether. Some investigators report complete remission of tics in as many as 8% of patients.[27]

Chronic motor or vocal tic disorder is probably related to TD and tends to follow a similar clinical course. Unfortunately, to date, no systematic, long-term, prospective cohort studies have been performed in these populations. Most of the studies described as follow-up of tic and Tourette's disorder are actually retrospective, follow-back, clinical-treatment studies, so that reliable information on the long-term course is lacking.[13,27–33]

Epidemiology

Estimates of the prevalence of TD vary. Studies have found TD rates in non-referred populations between 2.87 of 10,000[34] and 9.3 to 10 of 10,000.[35] The best current estimate is approximately 4 of 10,000 for the full syndrome; if chronic motor tics are added, the prevalence increases to 1 in 200.[36] Recently, Apter, et al[37] conducted a population-based, epidemiologic study of lifetime prevalence of TD in Israel involving 28,037 16- and 17-year-old armed service recruits and found a point prevalence of 4.3 of 10,000.

Psychiatric Comorbidity

Most patients with TD also have nontic psychiatric symptoms, including obsessions, compulsions, attentional dysfunction, learning problems, impulsivity, and affective disturbance.[38–43] The nature of these symptoms and their relationship to TD is not well understood. For example, it is not known whether these symptoms represent biologic heterogeneity in a spectrum of Tourette's-related disorders, whether they are genetically related or secondary reactions to having TD.[44]

The association between TD and OCD is discussed in more detail in the next section. Other associated problems include attention deficit hyperactivity disorder (ADHD); anxiety disorders (non–OCD); mood disorders; and primary and secondary behavior problems, such as failure to inhibit aggressive or self-injurious behaviors.[44]

Significant attentional problems (e.g., distractibility, restlessness, and poor concentration), with or without hyperactivity, occur in approximately 50% of patients with TD.[45,46] When ADHD is present, it may either precede the onset of motor and vocal tics by several years or occur after the tics have begun.[26,42]

Patients with TD score higher than normal controls on measures of psychopathology, such as depression.[43] Although this may be the result of the effects of having a chronic stigmatizing illness, a possible genetic vulnerability in a subgroup of patients with TD must be considered. Medication effects on a patient's mood also have to be assessed, because the commonly prescribed neuroleptics have been reported to produce dysphoria in some patients.[43]

Non–OCD anxiety disorders may be more frequent in TD patients than in the general population. Some authors have reported an increased incidence of panic disorders and phobias in TD patients when compared with normal controls.[39]

We have found that of the first 100 children and adolescents with TD evaluated in our specialty clinic, 76% met DSM-III-R criteria for lifetime history of any mood disorder, 25% met full criteria for OCD, 52% met criteria for subthreshold OCD, and 64% met criteria for any non–OCD anxiety disorder (Table 8-1).

Failure to inhibit aggressive behavior is frequently described in TD. This may be expressed in numerous ways (e.g., throwing or destroying objects, hitting, biting, scratching, or kicking). This is an especially disabling problem for adult TD patients, because it often results in secondary difficulties, such as social isolation and depression.[47]

Clinical Phenomenology

Studies of TD patients have reported obsessive-compulsive symptoms and OCD in 20% to 60% of patients,[37,48–52] and studies of OCD patients have described motor tics in more than 50% and TD in 15%.[50–52]

Bliss,[53] describing his 35 years of self-observation of TD, was the first to emphasize the importance of distinct and discrete focal sensations preceding tics. Shapiro, et al[24] used the term "sensory tics" to describe these sensations. In 1993, the Tourette Syndrome Classification Study Group defined sensory tics as focal, localized, or general uncomfortable sensations relieved by movement of the affected body region.[54] Recently, several studies have reported a high frequency of sensory phenomena immediately preceding tics.[55–57] The relationship between these sensory phenomena and tics in TD may be analogous to the relationship between obsessions and compulsions in OCD.

Despite clinical similarities, obsessive-compulsive symptoms seem to present a distinct phenomenology when patients with OCD without tics are compared with patients who have both OCD and TD. For example, checking, ordering, arranging, tapping, rubbing, blinking, compulsive touching, and searching for symmetry seem to be more common in TD patients than in OCD patients; in contrast, behaviors concerning contamination are more frequent in OCD patients.[50,58] Obsessive-compulsive disorder patients with tics have more ticlike compulsions (e.g., touching, tapping, rubbing, blinking, and staring) than OCD patients without tics.[59] Finally, patients who have OCD without tics are more likely to have cognitions preceding compulsions than patients with both TD and OCD.[60]

To clarify some of the phenomenologic differences observed in the spectrum of compulsions and complex motor tics observed in these two disorders, our group recently studied intentional repetitive behaviors (i.e., behaviors always performed intentionally and in a stereotyped manner) in patients with TD without OCD and patients with OCD without tics. Results indicated that intentional repetitive behaviors in OCD and TD are differentially associated with cognitive and autonomic phenomena. Sensory phenomena (generalized and localized uncontrollable sensations) preceded intentional repetitive behaviors in TD but not in OCD patients, and cognitive phenomena (ideas, thoughts, images) and physiologic symptoms of anxiety preceded such behaviors in OCD but not in TD.[61] We speculated that the dimensions examined in this study (cognition, sensory phenomena, and autonomic anxiety) may represent valid clinical indices for characterization of complex, stereotyped repetitive behaviors in OCD and TD.

ETIOLOGY AND NEUROBIOLOGY OF TOURETTE'S DISORDER
Genetics

There is growing scientific evidence of an association between TD and OCD. Family studies have indicated that at least some forms of OCD may represent a variant expression of TD.[62] Genetic data have accumulated through family pedigree and twin studies. Tourette's disorder, chronic motor tic disorders, and OCD show a familial concentration. For example, twin studies have found 53% concordance for monozygotic (MZ) twin pairs versus 8% concordance with dizygotic (DZ) twin pairs of patients with TD. When chronic motor tic disorders were also included, concordance increased to 77% for MZ and 23% for DZ pairs.[63]

Family pedigree studies by Pauls, et al[63] have shown that first-degree relatives of TD patients have a higher prevalence of TD (10%), chronic motor tics (18%), and OCD (30%) than controls, and segregation analyses indicate an autosomal dominant inheritance pattern with incomplete penetrance. Among those with the putative gene, men are likely to show 99% penetrance and women approximately 70%.

Nongenetic factors may also contribute to TD; for example, men may be at higher risk because of prenatal exposure to androgenic hormones.[64] Similarly, birth weight may contribute. Hyde, et al[65] studied 16 MZ twin pairs and found that concordance for TD was 54%, and for all tic disorders the concordance was 94%. Thirteen of the 16 pairs had differing birth weights; in 12 of the 13 pairs, the twin with the lower birth weight had a higher tic severity score.

Nongenetic theories of the etiology of tics also have been tested. Allen, et al[66] and Kiessling, et al[67] described a subgroup of children with movement disorders and obsessive-compulsive symptoms with a history of group A β-hemolytic streptococcal infection who developed antineuronal antibodies in their sera following infection.

Neurobiologic Models of Obsessive-Compulsive Disorder and Tourette's Disorder

The etiology and pathophysiology of TD and related disorders such as OCD are unknown. Studies of the neuroanatomy and neurochemistry of TD conducted in the past decade point to a diffuse process in the brain involving multiple pathways in the basal ganglia and frontal lobes.[68] Several neurotransmitters and neuromodulators have been implicated, including dopamine, serotonin, and endogenous opioids. Although a specific animal model has not been identified, promising candidates include dogs with acral lick dermatitis and horses with crib biting.[69,70]

Proposed neurobiologic models have been based on a comparison between TD and OCD. In 1990, Baxter, et al proposed a model incorporating previous theories of TD and OCD centered around the concept of multiple parallel segregated corticostriatal circuits in the basal ganglia.[23,71] Baxter's group suggested that the range of symptoms across the OCD-TD spectrum could be explained by the distribution of dysfunction within the striatum. A recent study in monozygotic twins concordant for Tourette's disorder but discordant for severity demonstrated abnormalities in D2 receptors in the caudate area in the more severely afflicted twin.[72]

Neuroimaging studies of the pathophysiology of TD have yielded data consistent with a role for corticostriatal circuits, including sensorimotor cortex and the putamen, as well as ventral striatum.[73,74] Recently, morphometric studies have suggested that the striatum may lack normal asymmetry in TD.[73–76] A dopaminergic theory of TD is supported by four lines of research: (1) the apparent efficacy of dopaminergic antagonists in the treatment of tics;[77–79] (2) the exacerbating effects of functional dopamine agonists such as amphetamines;[80–82] (3) postmortem findings of increased dopamine presynaptic carrier sites in the striatum of TD subjects;[83] and (4) PET data suggesting an increased Bmax for D2 receptors in the striatum of subjects with TD.[84]

Although it is unlikely that dysregulation of a single neurotransmitter system mediates the full scope of either OCD or TD,[68,83,85–87] current neurochemical models of OCD have largely been limited to hypotheses regarding dysfunctional serotonergic transmission (derived from the observed antiobsessional efficacy of serotonergic reuptake inhibitors in OCD).[85] Despite a great deal of literature on probes of serotonergic function in OCD subjects, both pretreatment and posttreatment, as well as compared with non–OCD controls, there is little evidence to support a strictly serotonergic theory of OCD. Some patients with TD also respond positively to serotonergic agents.[14,88–90] Because some patients with OCD respond to dopamine antagonists such as neuroleptics, investigators also have sought evidence for dopaminergic dysfunction in OCD, but without impressive results.[91,92]

Neuropsychology of Tourette's Disorder and Obsessive-Compulsive Disorder

Neuropsychologic studies of TD have used standardized instruments from clinical neuropsychology to identify general domains of cognitive dysfunction. These studies have found preserved intellectual, memory, and language functions in TD subjects.[93–97] Impairment has been reported in motor speed, and coordination and tactile sensory perceptual functions.[95–97] Mild, nonspecific deficits in executive functioning also have been documented, primarily with the Category Test.[95–97] Recent evidence suggests that the findings of such "cognitive deficits" in TD may not be the result of TD per se, but rather may be related to the comorbid problems such as ADHD.[98]

In general, cognitive abnormalities have been reported more frequently in OCD patients than in those with TD. For example, studies of OCD have reported impairment of selected visuospatial, executive, and visual memory functions in the presence of normal language, motor, and intellectual abilities.[99–105] Executive functions have been studied primarily with the Wisconsin Card Sort Test[106] and several studies have identified increased perseverative responses among some OCD subjects (interpreted as difficulty in shifting mental set).[101,102,107] Regarding memory in OCD, there is consistent evidence of abnormal encoding and immediate memory for visual and spatial stimuli.[99]

Thus, there is at least preliminary evidence that patients with OCD are more "cognitively" impaired, whereas those with TD are more impaired on tactile and motor functions. Tourette's disorder studies have been conducted, however, primarily on children and OCD studies mainly on adults.

EVALUATION

The diagnosis of TD is made on clinical grounds based on the characteristic history of multiple tics beginning in early childhood. A detailed history with documentation from multiple sources is the cornerstone of clinical evaluation of tic disorders, because patients often suppress tics during office examinations. Family history of related problems such as tics, TD, and OCD should be obtained.

Psychiatric evaluation should include a systematic assessment of the behavioral and emotional problems that are known to be associated with TD, including (1) obsessive-compulsive symptoms; (2) attentional dysfunction; (3) hyperactivity; (4) learning problems; (5) anxiety; and (6) affective dysfunction (including aggressivity). The use of structured or semistructured interviews, such as the children's version of the Schedule for Affective Disorders and Schizophrenia (Kiddie-SADS)[108] and the Diagnostic Interview Schedule for Children (DISC),[109] can improve classification and comorbidity assessment.[110] Videotaped standardized interviews may be used to quantify frequency, severity, and complexity of symptoms.

Standardized global rating scales developed specifically for TD, such as the Yale Global Tic Severity Scale (YGTSS),[111] can be useful in the clinic and in research settings. This scale rates tics, compulsions, and other associated features. Specific rating scales for OCD (Yale-Brown Obsessive Compulsive Scale[112,113]) and ADHD (Conners Checklist[114–116]) also can be used to assess severity of these symptoms.

Auxiliary data from outside sources such as pediatric, medical, and educational records are often extremely useful.

TREATMENT

General Principles

Treatment should be individualized to best achieve the goals of (1) maximal symptom control; (2) support of adaptive functioning and strengths; and (3) promotion of optimal developmental progress.

Education about the phenomenology, course, and treatment options for tics and OCD is essential. Referrals to the National Tourette's Syndrome Association (TSA) and to local chapters of the TSA* can provide ongoing support and a source of advocacy for families.

The decision to treat tics should be based on a thorough appraisal of benefits and risks after a comprehensive evaluation. Patients with mild symptoms usually require only monitoring, education, guidance, and support. Patients with moderate to severe symptoms are candidates for more aggressive management. Patients who have symptoms that significantly interfere with optimal adaptation or who are greatly distressed by mild symptoms should be treated.

Pharmacotherapy is the cornerstone of treatment for TD. Generally, patients should be started on the lowest possible dose of medication with gradual increases over several weeks. It is best initially to use monotherapy, but typically combinations of medications (targeted combined pharmacotherapy) are necessary, particularly in the presence of other disorders, such as OCD or ADHD.

Determining what constitutes an adequate trial in tic patients is challenging, because the symptoms naturally wax and wane. It is generally best to wait several weeks after changing a dose to evaluate the response. External stressors must be taken into account as potential causes of increased symptoms at any one time point.

Pharmacotherapy

Neuroleptics

Neuroleptics are the only medications formally approved (for advertising) for the treatment of tic disorders. The neuroleptics, including haloperidol (Haldol) and pimozide (Orap), reduce tics by blocking D2 receptors in the basal ganglia. Both agents are effective and relatively safe; however, long-term risk for tardive dyskinesia and other extrapyramidal side effects must be weighed against potential efficacy for tics.[117] Patients who refuse neuroleptic treatment because of concern about risks should try other nonneuroleptic treatment.

Pimozide may cause fewer side effects than haloperidol. However, because it can produce quinidine-like cardiac effects, including prolongation of the QTc interval, normal cardiac function and baseline cardiac assessment and electrocardiogram (ECG) are prerequisites. Children or adults with preexisting

---

* 42-40 Bell Boulevard, Bayside, NY, 11361, (212) 224-2480

arrhythmias and/or prolonged QTc intervals and adults with a history of ischemic disease may require cardiology consultation before use of this drug.[118]

Of the other neuroleptics used to treat tic disorders, fluphenazine (Prolixin) has received the most attention. Potentially, however, any higher-potency neuroleptic could be effective.[119] A newer, atypical neuroleptic called risperidone (Risperdal) has been found to reduce tics and may carry less risk for the development of tardive dyskinesia than the typical neuroleptics.[7,120]

The most common side effects of neuroleptics include extrapyramidal and anticholinergic symptoms, weight gain, sedation, and dysphoria syndromes. Although the neuroleptics are reasonably effective in the treatment of moderate to severe tic disorders, they have the potential to cause serious sequelae in the form of tardive dyskinesia. Neuroleptics are not specifically indicated when comorbid conditions, such as OCD or ADHD, are the primary target of psychopharmacologic intervention instead of tics. Some studies have reported effective use of neuroleptics to augment selective serotonin reuptake inhibitors (SRIs) in OCD patients with tics.[121]

Clonidine

Clonidine (Catapres), an α-2 presynaptic norepinephrine agonist, has been used for over a decade in the treatment of TD. This medication is believed to act by reducing presynaptic norepinephrine. Clonidine also ameliorates the disinhibition, impulsivity, hyperarousal, and motoric overactivity that can be seen in TD patients,[12] and may attenuate anxiety. Common side effects include sedation, headaches and stomachaches, and occasionally dysphoria, particularly in younger children. Sedation, which is most common, may be mitigated by initiating therapy at low doses and gradually increasing the dose over time. Although the risk of hypotension is minimal, blood pressure should be monitored.[122] Guanfacine, a newer α-2 adrenergic agonist, may also reduce motoric hyperactivity, inattention, and tics.[8]

Tricyclic Antidepressants

Patients with comorbid ADHD may be candidates for treatment with a tricyclic antidepressant, such as desipramine or nortriptyline. Recent studies also indicate potential therapeutic effects on tics.[16,123] Anticholinergic side effects, such as dry mouth and constipation, usually diminish over time; potential cardiotoxicity necessitates normal baseline cardiac function and ECG monitoring.[124] Although there have been several reports of sudden death of children treated with desipramine, the number of sudden deaths did not increase from 1986 to 1992, despite a marked increase in exposure.[125] With an estimated 2.1 to 3.1 relative risk for sudden death in 5- to 14-year-old children, careful assessment of the risk-to-benefit ratio is indicated. Nevertheless, this association has occurred in the context of the safe and effective treatment of thousands of children with this medication.

Serotonin Reuptake Inhibitors

Serotonergic drugs, such as clomipramine (Anafranil) and fluoxetine (Prozac), are options for some target symptoms in TD; because many patients with TD also have obsessions and compulsions, and neuroleptics and clonidine do not usually control these symptoms, specific antiobsessional agents may be useful in their treatment. Indeed, complex motor tics such as squatting and touching are often difficult to differentiate from compulsions and may be more responsive to a serotonergic medication than a dopamine blocker.

In general, serotonergic agents should be used in TD only if obsessions and compulsions are moderate to severe or are impairing adaptive functioning. Recent studies indicate both positive (ameliorating) and negative (exacerbating) effects of these agents on tics in patients with comorbid OCD and tic disorders.[88,89,126,127]

Clomipramine has been investigated in OCD and fluoxetine has been investigated in TD. Fluoxetine has been found to be useful for obsessive-compulsive symptoms in TD and may decrease such symptoms in at least 50% of patients.[14,89] Efficacy of these two drugs for OCD is probably similar. Medication may be chosen based on side-effect profiles. Newer selective SRIs such as sertraline (Zoloft), paroxetine (Paxil), and fluvoxamine (Luvox) also are options in TD, although systematic investigation has not occurred.

Dosage ranges for use of SRIs in TD have not been established. Common side effects of these medications include behavioral activation, insomnia, headaches, gastrointestinal distress, and sexual dysfunction.[128] Cardiac assessment including baseline ECG and blood pressure should be obtained for patients who are candidates for treatment with clomipramine. Patients with a personal or family history of seizures should have appropriate neurologic consultation including electroencephalogram before treatment with clomipramine.

Other Medications

Many other agents have been tried in patients with TD, including case reports and open trials. Clonazepam, a benzodiazepine, has shown some efficacy for tics in case reports.[129] In addition, benzodiazepines can be used to treat the phobic anxiety or panic attacks that can occur in TD. Traditionally, stimulants have infrequently been used because of their potential to increase tics. However, recent studies have reported that some patients with moderate to severe comorbid ADHD improve in attentional functioning on stimulants without a significant increase in their tics.[130,131] Although caution is still advised, children with TD and ADHD who have been unresponsive to other medications may be candidates for stimulants if the risk-to-benefit ratio is considered acceptable.

Other Treatments

There has been relatively little systematic investigation of nondrug treatments for TD. Behavioral treatments have been reported (e.g., relaxation techniques for anxiety, habit reversal, isometric muscle tensing to oppose motor tics, substitution of a socially acceptable tic for a socially unacceptable one, or contingency management emphasizing positive reinforcement and massed negative practice)[132,133] but need further controlled investigation.

Psychotherapy (dynamic or cognitive) may be useful as adjunctive treatment of patients with TD. For example, psychotherapy may be indicated for patients with adjustment difficulty, moderate stress or anxiety, or other comorbid psychiatric conditions, such as depression.[128]

Family therapy is indicated for maladaptive reactions in family members and for disturbing symptoms that affect them.

Learning problems and classroom difficulties secondary to the tics or comorbid problems are seen frequently in children with TD. Specific developmental disorders, ADHD, and obsessional symptoms can interfere with academic functioning. Education, consultation, and guidance for teachers and employers of patients with TD is frequently indicated. Tutoring and special education techniques are sometimes necessary.

SUMMARY

Tourette's disorder is a complex condition representing one end of a continuum of dysfunction mediated by the corticostriatothalamocortical circuits in the central nervous system, with involvement of dopaminergic and other neurotransmitter systems. A heterogeneous condition, Tourette's disorder is genetically determined in most cases, but also may arise *de novo* (as in relation to prenatal or perinatal trauma or infection). There is significant clinical overlap between TD and OCD, including (1) juvenile or young-adult onset; (2) chronic waxing and waning course; (3) familial occurrence; (4) involuntary, intrusive repetitive behaviors; (5) aggressive, sexual, or scatologic themes in the content of thoughts and behaviors; (6) exacerbation of symptoms by stress or anxiety; and (7) neuroanatomic sites of dysfunction in the basal ganglia and related structures (e.g., corticostriatothalamocortical tracts and frontal lobes). Current theoretic paradigms suggest that TD may be part of a spectrum, with simple tics and pure obsessions at the extremes, and complex sensorimotor behaviors of TD, including complex motor tics and compulsions, in between.

Future investigation should focus on phenomenologic similarities and differences between TD and OCD and delineation of clinical phenotypes. Longitudinal follow-up studies are needed to provide data regarding the developmental psychopathology of tics and their relationship to other comorbid conditions.

REFERENCES

1. de la Tourette G: Etude sur une affection nerveous, characterisie par de l'incoordination motric accompagnee d'echolalie et de coprolalie, *Arch Neurol* 9:19–42, 158–200, 1885.

2. Freud S: Studies in hysteria. In *Standard edition of the complete psychological works*, vol II, London, 1955, Hogarth Press, pp. 48–105.
3. American Psychiatric Association: *Diagnostic and statistical manual of mental disorders*, ed 3, Washington, 1980, American Psychiatric Press.
4. American Psychiatric Association: *Diagnostic and statistical manual of mental disorders,* third edition-revised, Washington, 1987, American Psychiatric Press.
5. Shapiro A, Shapiro E: *Samples, procedures, variables in Gilles de la Tourette syndrome*, ed 2, New York, 1988, Raven Press.
6. Bhatia MS, Balkrishna, Singhal PK, Kaur N: Tourette syndrome treated with nifedipine, *Ind J Pediatr* 56:300–301, 1989.
7. Bruun R, Budman C: Risperidone as a treatment for Tourette's syndrome, *J Clin Psychiatry* 57:29–32, 1996.
8. Chappell P, Riddle M, Scahill L, et al: Guanfacine treatment of comorbid attention-deficit hyperactivity disorder and Tourette's syndrome: Preliminary clinical experience, *J Am Acad Child Adolesc Psychiatry* 34:1140–1146, 1995.
9. Chappell PB: Sequential use of opioid antagonists and agonists in Tourette's syndrome (comment), *Lancet* 343:556, 1994.
10. Cohen DJ, Riddle MA, Leckman JF: Pharmacotherapy of Tourette's syndrome and associated disorders (review), *Psychiatr Clin North Am* 15:109–129, 1992.
11. Delgado PL, Goodman WK, Price LH, et al: Fluvoxamine/pimozide treatment of concurrent Tourette's and obsessive-compulsive disorder, *Br J Psychiatry* 157:762–765, 1990.
12. Leckman J, Hardin M, Riddle M, et al: Clonidine treatment of GTS, *Arch Gen Psychiatry* 48:324–328, 1991.
13. Regeur L, Pakkenberg B, Fog R, Pakkenberg H: Clinical features and long-term treatment with pimozide in 65 patients with Gilles de la Tourette's syndrome, *J Neurol Neurosurg Psychiatry* 49:791–795, 1986.
14. Riddle MA, Leckman JF, Hardin MT, et al: Fluoxetine treatment of obsessions and compulsions in patients with Tourette's syndrome, *Am J Psychiatry* 145:1173–1174, 1988 (letter).
15. Robertson MM, Schnieden V, Lees AJ: Management of Gilles de la Tourette syndrome using sulpiride, *Clin Neuropharmacol* 13:229–235, 1990.
16. Spencer T, Biederman J, Kerman K, et al: Desipramine treatment of children with attention deficit hyperactivity disorder and tic disorder or Tourette's syndrome, *J Am Acad Child Adolesc Psychiatry* 32:354–360, 1993.
17. Leckman JF, Walker DE, Goodman WK, et al: "Just right" perceptions associated with compulsive behavior in Tourette's syndrome, *Am J Psychiatry* 151:675–680, 1994.
18. Swedo S, Rapoport J, Leonard H, et al: Obsessive compulsive disorder in children and adolescents, *Arch Gen Psychiatry* 46:335, 1989.
19. Steingard R, Dillon-Stout D: Tourette's syndrome and obsessive compulsive disorder: Clinical aspects (review), *Psychiatr Clin North Am* 15:849–860, 1992.
20. Swedo SE, Leonard HL: Childhood movement disorders and obsessive compulsive disorder, *J Clin Psychiatry* 55:32–37, 1994.
21. Karno M, Golding JM, Sorenson SB, Burnam MA: The epidemiology of obsessive compulsive disorder in five U.S. communities, *Arch Gen Psychiatry* 45:1094, 1988.

22. Cummings JL, Frankel M: Gilles de la Tourette syndrome and the neurological basis of obsessions and compulsions, *Biol Psychiatry* 20:117–126, 1985.
23. Baxter L, Schwartz J, Guze B, et al: Neuroimaging in obsessive compulsive disorder seeking the mediating neuroanatomy. In Jenike M, Baer L, Minichiello W, editors: *Obsessive compulsive disorder: Theory and management*, ed 2, Chicago, 1990, Year Book Medical Publishers.
24. Shapiro A, Shapiro E: Nosology, criteria and diagnosis. In Shapiro A, Shapiro E, Young J, Feinberg T, editors: *Gilles de la Tourette's syndrome*, ed 2, New York, 1988, Raven Press.
25. American Psychiatric Association: *Diagnostic and statistical manual of mental disorders*, ed 4, Washington, 1994, American Psychiatric Press.
26. Bruun RD, Budman CL: The natural history of Tourette syndrome (review), *Adv Neurol* 58:1–6, 1992.
27. Shapiro A: Signs, symptoms, and clinical course. In Shapiro A, Shapiro E, Feinberg T, Young JG, editors: *Gilles de la Tourette syndrome*, ed 2, New York, 1988, Raven Press, pp 127–193.
28. Bruun RD, Shapiro AK, Shapiro E, et al: A follow-up of 78 patients with Gilles de la Tourette's syndrome, *Am J Psychiatry* 133:944–947, 1976.
29. Erenberg G, Cruse RP, Rothner AD: The natural history of Tourette syndrome: A follow-up study, *Ann Neurol* 22:383–385, 1987.
30. Lucas AR, Kauffman PE, Morris EM: Gilles de la Tourette's disease: A clinical study of fifteen cases, *J Am Acad Child Psychiatry* 6:700–722, 1967.
31. Mak FL, Chung SY, Lee P, Chen S: Tourette syndrome in the Chinese: A follow-up of 15 cases, *Adv Neurol* 35:281–283, 1982.
32. Zausmer DM: The treatment of tics in childhood: A review and followup study, *Arch Dis Child* 29:537–542, 1954.
33. Corbett JA, Mathews AM, Connell PH, Shapiro DA: Tics and Gilles de la Tourette's syndrome: A follow-up study and critical review, *Br J Psychiatry* 115:1229–1241, 1969.
34. Caine ED, McBride MC, Chiverton P, et al: Tourette's syndrome in Monroe County school children, *Neurology* 38:472–475, 1988.
35. Burd L, Kerbeshian J, Wikenheiser M, Fisher W: A prevalence study of Gilles de la Tourette syndrome in North Dakota school-age children, *J Am Acad Child Psychiatry* 25:552–553, 1986.
36. Zahner G, Clubb M, Leckman J, Biels D: Epidemiology of Tourette's syndrome. In Cohen D, Bruun R, Leckman J, editors: *Tourette's syndrome and tic disorders: Clinical understanding and treatment*, New York, 1988, J Wiley, pp 79–90.
37. Apter A, Pauls DL, Bleich A, et al: An epidemiologic study of Gilles de la Tourette's syndrome in Israel, *Arch Gen Psychiatry* 50:734–738, 1993.
38. Coffey B, Miguel E, Savage C, Rauch S: Tourette's disorder and related problems: A review and update, *Harv Rev Psychiatry* 2:121–132, 1994.
39. Comings DE, Comings BG: A controlled study of Tourette syndrome: III. Phobias and panic attacks, *Am J Hum Genet* 41:761–781, 1987.
40. Comings DE, Comings BG: A controlled study of Tourette syndrome. II. Conduct, *Am J Hum Genet* 41:742–760, 1987.
41. Comings DE, Comings BG: A controlled study of Tourette syndrome: I. Attention-

deficit disorder, learning disorders, and school problems, *Am J Hum Genet* 41: 701–741, 1987.

42. Shapiro A, Shapiro E, Young J, Feinberg T: Psychology, psychopathology, and neuropsychology. In Shapiro A, Shapiro E, Young J, Feinberg T, editors: *Gilles de la Tourette syndrome*, New York, 1988, Raven Press, pp 195–252.

43. Robertson MM, Channon S, Baker J, Flynn D: The psychopathology of Gilles de la Tourette's syndrome: A controlled study, *Br J Psychiatry* 162:114–117, 1993.

44. Riddle MA, Leckman JF, Anderson GM, et al: Tourette's syndrome: Clinical and neurochemical correlates, *J Am Acad Child Adolesc Psychiatry* 27:409–412, 1988.

45. Pauls DL, Hurst CR, Kruger SD, et al: Gilles de la Tourette's syndrome and attention deficit disorder with hyperactivity: Evidence against a genetic relationship, *Arch Gen Psychiatry* 43:1177–1179, 1986.

46. Comings D, Comings B: Tourette's syndrome and attention deficit disorder. In Cohen D, Bruun R, Leckman J, editors: *Tourette's syndrome and tic disorders: Clinical understanding and treatment*, New York, 1988, J Wiley, pp 119–135.

47. Robertson MM: Self-injurious behavior and Tourette syndrome (review), *Adv Neurol* 58:105–114, 1992.

48. Grad LR, Pelcovitz D, Olson M, et al: Obsessive-compulsive symptomatology in children with Tourette's syndrome, *J Am Acad Child Adolesc Psychiatry* 26:69–73, 1987.

49. Frankel M, Cummings JL, Robertson MM, et al: Obsessions and compulsions in Gilles de la Tourette's syndrome, *Neurology* 36:378–382, 1986.

50. Pitman RK, Green RC, Jenike MA, Mesulam MM: Clinical comparison of Tourette's disorder and obsessive-compulsive disorder, *Am J Psychiatry* 144: 1166–1171, 1987.

51. Leonard H, Lenane M, Swedo S, et al: Tics and Tourette's disorder: A two- to seven-year followup of 54 obsessive compulsive children, *Am J Psychiatry* 149: 1244–1251, 1992.

52. Leonard HL, Swedo SE, Rapoport JL, et al: Tourette syndrome and obsessive-compulsive disorder (review), *Adv Neurol* 58:83–93, 1992.

53. Bliss J: Sensory experiences of Gilles de la Tourette syndrome, *Arch Gen Psychiatry* 37:1343–1347, 1980.

54. Tourette Syndrome Classification Study Group: Definitions and classifications of tic disorders, *Arch Neurol* 50:1013–1016, 1993.

55. Shapiro AK, Shapiro E: Evaluation of the reported association of obsessive-compulsive symptoms or disorder with Tourette's disorder (review), *Compr Psychiatry* 33:152–165, 1992.

56. Cohen AJ, Leckman JF: Sensory phenomena associated with Gilles de la Tourette's syndrome, *J Clin Psychiatry* 53:319–323, 1992.

57. Leckman JF, Walker DE, Cohen DJ: Premonitory urges in Tourette's syndrome, *Am J Psychiatry* 150:98–102, 1993.

58. Robertson M: The Gilles de la Tourette syndrome: The current status, *Br J Psychiatry* 154:147–169, 1989.

59. Holzer JC, Goodman WK, McDougle CJ, et al: Obsessive-compulsive disorder with and without a chronic tic disorder: A comparison of symptoms in 70 patients, *Br J Psychiatry* 164:469–473, 1994.

60. George MS, Trimble MR, Ring HA, et al: Obsessions in obsessive-compulsive dis-

order with and without Gilles de la Tourette's syndrome, *Am J Psychiatry* 150: 93–97, 1993.

61. Coffey B, Miguel E, Savage C, et al: Phenomenology of symptoms in obsessive compulsive disorder and Tourette's disorder, *Proc Am Acad Child Adolesc Psychiatry*, 2631, 1993.

62. Pauls DL, Towbin KE, Leckman JF, et al: Gilles de la Tourette's syndrome and obsessive-compulsive disorder: Evidence supporting a genetic relationship, *Arch Gen Psychiatry* 43:1180–1182, 1986.

63. Pauls D, Leckman J: Genetics of Tourette's syndrome. In Cohen D, Bruun R, Leckman J, editors: *Tourette's syndrome and tics disorders: Clinical understanding and treatment*, New York, 1988, J Wiley, pp 91–102.

64. Cohen DJ, Leckman JF: Developmental psychopathology and neurobiology of Tourette's syndrome (review), *J Am Acad Child Adolesc Psychiatry* 33:2–15, 1994.

65. Hyde TM, Aaronson BA, Randolph C, et al: Relationship of birth weight to the phenotypic expression of Gilles de la Tourette's syndrome in monozygotic twins, *Neurology* 42:652–658, 1992.

66. Allen AJ, Leonard H, Swedo S: Case study: A new infection-triggered, autoimmune subtype of pediatric OCD and Tourette's syndrome, *J Am Acad Child Adolesc Psychiatry* 34:307–311, 1995.

67. Kiessling L, Marcotte A, Culpepper L: Antineural antibodies in movement disorders, *Pediatrics* 92:39–43, 1993.

68. Singer HS, Walkup JT: Tourette syndrome and other tic disorders: Diagnosis, pathophysiology, and treatment (review), *Medicine* 70:15–32, 1991.

69. Dodman N, Shuster L, Court M, Dixon R: Investigation into the use of narcotic antagonists in the treatment of stereotypic behavior pattern (crib-biting) in the horse, *Am J Vet Res* 48:311–319, 1987.

70. Dodman N, Shuster L, White S, et al: Use of narcotic antagonists to modify stereotypic self-licking, self-chewing and scratching behavior in dogs, *J Am Vet Med Assoc* 193:815–819, 1988.

71. Alexander G, DeLong M, Strick P: Parallel organization of functionally segregated circuits linking basal ganglia and cortex, *Ann Rev Neurosci* 9:357–381, 1986.

72. Wolf SS, Jones DW, Knable MB, et al: Tourette syndrome: Prediction of phenotypic variation in monozygotic twins by caudate nucleus D2 receptor binding, *Science* 273:1225–1227, 1996.

73. Chase T, Foster N, Fedio P, et al: Gilles de la Tourette's syndrome: Studies with the fluorine-18-labeled fluorodeoxyglucose positron emission tomographic method, *Ann Neurol* 15, 1984.

74. Peterson B, Riddle MA, Cohen DJ, et al: Reduced basal ganglia volumes in Tourette's syndrome using three-dimensional reconstruction techniques from magnetic resonance images, *Neurology* 43:941–949, 1993.

75. Singer HS, Reiss AL, Brown JE, et al: Volumetric MRI changes in basal ganglia of children with Tourette's syndrome, *Neurology* 43:950–956, 1993.

76. Witelson SF: Clinical neurology as data for basic neuroscience: Tourette's syndrome and the human motor system (review), *Neurology* 43:859–861, 1993.

77. Shapiro AK, Shapiro E: Treatment of Gilles de la Tourette's syndrome with haloperidol, *Br J Psychiatry* 114:345–350, 1968.

78. Shapiro AK, Shapiro E, Fulop G: Pimozide treatment of tic and Tourette disorders (review), *Pediatrics* 79:1032–1039, 1987.
79. Shapiro E, Shapiro AK, Fulop G, et al: Controlled study of haloperidol, pimozide and placebo for the treatment of Gilles de la Tourette's syndrome, *Arch Gen Psychiatry* 46:722–730, 1989.
80. Feinberg M, Carrol B: Effects of dopamine agonists and antagonists in Tourette's disease, *Arch Gen Psychiatry* 36:979–985, 1979.
81. Golden G: The relationship between stimulant medication and tics, *Pediatr Ann* 17:405–408, 1988.
82. Klempel K: Gilles de la Tourette's symptoms induced by L-dopa, *South Afr Med J* 48:1379–1380, 1974.
83. Singer HS: Neurochemical analysis of postmortem cortical and striatal brain tissue in patients with Tourette syndrome (review), *Adv Neurol* 58:135–144, 1992.
84. Wong D, Pearlson G, Young L, et al: D2 dopamine receptors are elevated in neuropsychiatric disorders other than schizophrenia, *J Cereb Blood Flow Metab* 9: S593, 1989.
85. Rauch S, Jenike M: Neurobiological models of obsessive compulsive disorder, *Psychosomatics* 34:20–32, 1993.
86. Haber SN, Wolfer D: Basal ganglia peptidergic staining in Tourette syndrome: A follow-up study (review), *Adv Neurol* 58:145–150, 1992.
87. Anderson GM, Pollak ES, Chatterjee D, et al: Postmortem analysis of subcortical monoamines and amino acids in Tourette syndrome, *Adv Neurol* 58:123–133, 1992.
88. Kurlan R, Como PG, Deeley C, et al: A pilot controlled study of fluoxetine for obsessive-compulsive symptoms in children with Tourette's syndrome, *Clin Neuropharmacol* 16:167–172, 1993.
89. Riddle MA, Hardin MT, King R, et al: Fluoxetine treatment of children and adolescents with Tourette's and obsessive compulsive disorders: Preliminary clinical experience, *J Am Acad Child Adolesc Psychiatry* 29:45–48, 1990.
90. Barr L, Goodman W, Price L, et al: Serotonin hypothesis of obsessive compulsive disorder: Implications of pharmacologic challenge studies, *J Clin Psychiatry* 53: 17–28, 1992.
91. Goodman W, McDougle C, Price L, et al: Beyond the serotonin hypothesis: A role for dopamine in some forms of obsessive compulsive disorder? *J Clin Psychiatry* 51:36–43, 1990.
92. Sawle G, Hymas N, Lees A, Fraonckowiak R: Obsessional slowness: Functional studies with positron emission tomography, *Brain* 114:2191–2202, 1991.
93. Golden GS: Tourette syndrome: Recent advances (review), *Neurol Clin* 8:705–714, 1990.
94. Golden GS: Psychologic and neuropsychologic aspects of Tourette's syndrome, *Neurol Clin* 2:91–102, 1984.
95. Bornstein RA: Neuropsychological performance in adults with Tourette's syndrome, *Psychiatry Res* 37:229–236, 1991.
96. Bornstein RA: Neuropsychological performance in children with Tourette's syndrome, *Psychiatry Res* 33:73–81, 1990.
97. Bornstein RA, Baker GB, Bazylewich T, Douglass AB: Tourette syndrome and neuropsychological performance, *Acta Psychiatr Scand* 84:212–216, 1991.

98. Yeates K, Bornstein R: Attention deficit disorder and neuropsychological functioning in children with Tourette's syndrome, *Neuropsychology* 8:65–74, 1994.

99. Boone K, Ananth J, Philpott L, et al: Neuropsychological characteristics of nondepressed adults with obsessive-compulsive disorder, *Neuropsychiat Neuropsychol Behav Neurol* 4:96–109, 1991.

100. Christensen K, Kim S, Dysken M, Hoover K: Neuropsychological performance in obsessive-compulsive disorder, *Biol Psychiatry* 31:4–18, 1992.

101. Harvey N: Impaired cognitive set-shifting in obsessive-compulsive disorder, *Med Sci* 14:936–937, 1986.

102. Head D, Hymas N: Deficit in cognitive shifting ability in patients with obsessive-compulsive disorder, *Biol Psychiatry* 25:929–937, 1989.

103. Insel T, Donnelly E, Lalakea M, et al: Neurological and neuropsychological studies of patients with obsessive-compulsive disorder, *Biol Psychiatry* 18:741–751, 1983.

104. Zielinski C, Taylor M, Juzwin K: Neuropsychological deficits in obsessive compulsive disorder, *Neuropsychiatr Neuropsychol Behav Neurol* 4:110–126, 1991.

105. Hollander E, Cohen L, Richards M, et al: A pilot study of the neuropsychology of obsessive compulsive disorder and Parkinson's disease: Basal ganglia disorders, *J Neuropsychiatr* 5:104–107, 1993.

106. Grant DA, Berg EA: *Wisconsin card sort test*, Odessa, 1948, Psychological Assessment Resources.

107. Malloy P: Frontal lobe dysfunction in obsessive-compulsive disorder. In Perecman E, editor: *The frontal lobes revisited*, ISBN Press, 1987, pp 207–223.

108. Orvaschel H, Puig-Antich J: *Schedule for affective disorders and schizophrenia for school-age children: Epidemiologic 4th version*, Ft. Lauderdale, 1987, Nova University, Center for Psychological Study.

109. Shaffer D, Fisher P, Dulcan M, et al: The NIMH Diagnostic Interview Schedule for children version 2.3 (DISC-2.3): Description, acceptability, prevalence rates, and performance in the MECA study, *J Am Acad Child Adolesc Psychiatry* 35:865–877, 1996.

110. Young G, O'Brien J, Gutterman E, Cohen P: Research on the clinical interview, *J Am Acad Child Adolesc Psychiatry* 26:613–620, 1987.

111. Leckman JF, Riddle MA, Hardin MT, et al: The Yale Global Tic Severity Scale: Initial testing of a clinician-rated scale of tic severity, *J Am Acad Child Adolesc Psychiatry* 28:566–573, 1989.

112. Goodman WK, Price LH, Rasmussen SA, et al: The Yale-Brown Obsessive Compulsive Scale (Y-BOCS): Part I. Development, use and reliability, *Arch Gen Psychiatry* 46:1006–1011, 1989.

113. Goodman WK, Price LH, Rasmussen SA, et al: The Yale-Brown Obsessive Compulsive Scale II. Validity, *Arch Gen Psychiatry* 46:1012–1016, 1989.

114. Conners C: Conners rating scales manual. In Conners C, editor: *Instruments for use with children and adolescents*, North Tonananda, 1990, Multihealth Systems.

115. Conners C: Conners teachers rating scales. In Conners C, editor: *Instruments for use with children and adolescents*, North Tonananda, 1990, Multihealth Systems.

116. Conners C: Conners parent rating scales. In Conners C, editor: *Instruments for use with children and adolescents*, North Tonananda, 1990, Multihealth Systems.

117. Shapiro A, Shapiro E: Treatment of tic disorders with haloperidol. In Cohen D,

Bruun R, Leckman J, editors: *Tourette's syndrome and tic disorders: Clinical understanding and treatment*, New York, 1988, J Wiley, pp 267–280.

118. Moldofsky H, Sandor P: Pimozide in the treatment of Tourette's syndrome. In Cohen D, Bruun R, Leckman J, editors: *Tourette's syndrome and tic disorders: Clinical understanding and treatment*, New York, 1988, J Wiley, pp 281–290.

119. Singer H, Trifiletti R, Gammon K: The role of "other" neuroleptic drugs in the treatment of Tourette's syndrome. In Cohen D, Bruun R, Leckman J, editors: *Tourette's syndrome and tic disorders: Clinical understanding and treatment*, New York, 1988, J Wiley, pp 303–316.

120. Lombroso P, Scahill L, King R, et al: Risperidone treatment of children and adolescents with chronic tic disorders: A preliminary report, *J Am Acad Child Adolesc Psychiatry* 34:1147–1152, 1995.

121. McDougle C, Goodman W, Price L, et al: Neuroleptic addition in fluvoxamine-refractory obsessive-compulsive disorder, *Am J Psychiatry* 147:652–654, 1990.

122. Hunt R, Capper L, O'Connell P: Clonidine in child and adolescent psychiatry, *J Child Adolesc Psychopharmacol* 1:87–102, 1990.

123. Riddle M, Hardin M, King R, et al: Desipramine treatment of boys with attention deficit disorder and tics: Preliminary clinical experience, *J Am Acad Child Adolesc Psychiatry* 27:811–814, 1988.

124. Biederman J: Sudden death in children treated with a tricyclic antidepressant: A commentary, *J Am Acad Child Adolesc Psychiatry* 30:495–498, 1991.

125. Biederman J, Thisted R, Greenhill L, Ryan N: Estimation of the association between desipramine and the risk for sudden death in 5- to 14-year-old children, *J Clin Psychiatry* 56:87–93, 1995.

126. Leonard H, Swedo S, Rapoport J: Treatment of childhood obsessive compulsive disorder with clomipramine and desmethylimipramine: A double blind crossover comparison, *Psychopharmacol Bull* 24:93–95, 1988.

127. McDougle C, Goodman W, Leckman J, et al: The efficacy of fluvoxamine in obsessive-compulsive disorder: Effects of comorbid chronic tic disorder, *J Clin Psychopharmacol* 16:167–172, 1993.

128. Wulff E: Psychosocial interventions in Tourette syndrome. In Cohen D, Bruun R, Leckman J, editors: *Tourette's syndrome and tic disorders: Clinical understanding and treatment*, New York, 1988, J Wiley, pp 207–222.

129. Gonce M, Barbeau A: Seven cases of Gilles de la Tourette's syndrome: Partial relief with clonazepam: A pilot study, *Can J Neurol Sci* 4:279–83, 1977.

130. Gadow KD, Sverd J: Stimulants for ADHD in child patients with Tourette's syndrome: The issue of relative risk (review), *J Dev Behav Pediatr* 11:269–271, 1990.

131. Gadow KD, Nolan EE, Sverd J: Methylphenidate in hyperactive boys with comorbid tic disorder: II. Short-term behavioral effects in school settings, *J Am Acad Child Adolesc Psychiatry* 31:462–471, 1992.

132. Azrin NH, Peterson AL: Habit reversal for the treatment of Tourette syndrome. *Behav Res Ther* 26:347–351, 1988.

133. Azrin N, Peterson A: Behavior therapy for Tourette's syndrome and tic disorders. In Cohen D, Bruun R, Leckman J, editors: *Tourette's syndrome and tic disorders: Clinical understanding and treatment*, New York, 1988, J Wiley, pp 237–276.

9

Trichotillomania: Clinical Concepts and Treatment Approaches

Nancy J. Keuthen, Ph.D., Richard L. O'Sullivan, M.D., Donald E. Jefferys, Ph.D.

Trichotillomania (TTM) is a disorder characterized by chronic, repetitive hair pulling resulting in alopecia. It is relatively underdiagnosed and only recently has begun to receive recognition from both the medical community and the lay public. Historically, it was conceptualized as a symptom of obsessive-compulsive disorder (OCD);[1-3] more recent studies have identified possible links to other OCD spectrum candidates[4] and other psychiatric disorders.[5]

Heterogeneity in its phenomenologic and behavioral patterns,[6-9] bimodal distribution of onset,[7,10] and conflicting treatment outcome data[6,11] have prompted researchers to question whether a unitary disorder exists, or conversely, whether hair pulling can be symptomatic of multiple etiologies.[12] High rates of psychiatric comorbidity[7,13] and compelling physical and psychosocial sequelae[14,15] underscore its significance as a psychiatric condition. Unfortunately, however, it continues to present a treatment challenge with some sufferers failing to report substantial relief from current treatments.

DIAGNOSTIC CRITERIA

Despite historic references dating back to the past century,[16] TTM was first included in the psychiatric nomenclature in the *Diagnostic and Statistical Manual of Mental Disorders* (DSM-III-R).[17] In both DSM-III-R and DSM-IV,[18] trichotillomania is classified as an "impulse control disorder not elsewhere classified." Minor modification in diagnostic criteria with DSM-IV resulted in the following current criteria:

1. A recurrent pulling out of one's hair resulting in noticeable hair loss.
2. An increasing sense of tension immediately before pulling out the hair or when attempting to resist the behavior.
3. Pleasure, gratification, or relief when pulling out the hair.

4. The disturbance is not better accounted for by another mental disorder and is not the result of a general medical condition (e.g., a dermatologic condition).
5. The disturbance causes clinically significant distress or impairment in social, occupational, or other important areas of functioning.[18]

EPIDEMIOLOGY
Prevalence

Early evidence from pediatric clinical samples suggested that TTM was very rare. Mannino and Delgado[19] reported only 0.5% of patients in a mental health center had TTM and cited rates of 0.05% to 0.6% from other earlier studies. More recent evidence, however, indicates that this disorder may be much more common. Azrin and Nunn,[20] for example, proposed a prevalence rate as high as 2% to 3%, which would make TTM as common as OCD.[21] Unfortunately, epidemiologic studies of the incidence and prevalence of TTM are still lacking.

Several researchers have estimated prevalence rates by surveying nonclinical groups of college students. Christenson, Pyle, and Mitchell,[22] in a survey of 2,534 college students, reported a lifetime prevalence rate of 0.6% satisfying full DSM-III-R criteria for TTM. Gender differences in prevalence rates were not reported when full diagnostic criteria were applied. However, 3.4% of women and 1.5% of men endorsed lifetime prevalence excluding the criteria of tension prior to pulling and gratification/relief after pulling. Stanley, et al[23] surveyed 243 undergraduates and reported that 14.8% had hairpulling unrelated to grooming in the prior year. Rothbaum, et al[24] found that 10.8% of 711 college freshmen pulled out hair; of this sample, 1.7% reported baldness, 1.4% reported distress, and 1.0% reported both baldness and distress.

Recently King, et al[25] surveyed 794 nonreferred Israeli adolescents and reported a 1% lifetime prevalence of hair pulling. None of the pullers, however, met full DSM-III-R criteria for TTM.

The prevalence of TTM may continue to be underestimated since many sufferers are secretive about their condition and avoid treatment. Others are unaware of their diagnosis and do not know where to seek treatment. Male hair pullers can account for hair loss in a tonsure distribution as male pattern baldness, whereas other individuals with TTM pull from sites not easily visible. In addition, few medical and psychiatric professionals inquire about hair pulling.

Onset and Course

Onset of TTM generally occurs in childhood or adolescence, although cases have been documented with onset from the first year of life up until middle age.[7] Christenson and colleagues reported a mean age of onset of 13 years (standard deviation [SD] = 8 years, median = 12 years) for their sample of 60 adult chronic hairpullers. Onset of TTM in middle age or later is rarely observed.

Swedo and colleagues[10] at the National Institute of Mental Health reported a subgroup of hair pullers with onset before 5 years of age ("baby trichs"). Differences in reported gender ratios, associated symptoms, and course of illness have been noted between hair pullers with early and later onset. Muller[26] reported a higher predominance of boys in a group of preschool hair pullers. Swedo and her associates[10] reported that younger children fail to endorse anxiety-driven pulling or relief subsequent to the behavior. There has also been some suggestion that early-onset TTM does not continue into adolescence and adulthood.[27]

Trichotillomania is believed to be a chronically waxing and waning disorder, although no longitudinal studies yet exist. Our anecdotal clinical experience suggests that symptom course is highly variable from one hairpuller to another.

Gender Distribution

The majority of studies on adolescent and adult hair pullers have reported an overwhelming female preponderance. Swedo, et al[10] studied hairpulling in older children, adolescents, and adults and reported 70% women sufferers. Christenson and colleagues[7] reported that 93% of their sample of adult chronic hairpullers were women. In contrast, the gender ratio for very early onset TTM has been reported to be gender equivalent.[28] Although most studies on childhood onset document a female preponderance,[19,29,30] others report no gender difference or male predominance.[26,31]

Various hypotheses have been postulated to account for unequal gender distribution in TTM as a function of age. Swedo and coworkers[10] questioned whether hair pulling in young men is more likely to resolve than hair pulling in young women. Christenson, et al[32] report that women hair pullers were nearly twice as likely to have had major depression, which may contribute to increased efforts to seek treatment. One might also question whether the higher incidence of major depressive disorder in adult women lowers the threshold for development of hair pulling, or, conversely, lowers motivation to address this problem.

CLINICAL CHARACTERISTICS

Hairpulling can be focused on any body region and can occur from single or multiple sites. In their classic study, Christenson, et al[7] reported that 38% of subjects pulled from one site, 62% from two or more sites, 33% from three or more sites, and 10% from four or more sites. The scalp was reported to be the most common area for hair pulling (75%), with other sites including the eyelashes (53%); eyebrows (42%); pubic area (17%); beard and face (10%); arms (10%); and legs (7%). In addition to using the fingers to pull hair, implements such as tweezers can be used. Some pullers acknowledge pulling hair from the scalp of a child, spouse, or pet.

The number of hairs extracted, amount of time engaged in the behavior, and pattern of pulling vary considerably among sufferers, as well as over time in the individual hair puller. Some pull out single hairs, whereas others pull out tufts of hair. Many select specific hairs to pull on the basis of hair length (e.g., early growth hairs), color (e.g., gray or white), or texture (e.g., coarse, thick or kinky). Oral behaviors, including licking and/or sucking the hair, rubbing the hair around the mouth, and chewing the hair followed by ingestion (trichophagy), are reported by 48% to 64% of sufferers.[7,13] Ingestion of hair may result in trichobezoars (hairballs) although this result is historically believed to be uncommon. However, a recent report by Bhatia, et al[33] cited a 37.5% rate of occurrence of trichobezoars or trichophytobezoars (hairballs including vegetable matter), suggesting that more careful consideration of this problem is warranted.

Individuals who pull hair from their scalp often use wigs, hairpieces, scarves, and disguising hairstyles to hide their problem. Those who pull their eyelashes may use false eyelashes, wear glasses, or use make-up.[7,13] Most pullers have also tried self imposed barriers to pulling, including making fingernail length longer or shorter; taping fingers together; lubricating or washing their hair to alter tactile sensations; wearing hats, gloves, scarves; and avoiding activities that trigger the behavior.

A high frequency of other repetitive body-focused behaviors has been reported as comorbid with TTM. As many as 85% of chronic pullers report onychophagia (nail biting), tongue chewing, head banging, and cheek chewing.[7] It has been our anecdotal experience that many hair pullers also pick at their skin or lesions (e.g., scabs and pimples) on their body.

PHENOMENOLOGY OF HAIRPULLING

The experience of tension prior to pulling and gratification or relief after hair extraction is not universal. As a result, controversy exists regarding whether these phenomenologic features are nosologically important. Christenson and coworkers[7] reported that 95% of pullers experienced increasing tension before pulling, and 88% reported gratification or relief after pulling. Although all pullers acknowledged one or both of these experiences, 17% failed to endorse both criteria. In contrast, Schlosser, et al[13] found that only 50% of subjects reported tension prior to hair pulling and 50% reported feelings of gratification and relief subsequent to pulling.

Subtypes of hair pulling have been proposed as a function of emotional and environmental cue profiles.[8] One postulated subtype is characterized by the association of negative affective states with hair pulling. These hair pullers generally endorse tension buildup before hair pulling and tension release afterward. Twenty-five percent of pullers endorse this pattern as their primary style of pulling. A second subtype of hair pulling occurs in the presence of "sedentary" activities involving "contemplative attitudes" (e.g., reading, studying). In the sedentary hair pulling, attention is directed toward the ongoing activity and awareness of pulling behavior is diminished. Most pullers report a combination of both styles of hair pulling.

A recent retrospective study of women hairpullers by our group found self-reported changes in hair pulling phenomenology as a function of menstrual cycle phase.[34] Premenstrual symptom exacerbation was reported for hair pulling, urge intensity and frequency, and the ability to control pulling but not for efforts to resist hair pulling. Alleviation of symptom exacerbation was reported to occur during menstruation and immediately afterward. Christenson and colleagues[7] also reported that 20% of their women cohort endorsed symptom exacerbation premenstrually (and one subject pulled only during this time).

Although most pullers deny experiencing pain upon hair extraction,[7] pain tolerance and thresholds for noxious stimuli have not been found to differ significantly between hairpullers and nonclinical subjects.[35]

COMORBIDITY

Trichotillomania is historically believed to be associated with many psychiatric disorders, including mental retardation, schizophrenia, borderline personality disorder, and OCD.[36] More recent studies, employing structured diagnostic interviews with clinical samples, have confirmed high rates of psychiatric comorbidity in TTM patients.

In a study of 43 older children, adolescents, and adults with TTM, 78% currently had an additional axis I diagnosis.[10] Similarly, in another report, 82% of adults with TTM had one or more lifetime psychiatric diagnoses.[7] Schlosser and colleagues[13] also studied adults with TTM and reported lifetime prevalence of comorbid psychiatric diagnoses of 64% and current prevalence of 55%.

The most common comorbid psychiatric conditions are affective and anxiety disorders, with lifetime prevalence rates of 65% and 41% reported for affective disorders (most commonly major depression).[7,13] For anxiety disorders, lifetime prevalence rates have ranged from 55% to 57%.[7,13]

Early reports of TTM noted the comorbid occurrence of eating disorders along with overconcern about weight in women hair pullers.[37] Twenty percent of hair pullers have been diagnosed by structured interview to have current or past eating disorders.[7] Lifetime prevalence rates of alcohol and drug abuse were reported as 18% to 20%.[7,13] Rates of attention deficit disorder (ADD) approaching 25% have been reported in two series of adolescents with TTM.[11,30]

A significantly higher rate of hair pulling was observed in a cohort of subjects with both Tourette disorder (TD) and OCD, as compared with subjects with either TD or OCD alone.[38] This suggests that comorbid TD and OCD may confer an elevated risk for hair pulling. Finally, comorbid body dysmorphic disorder (BDD) was reported in nearly 26% of a recent series of 23 patients with TTM in our clinic, suggesting that BDD may be more common than previously recognized in hair pullers.[39] Studies have yet to determine the age at which comorbid diagnoses develop in hair pullers.[40,41]

Obsessional, hysterical, aggressive, borderline, and schizoid personality characteristics were emphasized in early descriptions of hairpullers.[42-44] Recent studies with structured interviews for DSM-III-R personality disorders have also found a wide range of personality diagnoses associated with TTM. Swedo, et al[10] reported that 38% of TTM sufferers had a comorbid axis II diagnosis, including histrionic, borderline, and passive-aggressive personality disorders. Personality disorders were diagnosed in 66.7% of a sample of women outpatients with TTM.[40] In this study, histrionic personality was the most common axis II diagnosis (14.6%), followed by avoidant, OCD, and dependent personality disorders (10.4%, 8.3%, 8.3%, respectively). A 55% prevalence rate of axis II disorders was reported by Schlosser and coworkers,[13] with obsessive-compulsive personality disorder (27%) followed by avoidant, schizoid, borderline, passive-aggressive, and self-defeating personality disorders (all 14%).

PHYSICAL AND PSYCHIATRIC SEQUELAE TO HAIRPULLING

In addition to alopecia secondary to hair pulling, the site of hair extraction may develop a localized infection, chronic inflammation and pruritus, or scarring. Future hair growth can be slowed or stopped, and hair regrowth may be different in texture or color. As described previously, hair ingestion may result in trichobezoars or trichophytobezoars. "Rapunzel syndrome," a particularly severe form of trichobezoars in which a twisted mass of hair stretches from the stomach to the colon, can also occur. Such conditions can result in stomach pain, anorexia, obstruction, peritonitis, or even death.[45]

The repetitive arm and hand movements involved in hair pulling have been noted to give rise to carpal tunnel syndrome[15] and may also result in other occult neuromuscular problems.

Shame secondary to hair pulling is common[46] and can result in avoidance of gynecologic, dental, and other medical care. A recent study by researchers in our group investigated the factors that predicted self-esteem difficulties in hair pullers.[39] Levels of depression and anxiety, hair pulling frequency, and body dissatisfaction unrelated to hairpulling were related to self-esteem in hairpullers, whereas onset and severity of hair loss were not.

Jefferys[14] documented significant psychosocial sequelae in a sample of 25 self-referred women. On the Sheehan Disability Scale, 50% to 55% of their sample reported a moderate impairment in work and family life. Seventy percent reported that their social life and leisure activities were moderately affected.

ETIOLOGY AND CONCEPTUAL MODELS

Consensus is lacking regarding the etiology of TTM. Psychoanalytic perspectives have historically prevailed, in which the behavior was interpreted as a maladaptive expression of either erotic or aggressive impulses.[47-49] Abnormal psychosexual development in hair pullers was attributed to family constellations characterized by domineering, aloof mothers and passive fathers.[50,51] Although many proposed that the onset of hairpulling is correlated with traumatic events,[37,51–53] little empirical evidence exists to substantiate this claim.

Neurobiologic models of TTM are currently receiving considerable attention.[54] For the most part, these models have derived from noted phenomenologic similarities between hair pulling and the compulsions of OCD,[55] that is, impulsive actions[56] and tics.[4,57,58] Further impetus derives from similarities between hairpulling and sterotypes, habit disorders and behaviors, described as "fixed action patterns."[59–61]

There has been growing evidence of differences in central nervous system (CNS) function and structure between hair pullers and normal controls. Furthermore, findings of CNS differences in TTM also overlap with reported abnormalities in putatively related disorders such as OCD and TD.

Two neuroimaging investigations have found significant differences in brain function and structure between TTM subjects and normal controls. Swedo and colleagues[62] compared resting brain metabolism in 10 women TTM subjects and 20 matched normal controls using positron emission tomography (PET). Differences in resting cerebral metabolism between groups were reported. Specifically, increased global, bilateral cerebellar, and right superior parietal metabolism was noted for hair pullers. Our group recently conducted a structural neuroimaging study using morphometric magnetic resonance imaging (mMRI) and found significant volume differences in the left putamen between 10 women with TTM and 10 matched normal controls.[4] Significantly smaller left putamen volumes were found in the TTM cohort. This finding is consistent with structural brain volume differences found in TD cohorts, rather than OCD patients, providing evidence for a neurobiologic link between TD and TTM.

Deficits in neuropsychologic functioning have been noted in two investigations of TTM subjects by our group and others.[63,64] However, in contrast to neurologic soft sign abnormalities found in OCD cohorts,[65] a TTM cohort did not exhibit soft sign abnormalities.[66]

Evidence of symptom worsening in OCD with administration of the mixed serotonin agonist m-chlorophenylpiperazine (m-CPP)[67] has resulted in its use as a pharmacologic probe in TTM. One report comparing women with TTM and normal controls failed to demonstrate worsening in TTM with m-CPP.[68] However, mild mood elevation in the TTM subjects was noted, similar to observations in patients with impulsive personalities when given m-CPP.[69] Biochemical investigations of cerebrospinal fluid (CSF) metabolite levels have found that pretreatment CSF levels of the serotonin metabolite 5-hydroxy indoleacetic acid (5-HIAA) were correlated with response to serotonin reuptake inhibitor (SRI) treatment in TTM.[70] Cerebrospinal 5-HIAA decreases from baseline were associated with symptom improvement.

Swedo and colleagues[10] have proposed an autoimmune theory to explain some cases of early-onset TTM. These researchers reported recurrent relapses in two early-onset hair pullers after documented streptococcal infections. Hair pulling remission subsequently occurred with resolution of the infection. These investigators suggested that induced autoantibodies crossreact with the CNS and release a "pathologic fixed action pattern" (e.g., hair pulling).

Attempts have been made to use dysregulated repetitive behavior syndromes in nonhuman species as conceptual models for OCD,[71] TTM, and other disorders[72] in humans. The use and limitations of these models, which include acral lick dermatitis and avian feature picking, have been recently reviewed[72] and is also described in detail in Chapter 16 of this book.

Lastly, anecdotal observations[73] have commented on the familial transmission of TTM. However, the results of empirical investigations have been inconclusive regarding this issue.[30,74]

TREATMENT INTERVENTIONS

Although psychoanalytic conceptualization remained the accepted theoretic model and treatment approach for years, empirical documentation of its efficacy has been virtually nonexistent. Current thinking in the field views behavioral treatment and pharmacotherapy as the treatment avenues of choice. There is also some indication that hypnosis may be effective. Although outcome data for these approaches remain sparse, sufficient data exist to support their use. The existing database, however, is insufficient to generate algorithms to guide treatment choice. The following is a summary of the state-of-the-art treatment methods for this disorder.

BEHAVIORAL TREATMENT

The behavioral literature on TTM includes a vast array of treatment approaches ranging from multicomponent treatment packages (e.g., habit reversal) to isolated techniques. Typically, however, individual techniques have been used in combination with other interventions, making it difficult to determine the relative contribution of single techniques to positive treatment outcomes.[75,76] In the following sections, we will group, albeit somewhat arbitrarily, the existing techniques and treatment packages for the purposes of illustration and discussion.

Habit Reversal

Habit reversal training (HRT)[77] is the most universally accepted and empirically researched behavioral therapy approach for TTM. To this day, it remains the only behavioral intervention studied through a randomized group treatment design.

HRT is a multimodal treatment approach comprised of 13 separate techniques.[78] Each individual treatment component will be briefly described.

Competing reaction training involves training patients to learn an incompatible response (often grasping or clenching hands) that they can use for 3 minutes when hair pulling has occurred or has a high probability of occurrence. *Awareness training* develops awareness of the motor movements associated with hairpulling, often through self-observation in a mirror. In *identifying response precursors*, the individual puller pinpoints responses that often precede their hair pulling (e.g., hair touching or stroking). Similarly, in *identifying habit-prone situations*, they identify those situations which often precede the behavior (e.g., watching television, talking on the phone, etc.). The technique of *relaxation training* instructs patients to use breathing and postural adjustment for the purposes of relaxation. During *prevention training*, pullers practice their competing response when they experience nervousness, exhibit a response precursor, or are in a habit-prone situation.

Through *habit interruption,* hair pullers are taught to use the competing response to immediately interrupt any hair pulling which has occurred. With *positive attention (overcorrection)*, the practice of positive hair care (e.g., hair brushing) or repair of eye makeup is recommended after every episode of pulling. The *daily practice of competing reaction* instructs the individual to implement the competing reaction at home on a preprogrammed schedule and exhibit routine positive hair care. Through *self-recording* of all hair pulls and urges, the individual acquires increased awareness as well as feedback on improvement. With *display of improvement*, previously avoided situations are purposefully sought out as an opportunity to practice competing responses. Significant others are instructed to prompt and reinforce the puller for habit control in *social support*. Lastly, all problems related to the hair pulling are catalogued in the *annoyance review* as a strategy to boost motivation and identify potential sources of reinforcement.

In their landmark study, Azrin, et al[78] randomly assigned subjects to either the habit reversal group (n = 19) or the negative practice group (n = 15). In the former group, pullers were instructed in the essentials of habit reversal in one 90-minute session. In the latter group, subjects were asked to mimic hair pulling (without actual hair extraction) when standing in front of a mirror for a 30-second period every hour. Negative practice exercises were continued for 4 days after total cessation of hair pulling. Subjects recorded hair pulling occurrence or duration (when the habit was more continuous). Both treatments showed rapid reductions on the first day posttraining (habit reversal, 99%; negative practice, 58%). At 3 months' follow-up, however, reductions in hair pulling in excess of 90% were reported for the habit reversal group versus 52% to 68% decrement in pulling for the negative practice group.

Early investigations of HRT can be criticized on numerous methodologic grounds. However, subsequent case studies and single subject experimental designs have corroborated these early findings of Azrin and his colleagues.[79-82] Tarnowski, et al[79] successfully used a modified habit reversal design with an

11-year-old girl with severe, refractory hair pulling. Rosenbaum and Ayllon[80] also demonstrated the efficacy of habit reversal in a case series of four hair-pullers. De Luca and Holborn[81] used relaxation techniques and competing response training to treat a 17-year-old girl. Although relaxation initially reduced pulling, lasting benefit did not occur; however, after instruction in competing response training, lasting benefit was noted at 2-year follow-up. More recently, Vitulano, et al[82] used a six-session program, modelled after Azrin and Nunn's habit reversal training, with three children. In this study, two of the three patients exhibited moderate improvement at posttreatment.

Self-Monitoring

The technique of self-monitoring can be simultaneously viewed as both a treatment tool and an assessment device. The recording of urges and actual hair pulling, as well as associated activities, emotions, physiologic experiences and motor behaviors, provides baseline and continuous data for assessment purposes. At the same time, however, the activity of self-monitoring enhances awareness of the relevant behavior(s) and engages reactivity effects.

Ottens[83] emphasized the importance of enhancing patient awareness of both the overt and covert precursors to pulling. Stanley, et al[84] suggested that self-monitoring of hair pulling behavior can enhance self-awareness, which consequently may reduce the behavior.

Anthony[85] documented hair pulling remission in a 9-year-old boy after only one session of instruction in self-monitoring. Some investigators[86] have combined self-monitoring with the mildly aversive technique of hair collection. The additive combination appears to enhance treatment outcome. Bayer[87] reported that the extent of therapist involvement in hair collection further determined the efficacy of the technique.

Reinforcement and Punishment Techniques

Several case studies and case series have highlighted the use of reinforcement and punishment strategies to reduce hair pulling. For the most part, these techniques have been implemented with children or with the developmentally delayed.

Reinforcement techniques have been either (1) directly applied contingent on reductions in the target behavior; or (2) used to differentially reinforce other more appropriate behaviors (differential reinforcement of other behavior [DRO] schedules of reinforcement). The primary reinforcers used in hair pulling research have included therapist praise,[88] parental praise,[89,90] and parental praise in conjunction with food.[91] Token economies have been used as well as primary reinforcers.[86,92–94]

Punishment paradigms have included self-administered contingencies such as aversive eyedrops,[95] rubber band snaps,[96,97] and rigorous exercise,[98] which have been implemented after pulling urges or pulling behavior. Therapist- or parent-administered contingencies have included hand slaps,[93] aromatic ammonia inhalation,[99] faradic shock when the patient views him- or herself extracting hair on a videotape,[100] electric shock contingent on hair pulling behavior,[101] and the application of a bad-tasting substance to the thumb when thumbsucking covaried with hair pulling.[88,102,103] Response cost techniques, in which privileges or positive stimuli are removed contingent on the target behavior, also have been used with some success.[95,104]

Overcorrection and facial screening are two aversive techniques that have been almost exclusively implemented with developmentally disabled patients.[105,106] By definition, overcorrection involves the repeated practice of "overly correct" behavior, which can repair damage incurred by the target behavior. For hairpullers, this could involve hair brushing/combing for extended periods after hair extraction has occurred. Although positive outcomes have been reported in these case studies, our clinical experience has suggested that this technique can often fail when contact with the hair actually triggers renewed urges to pull.

Facial screening, another aversive approach, involves covering the puller's face and hair with a soft bib for a predetermined amount of time contingent on pulling. Significant reductions in hair pulling were reported[107,108] when facial screening was used alone or in combination with other techniques with retarded children.

Cognitive-Behavioral Techniques

Cognitive-behavioral treatments for TTM target associated cognitive processes and actual hair pulling as areas for therapeutic intervention. In general, these approaches identify maladaptive thought patterns, develop awareness of the occurrence of these inner dialogues and the problematic behavior, and instruct patients in more adaptive, substitute thoughts and behaviors.

Ottens[83] proposed that "beliefs in self-efficacy, self-statements expressing futility and hopelessness, anxiety- and anger-engendering self-talk, decision-making processes, and irrational beliefs about hair pulling" are cognitive variables relevant to hair pulling. His comprehensive cognitive-behavioral treatment includes the strategies of calming self-talk, self-instruction, rational restructuring, covert assertion, and anticipatory strategies to control pulling. The successful use of these techniques in the reduction and subsequent elimination of hair pulling was reported in the case of an 18-year-old college freshman.[109]

Rothbaum[110] also recommends a multimodal treatment package designed as a 9-week program, including habit reversal, stimulus control, and stress management. In addition to habit reversal and relaxation/breathing training, the cognitive strategies of thought stopping, cognitive restructuring, guided self-dialogue, and covert modelling are included. Successful application of this program with several hairpullers has been reported.

More recently, Gluhoski[111] suggested a cognitive model for TTM adapted from an earlier model of addictive behavior. TTM is characterized as a cycle in which high-risk situations trigger negative affect, entrenched beliefs about the value of pulling (e.g., "Pulling will make me feel better"), and automatic thoughts about situations (e.g., "I can't handle this"). The urge to pull is experienced subsequent to the negative affect and dysfunctional cognitions and is often exacerbated by "permission-giving beliefs." This author provides anecdotal reports of the efficacy of this approach with several patients.

Other cognitive approaches were used early on with this disorder, including rational-emotive therapy and self-instructional training,[112] covert sensitization,[113] and cognitive desensitization.[114]

HYPNOSIS

Case reports and case series using hypnosis suggest that these techniques can be of benefit for some hair pullers. The hypnosis literature consists of treatment reports in which (1) habit awareness is enhanced and behavioral techniques are reinforced through hypnosis; and (2) age regression is used to uncover unconscious determinants of the disorder.

Gardner[115] used hypnosis to eliminate hair pulling in an 8-year-old girl. Suggestions of enhanced awareness and control over the habit were given and the patient was instructed in self-hypnosis. By report of her mother, she remained abstinent 2 months posttreatment. De Horne[100] cited a marked improvement in pulling in a 42-year-old man with hypnotic suggestion, relaxation, and self-monitoring until family discord precipitated a relapse. Hall and McGill[116] used a combination of hypnosis and behavioral techniques to successfully reduce hair pulling and terminate binge/purging behavior in a 22-year-old woman. At 6-month follow-up, no further episodes of either behavioral problem was reported.

Galski[117] reported that hypnotic suggestions of relaxation and heightened scalp sensitivity after pulling, coupled with autohypnosis, led to immediate cessation of pulling and no recurrence in a 26-year-old highly hypnotizable woman. Barabasz[118] found that hypnosis alone, or in combination with brief restricted environmental stimulation techniques, resulted in long-term abstinence from hair pulling in three out of four treatment cases.

Fabbri and Dy[119] successfully used hypnotherapy to significantly impact hair pulling in two different cases. The effectiveness of the treatment was attributed to anxiety management and habit substitution in one case and insight into etiologic factors in the other. Rowen[120] reports on the case of a 21-year-old prisoner with a history of hair pulling since 7 years of age. Initial treatment using hypnotic trances for covert sensitization (i.e., associating nauseous feelings with hair pulling behavior) and positive suggestions (e.g., desire to protect one's appearance) was successful. Relapse occurred, however, when self-hypnosis exercises were discontinued. Subsequently, hypnotic age regression with suggestions of physical discomfort accompanying hair pulling was used and proved to be successful. Hynes[121] reports on a series of five hair pulling patients in which age regression, abreaction of conflicts and emotions, and thought-stopping techniques were used. Highly hypnotizable patients were also instructed in autohypnosis. Three of the five hair pullers successfully ceased pulling for periods from 2.5 to 8 months at follow-up.

It is difficult to evaluate the hypnosis literature given the absence of experimentally controlled studies. A range of behavioral techniques have been successfully coupled with hypnosis for individual hair pullers. However, without control groups or reversal designs, it is too early to conclude what accounted for the noted improvement.

PHARMACOTHERAPY

The first report of successful medication treatment for TTM was published nearly 40 years ago.[122] Drug treatment data for TTM have expanded since then but are still relatively limited in comparison with the pharmacologic outcome data for OCD and other related disorders. Several reviews of pharmacotherapy for TTM have recently been published.[11,123]

Five controlled comparison medication trials (Table 9-1), several moderately sized open trials or case series, and numerous case reports have been published. Treatment results have been mixed. As is usually the case, open treatment data have typically been favorable and controlled data have been contradictory. The clinical heterogeneity of TTM, comorbidity, and methodologic limitations of the existing research contribute to these conflicting results.[123,124,128]

The efficacy of psychotropic medications for TTM was first reported in 1958 in a report of two women whose psychosis and hair pulling responded to chlorpromazine.[122]

The first controlled study of pharmacologic treatment for TTM occurred some four decades later when Swedo, et al[55] compared clomipramine with desipramine in a double-blind, cross-over design. Treatment with clomipramine was significantly better than desipramine in reducing hair pulling. Most subsequent pharmacologic trials in TTM have focused on antiobsessional serotonergic agents. Consequently, these medications are often considered the first-line drugs for treatment of this disorder.

Several open trials of fluoxetine found significantly decreased hair pulling in nearly 50 adults treated over 8 to 16 weeks.[129–133] Symptom recurrence after fluoxetine discontinuation was noted.[134] Positive open trials with other selective serotonin reuptake inhibitor (SSRI) antidepressants also have been reported. Fluvoxamine resulted in initial improvement of TTM, but these effects waned within 6 months of treatment.[6] Paroxetine[58,135] and sertraline[136,137] may be beneficial in some patients. Improvement in hair pulling symptoms was also reported in a naturalistic open-label study of 15 patients using the SSRI citalopram.[11]

Table 9-1 Pharmacotherapy of Trichotillomania-Controlled Trials

Study	Subjects	TTM Onset (yrs)	Method/Design	Treatment	Duration	Dose	Dose Interval	Baseline	Study Wash	Efficacy Ratings	Results
Swedo, et al[55]	14	13.8 ± 7.2	CMI vs DMI dbl-blind cross-over	CMI vs DMI	5 wks (each agent)	CMI-180 ± 56 mg DMI-173 ± 33 mg	50 mg incr over 3 wks to 250 mg	2 wks sing dbl PLB	None	TSS TIS PCS	CMI > DMI TIS, TSS, PCS
Christenson, et al[124]	15	Unknown	PLB controlled dbl-blind cross-over	FLX	18 wks Active 6 wks	≤80 mg	20 mg-2wks 40 mg-2wks 80 mg-2wks	1 wk	5 wks	Urges Wk assessment Estimated amount of HP	No sig drug by period Interaction Great baseline variability
Pigott, et al[125]	12	Unknown	Random dbl-blind crossover	CMI or FLX 10 wks	10 wks	CMI-200 ± 15 mg FLX-75 ± 5 mg	Unknown	2 wks PLB	4 wks PLB	Y-BOCS, Global OC, NIMH-OC, HDRS	Sig Imp for CMI & FLX on all measures
Christenson, et al[126]	17	Unknown	Dbl-blind PLB controlled parallel design	NAL	6 wks	50 mg	Unknown	Unknown	Unknown	TSS, PCS, TIS Estimate of # of hairs pulled	NAL > PLB 3 of 7 NAL subj with 50% reduction TSS
Streichenwein, et al[127]	16	21 ± 14	Dbl-blind PLB controlled crossover	FLX	12 wks	80 mg	20 mg-2wks 40 mg-2wks 60 mg-2wks 80 mg-6wks	2 wks	5 wks	HDRS, BDI, Self-Report HPS, Urges, Hair Counts, # of pull days	No sig difference btwn groups

FLX, Fluoxetine; CMI, Clomipramine; DMI, Desipramine; NAL, Naltrexone; PLB, Placebo; Y-BOCS, Yale-Brown Obsessive-Compulsive Scale; HDRS, Hamilton Depression Rating Scale; TSS, Trichotillomania Symptom Severity Scale; PCS, Physician's Change Scale; GOC, Global Obsessive Compulsive Symptom Scale; NIMH-OC, National Institute of Mental Health Obsessive Compulsive Scale.

Although reports of open treatment of TTM with various SSRI antidepressants have indicated efficacy, the results of controlled trials with fluoxetine have been mixed. Two reports found no significant difference compared with placebo[124,127] in contrast to a third report, which suggested efficacy with fluoxetine.[125]

Other antidepressants also show promise. Several anecdotal reports indicate symptom improvement with various tricyclic agents.[138,139] A retrospective review of 10 patients with TTM treated openly in our clinic with venlafaxine for 8 to 28 weeks showed significant improvement in hair pulling symptoms.[140] Lastly, additional reports with the monoamine oxidase inhibitor isocarboxazid[141] and other agents, including mianserin[142] and trazodone,[143] have been favorable.

It is surprising that more attention has not been paid to the study of mood stabilizers in the treatment of TTM, considering the mixed phenomenology of impulsiveness and compulsiveness in this disorder[5,56] as well as significant mood dysregulation in many hair pullers. Lithium carbonate, although not yet subjected to controlled study, shows promise in TTM treatment from both perspectives of percent responders (80%) and duration of effect (up to 14 months of follow-up) in a small retrospective review.[144,145]

Anxiolytics are commonly used as adjunctive treatments for hair pullers, but have yet to be subjected to controlled study. Buspirone[11,146] and clonazepam[6] have been anecdotally reported to be helpful.

Several reports describe the benefits of dopamine-blocking medications, both as monotherapy[122] and as augmenting agents to SSRI antidepressants, in cases refractory to SSRI treatment.[11,57,147] Some reports[11,122,148] describe hair-pulling responsive to neuroleptics, including clozapine, in populations with psychosis, mental retardation, or other developmental disabilities. These open clinical reports raise the possibility that neuroleptics may be indicated in circumscribed cases, perhaps similar to the use of neuroleptic augmentation in OCD patients with comorbid tics.[149]

The opiate antagonist naltrexone is the only nonantidepressant medication to have undergone controlled study in TTM.[126] Naltrexone was expected to decrease hair pulling through modulation of pain thresholds, but study results did not support this mechanism.[35] In comparison with placebo, however, naltrexone significantly improved hair pulling symptoms in a 6-week, double-blind, parallel design. Other investigators also have reported improvement in TTM with open naltrexone augmentation of fluoxetine.[150]

There has been little exploration of hormonal interventions for TTM, despite documentation of premenstrual symptom worsening.[34] A single report[151] documents the cessation of hair pulling in a woman treated with levonorgestrel, a progestin, in the form of a birth control pill.

Some evidence suggests that fenfluramine also may be a useful adjunct to SRIs in the treatment of TTM.[152]

Topical medications, including topical steroids, analgesics, and antibiotics, also have been used as anti-TTM agents. Topical agents have been used in an effort to diminish local sensations that precede bouts of hair pulling. The application of a topical steroid (flucinolone 0.01%) to pulling sites, in conjunction with clomipramine treatment, has been noted as successful.[153,154] Similarly, treatment of occult skin infections with topical antibiotics (tobramycin) resulted in remission of hair pulling symptoms.[11] Topical application of capsaicin, typically used as an analgesic, has also been successfully used as an adjunct to behavioral treatment.[155] Although its possible mechanism of action is unclear, after several days of use the patient reported greater awareness of hair pulling behavior.

In summary, there exists a range of medication treatment options for TTM that have some empirical documentation of efficacy. For the most part, existing studies address short-term treatment outcome, and long-term follow-up data are lacking. Pharmacologic interventions, however, are likely to be most successful when used in the context of a comprehensive treatment plan.

TREATMENT CONSIDERATIONS

The current state of the literature on TTM cannot yet provide algorithms to assist clinicians in the selection of treatment interventions. In addition to limited treatment outcome data, little is known about the natural long-term course of the disorder, including rates of spontaneous remissions and exacerbations. There exist no large-scale, long-term randomized drug studies and only one for behavioral treatment. Studies are needed which systematically compare behavioral treatment with pharmacotherapy, and single-treatment modalities (behavioral treatment or pharmacotherapy) with combined treatments (behavioral treatment and pharmacotherapy). Rates and predictors of relapse with treatment discontinuation are not known. Thus, though tentative treatment recommendations may be derived from available data, current thinking regarding treatment recommendations also derives from anecdotal experience and common sense.

At the present time, our guiding philosophy is that a combination of behavioral and medication therapy has the highest probability for the successful treatment of TTM. Important, yet unanswered, clincal questions include which treatment to begin with and when to augment one treatment with the other. An initial comprehensive assessment of coexisting psychiatric conditions and the psychosocial impact of the disorder is likely useful in making these determinations. Successful treatment of comorbid conditions may be necessary before the patient can focus on the hair pulling and, in some cases, TTM may be secondary to another psychiatric disorder.[5] We also strongly encourage medication trials when hair pulling results in significant functional impairment in social, professional, or academic functioning and a behavioral trial is not quickly effective.

In most cases, we initially recommend behavioral treatment with or without concomitant pharmacotherapy, depending on the patient's motivation and clinical status. The success of behavioral treatment may be compromised if the patient is cognitively limited in the ability to implement behavioral interventions and/or treatment motivation is low. Caution should be used in recommending behavioral treatment as a sole initial approach when significant comorbidity, particularly depression, is present. Thus, the timing of treatment initiation is an important consideration when recommending behavioral treatment.

Several factors should be noted when considering a drug trial, whether in combination with behavioral treatment or as monotherapy. Presently, there are no FDA-approved medications for TTM. Thus, use of these drugs is "off label" and patients should be advised of this. Pharmacotherapy is generally avoided in children and in pregnant patients, unless the potential benefits clearly outweigh careful consideration of the risks. For the most part, significant comorbidity that seriously limits functioning should be the only justification for pharmacotherapy in these cases. A trial of behavioral treatment should be implemented first, if feasible. Patients with significant medical instability or a history of medication intolerance will be less likely to initially be treated with medications.

In the presence of comorbid depression, mood instability, anxiety, or tic disorders, the selection of primary medications or augmenting agents may be altered. When impulsivity or mood instability is problematic, mood stabilizers, such as lithium or valproate, should be considered. Benzodiazepines, either alone or as augmentating agents, may be helpful when anxiety promotes pulling, particularly during premenstrual exacerbations. Neuroleptics may be helpful, particularly in the presence of a tic disorder, or refractoriness to SSRI and behavioral treatments. The severity and impact of TTM should be carefully weighed in considering potential risks of neuroleptics. Topical treatments with steroids, capsaicin, or possibly antibiotics also may be useful adjuncts. Finally, appreciation of the rare but important association of various medications with hair loss should be kept in mind.[156]

The issues of maintenance of treatment gain and relapse prevention must be addressed regardless of treatment modality. It is important that patients have reasonable expectations for the course of their disorder. With behavioral treatment, scheduled "booster" sessions may be useful to proactively prevent relapse. Individuals undergoing pharmacotherapy should have regular monitoring of their progress and "booster" sessions are thus built into their treatment. Both the short- and long-term benefits of pharmacotherapy must be considered. As stated earlier, results of investigation of the long-term benefits of treatment agents are mixed, with some reports suggesting a waning of effects over time.[157] In contrast, others suggest maintenance of improvement.[134,158,159]

An important clinical question often arises regarding whether failure to respond to one medication predicts failure to respond to another agent. Several case reports and clinical experience suggest that nonresponse to one agent does not necessarily mean that other agents, whether SSRI antidepressants or medications of different classes, will not prove helpful.[15,135]

We also strongly encourage involvement in support groups to help sustain active efforts to combat pulling and to address the shame and lowered self-esteem that often accompany this problem. At present, a comprehensive approach to treatment involving education, behavioral treatment, medications, and support groups may be most effective for the treatment of TTM.

SUMMARY

Trichotillomania is a perplexing and challenging psychiatric disorder, which occurs at higher prevalence rates than previously believed. It is often accompanied by significant psychiatric comorbidity and can have major physical, psychosocial, and emotional sequelae. Although previously viewed as a unitary disorder, recent evidence suggests heterogeneity in symptom profile, onset, and treatment response.

Existing treatment outcome data are limited and conflicting, most likely because of intraindividual and interindividual variability in symptom pictures, as well as methodologic limitations of existing research. Current treatment strategies include behavioral treatment, pharmacotherapy, and hypnosis. Because the empirical data offer limited guidance in the choice of treatment interventions, decisions regarding treatment strategies should follow comprehensive inital assessments and should preferably include combined treatment avenues.

REFERENCES

1. Jenike MA: Obsessive-compulsive and related disorders, *N Engl J Med* 321: 539–541, 1989.
2. Swedo SE, Leonard HL: Trichotillomania: an obsessive-compulsive spectrum disorder? *Psychiatr Clin North Am* 15:777–790, 1992.
3. Jenike MA: Reply to letters to the editor, *N Engl J Med* 322:472, 1990.
4. O'Sullivan RL, et al: Reduced basal ganglia volumes in trichotillomania measured via morphometric magnetic resonance imaging, *Biol Psychiatry* 42:39–45, 1997.
5. McElroy SL, et al: The DSM-III-R impulse control disorders not elsewhere classified: clinical characteristics and relationship to other psychiatric disorders, *Am J Psychiatry* 149:318–327, 1992.
6. Christenson GA, Crow SJ: The characterization and treatment of trichotillomania, *J Clin Psychiatry* 57(suppl 8):42–49, 1996.
7. Christenson GA, Mackenzie TB, Mitchell JE: Characteristics of 60 adult chronic hair pullers, *Am J Psychiatry* 148:365–370, 1991.
8. Christenson GA, Ristvedt SL, Mackenzie TB: Identification of trichotillomania cue profiles, *Behav Res Ther* 31:315–320, 1993.
9. Reeve EA, Bernstein GA, Christenson GA: Clinical characteristics and psychiatric comorbidity in children with trichotillomania, *J Am Acad Child Adolesc Psychiatry* 31:132–138, 1992.
10. Swedo SE, et al: Trichotillomania: a profile of the disorder from infancy through adulthood, *Int Pediatr* 7:144–150, 1992.
11. O'Sullivan RL, Christenson GA, Stein D: Pharmacotherapy of trichotillomania. In

Stein DJ, Christenson GA, Hollander E, editors: *Trichotillomania: new developments*, Washington, American Psychiatric Press, in press.

12. O'Sullivan RL, et al: Trichotillomania: behavioral symptom or clinical syndrome? *Am J Psychiatry* 154:1442–1449, 1997.

13. Schlosser S, et al: The demography, phenomenology, and family history of 22 persons with compulsive hair pulling, *Ann Clin Psychiatry* 6:147–152, 1994.

14. Jefferys D: Clinical comorbidity and social impact features of trichotillomania. Presentation at the 15th Annual Meeting, Anxiety Disorders Association of America, Pittsburgh, 1995 (abstract).

15. O'Sullivan RL, et al: Trichotillomania and carpal tunnel syndrome, *J Clin Psychiatry* 57:174, 1996.

16. Hallopeau H: Alopecie par grattage (trichomanie ou trichotillomanie), *Ann Dermatol Venereol* 10:440–441, 1889.

17. American Psychiatric Association: *Diagnostic and Statistical Manual of Mental Disorders*, ed 3, revised, Washington, 1987, American Psychiatric Association.

18. American Psychiatric Association: *Diagnostic and Statistical Manual of Mental Disorders*, ed 4, Washington, 1994, American Psychiatric Association.

19. Mannino FV, Delgado RA: Trichotillomania in children: a review, *Am J Psychiatry* 126:505–511, 1969.

20. Azrin NH, Nunn RG: *Habit control in a day*, New York, 1978, Simon and Schuster.

21. Karno M, et al: The epidemiology of obsessive compulsive disorder in five US communities, *Arch Gen Psychiatry* 45:1094–1099, 1988.

22. Christenson GA, Pyle RL, Mitchell JE: Estimated lifetime prevalence of trichotillomania in college students, *J Clin Psychiatry* 52:415–417, 1991.

23. Stanley MA, et al: Symptoms of trichotillomania in a general college population. Presentation at the 12th National Conference of the Anxiety Disorders Association of America, Houston, 1992.

24. Rothbaum BO, et al: Prevalence of trichotillomania in a college freshman population, *J Clin Psychiatry* 54:72, 1993.

25. King RA, et al: An epidemiological study of trichotillomania in Israeli adolescents, *J Am Acad Child Adolesc Psychiatry* 34:1212–1215, 1995.

26. Muller SA: Trichotillomania, *Dermatol Clin* 5:595–601, 1987.

27. Friman PC, et al: Hair pulling, *J Acad Child Adolesc Psychiatry* 29:489–490, 1990.

28. Swedo SE, Rapoport J: Annotation: trichotillomania, *J Child Psychol Psychiatry* 32:401–409, 1991.

29. Cohen LJ, et al: Clinical profile, comorbidity, and treatment history in 123 hair pullers: a survey study, *J Clin Psychiatry* 56:319–326, 1995.

30. King RA, et al: Childhood trichotillomania: clinical phenomenology, comorbidity, and family genetics, *J Am Acad Child Adolesc Psychiatry* 34:1451–1459, 1995.

31. Bartsch JE: Contribution towards the aetiology of trichotillomania in infancy, *Psychiatr Neurol Med Psychol* 8:173–182, 1956.

32. Christenson GA, MacKenzie TB, Mitchell JE: Adult men and women with trichotillomania, *Psychosomatics* 35:142–149, 1994.

33. Bhatia MS, et al: Clinical profile of trichotillomania, *J Indian Med Assoc* 89:137–139, 1991.

34. Keuthen NJ, et al: The relationship of menstrual cycle and pregnancy to compulsive hairpulling, *Psychother Psychosom* 66:33–37, 1997.

35. Christenson GA, et al: Pain thresholds are not elevated in trichotillomania, *Biol Psychiatry* 36:347–349, 1994.
36. Krishnan KRR, Davidson JRT, Guajardo C: Trichotillomania: a review, *Compr Psychiatry* 26:123–128, 1985.
37. Greenberg HR, Sarner CA: Trichotillomania: symptom and syndrome, *Arch Gen Psychiatry* 12:482–489, 1965.
38. O'Sullivan RL, et al: Trichotillomania—symptom and syndrome. American Psychiatric Association Annual Meeting, Scientific Proceeding Syllabus, Philadelphia, 1994, 299–300.
39. Soriano JL, et al: Trichotillomania and self-esteem: a survey of 62 female hair pullers, *J Clin Psychiatry* 57:77–82, 1996.
40. Christenson GA, Chernoff-Clementz E, Clementz BA: Personality and clinical characteristics in patients with trichotillomania, *J Clin Psychiatry* 53:407–413, 1992.
41. Kessler RC, et al: Lifetime and 12 month prevalence of DSM-III-R psychiatric disorders in the United States, *Arch Gen Psychiatry* 51:975–983, 1994.
42. Sorosky AD, Sticher MB: Trichotillomania in adolescence, *Adolesc Psychiatry* 8:437–454, 1980.
43. Schnurr RG: Psychological assessment and discussion of female adolescents with trichotillomania, *Adolesc Psychiatry* 15:463–470, 1988.
44. Chauhan S, Jaim RK, Dhir GG: Trichotillomania: a phenomenological study, *Indian J Clin Psychol* 2:47–50, 1985.
45. DeBakey M, Ochsner A: Bezoars and concretions, *Surgery* 4:934–967, 1938.
46. Averill PM, et al: Guilt, shame, and psychopathology in obsessive compulsive disorder and trichotillomania. Presentation at the 29th annual convention of the Association for the Advancement of Behavior Therapy, Washington, 1995.
47. Masserman J: *Dynamic psychotherapy*, Philadelphia, 1955, WB Saunders.
48. Zaidens S: The skin: psychodynamics and psychological concepts, *J Nerv Ment Dis* 113:388–394, 1951.
49. Fenichel O: *The psychoanalytic theory of neuroses*, New York, 1945, WW Norton.
50. Greenberg HR: Transactions of a hairpulling symbiosis, *Psychiatr Q* 43:662–674, 1969.
51. Monroe JT, Abse DW: The psychopathology of trichotillomania and trichophagy, *Psychiatry* 26:95–103, 1963.
52. Oguchi T, Miura S: Trichotillomania: its psychopathological aspect, *Compr Psychiatry* 18:177–182, 1977.
53. Orange AP, Peereboom-Wynia JDR, DeRaeymaecker DMJ: Trichotillomania in childhood, *J Am Acad Dermatol* 15:614–619, 1986.
54. Stein DJ, O'Sullivan, Hollander E: Neurobiology of trichotillomania. In Stein DJ, Christenson GA, Hollander E, editors: *Trichotillomania: new developments*, Washington, American Psychiatric Press, in press.
55. Swedo SE, et al: A double-blind comparison of clomipramine and desipramine in the treatment of trichotillomania (hair pulling), *N Engl J Med* 321:497–501, 1989.
56. Stein DJ, et al: Compulsive and impulsive symptoms in trichotillomania, *Psychopathology* 28:208–213, 1995.
57. Stein DJ, Hollander E: Low-dose pimozide augmentation of serotonin reuptake blockers in the treatment of trichotillomania, *J Clin Psychiatry* 53:123–126, 1992.

58. Minichiello WE, et al: Trichotillomania: clinical aspects and treatment strategies, *Harvard Rev Psychiatry* 1:336–344, 1994.
59. Demeret A: Onychophagia, trichotillomania and grooming, *Ann Med Psychol (Paris)* 1:235–242, 1973.
60. Dodman NH, et al: Use of narcotic antagonists to modify stereotypic self-licking, self-chewing, and scratching behavior in dogs, *J Am Vet Med Assoc* 193:815–819, 1988.
61. Swedo SE: Rituals and releasers: an ethological model of obsessive compulsive disorder. In Rapoport JL, editor: *Obsessive-compulsive disorder in children and adolescents*, Washington, 1989, American Psychiatric Press.
62. Swedo SE, et al: Regional cerebral glucose metabolism of women with trichotillomania, *Arch Gen Psychiatry* 48:828–833, 1991.
63. Rettew DC, et al: Neuropsychological test performance in trichotillomania: a further link with obsessive-compulsive disorder, *J Anx Dis* 5:225–235, 1991.
64. Keuthen NJ, et al: Neuropsychological functioning in trichotillomania, *Biol Psychiatry* 39:747–749, 1996.
65. Hollander E, et al: Neurological soft signs in obsessive-compulsive disorder, *Arch Gen Psychiatry* 48:278–279, 1991.
66. Stein DJ, et al: Neurological soft signs in female patients with trichotillomania, *J Neuropsychiatry Clin Neurosci* 6:184–187, 1994.
67. Zohar J, et al: Serotonergic responsivity in obsessive-compulsive disorder: comparison of patients and healthy controls, *Arch Gen Psychiatry* 44:946–951, 1987.
68. Stein DJ, et al: Serotonergic responsivity in trichotillomania: neuroendocrine effects of m-chlorophenylpiperazine, *Biol Psychiatry* 37:414–416, 1995.
69. Hollander E, et al: Serotonergic sensitivity in borderline personality disorder: preliminary findings, *Am J Psychiatry* 151:277–280, 1994.
70. Ninan PT, et al: CSF 5HIAA as a predictor of treatment response in trichotillomania, *Psychopharmacol Bull* 28:451–455, 1992.
71. Rapoport JL, Ryland DH, Kriete M: Drug treatment of canine acral lick: an animal model of obsessive-compulsive disorder, *Arch Gen Psychiatry* 49:517–521, 1992.
72. Moon-Fanelli A, Dodman N, O'Sullivan RL: Veterinary models of trichotillomania. In Stein DJ, Christenson GA, Hollander E, editors: *Trichotillomania: new developments*, Washington, American Psychiatric Press, in press.
73. Christenson GA, Mackenzie TM, Reeve EA: Familial trichotillomania (letter), *Am J Psychiatry* 149:283, 1992.
74. Lenane MC, et al: Rates of obsessive compulsive disorder in first degree relatives of patients with trichotillomania: a research note, *J Child Psychol Psychiatry* 33:925–933, 1992.
75. Keuthen NJ, et al: Behavioral treatment for trichotillomania: a review. In Stein D, Christenson GA, Hollander E, editors: *Trichotillomania: new developments*, Washington, American Psychiatric Press, in press.
76. Friman PC, Finney JW, Christophersen ER: Behavioral treatment of trichotillomania: an evaluative review, *Behav Res Ther* 15:249–265, 1984.
77. Azrin NH, Nunn RG: Habit reversal: a method of eliminating nervous habits and tics, *Behav Res Ther* 11:619–628, 1973.
78. Azrin NH, Nunn RG, Frantz SE: Treatment of hairpulling (trichotillomania): a comparative study of habit reversal and negative practice training, *J Behav Ther Exp Psychiatry* 11:13–20, 1980.

79. Tarnowski KJ, et al: A modified habit reversal procedure in a recalcitrant case of trichotillomania, *J Behav Ther Exp Psychiatry* 18:157–163, 1987.
80. Rosenbaum MS, Ayllon T: The habit reversal technique in treating trichotillomania, *Behav Res Ther* 12:473–481, 1981.
81. De Luca RV, Holborn SW: A comparison of relaxation training and competing response training to eliminate hair pulling and nail biting, *J Behav Ther Exp Psychiatry* 15:67–70, 1984.
82. Vitulano LA, et al: Behavioral treatment of children and adolescents with trichotillomania, *J Am Acad Child Adolesc Psychiatry* 31:139–146, 1992.
83. Ottens AJ: A cognitive-behavioral modification treatment of trichotillomania, *J Am Coll Health* 31:78–81, 1982.
84. Stanley MA, et al: Treatment of trichotillomania with fluoxetine (letter), *J Clin Psychiatry* 52:282, 1991.
85. Anthony WZ: Brief intervention in a case of childhood trichotillomania by self-monitoring, *J Behav Ther Exp Psychiatry* 9:173–175, 1978.
86. Wulfsohn D, Barling J: From external to self-control: behavioral treatment of trichotillomania in an eleven-year-old girl, *Psychol Rep* 42:1171–1174, 1978.
87. Bayer CA: Self-monitoring and mild aversion treatment of trichotillomania, *J Behav Ther Exp Psychiatry* 3:139–141, 1972.
88. Saper B: A report on behavior therapy with outpatient clinic patients, *Psychiatr Q* 45:209–215, 1971.
89. Altman K, Grahs C, Friman P: Treatment of unobserved trichotillomania by attention-reflection and punishment of an apparent covariant, *J Behav Ther Exp Psychiatry* 13:337–340, 1982.
90. Massong SR, et al: A case of trichotillomania in a three-year-old treated by response prevention, *J Behav Ther Exp Psychiatry* 11:223–225, 1980.
91. Sanchez V: Behavioral treatment of chronic hair pulling in a two-year-old, *J Behav Ther Exp Psychiatry* 10:241–245, 1979.
92. Evans B: A case of trichotillomania in a child treated in a home program, *J Behav Ther Exp Psychiatry* 7:197–198, 1976.
93. Gray JJ: Positive reinforcement and punishment in the treatment of childhood trichotillomania, *J Behav Ther Exp Psychiatry* 10:125–129, 1979.
94. Stabler B, Warren AB: Behavioral contracting in treating trichotillomania: a case note, *Psychol Rep* 34:293–301, 1974.
95. Epstein LH, Peterson GL: The control of undesired behavior by self-imposed contingencies, *Behav Ther* 4:91–95, 1973.
96. Mastellone M: Aversion therapy: a new use for the old rubber band, *J Behav Ther Exp Psychiatry* 5:311–312, 1974.
97. Stevens MJ: Behavioral treatment of trichotillomania, *Psychol Rep* 55:987–990, 1984.
98. MacNeil J, Thomas MR: The treatment of obsessive compulsive hairpulling by behavioral and cognitive contingency manipulation, *J Behav Ther Exp Psychiatry* 7:391–392, 1976.
99. Altman K, Haavik S, Cook W: Punishment of self-injurious behavior in natural settings using contingent aromatic ammonia, *Behav Res Ther* 16:85–96, 1978.
100. De Horne DJ: Behaviour therapy for trichotillomania, *Behav Res Ther* 15:192–196, 1977.

101. Corte HE, Wolf MM, Locke BJ: A comparison of procedures for eliminating self-injurious behavior of retarded adolescents, *JABA* 4:201–213, 1971.
102. Friman PC, Hove C: Apparent covariation between child habit disorders: effects of successful treatment for thumb sucking on untargeted chronic hair pulling, *JABA* 20:421–425, 1987.
103. Knell SM, Moore DJ: Childhood trichotillomania treated indirectly by punishing thumb sucking, *J Behav Ther Exp Psychiatry* 19:305–310, 1988.
104. McLaughlin JG, Nay WR: Treatment of trichotillomania using positive coverants and response cost: a case report, *Behav Ther* 6:87–91, 1975.
105. Barrett RP, Shapiro ES: Treatment of stereotyped hairpulling with overcorrection: a case study with long term follow-up, *J Behav Ther Exp Psychiatry* 11:317–320, 1980.
106. Nelson WM: Behavioral treatment of childhood trichotillomania: a case study, *J Clin Child Psychol* 11:227–230, 1982.
107. Barmann BC, Vitali DL: Facial screening to eliminate trichotillomania in developmentally disabled persons, *Behav Res Ther* 13:735–742, 1982.
108. Gross AM, Farrar MJ, Liner D: Reduction of trichotillomania in a retarded cerebral palsied child using overcorrection, facial screening, and differential reinforcement of other behavior, *Edu Treat Child* 5:133–140, 1982.
109. Ottens AJ: Multifaceted treatment of compulsive hair pulling, *J Behav Ther Exp Psychiatry* 12:77–80, 1981.
110. Rothbaum BO: The behavioral treatment of trichotillomania, *Behav Psychother* 20:85–90, 1992.
111. Gluhoski VL: A cognitive approach for treating trichotillomania, *J Psychother Pract Res* 4:277–285, 1995.
112. Bernard ME, Kratochwill TR, Keefauver LW: The effects of rational-emotive therapy and self-instructional training on chronic hair pulling, *Cogn Ther Res* 7:273–280, 1983.
113. Levine BA: Treatment of trichotillomania by covert sensitization, *J Behav Ther Exp Psychiatry* 7:75–76, 1976.
114. Bornstein PH, Rychtarik RG: Multicomponent behavioral treatment of trichotillomania: a case study, *Behav Res Ther* 16:217–220, 1978.
115. Gardner GG: Hypnotherapy in the management of childhood habit disorders, *J Pediatr* 92:838–840, 1978.
116. Hall JR, McGill JC: Hypnobehavioral treatment of a self-destructive habit: trichotillomania, *Am J Clin Hypn* 29:39–46, 1986.
117. Galski TJ: The adjunctive use of hypnosis in the treatment of trichotillomania: a case report, *Am J Clin Hypn* 23:198–201, 1981.
118. Barabasz M: Trichotillomania: a new treatment, *Int J Clin Exp Hypn* 35:146–154, 1987.
119. Fabbri R, Dy AJ: Hypnotic treatment of trichotillomania: two cases, *Int J Clin Exp Hypn* 22:210–215, 1974.
120. Rowen R: Hypnotic age regression in the treatment of a self-destructive habit: trichotillomania, *Am J Clin Hypn* 23:195–197, 1981.
121. Hynes JV: Hypnotic treatment of five adult cases of trichotillomania, *Austr J Clin Exp Hypn* 10:109–116, 1982.
122. Childers RT: Report of two cases of trichotillomania of longstanding duration and

their response to chlorpromazine, *J Clin Exp Psychopathol Q Rev Psychiatry Neurol* 19:141–144, 1958.

123. Christenson GA, O'Sullivan RL: Trichotillomania: rational treatment options, *CNS Drugs* 6:23–34, 1996.

124. Christenson GA, et al: A placebo-controlled double-blind crossover study of fluoxetine in trichotillomania, *Am J Psychiatry* 148:1566–1571, 1991.

125. Pigott TA, et al: Controlled comparison of clomipramine and fluoxetine in trichotillomania (abstract). In Abstracts of panels and posters of the thirty-first annual meeting of the American College of Neuropsychopharmacology, San Juan, 1992, 157.

126. Christenson GA, et al: A placebo controlled double-blind study of naltrexone for trichotillomania (abstract), New Research Program and Abstracts, the 150th annual meeting of the American Psychiatric Association, Philadelphia, 1994, 212.

127. Streichenwein SM, Thornby JI: A long-term, double-blind, placebo-controlled crossover trial of the efficacy of fluoxetine for trichotillomania, *Am J Psychiatry* 152:1192–1196, 1995.

128. Winchel RM, et al: The Psychiatric Institute Trichotillomania Scale (PITS), *Psychopharm Bull* 28:463–476, 1992.

129. Benarroche CL: Trichotillomania symptoms and fluoxetine response (abstract), New Research Program and Abstracts, American Psychiatric Association Annual Meeting, New York, 1990, 173.

130. Alexander RC: Fluoxetine treatment of trichotillomania, *J Clin Psychiatry* 52:88, 1991.

131. Stanley M, et al: Treatment of trichotillomania with fluoxetine, *J Clin Psychiatry* 52:282, 1991.

132. Koran LM, Ringold A, Hewlett W: Fluoxetine for trichotillomania: an open clinical trial, *Psychopharmacol Bull* 28:145–214, 1992.

133. Winchel RM, et al: Clinical characteristics of trichotillomania and its response to fluoxetine, *J Clin Psychiatry* 53:304–308, 1992.

134. Benarroche CL: Discontinuation of fluoxetine in trichotillomania (abstract), New Research Program and Abstracts, American Psychiatric Association Annual Meeting, New Orleans, 1991, 138.

135. Reid TL: Treatment of resistant trichotillomania with paroxetine (letter), *Am J Psychiatry* 151:290, 1994.

136. Bradford JMW, Gratzer TG: A treatment for impulse control disorders and paraphilia: a case report, *Can J Psychiatry* 40:4–5, 1995.

137. Rahman MA, Gregory R: Trichotillomania associated with HIV infection and response to sertraline, *Psychosomatics* 36:417–418, 1995.

138. Snyder S: Trichotillomania treated with amitriptyline, *J Nerv Ment Dis* 168:505–507, 1980.

139. Sachdeva JS, Sidhu BS: Trichotillomania associated with depression, *J Indian Med Assoc* 85:151–152, 1987.

140. O'Sullivan RL, et al: Venlafaxine treatment of trichotillomania: a review of ten cases (abstract). Anxiety Disorders Association of American Annual Meeting, New Orleans, 1997.

141. Krishnan RR, Davidson J, Miller R: MAO inhibitor therapy in trichotillomania associated with depression: case report, *J Clin Psychiatry* 45:267–268, 1984.

142. Hussain SH: Trichotillomania, *JPMA* 42:19–20, 1992.
143. Sunkureddi K, Markovitz P: Trazodone treatment of obsessive-compulsive disorder and trichotillomania, *Am J Psychiatry* 150:523–524, 1993.
144. Popkin MK: Impulse control disorders not elsewhere classified. In Kaplan HI, Sadock BJ, editors: *Comprehensive textbook of psychiatry*, ed 5, Baltimore, 1989, Williams & Wilkins.
145. Christenson GA, et al: Lithium treatment of chronic hair pulling, *J Clin Psychiatry* 52:116–120, 1991.
146. Reid TL: Treatment of generalized anxiety disorder and trichotillomania with buspirone, *Am J Psychiatry* 149:573–574, 1992.
147. VanAmerigen M, Mancini C: Treatment of trichotillomania with haloperidol (abstract). Anxiety Disorders Association of American Annual Meeting, Orlando, 1996.
148. Ghaziuddin M, Tsai LY, Ghaziuddin N: Haloperidol treatment of trichotillomania in a boy with autism and mental retardation, *J Autism Dev Disord* 21:365–371, 1991.
149. McDougle CJ, et al: Neuroleptic addition in fluvoxamine-refractory obsessive-compulsive disorder, *Am J Psychiatry* 147:652–654, 1990.
150. Carrion VC: Naltrexone for the treatment of trichotillomania: a case report, *J Clin Psychopharmacol* 15:444–445, 1995.
151. Perciaccante M, Perciaccante RG: Progestin treatment of obsessive-compulsive disorder, *Psychosomatics* 34:284–285, 1993.
152. Mahr G: Fenfluramine and trichotillomania, *Psychosomatics* 34:284, 1993.
153. Black DW, Blum N: Trichotillomania treated with clomipramine and a topical steroid, *Am J Psychiatry* 149:842–843, 1992.
154. Gupta S, Freimer M: Trichotillomania, clomipramine, topical steroids, *Am J Psychiatry* 150:524, 1993.
155. Ristvedt SL, Christenson GA: The use of pharmacological pain sensitization in the treatment of repetitive hair pulling, *Behav Res Ther* 34:647–648, 1996.
156. Warnock JK: Psychotrophic medication and drug-related alopecia, *Psychosomatics* 32:149–152, 1991.
157. Pollard CA, et al: Clomipramine treatment of trichotillomania: a follow-up report on four cases, *J Clin Psychiatry* 52:128–130, 1991.
158. Swedo SE, Lenane MC, Leonard HL: Long-term treatment of trichotillomania (hair pulling), *N Engl J Med* 329:141–142, 1993.
159. Keuthen NJ, et al: A retrospective review of treatment outcome in 63 hair pullers, *Am J Psychiatry*, in press.

10

Body Dysmorphic Disorder: Clinical Aspects and Treatment Strategies

Katharine A. Phillips, M.D.

"The dysmorphophobic patient is really miserable; in the middle of his daily routines, talks, while reading, during meals, everywhere and at any time, he is caught by the doubt of deformity. . . ."

Enrique Morselli, 1891*

Body dysmorphic disorder (BDD), a preoccupation with an imagined or slight defect in appearance, has until recently been an underrecognized and understudied disorder. Although BDD can easily be trivialized and considered an epiphenomenon of our appearance-focused society, this often-secret disorder has been reported around the world and consistently described for more than 100 years.[1] In severe cases, individuals with this disorder may be unable to work, socialize, or leave their house, and some commit suicide.[1,2]

Written in 1891, Enrique Morselli's description of BDD (previously known as dysmorphophobia) reflects the suffering that characterizes this disorder. Morselli was one of several early psychopathologists who considered BDD to be related to obsessive-compulsive disorder (OCD), noting the obsessive nature of the "idea of deformity" and the compulsive checking behaviors (such as mirror checking) that accompany the obsessional worry.[3,4] Janet[5] similarly classified BDD within a group of syndromes related to OCD, referring to BDD as *obsession de la honte du corps* (obsession with shame of the body). He noted the morbidity caused by this disorder in his description of a 27-year-old woman who worried that no one would ever love her because she was "ugly

---

* From Fava GA: Morselli's legacy: dysmorphophobia, *Psychother Psychosom* 58:117–118, 1992.

and ridiculous," and who for 5 years confined herself to a tiny apartment that she rarely left.

Although BDD is classified in the *Diagnostic and Statistical Manual of Mental Disorders* (DSM-IV) as a somatoform disorder, a number of researchers conceptualize it as an "OCD-spectrum disorder" (i.e., a disorder with similarities to OCD in a variety of domains).[6,7] During the development of the DSM-IV, it was considered whether BDD should be moved from the somatoform disorder section to the anxiety disorder section alongside OCD.[8] In addition, reflecting its similarities with OCD, BDD is included in the Symptom Checklist of the Yale-Brown Obsessive Compulsive Scale (Y-BOCS)[9,10] (although the checklist notes that BDD is not a *bona fide* symptom of OCD and should not be included in scoring the Y-BOCS).

BDD is defined as a preoccupation with an imagined or slight defect in appearance that causes clinically significant distress or impairment in functioning.[11] In addition, it must not be better accounted for by another psychiatric disorder, such as anorexia nervosa. The delusional variant of BDD is classified as a somatic type of delusional disorder. However, cases of delusional BDD can be double coded as both delusional disorder and BDD, reflecting the possibility that BDD delusional and nondelusional variants may actually be a single disorder spanning a spectrum of insight, rather than two distinct disorders.[12,13]

The following case illustrates many of the clinical features of BDD.

Case 1

A 40-year-old divorced, unemployed man presented with a chief complaint of "I must be an alien—from another planet—because I look so strange." He disliked "everything" about his appearance—in particular, his nose, which he believed was protuberant and misshapen, his supposedly thinning hair, "stuck-out" ears, small body build, large jaw, ugly teeth, and thick eyebrows. The patient thought about his perceived deformities "24 hours a day." He had covered his hair with a hat for the past 15 years, and he tinted his car windows so he couldn't be seen while driving. He also frequently checked his "defects" in mirrors, and sometimes became so anxious when doing so that he experienced full-fledged panic attacks. The patient also frequently sought reassurance about his appearance and often discussed his desire for cosmetic surgery with others, to the point where his wife could no longer tolerate his incessant discussions about surgery and threatened him with a knife.

The patient had dropped out of high school to avoid a required physical examination during which his body would have been seen by a physician. He subsequently performed poorly at several jobs because he believed others took special notice of and mocked his supposed defects, and he sometimes missed work on days when he believed he looked especially ugly. He was eventually unable to work at all and received disability insurance. He also avoided most social situations and sometimes became completely housebound for weeks at a time. Because of his symptoms, his wife eventually divorced him. He frequently felt suicidal and once made a suicide attempt after inspecting himself in the mirror and feeling devastated by what he perceived.

The patient sought treatment from three dermatologists, three dentists, and 16 plastic surgeons, all of whom refused to treat him. He did eventually obtain a rhinoplasty but was disappointed with the results and later sued the surgeon. To obtain further plastic surgery, he was considering either going to another country, where he believed surgery would be easier to obtain, or having a car accident so he could "destroy (his) face" and have his insurance pay for total facial reconstruction.

CLINICAL FEATURES

Phenomenology

Individuals with BDD are preoccupied with the belief that some aspect of their appearance is unattractive, deformed, or "not right" in some way. These preoccupations commonly involve the face or head, although any body part can be the focus of concern.[2,14] The skin, hair, and nose are most often disliked (e.g., acne, scarring, lines, spots, or pale skin; hair thinning; or a large or crooked nose).[13] Many people with BDD have some concern involving bodily asymmetry. "Muscle dysmorphia" is a type of BDD in which individuals (usually men) worry that their body build is small and puny, when in reality they are typically large and muscular.[15]

Another variant of BDD, "BDD by proxy," consists of an obsession with supposed flaws in another person's appearance. This form of BDD may lead to the insistence that the other person have surgery or dermatologic treatment to correct the perceived problem.[16]

BDD preoccupations are distressing, time consuming, and usually difficult to resist or control. Unlike OCD, insight is often poor or absent.[17] One study found that more than half of 100 patients with BDD were delusional for a significant period of time, a percentage far higher than that reported for OCD.[13,18] BDD also is more often accompanied by ideas or delusions of reference[17] (thinking that others are taking special notice of the supposed defect and perhaps talking about it or mocking it). For example, a man who sang in a choir believed the entire audience was staring at a barely visible scar on his neck, and a woman believed that other people stared at her minor skin blemishes through binoculars. This experience can exacerbate the social isolation often caused by this disorder. Low self-esteem, shame, and fear of rejection are other features commonly associated with BDD.[16]

Although compulsive behaviors are not included in the diagnostic criteria for BDD, more than 90% of patients in one series performed one or more repetitive and often time-consuming behaviors.[13] The usual intent of such behaviors is to examine, improve, or hide the perceived defect (e.g., excessive mirror checking; excessive grooming or shaving, hair styling, or washing; comparing with others; reassurance seeking or trying to convince others of the defect's ugliness; skin picking; or weight lifting in the case of muscle dysmorphia). Some people with BDD compulsively cut their hair, trying to make it exactly even or "just right," which can leave them with very little hair and lead to wearing of turbans or wigs (which also may be cut). Others with BDD repeatedly seek dermatologic or surgical treatment. In addition, a majority camouflage the perceived deformity with hair, clothing, make-up, or body position (as when wearing six layers of T-shirts to "build up" a supposedly small body or constantly jutting out a "wimpy-looking" jaw).

There is no limit to the strategies patients may devise to try to alleviate their suffering. One teenage boy who believed his facial features were asymmetrical tried to "straighten them out" by tying socks tightly around his head to the point of causing pain. To make his calves smaller, another man tied them up with rope when he slept. A man who worried about hair loss searched his pillow each morning for hair, saved those he found in a plastic bag, and developed complex math formulas to determine his rate of hair loss.

Many of these behaviors may actually increase, rather than decrease, anxiety. Many patients, for example, report increased anxiety after looking in the mirror, which sometimes even precipitates a suicide attempt. Although skin picking may temporarily relieve tension, most patients feel more anxious and depressed after performing this behavior when they survey the damage done to their skin.

Impairment Caused by Body Dysmorphic Disorder

Level of functioning is widely variable in BDD, as in OCD.[2] Some people, with effort, function well despite their distress, although often below their capacity. Preoccupation with appearance can impair concentration, and associated behaviors can consume significant amounts of time. Some BDD sufferers are severely impaired by their symptoms.[1,2] They may perform their job or school work poorly, drop out of school, quit their job, or go on disability.

Some degree of social impairment is nearly universal, and individuals with BDD may have few friends, avoid dating and other social interactions, or divorce because of their symptoms. They often avoid specific situations, such as restaurants, beaches, or shopping, in which they feel particularly self-conscious about their appearance. In one series, 30% of patients had been housebound for at least 1 week, more than 50% had been psychiatrically hospitalized, and 25% had made a suicide attempt.[2]

Some BDD sufferers have gotten into car accidents as a result of checking the rearview mirror when driving. Some pick their skin so deeply that they require emergency surgery.[19,20] Yet others perform their own surgery, as did one man who cut his nose open and tried to replace his own cartilage with chicken cartilage.[16]

Demographic Features and Course of Illness

The reported gender ratio of BDD has varied, with some studies reporting a preponderance of men[14,21] and others a preponderance of women.[22,23] In the largest series to date of DSM-IV BDD (n = 188), we found that 51% were men.[24] The clinical features of BDD in men and women appear generally similar.[24] Nearly 75% of BDD patients have never been married.[13]

BDD usually begins during adolescence[25] and can also occur in childhood,[26] although the condition remains underrecognized in these age groups. Available data suggest that the disorder is usually chronic, with waxing and waning symptoms over time,[13] although prospective studies are needed to confirm these impressions.

Comorbidity

Major depression appears to occur most often with BDD, with one study reporting a current rate of about 60% and a lifetime rate of more than 80%.[13] Other commonly comorbid disorders in this series were social phobia, substance use disorders, and OCD (all with lifetime rates of more than 30%). Similar comorbidity patterns were reported by another investigator,[14] although a report from England found notably lower rates of comorbid disorders.[22]

Rates of BDD ranging from 8% to 78% have been reported among patients with OCD.[14,27–29] BDD also has been found to occur at a relatively high rate (14%) among patients with atypical major depression.[30]

Family History

Hollander and colleagues[14] reported that OCD was the most common disorder in relatives of 50 patients with BDD. Although the presence of comorbid OCD in a high percentage of probands (78%) could account for this finding, it also may indicate that BDD and OCD are related disorders. We found that 4% of 172 first-degree relatives of BDD probands had OCD—a rate approximately twice that in the general population.[31] Major depression and substance use disorders were more common in relatives, both present in 17%. The family history method used in this study probably underestimated the rate of psychiatric disorders in relatives. BDD may occur in multiple generations of some families, as in one family in which both of the proband's parents and both maternal grandmothers appeared to have BDD.

Diagnosing Body Dysmorphic Disorder

BDD can be difficult to diagnose because sufferers often keep their symptoms secret because of embarrassment or shame. Other common reasons for underdiagnosis or misdiagnosis are pursuit of surgical and dermatologic treatment and clinicians' lack of familiarity with BDD.[1] Because of shame over their BDD symptoms, patients may volunteer only their depression, anxiety, or discomfort in social situations. Consequently, BDD may be misdiagnosed as social phobia or agoraphobia (because of secondary social anxiety and isolation), panic disorder (because situational panic attacks may occur, for example, after looking in the mirror), trichotillomania (in patients who cut or pluck their hair for the sake of appearance), or OCD (because of the similar obsessional preoccupation and compulsive behaviors). Delusional patients with BDD are sometimes misdiagnosed with schizophrenia or psychotic depression. In general, to diagnose BDD, clinicians typically need to ask specifically about BDD symptoms.

TREATMENT STRATEGIES

Surgical, Dermatologic, and Other Nonpsychiatric Medical Treatment

Because patients with BDD think they have a physical problem, and because their insight is often poor, most seen in a psychiatric setting have sought often-costly nonpsychiatric treatment.[13,14] Dermatologists and surgeons are most often consulted, although ophthalmologists may be asked to correct "cross-eyed" eyes; endocrinologists to evaluate "excessive" body hair; and urologists to enlarge "small" genitals. One author referred to patients with BDD as "polysurgery addicts."[21]

Although prospective studies are lacking, it appears that most patients with BDD are dissatisfied with such treatment; many dislike their appearance even more or develop new preoccupations with their appearance.[1,13] Multiple procedures may be received in the search for a cosmetic solution to this psychiatric problem. One author noted that patients who have cosmetic surgery "will often then find a new 'defect,' which needs correction; they may eventually become synthetic creations of artificial noses, breasts, ears, and hips."[32] Some dissatisfied patients have sued their physicians or become violent.[33]

Pharmacotherapy and Other Somatic Treatments

Although BDD has been said to be "extremely difficult" to treat,[34] preliminary data suggest that serotonin reuptake inhibitors (SRIs) and cognitive-behavioral therapy may be effective for many patients. Early reports noted response of one patient to clomipramine,[35] three patients to fluoxetine,[36] and five patients to fluoxetine or clomipramine after failing a variety of medications.[37] In a series of 130 patients (who had received a total of 316 medication trials) in whom treatment was assessed retrospectively, 42% of 65 SRI trials (fluoxetine, clomipramine, fluvoxamine, sertraline, or paroxetine) resulted in "much" or "very much" improvement, compared with 30% of 23 trials with monoamine oxidase inhibitors (MAOIs), 15% of 48 trials with non–SRI tricyclics, 3% with neuroleptics, 6% with a variety of other medications (e.g., benzodiazepines and mood stabilizers), and 0% of electroconvulsive therapy (ECT) trials.[38] Similarly, another retrospective study of 50 patients with BDD found that 35 SRI trials resulted in "much" improvement, whereas 18 non–SRI tricyclic trials resulted in no overall improvement in BDD symptoms.[14,39] In a study of 45 patients openly treated in a clinical practice with an SRI, 70% (43 of 61) of SRI trials resulted in "much" or "very much" improvement.[38]

Two open-label studies of the SRI fluvoxamine have been performed. In one, 19 (63%) of 30 subjects with DSM-IV BDD responded,[40] based on a version of the Yale-Brown Obsessive Compulsive Scale modified for BDD (the BDD-YBOCS).[41] The mean dose of fluvoxamine was approximately 240 mg/day and mean time to response was approximately 6 weeks, with one patient requiring as long as 14 weeks. Five responders discontinued fluvoxamine after completing the study, all of whom relapsed, with BDD symptoms significantly improving when an SRI was restarted. Of note, among subjects with comorbid OCD, change in severity of BDD and OCD was not significantly correlated. In another open-label study of fluvoxamine, two thirds of 15 subjects were considered responders based on the Clinical Global Impressions Scale.[42] These data, although promising, are limited by their uncontrolled nature. Prospective, controlled pharmacotherapy studies are needed to confirm these findings.

Available data indicate that response to medication usually results in decreased distress and time preoccupied with the "defect," decreased performance of associated compulsive behaviors, and improvement in functioning (all items on the BDD-YBOCS generally improve).[40] Many responders to SRIs also experience improved insight and a decrease in referential thinking. However, insight does not always improve with treatment, and in some cases in which it does improve, the patient still maintains that the defect was present and ugly prior to treatment. Improved insight with an SRI sometimes appears to be the result of resolution of an apparent visual illusion (i.e., patients' reports that they can no longer visually detect the defect). This outcome is interesting, given that serotonin appears to modulate the visual system.[38]

Of note, available data suggest that patients with delusional BDD (delusional disorder, somatic type) are as likely as those patients with nondelusional BDD to respond to SRIs.[13] Although requiring confirmation in controlled studies, this intriguing finding suggests that SRIs may be effective for some types of psychosis. It also raises the question of whether certain other types of delusional disorder with similarities to OCD (e.g., the jealous type of delusional disorder or olfactory reference syndrome) might also respond to SRIs.

Patients with BDD should receive an SRI for 12 weeks or longer before concluding that the medication is ineffective. Although dose-finding studies have not yet been performed, our experience is that some patients require relatively high SRI doses (either the highest dose tolerated or recommended by the manufacturer should be reached before concluding the medication is ineffective).

Although formal medication discontinuation studies have not been performed, we have found that most patients relapse after SRI discontinuation and that long-term treatment is often needed, with efficacy usually sustained over time. Some patients, however, do not experience recurrence of their symptoms (or experience only a partial relapse) after medication discontinuation.

Augmentation of an SRI with buspirone or pimozide (or perhaps other neuroleptics such as risperidone or olanzapine) is a promising strategy for patients who do not respond or respond only partially to an SRI. In an open study (n = 13), buspirone was added to fluoxetine or clomipramine (after reaching the highest dose tolerated or recommended by the manufacturers of these drugs and at least 10 weeks of treatment).[43] Six subjects (46%) were considered "much" or "very much" improved with buspirone augmentation (mean buspirone dose: 48.3 ± 14.7 mg/day; mean time to response = 6.4 weeks). Three of these responders later relapsed with decrease or discontinuation of buspirone.

Another option is to combine clomipramine with a selective SRI when an adequate trial of one of these medications alone has been ineffective. This approach is most rational when attempting to improve on a partial response to an adequate trial of one of these agents. Clomipramine blood levels should always be monitored when combined with a selective SRI because of the potential of SRI to increase clomipramine levels. In addition, patients who fail one adequate SRI trial may respond to another SRI. If none of these strategies are effective, MAOI may be worth trying.

Other medications used as single agents have not been well studied in BDD, although in the two retrospective studies previously noted, agents other than SRIs were not often effective (although MAOIs were of intermediate effectiveness). The question of whether non–SRI antidepressants are effective for BDD is interesting and important; if they are not, as retrospective data suggest, this would give strong support to the hypothesis that BDD is related to OCD. Another important question is whether antipsychotics alone are effective for delusional BDD, as might be expected. Although retrospective data suggest they are rarely effective, this question, too, requires controlled investigation. Pimozide, in particular, has been noted as particularly effective for monosymptomatic hypochondriacal psychosis[34] (the precursor of DSM-IV delusional disorder, somatic type) and deserves further study.

Available uncontrolled evidence suggests that ECT is generally ineffective for BDD. ECT was ineffective in six published case reports[1] and effective in two.[44,45] In the author's series of 130 cases, zero of eight ECT trials were successful (although the data were largely retrospective).[38]

Regarding psychosurgery, one published case report noted improvement in BDD symptoms with a modified leucotomy.[44] In another case, significant improvement occurred with a capsulotomy (Mindus P, personal communication), and another patient improved with a bilateral anterior cingulotomy and subcaudate tractotomy (Cassem E, personal communication).

Cognitive-Behavioral Therapy

Preliminary data suggest that cognitive-behavioral therapy (CBT) may be effective for BDD. Although earlier case reports noted an unsuccessful outcome with behavioral approaches,[1] one reported improvement using systematic desensitization[46] and another with exposure therapy.[47] More recently, several investigators have reported that strategies such as cognitive restructuring, exposure (e.g., exposing the defect in social situations and preventing avoidance behaviors), and response prevention (avoiding compulsive behaviors, such as mirror checking and reassurance seeking) are effective for a majority of patients.[22,23,48] In one report of five patients with BDD, four improved using such approaches in 90-minute sessions 1 day or 5 days per week (with the total number of sessions ranging from 12 to 48).[48] Techniques included having patients cover or remove mirrors, limiting grooming time, and stopping the use of make-up. Exposure techniques were used after developing an anxiety hierarchy that included having patients go to avoided restaurants or stores, sitting in crowded waiting rooms, and messing up their hair before interacting with other people.

Another study found that exposure and response prevention plus cognitive techniques were effective in 77% of 27 women who received this treatment in eight weekly 2-hour group sessions.[23] This study used similar techniques (e.g., exposure to social situations and avoiding camouflage, resisting body-checking behaviors, and changing negative self-statements about appearance). Subjects in the treatment group improved more than those in a no-treatment, waiting-list control group. Although this result is promising, the subjects appeared to have had relatively mild BDD, and many seemed to be in a "diagnostic gray zone" between BDD and eating disorders.

In a pilot study of 19 patients (primarily women) who were randomly assigned to a CBT group or a no-treatment, waiting-list control group, there was significantly greater improvement in BDD symptoms in the group that received CBT, and seven of nine patients who received CBT no longer met criteria for BDD at the end of the study.[22]

As is the case for pharmacotherapy, well-controlled studies are needed to confirm the effectiveness of CBT for BDD (only waiting-list controls have been used). Unanswered questions are the length and number of sessions needed, and whether response is maintained after treatment ends; no follow-up studies of CBT have been performed. An additional question is how effective is this treatment for more severely ill patients, who are often delusional, severely depressed, and suicidal?

No studies have been performed on the effectiveness of combining CBT and pharmacotherapy, although clinical experience suggests that some patients benefit from combining these treatments and that the combination is worth trying for patients who do not respond to CBT or medication alone.

Other Treatment Approaches

Although adequate data are lacking, it appears that BDD symptoms are unlikely to significantly improve with supportive or insight-oriented psychotherapy alone.[2] Most patients report that such treatments do not diminish their obsessional preoccupation with the defect or associated compulsive behaviors. Nonetheless, some patients do benefit from the addition of such treatments to CBT or medication. Insight-oriented or supportive therapy may be helpful for other disorders or problems that the patient may have, and most patients benefit from support in coping with their illness, whether from more formal supportive psychotherapy or as part of CBT or medication treatment.

Psychoeducation is an important element of any treatment, because patients benefit from learning what is known about BDD and what treatments may be helpful.[16] Educating family members and significant others also can facilitate treatment. Family members should be advised not to help perform BDD rituals (e.g., they should be asked to take down mirrors and avoid holding mirrors or lights for the patient, providing reassurance, or participating in grooming rituals). Family members also should not allow their lives to be severely disrupted by BDD symptoms, and they should encourage the patient to function at as high a level as possible while recognizing the person's limitations resulting from illness.

SUMMARY

Current data suggest that BDD patients' treatment response may be similar to that of OCD patients, with a possible preferential response to SRIs and CBT. However, treatment data are preliminary at this time, and the efficacy of these treatments requires confirmation in well-controlled studies.

It is sometimes difficult to persuade patients with BDD (especially those who are delusional) to accept psychiatric treatment. Some refuse treatment because they are convinced that surgical, dermatologic, or other medical treatment is needed to fix the perceived defect. A useful approach is to emphasize that psychiatric treatment can be helpful for their distress and suffering and may improve their functioning. Trying to convince delusional patients that psychiatric treatment is needed because their view of the defect is inaccurate or "imagined" is unlikely to be successful.

CONCLUSIONS

In the past few years, BDD has gone from being a neglected psychiatric disorder to one that is becoming better recognized and understood. Nonetheless, research on this disorder is still in its early stages, and much more investigation of BDD is needed. In addition to further research on its clinical features and treatment response, studies are needed that will shed light on its etiology and pathophysiology.

Another mystery that has yet to be solved is the nature of the BDD relationship to OCD. Is this condition a form of OCD, a related but distinct disorder, or a separate disorder? Available evidence suggests that BDD has many similarities to OCD, but also some important differences, such as poorer insight, higher comorbidity with major depression and social phobia, and possibly a higher suicide attempt rate.[29] BDD also has some features in common with social phobia.[48] Further complicating this issue is the likelihood that BDD is a heterogeneous disorder, with some forms more closely related to OCD or social phobia, and others more closely related to other disorders, such as the eating disorders. When more is understood about the underlying neurobiology of BDD, the answers to these questions will become clearer.

In the meantime, it is important that clinicians screen patients for BDD and accurately diagnose this condition, because available treatments are very promising for patients who suffer from this distressing and sometimes disabling disorder.

REFERENCES

1. Phillips KA: Body dysmorphic disorder: The distress of imagined ugliness, *Am J Psychiatry* 148:1138–1149, 1991.
2. Phillips KA, McElroy SL, Keck PE Jr, et al: Body dysmorphic disorder: 30 cases of imagined ugliness, *Am J Psychiatry* 150:302–308, 1993.
3. Morselli E: Sulla dismorfofobia e sulla tafefobia, *Bolletinno Della R Accademia di Genova* 6:110–119, 1891.
4. Fava GA: Morselli's legacy: Dysmorphophobia, *Psychother Psychosom* 58:117–118, 1992.
5. Janet P: *Les obsessions et la psychasthenie,* Paris, 1903, Felix Alcan.
6. Hollander E, Phillips KA: Body image and experience disorders: Body dysmorphic and depersonalization disorders. In Hollander E, editor: *Obsessive compulsive-related disorders*, Washington, 1993, American Psychiatric Press.
7. McElroy SL, Phillips KA, Keck PE Jr: Obsessive-compulsive spectrum disorders, *J Clin Psychiatry* 55(suppl):33–51, 1994.
8. Phillips KA, Hollander E: Body dysmorphic disorder. In Widiger TA, Frances AJ, Pincus HA, et al, editors: *DSM-IV sourcebook*, vol 2, Washington, 1996, American Psychiatric Association.
9. Goodman WK, Price LH, Rasmussen SA, et al: The Yale-Brown Obsessive Compulsive Scale (Y-BOCS): Part I. Development, use, and reliability, *Arch Gen Psychiatry* 46:1006–1011, 1989.
10. Goodman WK, Price LH, Rasmussen SA, et al: The Yale-Brown Obsessive Compulsive Scale (Y-BOCS): Part II. Validity, *Arch Gen Psychiatry* 46:1012–1016, 1989.
11. American Psychiatric Association: *Diagnostic and statistical manual of mental disorders*, ed 4, Washington, 1994, American Psychiatric Association.
12. Phillips KA, McElroy SL: Insight, overvalued ideation, and delusional thinking in body dysmorphic disorder: Theoretical and treatment implications, *J Nerv Ment Dis* 181:699–702, 1993.

13. Phillips KA, McElroy SL, Keck PE Jr, et al: A comparison of delusional and non-delusional body dysmorphic disorder in 100 cases, *Psychopharmacol Bull* 30: 179–186, 1994.
14. Hollander E, Cohen LJ, Simeon D: Body dysmorphic disorder, *Psychiatric Ann* 23:359–364, 1993.
15. Pope HG Jr, Gruber AJ, Choi P, et al: "Muscle dysmorphia": An underrecognized form of body dysmorphic disorder, *Psychosomatics* 38(6):548–557, 1997.
16. Phillips KA: *The broken mirror*, New York, 1996, Oxford University Press.
17. Eisen JL, Phillips KA, Rasmussen SA: Delusionality in OCD, body dysmorphic disorder, and mood disorders. Syllabus and Proceedings Summary, American Psychiatric Association 149th Annual Meeting. New York, 1996, American Psychiatric Association, p 165.
18. Eisen JL, Rasmussen SA: Obsessive compulsive disorder with psychotic features, *J Clin Psychiatry* 54:373–379, 1993.
19. O'Sullivan RL, Phillips KA, Keuthen NJ, et al: Near fatal skin picking from delusional body dysmorphic disorder responsive to fluvoxamine, *Psychosomatics,* in press.
20. Phillips KA, Taub SL: Skin picking as a symptom of body dysmorphic disorder, *Psychopharmacol Bull* 31:279–288, 1995.
21. Fukuda O: Statistical analysis of dysmorphophobia in out-patient clinic, *Japan J Plast Reconstr Surg* 20:569–577, 1977.
22. Veale D, Boocock A, Gournay K, et al: Body dysmorphic disorder: A survey of fifty cases, *Br J Psychiatry* 169:196–201, 1996.
23. Rosen JC, Reiter J, Orosan P: Cognitive-behavioral body image therapy for body dysmorphic disorder, *J Consult Clin Psychol* 63:263–269, 1995.
24. Phillips KA, Diaz S: Gender differences in body dysmorphic disorder, *J Nerv Ment Dis* 185:570–577, 1997.
25. Phillips KA, Atala KD, Albertini RS: Body dysmorphic disorder in adolescents, *J Am Acad Child Adolesc Psychiatry* 34:1216–1220, 1995.
26. Albertini R, Phillips KA, Guvremont D: Body dysmorphic disorder in a young child (letter), *J Am Acad Child Adolesc Psychiatry* 35:1425–1426, 1996.
27. Brawman-Mintzer O, Lydiard RB, Phillips KA, et al: Body dysmorphic disorder in patients with anxiety disorders and major depression: A comorbidity study, *Am J Psychiatry* 152:1665–1667, 1995.
28. Simeon D, Hollander E, Stein DJ, et al: Body dysmorphic disorder in the DSM-IV Field Trial for obsessive compulsive disorder, *Am J Psychiatry* 152:1207–1209, 1995.
29. Phillips KA, McElroy SL, Hudson JI, et al: Body dysmorphic disorder: An obsessive compulsive spectrum disorder, a form of affective spectrum disorder, or both? *J Clin Psychiatry* 56(suppl):41–51, 1995.
30. Phillips KA, Nierenberg AA, Brendel G, et al: Prevalence and clinical features of body dysmorphic disorder in atypical major depression, *J Nerv Ment Dis* 184: 125–129, 1996.
31. McElroy SL, Phillips KA, Keck PE Jr, et al: Body dysmorphic disorder: does it have a psychotic subtype? *J Clin Psychiatry* 54:389–395, 1993.
32. Andreasen NC, Bardach J: Dysmorphophobia: Symptom or disease? *Am J Psychiatry* 134:673–675, 1977.

33. Phillips KA, McElroy SL, Lion JR: Body dysmorphic disorder in cosmetic surgery patients, *J Plast Reconstr Surg* 90:333–334, 1992 (letter).
34. Munro A, Chmara J: Monosymptomatic hypochondriacal psychosis: A diagnostic checklist based on 50 cases of the disorder, *Can J Psychiatry* 27:374–376, 1982.
35. Sondheimer A: Clomipramine treatment of delusional disorder, somatic type, *J Am Acad Child Adolesc Psychiatry* 27:188–192, 1988.
36. Brady KT, Austin L, Lydiard RB: Body dysmorphic disorder: The relationship to obsessive-compulsive disorder, *J Nerv Ment Dis* 178:538–540, 1990.
37. Hollander E, Liebowitz MR, Winchel R, et al: Treatment of body-dysmorphic disorder with serotonin reuptake blockers, *Am J Psychiatry* 146:768–770, 1989.
38. Phillips KA: Pharmacologic treatment of body dysmorphic disorder, *Psychopharmacol Bull* 32:597–605, 1996.
39. Hollander E, Cohen L, Simeon D, et al: Fluvoxamine treatment of body dysmorphic disorder, *J Clin Psychopharmacol* 14:75–77, 1994 (letter).
40. Phillips KA, Dwight M, McElroy SL: Efficacy and safety of fluvoxamine in body dysmorphic disorder, *J Clin Psych,* in press.
41. Phillips KA, Hollander E, Rasmussen SA, et al: A severity rating scale for body dysmorphic disorder: Development, reliability, and validity of a modified version of the Yale-Brown Obsessive Compulsive Scale, *Psychopharmacol Bull* 33:17–22, 1997.
42. Perugi G, Giannotti D, Di Vaio S, et al: Fluvoxamine in the treatment of body dysmorphic disorder (dysmorphophobia), *Int Clin Psychopharmacol* 11:247–254, 1996.
43. Phillips KA: An open study of buspirone augmentation of serotonin-reuptake inhibitors in body dysmorphic disorder, *Psychopharmacol Bull* 32:175–180, 1996.
44. Hay GG: Dysmorphophobia, *Br J Psychiatry* 116:399–406, 1970.
45. Carroll BJ: Response of major depression with psychosis and body dysmorphic disorder to ECT, *Am J Psychiatry* 151:288–289, 1994 (letter).
46. Munjack J: The behavioral treatment of dysmorphophobia, *J Behav Ther Exp Psychiatry* 9:53–56, 1978.
47. Marks I, Mishan J: Dysmorphophobic avoidance with disturbed bodily perception: A pilot study of exposure therapy, *Br J Psychiatry* 152:674–678, 1988.
48. Neziroglu FA, Yaryura-Tobias JA: Exposure, response prevention, and cognitive therapy in the treatment of body dysmorphic disorder, *Behav Res Ther* 24:431–438, 1993.
49. Kasahara Y: Social phobia in Japan. In *Social phobia in Japan and Korea: Proceedings of the first cultural psychiatry symposium between Japan and Korea*, Seoul, 1987, Academy of Cultural Psychiatry.

Part III

Pathophysiology and Assessment

11

Theories of Etiology

Michael A. Jenike, M.D.

Early theories concerning the etiology of obsessive-compulsive disorders (OCD) involved possession by outside forces, and treatment involved exorcism of some sort. Janet and Freud presented some of the first rational hypotheses. Janet[1] considered the disorder as arising from psychic fatigue and diminution of available mental energy, causing a lack of control over an individual's thoughts and thereby precipitating obsessional ideas and compulsive acts (see Pitman[2] for review). Janet was also the first to use exposure techniques in the treatment of these patients.

There are currently more than 20 different ideas on what might be the cause of OCD and the only statement we can say with certainty is that we still have no idea of the etiology of this mysterious but treatable disorder. If we knew the cause, there would only be one theory.

Because virtually no researchers still view this disorder as solely psychologic in nature, investigators have been looking for chemical, structural, or functional abnormalities in these patients. With most of the modern studies, matched control groups have been used and quite careful and accurate measurements are now being reported. The future of these research efforts appears bright. Some of the neurologic and neurochemical etiologic hypotheses are reviewed in Chapter 12 on the neurobiology of OCD. This chapter will review some of the other speculations on etiology.

PSYCHODYNAMIC THEORY

Freud's earliest theory, abandoned when he altered his ideas on the role of sexual trauma, held that obsessional thoughts were the result of an actual genital experience during childhood in which the child was an active participant.[3] His later theories defined obsessions as defensive psychologic responses to unconscious impulses. He focused his attention on the mother-infant interaction and considered issues of aggression and autonomy to be paramount around the time of toilet training, when the child strives to hold on to valuable feces and the mother requests that he give them up to please her. Freud developed concepts of anality and anal sadism and proposed that hostile impulses against the parents were controlled by obsessive-compulsive behavior. In light of these theories, one might wonder why the disorder does not begin around the time of toilet training. Freud felt that the development of obsessional symptoms later in life could be explained as a regression to the earlier anal-sadistic era with the ego, superego, and id functioning in a manner appropriate to that phase. He theorized that these patients used ego defenses of reaction formation, isolation, displacement, and undoing to control their internal anxious state (see Chapter 27). In other words, the obsessional symptom, regardless of how revolting or uncomfortable, is still less distressing than the idea it is masking.

Any therapist who has worked in psychodynamic psychotherapy with obsessional patients cannot dispute the wisdom of Freud's observations—at least as they apply to some patients where issues of control, aggression, and sexuality persistently arise (see Chapter 27). Such issues are close to the surface and such patients are strikingly useful in teaching psychodynamic concepts. Unfortunately, understanding their psychologic workings leads to little change in obsessive or compulsive symptoms.

In contrast to patients with obsessive-compulsive *personality* disorder (i.e., similar to Freud's obsessional character) and other disorders with obsessional symptoms, OCD is generally believed to be refractory to traditional psychotherapeutic maneuvers. To our knowledge, there is not a single case report in the modern psychiatric literature of the efficacy of psychodynamic or psychoanalytic psychotherapy alone in OCD. These patients may well benefit in other areas from traditional psychotherapy, but obsessive-compulsive symptoms will likely persist.

LEARNING THEORY

In view of the success of behavioral treatments in OCD patients (see Chapters 17, 19, and 20), learning theories are particularly important.[4–6] According to these theories, obsessions or compulsions are conditioned responses that lower anxiety (see Chapters 17 and 19); these responses become established when a person learns that anxiety can be reduced by this mechanism. The relief brought about by the performance of a compulsive act reinforces that act. Gradually, because of its usefulness in reducing anxiety, the act becomes fixed in a learned pattern of behavior.

Learning theories of OCD are covered in detail in Chapter 17. Behaviorists concentrate predominantly on the symptoms themselves (i.e., compulsive behaviors) and are largely unconcerned with underlying psychodynamic hypotheses.

MEDICAL AND NEUROLOGIC ETIOLOGIES

Until the last few years, OCD was widely viewed as psychologic in genesis. However, the intractability of these states to traditional psychotherapeutic intervention and the often dramatic response to medication[4-8] or surgical intervention[9-16] suggest a cerebral basis for this disorder.[17-19]

Association with Infections

The first reported connection between a neurologic illness and OCD was made in the early part of the twentieth century, when von Economo's encephalitis swept across the United States in successive epidemics. No organism was ever isolated, but neurologic sequelae in survivors were common. The natural history of the illness had the characteristics of an encephalitic disorder caused by a neurotropic virus, and more recent epidemiologic studies confirm von Economo's[20] original suspicion that the illness was related to influenza.[21] The illness was established as an entity by its neuropsychiatric sequelae, particularly parkinsonism, oculogyric crises, movement disorders, and a wide range of chronic psychiatric illnesses, especially psychopathic and psychotic states.[22] There also were frequent case reports of patients who developed OCD after recovery from the encephalitis.[23-26] Some experts[22] hypothesize that sporadic cases of this infection still occur, and that these cases may be the antecedent of much chronic psychiatric illness.[27] There also is one case report of a previously healthy man who developed severe OCD in combination with various tics and dyskinesias after encephalitis, presumably induced by a wasp sting. A computed tomography (CT) scan demonstrated bilateral pallidostriatal necrosis.[28]

In 1938, Schilder noted this relationship between OCD and encephalitis and wondered if all obsessions and compulsions had an underlying neurologic cause. He attempted to link psychoanalytic theory with clinical neurology and theorized that encephalitis may produce a structural or chemical change releasing underlying hostile impulses, which the patient then tries to control through obsessional behavior. Noting that most obsessive patients did not have a history of encephalitis, he found seven OCD patients with mild neurologic abnormalities, including very mild tremor, decreased movement of arms, rigid face, akinesia, and hyperkinesis. Schilder concluded that two thirds of OCD patients had a neurologic cause for their disorder and that psychologic factors alone were important in one third of patients. He stated that most cases were not caused by subclinical epidemic encephalitis, but rather were caused by "lesions in fetal life, to birth trauma or to toxic and infectious processes of unknown etiology." Schilder was one of the first to speculate on the role of organic etiologies of OCD.

Grimshaw[29] wondered about a relationship between neurologic illness and obsessional disorders. He studied 103 obsessional patients and reported that 19.4% had a history of neurologic illness compared with only 7.6% of a control group of 105 normal subjects (a significant difference; $p = 0.05$). Six OCD patients had serious central nervous system infections: three had meningitis, two had epidemic encephalitis, and one patient had polio encephalitis. Eight patients had a history of convulsive disorder: five had infantile seizures, two had grand mal epilepsy, and one patient had eclampsia. Six patients had a history of chorea consistent with Sydenham's chorea. An important limitation of this study was the fact that the majority of the reports came solely from patient history and were not verified either clinically or by hospital records. All of the patients were subject to neurologic examination, but none of Schilder's signs were found.

Grimshaw's finding that some OCD patients had a history of Sydenham's chorea is of interest in light of a more recent study by Rapoport[30] who, noting that there recently had been a resurgence of rheumatic fever in parts of the United States, conducted a survey of 37 patients with rheumatic fever. Approximately 20% of rheumatic fever patients develop Sydenham's chorea, probably as the result of an autoimmune response to the basal ganglia, leading to potential damage in that area.[30] In her survey, 23 of the rheumatic fever patients had developed Sydenham's chorea and 14 did not have chorea. In blind evaluations, in which the interviewer did not know the medical diagnosis, scores for obsessional symptoms were significantly higher among those patients with Sydenham's chorea. In addition, three chorea patients, but no rheumatic fever patients without chorea, met diagnostic criteria for full-fledged OCD. This has been considered as evidence that, at least in some patients, dysfunction of the basal ganglia may be involved in OCD.

In children, such symptoms have been called *pediatric autoimmune neuropsychiatric disorders associated with streptococcal infections (PANDAS),* which may arise when antibodies directed against invading strep bacteria crossreact with basal ganglia structures, resulting in onset or exacerbation of OCD or tic disorder. There is a report[31] of severe worsening of obsessive-compulsive symptoms in an adolescent boy following infection with group A β-hemolytic streptococci for whom serial magnetic resonance imaging scans of the brain were acquired to assess the relationship between basal ganglia size, symptom severity, and treatment with plasmapheresis. OCD symptoms were associated with acute basal ganglia enlargement. These data provide further support for basal ganglia–mediated dysfunction in OCD and the potential for immunologic treatment in PANDAS patients.

Why do some patients develop OCD symptoms as a consequence of streptococcal infection and Sydenham's chorea and others do not? Intriguing recent findings[32] suggest that D8/17, a B lymphocyte antigen, may serve as a marker for susceptibility to some forms of childhood-onset OCD and Tourette's disorder (TD), as well as rheumatic fever or Sydenham's chorea. The average percentage of B cells expressing the D8/17 antigen was significantly higher in patients (mean = 22%; standard deviation [SD] = 5%) than in comparison subjects (mean = 9%; SD = 2%). When classified categorically, all patients but only one comparison subject were D8/17 positive. Patients with childhood-onset obsessive-compulsive disorder or TD syndrome had significantly greater B-cell D8/17 expression than comparison subjects, despite the absence of documented Sydenham's chorea or rheumatic fever.

Along the same research lines, Swedo, et al[33] wanted to further study whether this trait marker of rheumatic fever susceptibility (D8/17) could identify children with PANDAS. They obtained blood samples from 27 children with PANDAS, nine children with Sydenham's chorea, and 24 healthy children, which were evaluated for D8/17 reactivity. Individuals were defined as D8/17 positive if they had 12% or more D8/17+ cells. They found that the frequency of D8/17–positive individuals was significantly higher in both patient groups than it was among the healthy volunteers—85% of the children with PANDAS and 89% of the children with Sydenham's chorea, compared with 17% of the healthy children, were D8/17 positive. Further, the mean number of D8/17–positive cells was similar in the two patient groups and was significantly higher in these groups than in the group of healthy children. These results suggest that there may be a subgroup of D8/17–positive children who present with clinical symptoms of OCD and Tourette's disorder, rather than Sydenham's chorea, but who have similar poststreptococcal autoimmunity.

There are treatment implications of these findings. Researchers at the National Institute of Mental Health[34] (NIMH) reported that a boy who had tested positive for a strep infection was enrolled in an experimental study in which he received intravenous gammaglobulin, a treatment that removes circulating strep antibodies from the body. Within 3 weeks, the child's obsessions had lessened, and within 6 weeks, the obsessions had disappeared. So far 17 children—including the above 5-year-old boy—have been enrolled in a NIMH treatment trial being conducted during the past several years. In a presentation of the data at the American Psychiatric Association meeting, Dr. Susan Swedo[35] told psychiatrists that the results were dramatic. In a double-blind, placebo-controlled trial, there was virtually no change in either OCD or tics in those who received a placebo in an intravenous solution, but there was a 45% decrease in behavioral symptoms in the majority of those who received gammaglobulin.

Association with Hypothalamic Lesions

In rats, bilateral hippocampal lesions produce repetitive behaviors, invariability, excessiveness, retarded extinction, and improved shuttle-box avoidance.[36,37] Pitman believes that the similarities between the symptoms and behavior of OCD individuals and neurobehavioral findings in animals with damage to this limbic structure are too close to be coincidental and must be taken into account in any theory of causation of OCD.[37]

One group of researchers described nine patients with a syndrome of diabetes insipidus and obsessional neurosis.[38,39] The time relationship of the onset of symptoms in diabetes insipidus and obsessional disorder in these patients showed that each condition developed independently. The authors believed that the occurrence of these two disorders simultaneously could not be a coincidence and that this was strong evidence that OCD may be secondary to hypothalamic disturbance. In further support of this hypothesis, Barton[38] noted a similar case in which a patient developed long-standing obsessional illness following encephalitis at age 13. Diabetes insipidus appeared 5 years after the onset of the mental disturbance. As noted previously, obsessional illness is well recognized as a sequel to encephalitis lethargica (von Economo's encephalitis), as is diabetes insipidus.

Septohippocampal System

Gray[40] developed a model of septohippocampal function in which he suggested that the septohippocampal system (SHS) has two important and interrelated functions: (1) it acts as a checking system or comparator; and (2) it functions as a control system acting as a behavioral inhibition system. In discussing these concepts, Drummond and Matthews[41] noted that this model suggests that the SHS has multiple connections with higher cortical functions and, as well as receiving information from sensory structures, it functions as a checking system that constantly compares the actual stimuli and events perceived by an organism in its surroundings with the expected or predicted stimuli and events. However, if there is a discordance between the predicted and actual stimuli, then the SHS moves into its control mode and functions as a behavioral inhibitor. In other words, novel stimuli, signals of punishment, or signals of nonreward, activate the behavioral inhibition system, which results in behavioral inhibition, increase in arousal, and increased attention of the organism to its surroundings. Gray suggested that in OCD, the SHS becomes oversensitive and labels too many stimuli as "important," and thus leads to persistent searching for those stimuli with resultant checking and ritualizing.

Head Trauma

The association of OCD with head trauma has been noted occasionally in the literature.[42-45] Because there are few reports, the finding of patients in whom the onset of OCD followed head injury is of considerable interest, and careful study of such cases may help shed light on associations between injury and OCD. The following is a detailed account of one such patient:[45]

Case 1

Clinical History: A 24-year-old, right-handed man had been in a coma for approximately 1 month following a severe head injury sustained in a motorcycle accident when he was 17 years of age. At the time of the initial accident, medical evaluation revealed swelling in the left frontotemporal region and in the right temporal area. He was comatose, but responded to deep pain with withdrawal on both sides. Skull radiographs revealed a severe fracture of the right frontal region, and there was some evidence of a left frontoparietal fracture and bilateral middle fossa basilar fractures. A CT scan showed a hematoma in the left middle fossa with a left-to-right shift of brain tissue. At angiogram, there was a left middle fossa mass effect consistent with either a subtemporal-subdural, middle fossa epidural, or intracerebral left temporal lobe hematoma and contusion. He developed a focal motor seizure on the right side of his face and was given phenobarbital.

Frontotemporal craniotomy revealed a massive left middle fossa epidural hematoma extending into the frontal region and a marked amount of bleeding coming from multiple fractures along the left sphenoid wing. There was also evidence of disruption of the left orbit roof. Following removal of the epidural hematoma, the dura was opened, revealing a macerated left temporal lobe. Temporal lobe resection was extended back approximately 5 cm and was carried medically to the tentorial incisura where frank temporal lobe herniation was noted. This portion of the temporal lobe and hippocampus was then removed, relieving pressure from the brain stem and third nerve.

On eventual discharge from the hospital, the patient was reported to be severely aphasic, with right facial weakness and mild right upper-extremity paresis. These neurologic symptoms were noted to be gradually improving. Four months after the accident, his parents noted "spells" lasting from minutes to hours in which he would drool, mix up words, gaze into space, and follow simple but not complex commands. Also, during the spells, the right hemiparesis, which had resulted from the accident, became noticeably more severe. His neurologist observed one of the spells and believed that they were consistent with temporal lobe epilepsy. In addition, an abnormal electroencephalogram (EEG) was obtained, showing irregular slow wave activity appearing maximally in the left posterior temporal region but spreading to adjacent areas of the hemisphere. He was started on Depakene 250 mg, five times a day, and had no more spells. Six months after the accident, his major disabilities were residual language dysfunction, mild spastic right hemiparesis, and difficulties with thinking and impulse control.

He was referred to a large OCD clinic because of severe intrusive obsessive thoughts that began, according to his family, immediately after awakening from the coma after the accident; he reported severe intrusive thoughts that he might contract some severe illness, such as cancer. Later, other obsessive thoughts developed, such as an overwhelming fear of AIDS and of environmental pollutants. In addition, he could not rid his mind of negativistic news stories (e.g., war, pollution, accidents). These thoughts had the same quality as other OCD patients who did not have a history of head injury and resulted in significant impairment of all areas of this life, including social, vocational, and interpersonal pursuits. The thoughts were not experienced as being voluntarily produced, but rather as thoughts that invaded his consciousness; they were experienced as being senseless and repugnant. Although varying in intensity, these thoughts persisted for 7 years after the time of the accident. The obsessions had become so pervasive that he expressed significant self-depreciation, with concomitant feelings of hopelessness and helplessness. He unsuccessfully attempted to control the thoughts by excessive exercise. He denied checking rituals, but would frequently spend hours washing his hair and then combing it for more than 1 hour so that it was perfectly symmetrical.

By his parents' report, prior to the accident he was completely well, socially outgoing, and an excellent student and athlete. No previous obsessive-compulsive symptoms, head injuries, seizure disorder, or neurologic diseases were noted. Since the accident, he did quite well academically, graduated from high school on time, and completed college on the Dean's List.

Previous Treatments: Over the 7 years since the accident, the patient was hospitalized on two occasions for severe depression, which he believed resulted from his persistent need to fight the obsessions. Since the accident, he had been treated with adequate dosages of phenytoin, clonazepam, chlorpromazine, trimipramine, amitriptyline, amoxapine, trazodone, methylphenidate, imipramine, doxepin, and haloperidol. A trial of carbamazepine had to be cut short because of the onset of thrombocytopenia. The patient and his parents believed that none of these medications had helped his obsessional symptoms but had, on occasion, improved his mood.

Family History: There was no family history of schizophrenia, manic-depressive illness, depression, TD, alcoholism, or phobias. His maternal grandfather, however, had OCD with excessive handwashing associated with a fear of germs. His mother had a history of panic attacks and mitral valve prolapse.

Mental Status and Neuropsychiatric Evaluation: At interview, there was no evidence of psychosis, and the patient and his family specifically denied that he had a history of auditory, tactile, olfactory, gustatory, or visual hallucinations; ideas of reference; thought insertion or withdrawal; or paranoia. Testing performed just prior to coming to the OCD clinic found that the patient was functioning within the average range of general intellectual ability, as exhibited by performance on the WAIS-R (a Full Scale IQ of 108 with a Verbal IQ of 112 and a Performance IQ of 102). On the Verbal-Comprehension Factor, the patient exhibited intersubtest scatter that ranged from the average to a very superior level. For example, he performed within the high average range in his knowledge of vocabulary words (84th percentile), whereas average performance was evidenced in his ability to identify commonalities between two objects (verbal abstract reasoning, 63rd percentile). Exceptional performance was demonstrated on a measure of social comprehension (Satz-Mogel Short Form). High average performance was demonstrated in his general fund of long-term informational knowledge (75th percentile).

His attentional and concentration skills were variable, with Digit Span of 5 forward and 5 backward for a total of 10 (37th percentile). He evidenced generally intact performance on the Wechsler Memory Scale Mental Control. He generated 20 words beginning with the letter "F," 16 words beginning with the letter "A," and 22 words beginning with the letter "S," within 3 minutes. He was able to name 25 animals in 1 minute. On the Boston Naming Test, he performed generally within normal limits. He also performed extremely well (91st percentile) on a WAIS-R task involving alertness to details (Picture Completion) and exhibited average performance on constructional tasks with blocks (Block

Design, 50th Percentile). He completed the Rey-Osterrieth Complex Figure Drawing within normal limits on both an immediate copy and delayed recall format.

Performance on verbal memory tasks was generally efficient, although it was noted that across tasks (e.g., word pairs, isolated/unstructured words, and logical prose), he needed several initial attempts to implement and assess effective memory strategies before performing at an optimal level. Learning and recall of nonverbal material was generally within an expected range. His performance on the Minnesota Multiphasic Personality Inventory (MMPI) was similar to individuals who are generally described as withdrawn, confused, inefficient, anxious, and depressed. Patients with similar profiles typically evidence considerable difficulty in concentrating and thinking and may become agitated and exhibit a fear of losing control. Responses on the Rotter Sentence Completion Test generally corroborated findings on the MMPI.

Follow-up: Ten months after initial evaluation in the OCD clinic, both the patient and his mother stated that he was "about 80% better" when taking the monoamine oxidase inhibitor, phenelzine. He was working and dating and felt quite happy about his life situation. He felt well enough that he did not wish to discontinue phenelzine and undergo a trial of clomipramine at that point.

Elsewhere in this chapter we have reviewed some of the evidence that neurologic disorders may be associated with OCD. As noted previously, the association of OCD with head trauma specifically is infrequently noted.[42-45]

McKeon and associates[44] reported four cases of OCD following head injury. The first was an 18-year-old woman who sustained a head injury after an automobile accident and was unconscious for 2 or 3 minutes with resultant amnesia for 6 hours. Neurologic examination and skull radiographs were normal. Within 24 hours, she reported feeling anxious and developed an irrational conviction that she was "unclean" and that her nose was "dripping" (there was no evidence of cerebrospinal fluid leakage). These feelings caused her to wash and bathe repetitively. Subsequent compulsive rituals regarding contamination dominated her life and greatly curtailed her capacity to work. An EEG performed 1 year later showed slow waves, which were more prominent in the right temporooccipital area. A CT scan was normal, and thorough psychometric testing did not show impairment of intelligence or memory.

The second case was similar: a 37-year-old woman was unconscious for a few minutes following head trauma suffered in a car accident, with resultant 16 hours of transient amnesia. Again, neurologic examination and skull radiographs were normal. During her hospital stay, she began to feel "dirty" and believed that everything she touched became contaminated. Following discharge, this dirty feeling persisted, and she began lengthy cleaning rituals. She realized that these ideas were ridiculous and initially tried to resist them, but became increasingly depressed. Psychometric testing was normal, and a CT scan did not show evidence of brain damage. Four years later, she was reported to be free of obsessions. The report did not discuss whether or not she had received specific treatments for the disorder.

McKeon and associates' third patient was a 16-year-old girl who first developed symptoms of OCD after she was hit on the back of her head with a hair brush. Although dazed and bleeding from a laceration on her scalp, she did not seek medical attention. On awakening the following day, she felt anxious and, on her way to school, found she was searching for something she had lost. The idea of having dropped her handkerchief or money on the ground resulted in lengthy periods of searching on the streets and in late arrival at school. The compulsive searching later extended to her house, although she realized her obsessions were irrational and resisted them intensely for a few weeks. Eight years later, she was hospitalized in a depressed state, with obsessions and compulsions to search. Psychometric testing, EEG, and CT scan were all normal.

McKeon and associates' fourth patient was a 23-year-old man who was hit by a car when walking and was unconscious for 10 days. Investigations (type unspecified) showed evidence of cerebral fat embolism from fractured tibiae. When in the hospital, he developed rituals involving repeated checking of his clothing, brushing this teeth, and taking extensive precautions to avoid contamination in the bathroom. This behavior occupied most of his day and continued unchanged for 4 years from the time of the accident. CT scan showed mild generalized cortical atrophy, and EEG showed spikes in both posterior quadrants and "an excess of slow activity on over-breathing." Interestingly, this patient was a monozygotic twin (confirmed by blood typing) whose twin was discordant for OCD and who had a normal CT scan and EEG.

McKeon, et al[44] reported that each of these four patients developed obsessive-compulsive symptoms within 24 hours of a head injury. In each case, increased emotional arousal was reported following injury and preceded the onset of obsessions. They hypothesized that head injury may exert its role in some way other than as a perceived stress and that a possible physical mechanism may first produce heightened emotional arousal before obsessions intrude.

Lishman[43] reviewed the Oxford collection of head injury records in an effort to relate specific sites of injury to psychiatric symptoms. He restricted his study to 345 patients who were studied in special detail. Of these, 93 patients had no psychiatric disability, 108 had mild psychiatric disability, and 144 were severely ill. Left hemisphere lesions were more closely associated with psychiatric disability than those in the right, and the relationship between psychiatric disability and extent of brain damage was closer within the left hemisphere than the right. Of particular relevance to the case reported in detail previously, temporal lobe wounds were more closely associated with psychiatric disability than frontal, parietal, or occipital lobe wounds. This association was very largely the result of injuries of the left temporal lobe. He also noted that lesions that produced dysphasia were significantly related to psychiatric disability. Lishman[43] reported that only 1.4% of those patients with severe head injuries developed obsessive-compulsive neurosis and concluded that this was an uncommon variety of posttraumatic neurosis.

Hillbom[42] reviewed 414 cases of war-related head injuries and found a 3.4% prevalence of obsessional neurosis. Interestingly, obsessional neurosis was more common after severe trauma, whereas other neuroses were more frequent after milder injuries. He was unable to relate particular structural lesions with the type of neurosis.

The previous case reported in detail suggests an association between damage to a temporal lobe and the onset of OCD. This patient also developed quite classical clinical findings associated with temporal lobe epilepsy a few months after head injury, suggesting that an irritative focus had developed. The OCD symptoms, however, preceded the development of frank temporal lobe seizures. Clinical similarities exist between patients with temporal lobe epilepsy and those with OCD, and as noted in the later section in this chapter on EEG abnormalities, several authors[46-48] have described involuntary forced thinking in patients with temporal lobe epilepsy documented by EEG evidence of temporal spiking or slowing.

In an attempt to quantify the association between head injury and OCD onset, we reviewed the medical histories of 60 consecutively evaluated OCD patients in our clinic and found only one patient who had a history of significant head trauma that occurred some time before the onset of symptoms. One other patient reported the repair of a superficial left temporoparietal brain vascular lesion years before the onset of symptoms, and another had a calcified right parietal meningioma—again, present many years before the onset of her illness. From this small sample, it does not appear that head injury is a frequent precipitant of OCD symptoms. Further study of head-injured patients who subsequently develop OCD is warranted. In addition, it remains to be determined whether this subgroup of OCD patients will consistently respond to standard treatment techniques involving pharmacologic agents and behavior therapy.

Brain Tumors

Minski[49] found that in 58 patients with brain tumors, 25 patients had functional psychiatric illness; only one of these, however—a patient with a left-frontal tumor—developed an obsessional disorder.

Cambier, et al[50] reported one patient with a frontocallosal glioma who developed "affective indifference, severe disorders of attention and dynamic aphasia with marked reduction in spoken expression." The patient wrote spontaneously and in large amounts (compulsively). The authors noted that the writing showed "meticulous production and formal correction contrasted with its semantic incoherence." They felt that this behavior was comparable with the compulsive activity and they used the term *graphomania* to describe this clinical presentation. Apparently, the patient did not suffer from temporal lobe epilepsy.

Association with Drugs

Central nervous system stimulants administered chronically to animals predictably cause stereotypic behavior,[51] and there are a few case reports of drug-induced compulsive behavior in humans. Rylander[52] reported compulsions in phenmetrazine (hydrochloride) addicts, and Ellinwood[53] described them in association with amphetamine psychosis. Anden[54] reported one case in which high doses of L-dopa caused a patient to compulsively hammer nails.

Drummond and Matthews[41] reported a 32-year-old woman who developed OCD after diazepam withdrawal. The patient had been taking 6 mg/day of diazepam for 7 years and had a history of recurrent episodes of depression and chronic anxiety. She also had intermittently been treated with antidepressants, but she had no history of obsessive-compulsive symptoms and had no family history of any psychiatric disorder. She abruptly discontinued diazepam on her general practitioner's advice because she was planning to become pregnant; 2 weeks later, she developed symptoms of anxiety, hyperacusis, insomnia, and nightmares similar to those described as part of the benzodiazepine withdrawal syndrome. These symptoms persisted for several weeks but were overshadowed by an OCD that developed 4 weeks after stopping the benzodiazepine. Her symptoms were manifested as an overwhelming fear that she might inadvertently throw away something written, which would result in her home and family being removed from her by the authorities. Although viewing her fear as irrational, she was unable to resist performing a series of checking and avoidance rituals. Her symptoms responded well to a combination of clomipramine and behavior therapy. Apparently, the authors did not try to rechallenge the patient with diazepam to see if her symptoms improved. The authors of this report postulated that benzodiazepine withdrawal led to rebound hyperactivity in the brain as a result of a rapid reduction in γ-aminobutyric acid (GABA)—the main inhibitory neurotransmitter in the brain that is facilitated by diazepam; during the 7 years of benzodiazepine administration, tolerance to diazepam may have led to a reduction in benzodiazepine receptors, thus reducing the effects of the neurotransmitter GABA.

Insel and Pickar[55] performed a double-blind, placebo-controlled trial of naloxone hydrochloride in two patients with OCD. They hypothesized that if obsessional patients with ruminative doubt had a deficit in an opiate-mediated capacity to register reward, this deficit would be manifested cognitively as a difficulty in reaching certainty. The opiate system has been suggested as a mediator of reward systems. The two subjects in this study specifically described their obsessional symptoms as spontaneous doubts that required repeated checks until a point of certainty was reached. The opiate antagonist naloxone was administered intravenously at 0.3 mg/kg, a dose that is generally free from behavioral effects in normal subjects. On a separate day, saline was similarly administered, and both patients and raters were blind to the experimental condition. The first patient noticed no change after placebo administration, but became acutely absorbed in checking rituals when on naloxone and was unable to reach certainty about the physical relationships of objects in the protocol room. He had considerable difficulty completing the ratings, and this acute exacerbation continued for 24 hours. Similarly, the second patient noted no change with placebo, but became abruptly worse after naloxone with feelings that he could not reach a point of mastery with his intruding thoughts. In both cases, blind self- and observer ratings corroborated spontaneous self-reports. This report implicates the endogenous opiates in the pathophysiology of obsessive doubt and resultant checking, and it may have further implications in terms of future research on opiate agonists as therapeutic agents in OCD. As mentioned earlier in this chapter, clomipramine has been demonstrated to improve obsessional symptoms in at least some OCD patients; it has also been reported to potentiate the antinociceptive actions of opiates.[57] In addition, D-amphetamine has been reported to provide brief but significant relief to patients with severe obsessions[58,59] and may involve the opiate system, because naloxone blocks D-amphetamine increases in activation and self-stimulation.[60]

Association with Blood Types

Rinieris and associates[61] reported a lower incidence of phenotype "O" and a higher incidence of phenotype "A" in 38 OCD patients compared with those of a control sample. In a follow-up study[62] of 600 *normal* individuals, the authors looked at the relation of "ABO" blood types to obsessional personality traits, as measured by the Leyton Obsessional Inventory (LOI; see Chapter 6). High scorers on the LOI trait portion also demonstrated a significantly lower incidence of phenotype "O" and a significantly higher incidence of phenotypes "AB," "A," and "B," taken together, compared with those of a general population sample and the entire study group.

The authors concluded that the findings of these studies concerning a lower incidence of phenotype "O" and a higher incidence of phenotype "A" in obsessional patients could be interpreted as indicating that phenotype "O" may be associated with personality traits that hinder the development of obsessive-compulsive symptomatology.

ELECTROENCEPHALOGRAPHIC STUDIES

If we hypothesize that neurologic illness may account for at least some cases of OCD, EEG studies in these patients are of interest. Unfortunately, most of the literature on the EEG in obsessive patients is old, and diagnostic criteria for OCD were not clearly defined, so that patients with other serious forms of psychopathology, who had associated obsessional symptoms, were included with patients with pure OCD, as now defined by DSM-III. In addition, EEG leads were not standardized and abnormalities were not clearly defined. One group[63] reported that 22 of 31 "obsessional patients" had abnormal EEGs.

The EEG abnormalities were generally nonspecific, none were localized to the temporal lobes, and some patients in this study actually suffered from major motor seizures, indicating that this was not a population of patients with pure OCD.

Rockwell and Simons[64] reported that 10 of 11 obsessive patients with "stable and well-organized personalities" had normal EEGs. Ingram and McAdam[65] later reported that only 1 of 18 hospitalized patients who had obsessive personality traits had an abnormal EEG. Many of these patients were hospitalized for primarily affective illness and some were probably schizophrenic. Rapoport, et al[66] reviewed the awake EEGs of nine adolescents with primary OCD and found no abnormalities. Their sleep EEGs, however, were similar to those previously described in middle-aged depressed patients with short rapid eye movement (REM) latency and decreased total sleep time. Insel and colleagues[67] hypothesized a biologic link between OCD and affective illness in 14 well-characterized OCD patients; they reported all-night sleep EEG recordings which showed decreased REM efficiency and shortened REM latency, as well as decreased total sleep time with more awakenings. These abnormalities generally resembled those of age-matched depressed patients.

Clinical similarities exist between patients with temporal lobe epilepsy and those with OCD. Several authors[46-48,68] have described involuntary forced thinking in patients with temporal lobe epilepsy (partial complex seizures) documented by EEG evidence of temporal spiking, slowing, or both. Epstein and Bailine[69] reported that there were similarities between the all-night EEG findings of three patients studied and those EEG findings of temporal lobe epileptics. Each of their three OCD patients had EEG abnormalities consisting of spiking and theta slowing in the waking state; these were also present during sleep where they became more localized, appearing over the temporal lobes. They made no mention of medication trials in their patients.

In one report, 4 of 12 patients with well-documented OCD had EEG abnormalities over the temporal lobes.[70] Each of these patients was given a trial of antiseizure medication, but only one partially improved. These patients were very ill; in fact, three of the four patients were referred for cingulotomy because of the serious and refractory nature of their illness. These case reports were uncontrolled and retrospective, but the high percentage of temporal lobe abnormalities is consistent with the idea that OCD reflects cerebral abnormality. In this study, possibly more EEG abnormalities over the temporal lobes would have been demonstrated if sleep studies with nasopharyngeal leads had been performed.

Evidence from EEG studies and surgical lesion procedures points to the involvement of structures in the limbic system. Some patients have EEG findings consistent with temporal lobe epilepsy and also fit the interictal behavioral syndrome, which has been described in patients with temporal lobe epilepsy. This syndrome includes affective variability, irritability, religiosity, hyposexuality, viscosity, hypergraphia, and excessive concern with trivial events.[71] Bear and Fedio,[72] in studying 48 temporal lobe epileptics, reported that some patients rated high on measures of obsessionalism, viscosity, emotionality, and sadness and could be distinguished from normal controls by these traits. The use of anticonvulsants in patients with OCD merits further study. Perhaps, if temporal lobe abnormalities are detected early in the course of the illness, they may be reversed by anticonvulsant medication, with subsequent improvement or resolution of the clinical symptoms. Long-standing temporal lobe seizures may damage brain structures irreversibly.

Because temporal epileptic discharges may be intermittent, it is likely that a true seizure disorder could be missed with a single EEG sample. The possible interrelationships between OCD, temporal lobe epilepsy, and the cingulum remain largely speculative. Symptomatically, obsessive and compulsive states are typified by repetition or fixedness of thoughts and actions. It does not seem unreasonable to consider the hypothesis that such clinical states reflect repetitive and fixed neuronal activity—a physiologic process that is, supposedly, a normal property of either neurons or neuronal chains.[47] Papez,[73] in attempting to provide an anatomic basis for emotion, described a circuit that includes parts of the temporal lobe and the cingulate gyrus. He regarded the cingulate cortex as the receptive region for impulses concerned with emotion and suggested that radiation of impulses from the cingulate gyrus to other cortical regions added emotional coloring to the psychic process. He theorized that this circuit may be reverberatory and that it may be possible for impulses to circulate continually and, by reinforcement, that may cause an emotional experience to be intensified. Perhaps a "lesion" lies within this circuit for some patients with OCD.

SUMMARY

Since the last edition of this book, there have been major strides in the treatment and management of OCD patients, but our understanding of the cause of this disorder remains in its infancy. Nonetheless, we now have a number of leads that must be carefully evaluated.

Cerebral disorders appear to be associated with at least some cases of OCD. The fact that OCD is refractory to nonbehavioral psychotherapeutic maneuvers but is responsive to certain medications and surgical techniques lends support to a neurologic hypothesis for OCD. It may be revealed that there are many ways, however, to develop OCD; it may be a syndrome like dementia that can result from diverse etiologies, including genetic, infectious, traumatic, metabolic, or degenerative causes. There are indeed some OCD patients who seemed to develop the disorder secondary to medical and neurologic disorders. The association with von Economo's encephalitis and Sydenham's chorea has been discussed. At least some OCD cases develop after head injury.

The serotonergic theory (see Chapter 12) has been the most discussed over the past 10 years, and much work continues in this area. The development of drugs selective for various serotonergic receptors may help clarify which parts of this system are involved. Because serotonergic receptor subtypes have now been cloned, great strides can be expected in our understanding of this complex system and its relationship to psychiatric illnesses.

A possible link between OCD and temporal lobe epilepsy has been discussed. Areas of the brain that may be involved in OCD patients include the frontal lobes, cingulate gyri, septohippocampal system, hypothalamus, limbic system, and basal ganglia; sophisticated new techniques (see Chapters 12 and 15) that allow us to look at both structure and function simultaneously likely will make the next 10 years of study especially productive. Correlations of alterations with neuropsychologic findings are important.

Psychodynamic theories may well prove true in some patients, and the fact that treatments derived from these theories are ineffective does not prove these theories wrong. Learning hypotheses have led to promising and effective treatments, but they do not explain in total why some patients are predisposed to the development of this disorder and why metabolic and structural variances from normal control patients exist.

REFERENCES

1. Janet P: Les obsessions et la psychasthenie, vol 1, Paris, 1903, Felix Alcan.
2. Pitman RK: Pierre Janet on obsessive-compulsive disorder, *Arch Gen Psychiatry* 44:226–231, 1987.
3. Freud S: Notes upon a case of obsessional neurosis. In *Standard edition of the complete works of Sigmund Freud,* vol 10, London, 1955, Hogarth Press, p 153.
4. Salzman L, Thaler FH: Obsessive-compulsive disorder: a review of the literature, *Am J Psychiatry* 138:286–296, 1981.
5. Ncmiah J: Obsessive compulsive neurosis. In Freedman A, Kaplan H, Sadock B, editors: *A comprehensive textbook of psychiatry,* Baltimore, 1975, Williams & Wilkins, pp 1241–1255.
6. Nemiah J: Obsessive compulsive neurosis. In Nicoli AM, editor: *Harvard guide to modern psychiatry,* Cambridge, 1978, Belknap Press.
7. Insel RI, Murphy DL: The psychopharmacological treatment of obsessive-compulsive disorder: a review, *J Clin Psychopharmacol* 1:304–311, 1981.
8. Jenike MA: Obsessive-compulsive disorder, *Compr Psychiatry* 24:99–115, 1983.
9. LeBeau J: The cingular and precingular areas in psychosurgery (agitated behavior, obsessive-compulsive states, epilepsy), *Acta Psychiatr Neurol Scand* 27:305–316, 1952.
10. Kelly DHW, Walter C, Mitchell-Heggs N, et al: Modified leucotomy assessed clinically, physiologically and psychologically at six weeks and eighteen months, *Br J Psychiatry* 120:1929, 1972.
11. Tan E, Marks I, Marset P: Bimedial leucotomy in obsessive-compulsive neurosis: a controlled serial enquiry, *Br J Psychiatry* 118:155–164, 1971.
12. Sykes M, Tredgold R: Restricted orbital undercutting: a study of its effects on 350 patients over the ten years 1951–60, *Br J Psychiatry* 110:609, 1964.

13. Miller A: The lobotomy patient—a decade later: a follow-up study of a research project started in 1948, *Can Med Assoc J* 96:1095–1103, 1967.
14. Mitchell-Heggs N, Kelly D, Richardson A: Stereotactic limbic leucotomy: a follow-up at 16 months, *Br J Psychiatry* 128:226–240, 1976.
15. Lewin W: Selective leukotomy: A review. In Laitinen LV, Livingston KI, editors: *Surgical approaches in psychiatry,* England, 1973, Medical and Technical Publishing.
16. Tippin J, Henn FA: Modified leukotomy in the treatment of intractable obsessional neurosis, *Am J Psychiatry* 139:1601–1603, 1982.
17. Jenike MA: Obsessive-compulsive disorder: a question of a neurologic lesion, *Compr Psychiatry* 25:298–304, 1984.
18. Jenike MA, Baer L, Minichiello WE, editors: *Obsessive-compulsive disorders: theory and management,* ed 2, Chicago, 1990, Mosby.
19. Kettl PA, Marks IM: Neurological factors in obsessive compulsive disorder: two case reports and a review of the literature, *Br J Psychiatry* 149:315–319, 1986.
20. Newman KO: *Encephalitis lethargica: Its sequelae and treatment,* New York, 1931, Oxford University Press (Translated by C Von Economo).
21. Ravenholdt RT, Foege WH: 1918 influenza, encephalitis lethargica, Parkinsonism, *Lancet* 2:860–863, 1982.
22. Johnson J: Encephalitis lethargica, a contemporary cause of catatonic stupor: a report of two cases, *Br J Psychiatry* 151:550–552, 1987.
23. Jelliffe SE, Smith E: Psychopathology of forced movements in oculogyric crises of lethargic encephalitis, *Nerv Ment Dis Monogr Ser* 1–200, 1932.
24. Claude H, Bourk H, Lamache A: Obsessive-impulsions consecutives a l'encephalite epidemique, *Encephale* 22:716–722, 1927.
25. Schilder P: The organic background of obsessions and compulsions, *Am J Psychiatry* 94:1397, 1938.
26. Jenike MA: Behavioral aspects of neurotic syndromes, *Contemp Psychiatry* 1: 109–112, 1982.
27. Hunter R: Psychiatry and neurology, *Proc R Soc Med* 66:359–364, 1973.
28. Laplane D, Widlocher D, Pillon B, et al: Comportement compulsif d'allure obsessionnelle par necrose circonscrite bilaterale pallidopstriatale, *Rev Neurol* 137: 269–276, 1981.
29. Grimshaw L: Obsessional disorder and neurological illness, *J Neurol Neurosurg Psychiatry* 27:229, 1964.
30. Rapoport JL: The biology of obsessions and compulsions, *Sci Am* March:83–89, 1989.
31. Giedd JN, Rapoport JL, Leonard HL, et al: Case study: acute basal ganglia enlargement and obsessive-compulsive symptoms in an adolescent boy, *J Am Acad Child Adolesc Psychiatry* 35(7):913–915, 1996.
32. Murphy TK, Goodman WK, Fudge MW, et al: B lymphocyte antigen D8/17: a peripheral marker for childhood-onset obsessive-compulsive disorder and Tourette's syndrome? *Am J Psychiatry* 154(3):402–407, 1997.
33. Swedo SE, Leonard HL, Mittleman BB, et al: Identification of children with pediatric autoimmune neuropsychiatric disorders associated with streptococcal infections by a marker associated with rheumatic fever, *Am J Psychiatry* 154(1):110–112, 1997.
34. National Institute of Mental Health, oral communication, 1997.

35. Swedo S: Presentation at the meeting of the American Psychiatric Association, May 1997.
36. Davenport LD, Davenport JA, Holloway FA: Reward-induced stereotypy: modulation by the hippocampus, *Science* 212:1288–1289, 1981.
37. Pitman RK: Neurological etiology of obsessive-compulsive disorders? *Am J Psychiatry* 139:139–140, 1982.
38. Barton R: Diabetes insipidus, obsessional neurosis and hypothalamic dysfunction, *Proc R Soc Med* 47:276–277, 1954.
39. Barton R: Diabetes insipidus and obsessional neurosis: a syndrome, *Lancet* 1:133–135, 1965.
40. Gray JA: *The neuropsychology of anxiety: an enquiry into the functioning of the septohippocampal system,* New York, 1982, Oxford University Press.
41. Drummond LM, Matthews HP: Obsessive-compulsive disorder occurring as a complication in benzodiazepine withdrawal, *J Nerv Ment Dis* 176:688–691, 1988.
42. Hillbom E: After-effects of brain injuries, *Acta Psychiatr Neurol Scand* 35:(suppl 142), 1960.
43. Lishman WA: Brain damage in relation to psychiatric disability after head injury, *Br J Psychiatry* 114:373–410, 1968.
44. McKeon J, McGuffin P, Robinson P: Obsessive-compulsive neurosis following head injury: a report of four cases, *Br J Psychiatry* 144:190–192, 1984.
45. Jenike MA, Brandon AD: Obsessive-compulsive disorder and head trauma: a rare association, *J Anx Dis* 2:353–359, 1988.
46. Wilson SAD: *Modern problems in neurology,* New York, 1929, William Wood & Co.
47. Brickner RM, Rosen AA, Munro R: Physiological aspects of the obsessive state, *Psychosom Med* 2:369–383, 1940.
48. Hill D, Mitchell W: Epileptic amnesia, *Folia Psychiatry* 56:718, 1953.
49. Minski L: The mental symptoms associated with 58 cases of cerebral tumor, *J Neurol Psychopathol* 13, 1933.
50. Cambier J, Masson C, Benammou S, et al: La graphomanie, activite graphique compulsive manifestation d'un gliome fronto-calleux, *Rev Neurol (Paris)* 144: 158–164, 1988.
51. Ellinwood EH, Escalante O: Chronic amphetamine effect on the olfactory forebrain, *Biol Psychiatry* 2:189–203, 1970.
52. Rylander G: Clinical and medicocriminological aspects of addictions to central stimulating drugs. In Sjoquiste E, Tottie M, editors: *Abuse of central stimulants,* New York, 1969, Raven Press.
53. Ellinwood EH Jr: Amphetamine psychosis I. Description of the individuals and the process, *J Nerv Ment Dis* 144:273–283, 1967.
54. Anden NE: Oral L-dopa treatment of parkinsonism, *Acta Med Scand* 187:247–255, 1970.
55. Insel TR, Pickar D: Naloxone administration in obsessive-compulsive disorder: report of two cases, *Am J Psychiatry* 140:1219–1220, 1983.
56. Pickar D, Cohen MR, Naber D, et al: Clinical studies of the endogenous opioid system, *Biol Psychiatry* 17:1243–1276, 1982.
57. Sewell RDE, Lee RL: Opiate receptors, endorphins, and drug therapy, *Postgrad Med J* 56(suppl 1):25–30, 1980.

58. Insel TR, Hamilton J, Guttmacher L, et al: D-amphetamine in obsessive compulsive disorder, *Psychopharmacology* 80:231–235, 1983.
59. Insel TR, editor: *New findings in obsessive-compulsive disorder,* Washington, 1984, American Psychiatric Association Press.
60. Segal DS, Brown RG, Arnsten A, et al: Characteristics of beta endorphin–induced behavioral activation and immobilization. In Usdin E, Bunney WE Jr, Kline NS, editors: *Endorphins in mental health research,* New York, 1979, Oxford University Press.
61. Rinieris PM, Stefanis CN, Rabavilas AD, et al: Obsessive-compulsive neurosis, anacastic symptomatology and ABO blood types, *Acta Psychiatr Scand* 57: 377–381, 1978.
62. Rinieris P, Stefanis C, Rabavilas A, et al: Obsessional personality traits and ABO blood types, *Neuropsychobiology* 6:128–131, 1980.
63. Pacella BL, Polatin P, Nagler SH: Clinical and EEG studies in obsessive-compulsive states, *Am J Psychiatry* 100:830, 1944.
64. Rockwell FV, Simons DJ: The electroencephalogram and personality organization in the obsessive-compulsive reactions, *Arch Neurol Psychiatry* 57:71, 1947.
65. Ingram IM, McAdam WA: The electroencephalogram, obsessional illness and obsessional personality, *J Med Sci* 106:686, 1960.
66. Rapoport J, Elkins R, Langer DH, et al: Childhood obsessive-compulsive disorder, *Am J Psychiatry* 138:12, 1981.
67. Insel TR, Gillin C, Moore A, et al: The sleep of patients with obsessive-compulsive disorder, *Arch Gen Psychiatry* 39:1372–1377, 1982.
68. Ward CD: Transient feelings of compulsion caused by hemispheric lesions: three cases, *J Neurol Neurosurg Psychiatry* 51:266–268, 1988.
69. Epstein AW, Bailine SH: Sleep and dream studies in obsessional neurosis with particular reference to epileptic states, *Biol Psychiatry* 3:149–158, 1971.
70. Jenike MA, Brotman AW: The EEG in obsessive-compulsive disorder, *J Clin Psychiatry* 45:122–124, 1984.
71. Geschwind N, Shader RI, Bear DM, et al: Behavioral changes with temporal lobe epilepsy: assessment and treatment, *J Clin Psychiatry* 41:89–94, 1980.
72. Bear DM, Fedio P: Quantitative analysis of interictal behavior in temporal lobe epilepsy, *Arch Neurol* 34:454–467, 1977.
73. Papez JW: A proposed mechanism of emotion, *Arch Neurol Psychiatry* 38: 725–743, 1937.

12

Neurobiologic Models of Obsessive-Compulsive Disorder

Scott L. Rauch, M.D., Paul J. Whalen, Ph.D.,
Darin Dougherty, M.D., Michael A. Jenike, M.D.

Over the past decade, numerous reviews have been published regarding the pathophysiology of obsessive-compulsive disorder (OCD) and related disorders (hereafter referred to collectively as OCDs). In this chapter, we will present three different types of neurobiologic models: (1) corticostriatal circuitry models; (2) amygdalocentric models; and (3) neurochemical models. These constructs are not mutually exclusive. In fact, they are best viewed as potential elements of some larger scheme that should ideally integrate the three perspectives.

Much of the raw material out of which the current models have been fashioned is comprehensively presented elsewhere in this volume. Here, such data will be summarized briefly and only when necessary. Further, although the current presentation of these models represents an original synthesis, it necessarily relies heavily on previous contributions made by other investigators and theoreticians, as well as our own.[1–10]

Models of disease are intended to serve several purposes. First, they should serve an explanatory function that facilitates communication and education about the disorder in question. Second, they should provide a structure that aids in organizing existing as well as newly emerging data. Third, to be plausible, they should accommodate—or optimally, reconcile—currently available information. Finally, models of disease represent propositions rather than absolute truths, and thus advance science partly by prompting specific testable hypotheses.

WHAT DATA SHOULD MODELS OF OBSESSIVE-COMPULSIVE DISORDER ACCOMMODATE?

There is already a vast body of information regarding OCDs. Relevant domains of inquiry include phenomenology, epidemiology, genetics, neuropsychology, neuroanatomy, neurophysiology, and neuropharmacology, as well as data from clinical treatment trials. Optimal models of OCD should resonate with the data available from these various sources. Similarly, the pathophysiology of apparent human phenocopies of OCD (such as those arising from acquired lesions or documented medical causes) and animal models of repetitive behaviors can provide circumstantial supporting evidence as well.

Naturalistically, the clinical phenomenology of OCDs provided the initial impetus for considering them as related entities (also see Chapters 7 through 10).[11,12] It is worth examining what common theme among OCD, body dysmorphic disorder (BDD), Tourette's disorder (TD), and trichotillomania (TTM) has motivated investigators in this field to propose a spectrum of OCDs. One heuristic formulation suggests that OCDs are fundamentally characterized by intrusive events, which are accompanied by a drive to perform intentional (though unwanted) repetitive behaviors.[13,14] Conversely, OCDs also are distinguishable from one another. For instance, OCD and BDD involve intrusive cognitive events whereas TD and TTM involve primarily sensorimotor intrusions. Further, whereas the repetitive behaviors seen in OCD and BDD tend to be driven either by anxiety or some other affective impetus and often involve pseudorational attempts at neutralization of the cognitive intrusions, the repetitive behaviors in TD and TTM are typically driven by difficult-to-describe "urges" or attempts to relieve a sense of physical tension. Perhaps most perplexing is the fact that the specific content of the thoughts and behaviors varies among and between these different diagnoses. To date, no neurobiologic model has adequately explained the heterogeneity of content that these intrusions, affective accompaniments, and intentional repetitive behaviors embody. Thus, the face validity of any model depends on its ability to accommodate the rich and heterogeneous phenomenology of these disorders.

CORTICOSTRIATAL CIRCUITRY MODELS OF OBSESSIVE-COMPULSIVE DISORDER

Corticostriatal circuitry models of OCD focus on neuroanatomic relationships and the respective functions of various brain systems. Therefore, prior to elaborating these models, it is necessary to introduce the relevant neuroanatomy involved.

Relevant Normal Neuroanatomy

Prefrontal Cortex

The prefrontal cortex mediates a variety of cognitive functions, including response inhibition, planning, organizing, controlling, and verifying operations. Consequently, prefrontal dysfunction is associated with disinhibition, inflexibility, perseveration, stereotypy, or disorganization (also see Chapter 13).[15] The prefrontal cortex is divisible into several functional subterritories. The dorsolateral prefrontal cortex (DLPFC) plays an important role in learning and memory, as well as planning and other complex cognitive functions. The ventral prefrontal cortex, specifically orbitofrontal cortex, can be further subdivided into two functional domains. The posteromedial orbitofrontal cortex (PMOFC) is a component of the paralimbic system which plays a role in affective and motivational functions as discussed in the following paragraphs.[16,17] The anterior and lateral orbitofrontal cortex (ALOFC) represent the structural and functional intermediaries between the lateral prefrontal and paralimbic prefrontal zones. For instance, the ALOFC seems to play a role in response inhibition and regulation of behavior based on social context as well as, perhaps, other affectively tinged cognitive operations.[16,17]

The Paralimbic System

The paralimbic system is the name given to a contiguous belt of cortex that forms the functional conduit between other cortical areas and the limbic system proper. The constituents of the paralimbic belt include PMOFC, as well as cingulate, anterior temporal parahippocampal, and insular cortex.[16] This system is believed to integrate abstracted representations of the outside world with inner emotional states, so that appropriate meaning and priority can be assigned to information as it is processed. Convergent data from recent human neuroimaging studies, together with previous animal and human research, suggest that the paralimbic system plays a critical role in mediating intense emotional states or arousal. In particular, this system has been implicated in anxiety.[18–22] Further, it has long been appreciated that paralimbic elements serve to modulate autonomic responses, including heart rate and blood pressure, which represent the somatic manifestations of intense affects or heightened arousal.[16]

Corticostriatal Circuitry

The striatum comprises the caudate nucleus, putamen, and nucleus accumbens (also called the ventral striatum). Historically, the basal ganglia, including the striatum, were believed to play a circumscribed role, limited to the modulation of motor functions. More recently, however, a much more complicated scheme has been adopted, which recognizes the role of the striatum in cognitive and affective functions as well. In a series of landmark articles, Alexander and colleagues explicated the organization of multiple, parallel, segregated corticostriatal circuits.[23,24] There are several levels of complexity to be considered with regard to the anatomy and function of these circuits.

First, the circuits differ from one another on the basis of their distinct projection zones within the cortex, striatum, and thalamus, and thus the particular type of functions each subserves. For the purposes of this review, four of these corticostriatal circuits are emphasized (Figure 12-1): (1) the corticostriatal circuit involving projections from the paralimbic cortex via the nucleus accumbens subserves affective or motivational functions; (2) the circuit involving projections from the sensorimotor cortex via the putamen subserves sensorimotor

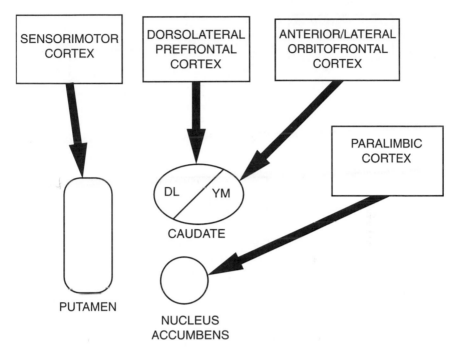

Fig. 12-1 Schematic illustration of the corticostriatal elements of relevant parallel segregated pathways.[23,24] Note the sensorimotor cortex projects to the putamen; the dorsolateral prefrontal cortex projects to the dorsolateral portion of the caudate (DL); anterior and lateral territories of the orbitofrontal cortex project to the ventromedial portion of the caudate (VM); and the paralimbic cortex projects to the nucleus accumbens.

functions; (3) projections from the ALOFC via the ventromedial caudate nucleus constitute the ventral cognitive circuit, which is believed to mediate context-related operations and response inhibition; and (4) projections from DLPFC via dorsolateral caudate nucleus constitute the dorsal cognitive circuit, which is believed to mediate working memory and other executive functions.

Second, each circuit has two major branches or arms (Figure 12-2): (1) The corticothalamic branch provides a reciprocal excitatory monosynaptic communication between cortex and thalamus that purportedly mediates consciously initiated output and consciously accessible input streams; and (2) the cortico-striatothalamic branch represents a collateral pathway that serves to modulate transmission at the level of the thalamus. Purportedly, the function of the striatum in this context is to process information automatically and without conscious representation. Hence, the healthy striatum serves to (1) filter out extraneous input; (2) ensure refined output; and (3) mediate stereotyped, rule-

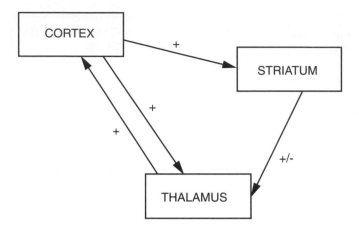

Fig. 12-2 Schematic illustration of the corticostriatothalamocortical loop. The corticothalamic connections are reciprocal and mutually excitatory (+). The corticostriatothalamic collateral has a modulating influence at the level of the thalamus (+/–), in which the gating of principal input and output occurs for this system.

based processes without necessitating the allocation of conscious resources.[25-30] In this way, the striatum regulates the content and facilitates the quality of information processing within the explicit (i.e., conscious) domain by fine tuning input and output. In addition, the striatum enhances the efficiency of the brain by carrying out some nonconscious functions, thereby reducing the computational load on conscious processing systems.

Third, each corticostriatothalamic collateral is composed of a "direct" and "indirect" system (Figure 12-3).[24,31] These two systems operate in parallel, with opposing ultimate influences at the level of the thalamus. The direct system is so-named because it involves direct projections from striatum to globus pallidus interna, with a net excitatory influence on the thalamus. Conversely, the indirect system involves indirect projections from the striatum via the globus pallidus externa to the globus pallidus interna, and has a net inhibitory effect at the level of the thalamus. Further, although these two systems share many features, they possess important neurochemical differences. In particular, although the direct system uses the neuropeptide substance P as a transmitter, and the indirect system uses enkephalin instead.

Fourth, within each striatal projection zone, there is heterogeneity with regard to striatal cellular characteristics. There are islands or "patches" of tissue called "striosomes," dotting the background or "matrix" called "matrisomes."[32,33] These different striatal compartments were initially discovered and defined on the basis of acetylcholinesterase (AChE)-sensitive staining assays; matrix is rich in AChE whereas striosomes are AChE-poor. Subsequently, it became

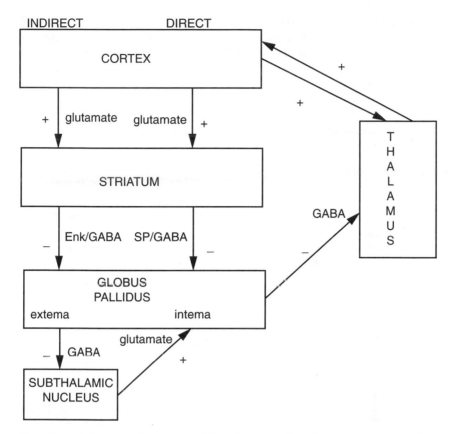

Fig. 12-3   Schematic illustration of the "direct" and "indirect" corticostriatotha-lamic pathways. The local influence of each projection is designated as excitatory (+) or inhibitory (–). From tracing the two systems in the diagram, it is evident that the direct pathway has a net excitatory influence on thalamus, whereas the indirect pathway, via the globus pallidus externa and subthalamic nucleus, has a net inhibitory influence. The principal neurotransmitters associated with each projection are indicated (enkephalin [Enk]; gamma aminobutyric acid [GABA]; substance P [SP]).

appreciated that there were many neurochemical as well as neuroanatomic differences between these two compartments. For instance, striosomes are characterized by a preponderance of D1-binding sites whereas matrix contains a greater density of D2 and 5-HT receptors. In addition, limbic and para-limbic areas project preferentially to striosomes, whereas other neocortical areas project to matrix. Likewise, striosomes project preferentially to ventral dopaminergic cells within the substantia nigra, whereas matrisomes project preferentially to dorsal dopaminergic cells. Thus, the patch-matrix level of organization belies the oversimplified scheme of a wholly segregated array of corticostriatal circuits. More specifically, the patch-matrix compartmentalization is woven throughout the caudate, putamen, and ventral striatum in a manner which could enable integration between the various circuits and most importantly may provide for an embedded limbic-paralimbic influence within each of the corticostriatal pathways.

The Corticostriatal Hypothesis of Obsessive-Compulsive Disorder

Since the late 1980s, several scientists have developed or modified neurobiologic models of OCD that emphasize the role of the frontal cortex and the striatum.[1–5,7–9,34] The scheme of corticostriatal circuitry fits well with emerging data implicating the elements of those circuits. Neuroimaging studies indicated hyperactivity of the orbitofrontal cortex, anterior cingulate cortex, and caudate nucleus at rest, and attenuation of these abnormalities with effective treatment (see Chapter 15). Neuropsychologic studies were consistent with subtle deficits involving frontostriatal functions (see Chapter 13). Neurosurgical procedures that interrupted this circuit appeared to reduce OCD symptoms (see Chapter 26). Further, cases of other diseases characterized by documented striatal pathology were noted to exhibit OCD symptoms or similar clinical manifestations.[7,34–36] As importantly, there was heuristic appeal to the hypothesis that positive feedback loops between the cortex and thalamus might mediate circular, repetitive thoughts, whereas the striatum might mediate fixed action patterns in the form of repetitive behaviors or compulsions.[2–5,8]

Appreciating that available data were not yet adequate to resolve the various possibilities, theoreticians tendered different versions of the model, although each of them accepted the notion of an overdriven corticothalamic reverberating circuit (Figure 12-4). Modell, et al[2] proposed that a hyperactive caudate nucleus might be the cause of net excitation of the thalamus; Baxter, et al[3] hypothesized that the apparent hyperactivity in caudate represented insufficient compensation for intrinsic striatal dysfunction, such that inhibition of the thalamus via the corticostriatothalamic collateral was inadequate. It is striking that Modell, et al based their model on the premise that the corticostriatothalamic collateral normally had a net positive influence on thalamus, whereas Baxter and colleagues' model indicated the exact opposite. As researchers became cognizant of the direct and indirect systems within the corticostriatothalamic collateral branch, this additional layer of complexity helped reconcile and advance the general proposition. A revised version suggested that in healthy individuals, an appropriate balance between the direct and indirect systems enabled the collateral to optimally modulate activity at the thalamus, whereas in OCD, a shift toward dominance of the direct system could result in excitation or disinhibition at the thalamus, thereby overdriving the corticothalamic branch. Insel[4] provided a complementary model of OCD, which focused on the role of orbitofrontal cortex as the prime mediator of a "worry circuit."

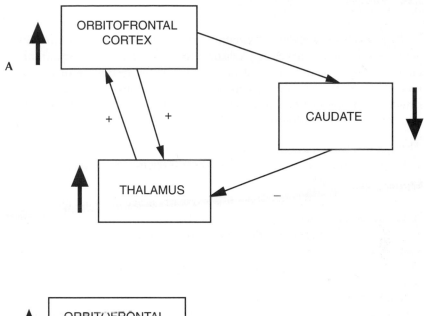

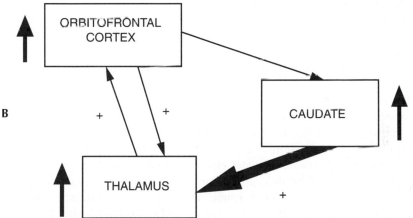

Fig. 12-4   Schematic illustration of pathologic activation within the corticostriato-thalamocortical circuit in obsessive-compulsive disorder. Two early models sought to explain hyperactivity found in orbitofrontal cortex, thalamus, and the caudate nucleus. The upper panel (A) reflects a model proposed by Baxter, et al,[3] in which hyperactivity in the caudate is insufficient to overcome inadequate function of the caudate in the service of inhibiting the thalamus. The lower panel (B) reflects a model proposed by Modell, et al,[2] in which hyperactivity in the caudate actually further excites the thalamus. Reconciliation of these two models was achieved via elaboration of the existence of the direct and indirect pathways (see Figure 12-3). Failure to achieve efficient gating at the level of the thalamus may result from an imbalance between the direct and indirect pathways. Specifically, pathologic dominance of the direct system would be consistent with disinhibition or excitation of the thalamus through the corticostriatothalamic collateral.

Thus, some early reviews treated the orbitofrontal cortex as a monolithic entity and further deemphasized a distinct functional role for the anterior cingulate cortex. Moreover, consistent with the spatial resolution of available imaging tools, the caudate nucleus was likewise treated as a homogeneous structure, whereas distinctions between the caudate and accumbens were also minimized or ignored. Nonetheless, the corticostriatal model of OCD accommodated much of the available data as of 1993.[2-5,8]

The Striatal Topography Hypothesis of Obsessive-Compulsive Disorders

Baxter and colleagues were the first to clearly articulate what has come to be known as the "striatal topography model" of OCDs.[3,6,9,10] As the phenomenologic, familial, and neurobiologic relationships between OCD and TD became appreciated, Baxter, et al hypothesized that the two disorders might share a fundamental pathophysiology, whereby the clinical manifestations of each disease are governed by the precise topography of dysfunction within the striatum. Again, by integrating a more sophisticated rendering of the normal functional anatomy, Baxter, et al suggested that different corticostriatal circuits might mediate different symptoms and therefore define a spectrum of different disease entities. Originally, they proposed that ventromedial caudate/accumbens involvement might mediate obsessions, dorsolateral caudate dysfunction might mediate compulsions, and that putamen involvement might mediate the tics of TD. Subsequently, based on results of symptom provocation studies, we have proposed that the paralimbic system (including PMOFC) mediates affective manifestions, including the anxiety of OCD or BDD and the "urges" of TD or TTM, whereas the ventral cognitive circuit comprising the ALOFC and the ventromedial caudate mediates obsessional symptoms (Figure 12-5) (see Chapter 15).[9,10,18–21,37] Further support for the striatal topography model comes from recent imaging studies that indicate structural abnormalities involving the caudate in OCD and the putamen in TD and TTM (see Chapter 15).

The Implicit Processing Deficit Hypothesis of Obsessive-Compulsive Disorders

The notion that striatal pathology causes OCDs, and that involvement of different striatal elements governs different phenomenologic characteristics is an incompletely developed concept. Elaboration of this model requires further consideration of corticostriatal function and is enriched via a cognitive neuroscience perspective. One scheme for understanding information processing, in the context of learning and memory, distinguishes between explicit (i.e., conscious) and implicit (i.e., unconscious) operations.[26,27,38–42] Apparently, these various information processing functions are performed by distinct and dissociable brain systems. Explicit learning and memory are primarily mediated via DLPFC and medial temporal structures, such as the hippocampus.[43–45] There

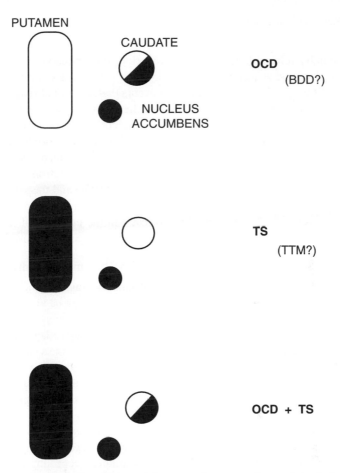

Fig. 12-5 Schematic illustration of the striatal topography model of obsessive-compulsive disorder (OCD). Shaded areas represent territories in which dysfunction or pathology is proposed to exist. In the case of pure OCD, the ventromedial caudate is primarily implicated; in Tourette's disorder (TD), the putamen is primarily implicated. Involvement across these two areas is implicated in comorbid OCD and TD. Because of phenomenologic correlates of limbic involvement, this figure suggests that the ventral striatum is involved in all three of these clinical phenotypes, although this aspect of the model is more speculative and controversial. Likewise, the hypothesis that trichotillomania (TTM) might reflect a pattern of involvement similar to TD, and body dysmorphic disorder (BDD) might reflect a pattern of involvement similar to OCD, remains to be tested.

are several types of implicit learning and memory. Classical conditioning (especially with regard to aversive stimuli) is mediated in part by the amygdala and is discussed in the subsequent section on amygdalocentric models. Implicit learning of procedures, skills, or stereotyped serial operations is purportedly mediated via corticostriatal systems.[26,42,46–48] Therefore, if OCDs are fundamentally referrable to striatal dysfunction, their phenomenology might best be understood as a consequence of implicit processing deficits.[48]

In fact, it is plausible that the intrusive events that are the hallmark of OCDs represent failures in filtering at the level of the thalamus, attributable to deficient modulation via the corticostriatothalamic collateral. Framed in another way, information that is normally processed efficiently via corticostriatal systems, outside of the conscious domain (i.e., implicitly), instead finds access to explicit processing systems as a result of striatal dysfunction. This theory could explain the cognitive intrusions of OCD and BDD and the sensorimotor intrusions of TD or TTM. Further, it makes sense that these symptoms persist or recur until they are effectively "put to rest"; in the presence of a dysfunctional corticostriatothalamic collateral, this end is not easily achieved.

Repetitive Behavior as a Means to Modulate Thalamic Overdrive

For the individual with some pattern of striatal dysfunction, the most adaptive means for producing striatothalamic modulation might be via performance of highly ritualized thoughts or behaviors that activate neighboring intact striatothalamic networks. In this way, compulsions or tics may represent the best available, although inefficient, method for recruiting the viable remnants of the corticostriatothalamic collateral, thereby ultimately quelling an otherwise unchecked corticothalamic reverberating circuit. This would explain why these behaviors sometimes require numerous repetitions before the precipitating intrusive symptoms are put to rest.

This model may also explain why the match between intrusive symptoms and the repetitive behaviors performed in response to them is so idiosyncratic. By this scheme, the two should principally be related according to the topography or interconnections of the neural systems involved. Within the putamen, it makes sense that these relationships would be somatotopic, such that sensory intrusions that involve a given somatic distribution (e.g., the right shoulder) should prompt repetitive behavior in the same or a nearby somatic distribution (i.e., a shoulder or arm tic). In the case of cognitions, this mapping is less obvious, and certainly has not yet been empirically established. It is plausible, however, that networks that mediate cognitive conceptualization of contamination, for instance, might be topographically nearby or linked with neural networks that mediate cleaning procedures. Further, this model would provide an explanation for why some patients develop mental rituals and also why some patients suffer from intrusions but never develop ritualistic behaviors because presumably in those cases no such behaviors evolve that effectively ameliorate the intrusive symptoms.

The current model is lacking an adequate explanation for the motivational and affective accompaniments of these symptoms. Presumably, the anxiety and/or urges that accompany intrusive symptoms and drive the repetitive behaviors are mediated via the limbic or paralimbic system. There are at least four possibilities regarding how these affective symptoms are precipitated: (1) the paralimbic belt is recruited "bottom up" as a consequence of thalamic filtering failures owing to accumbens dysfunction (just as with the symptoms mediated by caudate and putamen); (2) other limbic elements become involved and recruit paralimbic cortex via ascending influences (see the amygdalocentric models below); (3) the patch-matrix organization of the striatum allows caudate or putamen lesions to simultaneously influence the paralimbic corticostriatal collateral via the striosomal rests which are topographically imbedded within the neostriatum; or (4) corticocortical communications occur (i.e., between ALOFC or sensorimotor cortex and paralimbic cortex) after corticothalamic reverberation has already been initiated, thereby recruiting the paralimbic system at the cortical level.

AMYGDALOCENTRIC MODELS OF OBSESSIVE-COMPULSIVE DISORDER AND ITS TREATMENT

Thus far, we have emphasized corticostriatal systems and their role in supporting repetitive thoughts and behaviors. But, what is the neuroanatomic substrate of the affective accompaniments seen in OCD, and how might it relate to hallmark repetitive symptoms? These considerations have recently shifted our focus to the amygdala—a structure that has been implicated in emotional fear conditioning and that is intimately linked with the corticostriatal system.

The following discussion will (1) present the anatomy and connections of the amygdala; (2) present experimental evidence that the amygdala is the site of conditioned fear; (3) review the connectivity of the amygdala with corticostriatal regions; and (4) present plausible models that may elucidate the relationship between anxiety and repetitive behaviors, as well as the neurobiologic basis of behavior therapy.

Normal Anatomy and Function of the Amygdala

The amygdala is a complex of numerous subnuclei located within the medial temporal lobe (Figure 12-6).[49] Experimental evidence suggests that the amygdala responds to biologically relevant stimuli that evoke a state of increased arousal and emotional response.[50-53] Internal and external sensory stimuli access the amygdala through its lateral nucleus.[54] This information converges through the basolateral and accessory basal nuclei. The major output relay of the amygdala is the central nucleus.[51] Purportedly, it is during this intraamygdala processing that the emotional significance of a stimulus is assigned.[52,55]

The amygdala receives projections from unimodal and polymodal cortices, including all components of the paralimbic belt.[56] In addition, the amygdala receives projections from basal forebrain,[57,58] thalamus,[54,59] hippocampus,[49] and hypothalamus.[60] In turn, the amygdala projects to an even more extensive array of cortical areas.[49] These include direct projections to the orbitofrontal and prefrontal cortex,[61] and indirect projections to the cingulate, insular, temporal, and

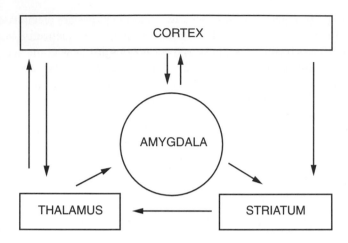

Fig. 12-6   Schematic diagram of the amygdala and its connections, emphasizing its interactions with elements of the corticostriatothalamocortical circuit. Note that incoming information can be rapidly transmitted from thalamus to amygdala, in which threat assessment is purported to occur. The amygdala is then well positioned to bias cortical activity via ascending projections, or promote stereotyped responses via projections to the striatum. Finally, descending projections from frontal (specifically medial or orbitofrontal) cortex can modulate amygdala activity in the context of habituation. Pathologic anxiety or misattribution of threat might result from excessive amygdala activation owing to (1) intrinsic pathology; (2) deficient gating at the level of the thalamus; or (3) insufficient inhibition from frontal cortex. Absent from this figure are other important connections between amygdala and territories of the basal ganglia (e.g., the ventral pallidum), basal forebrain (e.g., the substantia innominata), limbic system (e.g., the hippocampus), hypothalamus, and brain stem.

occipital cortex (including V1), via the thalamus.[49] In addition, the amygdala projects to striatum,[62,63] basal forebrain,[57,58] thalamus,[64] hippocampus,[63,65] hypothalamus,[66] and brain stem.[67,68]

Thus, the amygdala is situated between cortical sensory information processing areas (input) and brain stem autonomic and motor effector systems (output). The amygdala responds to biologically significant external and internal stimuli and then activates autonomic responses, potentiates motor reflexes, and possibly regulates the overall arousal level of the organism.[51,69] It is interesting to note that, generally, the amygdala's efferents are more influential than its afferents,[55] suggesting that once activated, the amygdala is not easily inhibited by the reciprocal projection from a given target area; consequently, this system appears biased for action. Moreover, incoming information from external sensory stimuli reaches the amygdala very rapidly, and well in advance of the cortex. This hardwiring probably serves a critical survival function, as potential threats are quickly acted on and communicated to all relevant brain regions,[52] often in advance of conscious awareness. The cost may be that fear and anxiety responses sometimes go unchecked and overgeneralize to inappropriate stimuli. This premise is critical to an amygdalocentric model of OCD or other anxiety disorders.

The Role of the Amygdala in Conditioned Fear and Anxiety

Conditioned fear describes experience-induced elicitation of autonomic and motor signs that are typical of a state of fear, in response to a previously neutral stimulus. For instance, a mild shock applied to the ear of a rabbit will produce a constellation of behaviors associated with what is presumed to be a state of fear.[51] These behaviors include heart rate changes,[70] respiration changes,[71] motor reflex potentiation,[68,72] and increased vigilance and arousal as measured by cortical electroencephalography.[69] When a previously neutral tone consistently predicts this ear shock, the tone will come to elicit these same autonomic and motor responses and, presumably, this same state of fear. At this point, fear is said to have been conditioned to the tone.

Considerable evidence now implicates the amygdala in the development and expression of conditioned fear in animals. Stimulation of the amygdala, and specifically the central nucleus of the amygdala (its major output relay) produces these same autonomic and motor fear responses.[68,70–76] Lesions of the amygdala administered prior to conditioning block the acquisition of these responses,[50,77–79] whereas lesions administered following acquisition block the expression of these responses.[80] Thus, the amygdala contributes to the acquisition and the expression of a variety of conditioned responses.[51]

Once the amygdala is actively responding to a source of threat, it can communicate this information via its massive efferent system to both brain stem effector systems and cortical processing systems. The vast majority of these connections are reciprocal,[49] suggesting the presence of feedback loops that serve to control the amount of amygdala activation. For example, a rat previously conditioned to freeze to a tone paired with shock will demonstrate extinction (i.e., disappearance) of this freezing behavior if the shock is no longer presented after the tone.[52] This fear response mediated by the amygdala is believed to be actively inhibited by feedback from the medial prefrontal cortex. The medial prefrontal cortex has reciprocal connections with the amygdala and receives projections from all sensory cortices.[49] If the medial prefrontal cortex is lesioned, the freezing response fails to extinguish in response to the tone no longer paired with the shock.[81,82] Thus, one way to conceptualize anxiety disorders is that the normal cortical to amygdala inhibition system that keeps the amygdala in check is malfunctioning and the anxiety response becomes more intrusive and chronic.[55] Thus, in humans, orbitofrontal dysfunction may well yield an analogous phenomenon.

The Relationship Between the Amygdala and Corticostriatal Systems

The amygdala has direct projections to striatum. The basolateral nucleus of the amygdala projects to both the dorsal and ventral striatum.[83–85] Amygdaloid projections terminate in the ventral and medial parts of the caudate nucleus and putamen, which border the nucleus accumbens, the body and tail of the caudate nucleus bordering the stria terminalis, and the caudal portion of the ventral putamen just dorsal to the amygdala. The basolateral nucleus actually has more in common anatomically with the adjacent temporal cortex than with other amygdaloid nuclei. Like other cortical areas, this nucleus has many reciprocal cortical connections, such as with premotor cortex;[86] the basolateral nucleus receives a direct cholinergic projection from nucleus basalis, it is reciprocally connected to thalamus, and it sends excitatory glutamate projections to striatum.[87,88] The amygdaloid projection to the striatum is considered one of its most substantial efferents.[49] Mogensen refers to these functional connections as the "limbic-motor interface,"[89] suggesting that the striatum is the site in which affective processes gain access to the subcortical motor system.

In addition, based on the pioneering neuroanatomic research of Johnston,[90] Alheid and Heimer[91] demonstrated that the amygdala and the striatum are much more anatomically proximate than had been previously appreciated. Anatomic studies of a portion of the basal forebrain referred to as "the sublenticular substantia innominata" demonstrate that this area of the brain (situated between the striatum and the amygdala) is composed of three separate forebrain structures: (1) the ventral striatopallidal system; (2) the "extended amygdala"; and (3) the magnocellular corticopetal system (or nucleus basalis). Simply put, the striatum and pallidum are now known to extend rostrally and ventrally to reach the base of the brain, forming a ventral striatum and ventral pallidum. Extending dorsally into this same region, the medial and central amygdala are continuous with the bed nucleus of the stria terminalis, the sublenticular substantia innominata, and the shell of the nucleus accumbens. The nucleus accumbens is, of course, continuous with the neostriatum immediately dorsal to it. It has definite striatal-like connections but, unlike the caudate and putamen, has many projections to brain stem that are more similar to the projection targets of the amygdala. Elements of the ventral striatum and extended amygdala actually may be intertwined at the shell of the accumbens.[92] In addition, the large cholinergic, cortically projecting cells of the nucleus basalis are interspersed throughout this basal forebrain region.

The Role of the Amygdala in Conditioned Fear and Anxiety in Obsessive-Compulsive Disorders

Given the amygdala's role in conditioned fear and anxiety and the anatomy linking it with corticostriatal systems, we propose that activation of the amygdala is a key neuroanatomic substrate of the anxiety that perpetuates compulsions in OCD. To support this argument, we will (1) present an experimental animal model of OCD; (2) describe how activation of the amygdala might functionally interact with corticostriatal systems to produce repetitive behaviors; and (3) describe how performing these behaviors might be anxiolytic by decreasing activity in the amygdala.

Most of what is known about the amygdala has been learned via animal research. Our knowledge of the anatomy of the amygdala in primates is based on studies of monkeys, and most of the relevant behavioral data have been obtained using rodents. OCD is a uniquely human disorder that is difficult to model in animals, partly because its essential elements involve subjective internal experiences. Nonetheless, rats have demonstrated that they will engage in repetitive behaviors to decrease fear in response to a cue associated with danger and not solely to the threat itself.[55,93] Rats in a box were trained to avoid a painful shock by jumping over a hurdle every time a buzzer sounded. The rats quickly learned to jump to the sound of the buzzer to avoid the shock. Mowrer[94] described this type of learning within the scope of two-factor learning theory. First, there is Pavlovian fear conditioning: the rat associates the buzzer with the shock and learns to fear the buzzer. Then, instrumental or operant conditioning: the rat learns that an overt response leads to avoidance of the shock. This example seems extremely relevant to a person who is assaulted on a subway train and consequently avoids subway trains. But how is this example relevant to the person with OCD who must wipe the kitchen counter exactly seven times with disinfectant? Here, the second part of Miller's[93] experiment is most intriguing: after the rats have learned the hurdle-jumping behavior, the shock is subsequently shut off. The rats are unaware of this fact, so they continue to jump. Next, the investigators modify the paradigm: suddenly, the buzzer continues to sound even when the rats perform the jumping response. The experimental contingency is changed, so that instead of jumping, the rats must press a lever to shut off the buzzer. In this setting, the rat rapidly learns the new repetitive behavior. In fact, even if the required operant continues to change, the rat quickly learns whatever is needed to shut the buzzer off. These animals are no longer avoiding shock, they are avoiding *fear*. Their behavior is expressly aimed at shutting off the buzzer—the new conditional source of fear. In this manner, behaviors that reduce fear and anxiety are reinforced and become habitual actions.[55] Wiping the counter seven times is no longer about avoiding disease, but rather about alleviating the anxiety associated with contracting disease.

From the above example, the compulsive actions observed in OCD can be thought of as avoidance responses that have become aimed more at reducing anxiety than at the avoidance of real danger. LeDoux[55] explains that avoidance responses are not quite emotional innate reactions or voluntary actions, but rather are somewhere in between. "Avoidance responses are instrumental responses that are learned because they are reinforced. They are then performed habitually, which is to say automatically, when the appropriate stimuli occur . . . These responses, once learned, prevent emotional arousal" (LeDoux, 1996, p. 261).

Given the proximate anatomy of the extended amygdala and ventral striatum and the direct amygdala-striatal excitatory projections from the basolateral nucleus, activation of the amygdala in a state of fear or anxiety could readily potentiate automated behavioral programs observed during striatal activation. One can easily imagine the survival advantage conferred by an automatic subcortical system that serves to potentiate an organism's most executed and practiced behaviors during a state of fear induced by some external stimulus which may be a threat to the organism. Presumably, continued activation of the striatum would serve to soothe the individual by (1) activating nucleus accumbens (a classic reward area of the brain) within the ventral striatum; and (2) inhibiting activation of the amygdala and, thus, decreasing fear and anxiety; and (3) successfully gating aversive input to the amygdala at the level of the thalamus via a striato-thalamic collateral. Given the data of Morgan, et al[81] and Morgan and LeDoux[82] presented previously, another plausible route from striatum to amygdala would be through the orbitofrontal cortex. This area directly projects to the basolateral[95] and lateral nuclei[96] of the amygdala—an area of the amygdala known to be richly innervated via the inhibitory transmitter gamma-aminobutyric acid (GABA)[97] and the proposed site of the anxiolytic actions of the benzodiazepines.[53,98] Interestingly, continued exposure to GABA antagonists injected into the basolateral nucleus produces a pathophysiologic "priming" effect in which experimental animals continually display physiologic and behavioral changes similar to symptoms of human anxiety states.[99]

Indeed, extinction-based behavior therapies such as exposure and response prevention might tap this very system (see Chapters 17, 19, and 20). During behavior therapy, the patient is incrementally exposed to a hierarchy of provocative stimuli. Although such stimuli activate the amygdala and lead to anxiety, careful titration, and coaching enable the patient to tolerate this state while preventing compulsive responses, despite the drive to engage in repetitive behaviors. These repetitive behaviors have been previously reinforced, in that they serve to decrease anxiety. But the compulsions have become sufficiently removed from the original source of anxiety that they are self-perpetuating. In a sense, the patient has not had an opportunity to "learn" that nothing bad will happen if he fails to perform the compulsions. By analogy to Miller's jumping rats, in the case of patients with OCD, the shock has long been turned off, and there is no reality-based threat. However, patients with OCD do not stop "jumping" long enough to develop this "limbic" equivalent of insight. In a third phase of Miller's study, a wall was placed between the two compartments, which prevented the rats from making the jumping response. Under these conditions, the repetitive behavior soon extinguished and did not return even when the wall was subsequently removed and the animal was given the opportunity to jump again.[100] Exposure and response prevention give the OCD patient who must cross the threshold just right, both the opportunity to learn that his mother does not die even if he does not perform the act, and the experience that his anxiety level ultimately declines even if the ritual is prevented. Presumably, such insight is not merely developed at some cognitive level, but more fundamentally within the system that mediates threat assessment and anxiety. Specifically, extinction-based behavior therapy may facilitate the process by which orbitofrontal cortex inhibits and controls amygdala activation.[55] Once amygdala activation decreases, so too does the drive to perform repetitive behaviors.

NEUROCHEMICAL MODELS OF OBSESSIVE-COMPULSIVE DISORDERS

The Serotonergic Hypothesis of Obsessive-Compulsive Disorder

Serotonin (5-hydroxytryptamine [5-HT]) is a neurotransmitter that is released from neurons in which cell bodies reside within the raphe nuclei of the midbrain. Serotonergic projections from the raphe are wide-ranging. Moreover, there are numerous different serotonergic receptor subtypes, each with their own profile in terms of distribution in brain, location on neurons, effector mechanisms (e.g., second messengers), and influences on neuronal firing (Table 12-1).[101] Consequently, dissection of the serotonergic system is a complex and challenging enterprise.

A serotonergic hypothesis of OCD was initially motivated by the observed differential efficacy of serotonergic reuptake inhibitors (SRIs) in alleviating OCD symptoms.[102–105] One obvious possibility is that SRIs might be having their antiobsessional effects by correcting some fundamental abnormality in the serotonergic system. Of course, the fact that medications with serotonergic action serve as effective antiobsessionals does not, however, imply that the serotonergic system is necessarily dysfunctional in OCD. To the contrary, SRIs may instead act via modulation of an intact system to compensate for the underlying pathophysiology in OCD. Therefore, research in this domain has sought to answer two basic questions: (1) Is there a primary serotonergic abnormality in patients with OCD? and (2) How and where do SRIs confer their beneficial antiobsessional effects?

Answering the first of these questions optimally requires methods for directly probing the salient elements of the serotonergic system. Recently, with the advent of functional imaging techniques that allow investigators to characterize receptor systems *in vivo,* such studies have become possible. Still, a full array of selective radioligands will be necessary to enable a comprehensive dissection of the serotonergic system in OCD and other disorders. No studies of this type have yet been published.

Over the past few years, a considerable literature has accrued based on indirect measurements of central serotonergic function. However, studies of peripheral receptor binding in the blood or concentrations of 5-HT metabolites in

Table 12-1   Serotonergic Receptors in Brain

Receptor	Brain Region	Neuronal Site	Effect
$5\text{-}HT_{1A}$	Dorsal raphe, hippocampus, cortex	Autoreceptor (somatodendritic) and postsynaptic	Hyperpolarizes
$5\text{-}HT_{1D}$	Substantia nigra, striatum, cortex	Autoreceptor (terminal) and postsynaptic	Inhibits release
$5\text{-}HT_{2A}$	Cortex	Postsynaptic	Increases phosphatidylinositol turnover
$5\text{-}HT_{2C}$	Substantia nigra, globus pallidus	Postsynaptic	Increases phosphatidylinositol turnover
$5\text{-}HT_{3}$	Brainstem, limbic system	Postsynaptic	Depolarizes
$5\text{-}HT_{4}$	Hippocampus	Postsynaptic	Increases cyclic adenosine monophosphate

5-HT, Serotonin.

cerebrospinal fluid, for instance, have been disappointingly inconsistent.[8,106,107] Further, it is acknowledged that these measures do not represent good indicators of serotonergic function within the brain. Pharmacologic challenge studies represent another indirect approach.[8,106–108] By administering various serotonergic agents and measuring endocrine or behavioral variables, investigators have attempted to assess central serotonergic sensitivities. These paradigms have likewise proven problematic because the pharmacologic probes are nonspecific and the dependent variables assayed are typically mediated by a complex interplay of different neurochemical systems. Therefore, the fundamental hypothesis that OCD is a manifestation of serotonergic dysfunction remains not only unproven but also essentially untested.

In contrast, basic and clinical pharmacologic research has begun to successfully elucidate possible therapeutic mechanisms of SRIs. There is convergent evidence from animal studies that antidepressants can potentiate serotonergic transmission.[109] In the case of SRIs, there is evidence that this potentiation occurs as a consequence of autoreceptor desensitization.[110,111] The time course of these receptor changes parallels the observed delay between initiation of SRIs and emergence of therapeutic response. More specifically, Mansari and colleagues[112] have shown that SRI–induced changes in serotonergic transmission occur more quickly in lateral frontal cortex than in medial frontal cortex of rodents. This converges beautifully with the observation that the antidepressant effects of SRIs tend to occur sooner than antiobsessional effects, because lateral prefrontal areas have been implicated in the pathophysiology of major depression whereas medial frontal (i.e., orbitofrontal) cortex has been implicated in the pathophysiology of OCD. The ultimate neuropharmacologic effects of SRIs on frontal cortex and other relevant territories, including paralimbic cortex, striatum, and the amygdala remain to be fully delineated. Further, the relative role of different receptor subtypes has not been determined.

In summary, there are not yet any compelling data to support the contention that OCD is fundamentally a disorder of serotonergic function. In contrast, serotonergic medications are clearly differentially effective as treatments for OCD. Hence, a serotonergic model of OCD pathophysiology remains untested, whereas the serotonergic model of antiobsessional pharmacotherapy finds substantial initial support. Emerging data suggest that SRIs might have their beneficial effects, following a delay of several weeks, by down-regulating terminal autoreceptors ($5HT_{1D}$) in orbitofrontal cortex, thereby facilitating serotonergic transmission in that region.[112] Functional imaging studies will provide the first opportunity to directly test the serotonergic hypothesis of OCD pathophysiology. Additional studies also are necessary to clarify the precise mechanisms that underlie the antiobsessional effects of SRIs, as well as other effective treatments, including nonpharmacologic modalities. Finally, it is unclear how this information generalizes to other OCDs. SRIs appear to be efficacious for BDD and TTM but are not typically effective for reducing the tics of TD (although they can be helpful for addressing other associated affective or behavioral manifestations). Thus, a serotonergic hypothesis of SRI action in OCDs should ultimately explain the observed differential efficacy across this spectrum of disorders.

The Dopaminergic Hypothesis of Tourette's Disorder

Paralleling the above discussion of serotonin and its role in OCD, dopamine antagonists have proven to be effective agents for reducing the tics of TD and the manifestations of other hyperkinetic movement disorders. Moreover, dopamine agonists are known to exacerbate tics and other adventitial movements. Unlike the serotonergic hypothesis of OCD, however, there are now concrete data that show dopaminergic abnormalities in TD.

The cell bodies of dopamine-containing neurons are principally concentrated in midbrain and tegmentum, and project forward forming a nigrostriatal pathway, as well as mesolimbic and mesocortical systems. It has long been presumed that the therapeutic effects of dopamine antagonists in hyperkinetic movement disorders follow logically from the well-established role of dopamine in mediating motor control via the nigrostriatal system. More recently, a series of studies have actually demonstrated striatal dopamine-receptor abnormalities in TD. A postmortem study revealed higher binding rates for a dopamine-transporter site ligand in the striatum of brains from people with TD versus comparison specimens.[113] An analogous *in vivo* neuroimaging study[114] has shown increased binding capacity for dopaminergic reuptake sites in the striatum of TD patients versus matched controls, indicating an elevated density of these transporter sites in TD. In a study of twins concordant for TD but discordant for tic severity, Wolf and colleagues[115] found decreased binding capacity for dopaminergic postsynaptic receptors in the striatum of the more severely affected twins. These results indicate that more severe TD is associated with either higher levels of ambient dopamine or a reduced density of postsynaptic dopamine-receptor sites. Taken together, the findings from these three studies suggest that patients with TD do exhibit abnormalities of the dopaminergic system within the striatum. One caveat to be acknowledged is that because the subjects in these studies were not neuroleptic naive, some of the observed abnormalities may be a consequence of past exposure to antidopaminergic medications. Nonetheless, the total body of evidence supports a dopaminergic hypothesis of TD. Specifically, TD may be associated with fundamental dopaminergic abnormalities within the striatum, and tic symptoms can be exacerbated by exposure to dopamimetic agents and ameliorated by treatment with dopamine anatagonist medications.

Synthetic Neurochemical Hypotheses

It is intriguing to consider that pathophysiologic heterogeneity may explain why some subtypes of OCD are responsive to SRIs alone and others are responsive to SRIs plus dopamine antagonists, whereas other subtypes are wholly unresponsive to either of these interventions. For instance, tic-related OCD appears to be relatively SRI–refractory and preferentially responsive to the combination of SRIs plus dopamine antagonists.[116] One possibility is that non–tic-related OCD and BDD involve primary orbitofrontal dysfunction or pathophysiology of the orbitofrontal-amygdalar axis, whereas tic-related OCD and TD involve primary striatal pathology. Hence, serotonergic modulation at the level of orbitofrontal cortex or the amygdala might be sufficient for antiobsessional effects in BDD or non–tic-related OCD, whereas dopaminergic modulation within the striatum synergizes with orbitofrontal serotonergic modulation to relieve tic-related OCD, and pure TD responds to dopamine modulation at the level of the striatum but not to serotonergic modulation at the orbitofrontal cortex.

SUMMARY AND INTEGRATION OF NEUROBIOLOGIC MODELS

In summary, we have reviewed three different models of OCDs, each of which speaks to different aspects of the phenomenology or neurobiology of these disorders. Presented together, these models can be seen as synergistic, rather than mutually exclusive.

Corticostriatal systems serve multiple normal functions, including processing and/or filtering information such that it does not reach the conscious domain, as well as the mediation of automated or stereotyped behaviors. Thus, it is intuitively appealing to suggest that dysfunction of corticostriatal systems could explain both the intrusive phenomena and the ritualized repetitive behaviors performed in response to obsessions that are the hallmarks of OCDs. This hypothesis finds extensive support in both the clinical and research literature. For instance, known lesions of the corticostriatal system can produce phenocopies of OCDs, and more importantly, studies of patients with OCDs demonstrate abnormalities in the structure and function of corticostriatal elements. Further, treatments that ameliorate the symptoms of OCDs appear to act, at least partly, by modulating activity within these same cortical or striatal territories. The striatal topography model of OCDs represents an extension of the basic corticostriatal concept. The striatal topography model represents three related hypotheses: (1) the fundamental site of pathology in OCD is within the striatum; (2) the analogous pathophysiologic substrates exist across the range of OCDs; and (3) the topography of striatal involvement corresponds with the clinical picture for each disorder (both with regard to presentation and treatment response profile). Finally, across the different variants of the cortico-striatal models of OCDs, there is agreement that effective treatments have the shared endpoint of reducing corticothalamic overdrive. It remains controversial as to whether intentional repetitive behaviors are more appropriately conceptualized as primary unwanted intrusive symptoms or pseudocompensatory behaviors. Regardless, there is good evidence to suggest that such behaviors are mediated via the striatum.

The amygdalocentric perspective enriches our understanding of the affective or motivational elements of OCDs. In one sense, the amygdala should be appreciated as a limbic structure which has unique influence over the paralimbic system and the striatum. The normal function of the amygdala involves a prominent role in the rapid assessment of danger, prioritization of information processing demands, assignment of significance to various stimuli, and facilitation of adaptive behavior. In particular, it is well established that the amygdala is critical to an organism's ability to modify the perceived danger value of a given stimulus, as well as the organism's behavior in response to that stimulus. This amygdala-mediated plasticity seems to rely heavily on its interconnections with medial frontal cortex. Moreover, the amygdala has dense connections with striatum that are presumed to support an efficient system for driving automated behaviors in response to danger; whereas reciprocal connections with the extended amygdala, including the ventral striatum and bed nucleus of the stria terminalis, may help to mediate the soothing or anxiolytic byproducts of repetitive behaviors. Thus, it is clear that future investigation of the amygdala and its interactions with medial frontal and striatal territories will be critical to understanding the neurobiology of behavioral therapies. Moreover, it is reasonable to suppose that the amygdala plays a critical role in other anxiety disorders and major affective illnesses. Therefore, a more thorough understanding of the amygdala also may help explain the high comorbidity of major affective disorders and other anxiety disorders with OCDs.

Neurochemical considerations must be superimposed over the anatomy described in the first two sections. Serotonergic medications modulate neurotransmission within frontal cortex in a manner that could explain their beneficial effects both as antiobsessionals and antidepressants.

Future research will be necessary to determine whether, in the case of OCDs, this represents correcting a fundamental serotonergic imbalance, or recruiting an intact system to compensate for pathophysiology of another kind. In contrast, TD appears to represent a disorder characterized by some primary dopaminergic abnormality within the striatum. However, although administration of dopamine antagonist medications may seem to represent the most logical and direct remedy for counteracting the pathophysiology of TD, more effective, nondopaminergic interventions still might be developed. Much work remains to be done in elucidating the normal brain chemistry of these various neural systems. Consequently, we should remain hopeful that new insights regarding pathophysiology and potential pharmacotherapies may emerge as research in this arena progresses. Further, the advent of new research tools, including neuroimaging receptor characterization methods and chemical compounds with selective receptor-binding properties, promise better means for testing neurochemical hypotheses as they emerge.

Future Research

In fact, as research regarding the neurobiology of OCDs ensues, the driving force must be a commitment to finding better means to relieve the suffering of individuals afflicted with these conditions. In this final section, we propose several lines of neuroscience research that might prove fruitful in advancing our understanding of OCDs and their treatment.

Corticostriatal models have given investigators discrete regions in which to focus their search for cellular or molecular abnormalities in OCDs. Morphometric and functional imaging studies that support the striatal topography concept for OCD and TD must be extended to BDD and TTM. Postmortem microscopic pathologic studies are long overdue but continue to await collection of adequate specimens for this type of research. In this regard, coordination of a postmortem brain banking initiative should be a top priority. As basic neuroscience studies advance our knowledge of cell biology, neurophysiology, and neurochemistry in the striatum, we will be better equipped to understand the underlying pathophysiology of OCDs and to discover innovative measures to counteract the disease process. For instance, our current understanding of differential neurochemistry in the direct and indirect pathways suggests that substance P antagonists might be effective antiobsessional agents by augmenting thalamic inhibition via the corticostriatothalamic branch. The implicit information-processing deficit model indicates that fundamental striatal pathology should lead to neuropsychologic deficits beyond the core symptoms of OCDs. Consequently, even when classical antiobsessional drugs reduce intrusions and repetitive phenomena, these drugs may not address the neuropsychologic information-processing deficits. Neuropsychologic studies and neuroimaging studies involving implicit learning tasks must be conducted to test such hypotheses.

We anticipate that the amygdala will also be a focus of OCD research in the future. First, human studies will likely take advantage of new neuroimaging techniques, perhaps especially functional magnetic resonance imaging (MRI). Recent studies have documented not only a capacity to detect gross amygdala activation in response to OCD symptom provocation,[37] but also in response to more subtle standardized stimuli in normal subjects.[117,118] Perhaps most importantly, we have demonstrated that MRI can be used to monitor subtle temporal changes in amygdala activity indicative of habituation.[117,118] Next, we propose to study the functional influence of the amygdala on medial frontal and striatal regions, in normal control subjects, patients with OCDs, and patients with other anxiety or affective disorders. We propose that, by employing subliminal and supraliminal stimuli, investigators will be able to tease out the top-down influence of cortical territories on the amygdala,[118] just as by using implicit and explicit learning paradigms we have begun to do the same for corticostriatal systems.[27,119] More practically, investigators should begin to explore pharmacologic means of augmenting or accelerating the extinction process that underlies behavior therapies. Ultimately, MRI probes of amygdala function may also serve to predict treatment response or guide treatment decisions. Animal models of fear-potentiated startle might represent one laboratory preparation that could serve to screen such candidate compounds.[120,121]

As already outlined, *in vivo* receptor characterization studies, which employ cutting edge imaging techniques, will allow investigators to test the serotonergic hypothesis of OCD. Likewise, studies of the serotonergic and the dopaminergic system should be extended across the full spectrum of OCDs. The true magnitude of such an undertaking is not evident until one considers the multitude of different receptor subtypes that must be independently assayed. Further, dopamine and serotonin are but two transmitters among many that dictate intercellular communication in these neural systems. Future studies will also begin to dissect the role of other transmitters, including neuropeptides. Simultaneously, animal research will continue to elucidate the receptor changes associated with short- and long-term pharmacotherapy; it will be intriguing to extend these methods to ascertain analogous changes that accompany conditioning and extinction which are analogous to behavior therapy.

Finally, we have intentionally foregone discussions of etiology, which are reviewed comprehensively elsewhere in this volume (see Chapters 11 and 14). Nonetheless, as clues about the genetics and pathogenesis of OCD emerge, they will undoubtedly prompt modifications to existing neurobiologic models and will stimulate novel ideas regarding potential strategies for prevention and cure. These are exciting times in psychiatric neuroscience, as new technologies and paradigms provide better opportunities for understanding the neurobiology of OCD and related disorders. More important still is the promise that such increased understanding can be translated into better diagnosis and treatment for those patients who suffer with these diseases.

ACKNOWLEDGMENT

Acknowledgment of support: Dr. Rauch is supported in part via the National Institute of Mental Health (grant MH01215) and a Young Investigator Award from the National Alliance for Research on Schizophrenia and Depression. Dr. Whalen is a fellow in the Harvard Clinical Research Training Program. Research in the Obsessive-Compulsive Disorders Clinic and Research Unit at the Massachusetts General Hospital is supported in part by the David Judah Research Fund.

REFERENCES

1. Rapoport JL, Wise SP: Obsessive-compulsive disorder: is it a basal ganglia dysfunction? *Psychopharmacol Bull* 24:380–384, 1988.
2. Modell J, Mountz J, Curtis G, et al: Neurophysiologic dysfunction in basal ganglia/limbic striatal and thalamocortical circuits as a pathogenetic mechanism of obsessive-compulsive disorder, *J Neuropsychiatry* 1:27–36, 1989.
3. Baxter LR, Schwartz JM, Guze BH, et al: Neuroimaging in obsessive-compulsive disorder: seeking the mediating neuroanatomy. In Jenike MA, Baer L, Minichiello WE, editors: *Obsessive compulsive disorder: Theory and management*, ed 2, Chicago, 1990, Mosby.
4. Insel TR: Toward a neuroanatomy of obsessive-compulsive disorder, *Arch Gen Psychiatry* 49:739–744, 1992.
5. Baxter LR Jr, Schwartz JM, Bergman KS, et al: Caudate glucose metabolic rate changes with both drug and behavior therapy for obsessive-compulsive disorder, *Arch Gen Psychiatry* 49:681–689, 1992.
6. Leckman JF, Pauls DL, Peterson BS, et al: Pathogenesis of Tourette syndrome: clues from the clinical phenotype and natural history, *Adv Neurol* 58:15–24, 1992.
7. Cummings JL: Frontal-subcortical circuits and human behavior, *Arch Neurol* 50:873–880, 1993.
8. Rauch SL, Jenike MA: Neurobiological models of obsessive-compulsive disorder, *Psychosomatics* 34:20–32, 1993.
9. Rauch SL, Jenike MA: Neural mechanisms of obsessive-compulsive disorder, *Curr Rev Mood Anx Dis* 1:84–94, 1997.
10. Rauch SL, Bates JF, Grachev ID: Obsessive compulsive disorder. In Peterson BF, editor: *Neuroimaging—child and adolescent. Psychiatric Clinics of North America*, Philadelphia, 1997, WB Saunders.
11. Hollander E, editor: Obsessive-compulsive spectrum disorders, *Psychiatr Ann* 23:355–407, 1993.
12. McElroy SL, Phillips KA, Keck PE: Obsessive compulsive spectrum disorder, *J Clin Psychiatry* 55(suppl):15–32, 1994.

13. Miguel EC, Coffey BJ, Baer L, et al: Phenomenology of intentional repetitive behaviors in obsessive-compulsive disorder and Tourette's syndrome, *J Clin Psychiatry* 56:246–255, 1995.
14. Rauch SL: Neuroimaging in obsessive-compulsive disorder and related disorders. In Jenike MA, chairman: Recent developments in neurobiology of OCD, *J Clin Psychiatry* 57:492–503, 1996.
15. Otto MW: Neuropsychological approaches to obsessive-compulsive disorder. In Jenike MA, Baer L, Minichiello WE, editors: *Obsessive compulsive disorder: theory and management*, ed 2, Chicago, 1990, Mosby.
16. Mesulam M-M: Patterns in behavioral neuroanatomy: association areas, the limbic system, and hemispheric specialization. In Mesulam M-M editor: *Principles of behavioral neurology*, Philadelphia, 1985, FA Davis.
17. Zald DH, Kim SW: Anatomy and function of the orbital frontal cortex II: function and relevance to obsessive-compulsive disorder, *J Neuropsychiatry* 8:249–261, 1996.
18. Rauch SL, Jenike MA, Alpert NM, et al: Regional cerebral blood flow measured during symptom provocation in obsessive-compulsive disorder using ^{15}O-labeled CO_2 and positron emission tomography, *Arch Gen Psychiatry* 51:62–70, 1994.
19. Rauch SL, Savage CR, Alpert NM, et al: A positron emission tomographic study of simple phobic symptom provocation, *Arch Gen Psychiatry* 52:20–28, 1995.
20. Rauch SL, van der Kolk BA, Fisler RE, et al: A symptom provocation study of posttraumatic stress disorder using positron emission tomography and script driven imagery, *Arch Gen Psychiatry* 53:380–387, 1996.
21. Rauch SL, Savage CR, Alpert NM, et al: The functional neuroanatomy of anxiety: a study of three disorders using PET and symptom provocation, *Biol Psychiatry* 42:446–452, 1997.
22. Rauch SL, Shin LM: Functional neuroimaging studies in PTSD, *Ann New York Acad Sci* 821:83–98, 1997.
23. Alexander GE, DeLong MR, Strick PL: Parallel organization of functionally segregated circuits linking basal ganglia and cortex, *Ann Rev Neurosci* 9:357–381, 1986.
24. Alexander GE, Crutcher MD, DeLong MR: Basal ganglia-thalamocortical circuits: parallel substrates for motor, oculomotor, "prefrontal" and "limbic" functions, *Prog Brain Res* 85:119–146, 1990.
25. Houk JC, Davis JL, Beiser DG, editors: *Models of information processing in the basal ganglia,* Cambridge, 1995, MIT Press.
26. Rauch SL, Savage CR, Brown HD, et al: A PET investigation of implicit and explicit sequence learning, *Hum Brain Mapping* 3:271–286, 1995.
27. Rauch SL, Savage CR, Alpert NM, et al: Probing striatal function in obsessive compulsive disorder: a PET study of implicit sequence learning, *J Neuropsychiatry* 9:568–573, 1997.
28. Rauch SL, Savage CR: Neuroimaging and neuropsychology of the striatum. In Miguel EC, Rauch SL, Leckman JF, editors: *Neuropsychiatry of the basal ganglia. Psychiatric Clinics of North America*, Philadelphia, 1997, WB Saunders.
29. Wise SP, Murray EA, Gerfen CR: The frontal cortex-basal ganglia system in primates, *Crit Rev Neurobiol* 10:317–356, 1996.
30. Graybiel AM: Building action repertoires: memory and learning functions of the basal ganglia, *Curr Opin Neurobiol* 5:733–741, 1995.

31. Albin RL, Young AB, Penney JB: The functional anatomy of basal ganglia disorders, *Trends Neurosci* 12:366–375, 1989.
32. Graybiel AM: Neurotransmitters and neuromodulators in the basal ganglia, *Trends Neurosci* 13:244–253, 1990.
33. Gerfen CR: The neostriatal mosaic: Multiple levels of compartmental organization in the basal ganglia, *Ann Rev Neurosci* 15:285–320, 1992.
34. Salloway S, Cummings JL: Subcortical structures and neuropsychiatric illness, *Neuroscientist* 2:66–75, 1996.
35. Williams AC, Owen C, Heath DA: A compulsive movement disorder with cavitation of caudate nucleus, *J Neurol Neurosurg Psychiatry* 51:447–448, 1988.
36. Weilburg JB, Mesulam MM, Weintraub S, et al: Focal striatal abnormalities in a patient with obsessive-compulsive disorder, *Arch Neurol* 46:233–235, 1989.
37. Breiter HC, Rauch SL, Kwong KK, et al: Functional magnetic resonance imaging of symptom provocation in obsessive compulsive disorder, *Arch Gen Psychiatry* 53:595–606, 1996.
38. Reber AS: Implicit learning and tacit knowledge, *J Exper Psychol Gen* 118:219–235, 1989.
39. Reber AS: The cognitive unconcious: an evolutionary perspective, *Consci Cogn* 1:93–133, 1992.
40. Reber PJ, Squire LR: Parallel brain systems for learning with and without awareness, *Learn Mem* 1:217–229, 1994.
41. Schacter DL, Tulving E, editors: *Memory systems 1994*, Cambridge, 1994, MIT Press.
42. Curran T: On the neural mechanisms of sequence learning, Psyche *2* (2), URL: http://psyche.cs.monash.edu.au/volume2-1/psyche-95-2-12-sequence-1-curran.html. 1995.
43. Squire LR: Memory and the hippocampus: a synthesis from findings with rats, monkeys, and humans, *Psychol Rev* 99:195–231, 1992.
44. Ungerleider LG: Functional brain imaging studies of cortical mechanisms for memory, *Science* 270:769–775, 1995.
45. Schacter DL, Alpert NM, Savage CR, et al: Conscious recollection and the human hippocampal formation: evidence from positron emission tomography, *Proc Natl Acad Sci U S A* 93:321–325, 1996.
46. Mishkin M, Malamut B, Bachevalier: Memories and habits: two neural systems. In Lynch G, McGaugh JL, Weinberger NM, editors: *Neurobiology of learning and memory*, New York, 1984, Guilford Press.
47. Mishkin N, Petri HL: Memory and habits: some implications for the analysis of learning and retention. In Squire LR, Butters N, editors: *Neuropsychology of memory,* New York, 1984, Guilford Press.
48. Rauch SL, Savage CR: Investigating cortico-striatal pathophysiology in obsessive compulsive disorders: Procedural learning and imaging probes. In Goodman WK, Rudorfer MV, Maser JD, editors: *Treatment resistant obsessive-compulsive disorder*, (in press).
49. Amaral DG, Price JL, Pitkanen A, et al: Anatomical organization of the primate amygdala. In Aggleton JP, editor: *The amygdala: neurobiological aspects of emotion, memory and mental dysfunction*, New York, 1992, Wiley-Liss.
50. Kapp BS, Frysinger RC, Gallagher M, et al: Amygdala central nucleus lesions:

Effects on heart rate conditioning in the rabbit, *Physiol Behav* 23:1109–1117, 1979.

51. Kapp BS, Whalen PJ, Supple WF, et al: Amygdaloid contributions to conditioned arousal and sensory information processing. In Aggleton JP, editor: *The amygdala: neurobiological aspects of emotion, memory and mental dysfunction*, New York, 1992, Wiley-Liss.

52. LeDoux JE: Emotion, memory and the brain, *Sci Am* 270:32–39, 1994.

53. Davis M: The role of the amygdala in conditioned fear. In Aggleton JP, editor: *The amygdala: neurobiological aspects of emotion, memory and mental dysfunction*, New York, 1992, Wiley-Liss.

54. LeDoux JE, Cicchetti P, Xagoraris A, et al: The lateral amygdaloid nucleus: sensory interface of the amygdala in fear conditioning, *J Neurosci* 10:1062–1069, 1990.

55. LeDoux JE: *The emotional brain*, New York, 1996, Simon and Schuster.

56. Aggleton JP, Burton MJ, Passingham RE: Cortical and subcortical afferents to the amygdala of the rhesus monkey (Macaca mulatta), *Brain Res* 109:347–368, 1980.

57. Mesulam M-M, Mufson EJ, Levey AI, et al: Cholinergic innervation of cortex by the basal forebrain: cytochemistry and cortical connections of the septal area, diagonal band nuclci, nucleus basalis (substantia innominata) and hypothalamus in the rhesus monkey, *J Comp Neurol* 214:170–197, 1983.

58. Russchen FT, Amaral DG, Price JL: The afferent connections of the substantia innominata in the monkey, Macaca fascicularis, *J Comp Neurol* 242:1–27, 1985.

59. Russchen FT: Amygdalopetal projections in the cat. I. Cortical afferent connections. A study with retrograde and anterograde tracing techniques, *J Comp Neurol* 206:159–179, 1982.

60. Amaral DG, Veazey RB, Cowan WM: Some observations on the hypothalamo-amygdaloid connections in the monkey, *Brain Res* 252:13–27, 1982.

61. Yeterian EH, van Hoesen GW: Cortico-striate projections in the rhesus monkey: the organization of certain cortico-caudate connections, *Brain Res* 139:43–63, 1978.

62. Nauta WJH: Neural associations of the amygdaloid complex in the monkey, *Brain* 85:505–520, 1962.

63. Krettek JE, Price DL: A description of the amygdaloid complex in the rat and cat with observations on intra-amygdaloid axonal connections, *J Comp Neurol* 178:255–280, 1978.

64. Price JL, Amaral DG: An autoradiographic study of the projections of the central nucleus of the monkey amygdala, *J Neurosci* 11:1242–1259, 1981.

65. Krettek JE, Price DL: A direct input from the amygdala to the thalamus and the cerebral cortex, *Brain Res* 67:169–174, 1974.

66. Holstege G, Meiners L, Tan K: Projections of the bed nucleus of the stria terminalis to the mesencephalon, pons, and medulla oblongata in the cat, *Exper Brain Res* 58:379–391, 1985.

67. Hopkins DA: Amygdalotegmental projections in the rat, cat and rhesus monkey, *Neurosci Lett* 1:263–270, 1975.

68. Whalen PJ, Kapp BS: Contributions of the amygdaloid central nucleus to the modulation of the nictitating membrane reflex in the rabbit, *Behav Neurosci* 105: 141–153, 1991.

69. Whalen PJ, Kapp BS, Pascoe JP: Neuronal activity within the nucleus basalis and conditioned neocortical electroencephalographic activation, *J Neurosci* 14: 1623–1633, 1994.

70. Kapp BS, Gallagher M, Underwood MD, et al: Cardiovascular responses elicited by electrical stimulation of the amygdala central nucleus in the rabbit, *Brain Res* 234:251–262, 1982.

71. Applegate CD, Kapp BS, Underwood M, et al: Autonomic and somatomotor effects of amygdala central n. stimulation in awake rabbits, *Physiol Behav* 31: 353–360, 1983.

72. Rosen JB, Davis M: Enhancement of acoustic startle by electrical stimulation of the amygdala, *Behav Neurosci* 102:195–202, 1988.

73. Kaada BR: Somatomotor, autonomic and electrophysiological responses to electrical stimulation of "rhinencephalic" and other structures in primates, cat and dog, *Acta Physiol Scand* (suppl 83)24:1–285, 1951.

74. Bonvallet M, Gary Bobo E: Changes in the phrenic activity and heart rate elicited by localized stimulation of the amygdala and adjacent structures, *Electroencephal Clin Neurophysiol* 32:1–16, 1972.

75. Gloor P: Amygdala. In Field J, editor: *Handbook of physiology: Sec. I. Neurophysiology,* Washington, 1960, American Physiological Society.

76. Kaada BR: Stimulation and regional ablation of the amygdaloid complex with reference to functional representations. In Eleftherlou BF, editor: *The neurobiology of the amygdala,* New York, 1972, Plenum Press.

77. Gentile CG, Romanski LM, Jarrell TW, et al: Ibotenic acid lesions in amygdaloid central nucleus prevent the acquisition of differentially conditioned bradycardic responses in rabbits, *Neurosci Abstr* 12:755, 1986.

78. Iwata J, LeDoux JE, Meeley MP, et al: Intrinsic neurons in the amygdaloid field projected to by the medial geniculate body mediate emotional responses conditioned to acoustic stimuli, *Brain Res* 383:195–214, 1986.

79. Hitchcock JM, Davis M: Lesions of the amygdala, but not of the cerebellum or red nucleus, block conditioned fear as measured with the potentiated startle paradigm, *Behav Neurosci* 100:11–22, 1986.

80. Gentile CG, Jarrell TW, Teich AH, et al: The role of the amygdaloid central nucleus in differential Pavlovian conditioning of bradycardia in rabbits, *Behav Brain Res* 20:263–276, 1986.

81. Morgan MA, Romanski L, LeDoux JE: Extinction of emotional learning: contribution of medial prefrontal cortex, *Neurosci Lett* 163:109–113, 1993.

82. Morgan MA, LeDoux JE: Differential contribution of dorsal and ventral medial prefrontal cortex to the acquisition and extinction of conditioned fear in rats, *Behav Neurosci* 109:681–688, 1995.

83. Russchen FT, Price JL: Amygdalostriatal projections in the rat. Topographical organization and fiber morphology shown using the lectin PHA-L as an anterograde tracer, *Neurosci Lett* 47:15–22, 1984.

84. Ragsdale CW, Graybiel AM: Fibers from the basolateral nucleus of the amygdala selectively innervate striosomes in the caudate nucleus of the cat, *J Comp Neurol* 269:506–522, 1988.

85. Russchen FT, Bakst I, Amaral DG, et al: The amygdalostriatal projections in the monkey. An anterograde tracing study, *Brain Res* 329:241–257, 1985.

86. Avendano C, Price JL, Amaral DG: Evidence for an amygdaloid projection to premotor cortex but not to motor cortex in the monkey, *Brain Res* 264:111–117, 1983.
87. Fuller TA, Russchen FT, Price JL: Sources of presumptive glutamergic/aspartergic afferents to the rat ventral striatopallidal region, *J Comp Neurol* 258:317–338, 1987.
88. Kelley AE, Domesick VB, Nauta WJH: The amygdalostriatal projection in the rat—an anatomical study by anterograde and retrograde horseradish peroxidase study, *Neuroscience* 7:615–630, 1982.
89. Mogensen GJ: Limbic and motor integration. In Sprague JN, Epstein AN, editors: *Progress in psychobiology and physiological psychology*, vol 12, New York, 1987, Academic Press.
90. Johnston JB: Further contributions to the study of the evolution of the forebrain, *J Comp Neurol* 35:337–481, 1923.
91. Alheid GF, Heimer L: New perspectives in basal forebrain organization of special relevance for neuropsychiatric disorders: the striatopallidal, amygdaloid and corticopetal components of substantia innominata, *Neuroscience* 27(1):1–39, 1988.
92. Alheid GF, Heimer L: The ventral striato-pallidal (VSP) system and the substantia innominata (SI) complex of the rat (abstract), *Appetite* 6:198, 1985.
93. Miller NE: Studies of fear as an acquirable drive: I. Fear as motivation and fear reduction as reinforcement in the learning of new responses, *J Exper Psychol* 38: 89–101, 1948.
94. Mowrer OH: A stimulus-response analysis of anxiety and its role as a reinforcing agent, *Psychol Rev* 46:553–565, 1939.
95. Brinely-Reed M, Mascagni F, McDonald AJ: Synaptology of prefrontal cortical projections to the basolateral amygdala: an electron microscope study in the rat, *Neurosci Lett* 202:45–48, 1995.
96. Carmichael ST, Price JL: Limbic connections of the orbital and medial prefrontal cortex in macaque monkeys, *J Comp Neurol* 363:615–641, 1995.
97. Sanders SK, Shekar A: Regulation of anxiety by GABAA receptors in the rat amygdala, *Pharmacol Biochem Behav* 52:701–706, 1995.
98. Sanders SK, Shekar A: Anxiolytic effects of chlordiazepoxide blocked by injection of GABAA and benzodiazapine receptor antagonists in the region of the anterior basolateral amygdala of rats, *Biol Psychiatry* 37:473–476, 1995.
99. Sanders SK, Morzorati SL, Shekhar A: Priming of experimental anxiety by repeated subthreshold GABA blockade in the rat amygdala, *Brain Res* 699: 250–259, 1995.
100. Seligman MEP: Phobias and preparedness, *Behav Ther* 2:307–320, 1971.
101. Hoyer D, Clarke DE, Fozard JR, et al: International Union of Pharmacology classification of receptors for 5-hydroxytryptamine (serotonin), *Pharmacol Rev* 46:157–203, 1994.
102. Thoren P, Asberg M, Cronholm B, et al: Clomipramine treatment of obsessive compulsive disorder. I. A controlled clinical trial, *Arch Gen Psychiatry* 37: 1281–1285, 1980.
103. Thoren P, Asberg M, Cronholm B, et al: Clomipramine treatment of obsessive compulsive disorder. II, *Arch Gen Psychiatry* 37:1286–1294, 1980.
104. Insel TR, Murphy DL, Cohen RM, et al: Obsessive compulsive disorder: a

double blind trial of clomipramine and clorgyline, *Arch Gen Psychiatry* 40: 605–612, 1983.

105. Greist JH, Jefferson JW, Kobak KA, et al: Efficacy and tolerability of serotonin transport inhibitors in obsessive-compulsive disorder: a meta-analysis, *Arch Gen Psychiatry* 52:53–60, 1995.

106. Barr LC, Goodman WK, Price LH, et al: The serotonin hypothesis of obsessive compulsive disorder: implications of pharmacologic challenge studies, *J Clin Psychiatry* 53(suppl):17–28, 1992.

107. Marazziti D, Zohar J, Cassano G: Biological dissection of obsessive compulsive disorder. In Berend B, Hollander E, Marazziti D, Zohar J, editors: *Current insights in obsessive-compulsive disorder*, Chichester, 1994, John Wiley and Sons.

108. Gross-Isseroff R, Kindler S, Kotler M, et al: Pharmacologic challenges. In Berend B, Hollander E, Marazziti D, Zohar J, editors: *Current insights in obsessive-compulsive disorder*, Chichester, 1994, John Wiley and Sons.

109. Blier P, de Montigny C: Current advances and trends in the treatment of depression, *Trends Pharmacol Sci* 15:220–226, 1994.

110. Blier P, Chaput Y, de Montigny C: Long-term 5HT reuptake blockade, but not monoamine oxidase inhibition, decreases the function of the terminal 5HT autoreceptors: an electrophysiological study in the rat brain, *Naunyn-Schmiedeberg's Arch Pharmacol* 337:246–254, 1988.

111. Blier P, Bouchard C: Modulation of 5HT release in the guinea pig brain following long-term administration of antidepressant drugs, *Br J Pharmacol* 113: 485–495, 1994.

112. Mansari ME, Bouchard C, Blier P: Alteration of serotonin release in the guinea pig orbito-frontal cortex by selective serotonin reuptake inhibitors: relevance to treatment of obsessive-compulsive disorder, *Neuropsychopharmacology* 13: 117–127, 1995.

113. Singer H, Hahn I, Moran T: Tourette's syndrome: abnormal dopamine uptake sites in postmortem striatum from patients with Tourette's syndrome, *Ann Neurol* 30:558–562, 1991.

114. Malison RT, McDougle CJ, van Dyck CH, et al: I-123-β-CIT SPECT imaging of striatal dopamine transporter binding in Tourette's disorder, *Am J Psychiatry* 152:1359–1361, 1995.

115. Wolf SS, Jones DW, Knable MB, et al: Tourette syndrome: prediction of phenotypic variation in monozygotic twins by caudate nucleus D2 receptor binding, *Science* 273:1225–1227, 1996.

116. McDougle CJ, Goodman WK, Price LH, et al: Neuroleptic addition in fluvoxamine refractory obsessive compulsive disorder, *Am J Psychiatry* 147:652–654, 1990.

117. Breiter HC, Etcoff NL, Whalen PJ, et al: Response and habituation of the human amygdala during processing of facial expression, *Neuron* 17:875–887, 1996.

118. Whalen PJ, Rauch SL, Etcoff NL, et al: Masked presentations of emotional facial expressions modulate amygdala activity without explicit knowledge, *J Neurosci* 18(1):411–418, 1998.

119. Rauch SL, Whalen PJ, Savage CR, et al: Striatal recruitment during an implicit sequence learning task as measured by functional magnetic resonance imaging, *Hum Brain Mapping,* (in press).

120. Davis M: Differential roles of the amygdala and bed nucleus of the stria terminalis in conditioned fear and startle enhanced by corticotropin releasing hormone. In Ono T, editor: *Perception, memory and emotion: Frontiers in neuroscience*, Oxford, 1996, Elsevier.
121. Davis M, Walker DL, Lee Y: Amygdala and bed nucleus of the stria terminalis: differential roles in fear and anxiety measured with the acoustic startle reflex. In Squire L, Schacter D, editors: *Biological and psychological perspectives on memory and memory disorder,* American Psychiatric Press, (in press).

13

Neuropsychology of Obsessive-Compulsive Disorder: Research Findings and Treatment Implications

Cary R. Savage, Ph.D.

When the previous edition of this book was published in 1990, there were only five original reports examining neuropsychologic functioning in obsessive-compulsive disorder (OCD), and the results had been somewhat inconsistent across studies. Since that time, at least 15 additional neuropsychologic studies have appeared in the literature, and some consistency is beginning to emerge. In addition, several neuroimaging studies have been conducted and much more is known regarding the neurobiology of OCD. We have, therefore, begun to better understand the specific nature of cognitive dysfunction in OCD and how this is related to changes in brain function.

This chapter begins by reviewing findings from the previous neuropsychologic studies, focusing on the most consistent results rather than describing each study in any detail. A brief overview is then provided concerning what is known about the neurobiology of the disorder and what can be learned from studying neurologic disorders that affect similar brain systems. Finally, this chapter describes results from studies attempting to reconcile neuropsychologic and neurobiologic theories, suggests ways of applying this knowledge to the treatment of the disorder, and proposes future directions for neuropsychologic research in OCD.

NEUROPSYCHOLOGIC FINDINGS IN OBSESSIVE-COMPULSIVE DISORDER

Neuropsychology is the branch of psychology focusing on brain–behavior interactions—that is, how the brain controls higher cognitive functions such as language, visuospatial ability, memory, and reasoning. Neuropsychology originated from investigations of patients with neurologic disorders, such as stroke, brain tumors, and degenerative diseases of aging. More recently, researchers have begun to apply neuropsychologic approaches to the study of psychiatric disorders, including OCD. These patients may not have "lesions" of the brain per se, but they nonetheless demonstrate consistent patterns of brain dysfunction that impact on cognition in predictable ways. This review is organized according to the domains of cognitive functioning most consistently affected in OCD sufferers: visuospatial skill, nonverbal memory, and executive abilities. The reader is referred to the original reports for a detailed description of individual tests; only one from each domain is described in detail, to provide an example.

Visuospatial Skill

One of the most consistent findings has been the presence of impaired visuospatial ability in OCD. The term *visuospatial ability* describes the patient's mental capacity to perceive and manipulate objects in two- and three-dimensional space.[1] An example is a test in which subjects are instructed to draw a three-dimensional cube. To do this, one must have the ability to perceive the components of the figure (the lines), appreciate the relationships between them, and assemble (i.e., draw) them in a way that preserves the overall contour and impression of depth from the original model. The reader can appreciate that this apparently simple task is actually composed of a number of individual cognitive components, all of which must be coordinated to reproduce the figure. Visuospatial tests may involve drawing figures or assembling two- and three-dimensional objects from models. Some tests do not even involve visual perception per se, but rather one's ability, while blindfolded, to appreciate and coordinate interactions between the body and objects in space. These are complex tests which require the integration of a number of abilities for successful performance; however, all share the element of spatial reasoning.

Patients with OCD have been found to be impaired on a number of tests which purport to measure visuospatial functioning, including the block designs subtest of the Wechsler Adult Intelligence Scale—Revised (WAIS-R),[2-4] Cube Copying,[5] Money's Road Map Test,[6] the Figure Matching Test,[7] the Tactual Performance Test,[3,8,9] the Hooper Visual Organization Test,[10] the Mental Rotations Test,[11] and the copy condition of the Rey-Osterrieth Complex Figure Test (RCFT).[6,10]

Nonverbal Memory

Obsessive-compulsive disorder subjects also have demonstrated consistent problems on tests of nonverbal memory. *Nonverbal memory* refers to the ability to learn and recall new visual objects and images,[1] preferably ones not easily described with words (e.g., ball and square, which lend themselves to verbal labelling). Understanding the nature of memory impairment requires an appreciation of the different components of memory. Memory is a complex process, entailing many distinct processes that are potentially dissociable in different patient populations.[12] For instance, memory can be described as either "immediate" or "long-term." *Immediate memory* (also called *short-term memory*) refers to the ability to keep information in active storage with constant rehearsal (i.e., without distraction). *Long-term memory* describes the ability to store and retrieve information after a period of distraction (i.e., the information can be retrieved even after some time has passed with attention focused on other things). Long-term memories can be further described according to at least three stages of processing: (1) encoding (learning); (2) storage (maintaining the representation over time); and (3) retrieval (accessing the stored representation). Impairment in any one of these component processes is associated with distinct types of neural system dysfunction. For example, the storage stage of long-term memory has been linked to systems in the medial temporal lobe, and patients with medial temporal dysfunction have difficulty maintaining new memories over time.[12] By comparison, impairment of encoding and retrieval processes is associated with dysfunction in prefrontal brain systems,[13,14] and patients with frontal system lesions have difficulty initially learning and later retrieving new memories.

The visual reproduction subtest of the Wechsler Memory Scale (WMS) provides a well-characterized example of nonverbal memory. In this test, subjects are shown figures, one at a time for 10 seconds each, and instructed to try to remember the figure. The model figure is then removed, and subjects are asked to draw as much of the figure as they can remember (i.e., immediate memory). Next, subjects are administered other cognitive tests, which serve to prevent rehearsal, and are later again instructed to draw as much as can be remembered of the figure (i.e., long-term memory).

Obsessive-compulsive disorder patient groups have shown consistent impairment on a number of tests of nonverbal memory, including the visual reproduction subtest of the WMS,[3,10] the Delayed Recognition Span Test,[15] the Benton Visual Retention Test,[7,16] the Recurring Figures Test,[17] Korsi's Block Test,[17] the Memory Efficiency Battery,[18] Stylus Maze Learning,[6] and the immediate and delayed recall conditions of the RCFT.[10,11]

Many of the tests of long-term memory used in studies of OCD require each of the encoding, storage, and retrieval processes for successful performance. Much of the research to date has examined memory in a general sense and has not attempted to differentiate between these component processes. However, it is important to differentiate these stages if one is to make reference to brain systems potentially underlying these difficulties. There are now some data on this issue indicating that OCD patients' problems specifically affect the ability to encode new nonverbal information.[7,10,11,16,17] However, another study has found that OCD patients were impaired exclusively on the delayed recall condition of the WMS,[3] findings which would appear to implicate either the storage or retrieval stage of memory.

One way to disentangle problems in storage and retrieval is to examine both recall and recognition at delayed recall. In recognition tests, subjects are presented with a number of stimuli—some of which were previously studied (targets), whereas others were not (distractors). Recognition of figures presumably has fewer retrieval demands, because the figures are provided and the subject simply has to discriminate between "targets" and "distractors." Savage, et al[15] recently examined recall and recognition memory and found that OCD patients were impaired on measures of nonverbal delayed recall but not delayed recognition. This suggests retrieval deficits rather than storage deficits; OCD patients may thus have difficulty retrieving new memories, but they do not appear to "forget" information.

In summary, results suggest that two nonverbal memory processes are selectively disrupted in OCD: encoding and retrieval. OCD patients appear to have difficulty learning new nonverbal material and later retrieving it on demand, whereas storage ability appears to be intact.

Executive Function

Patients with OCD also have been found to be impaired on measures of executive function. The term *executive function* describes the high-level control processes that modulate more elementary sensory, motor, cognitive, memory, and affective functions. Executive functioning requires the ability to take all aspects of a situation into account (i.e., overall context) and use this knowledge to prioritize goals and plans, implement behavior strategically, and monitor and shift behavior as the environmental context changes (e.g., see Lezak[1]). Consider as an example the Wisconsin Card Sorting Test (WCST), which is widely considered to be a prototypical measure of executive functioning. This test consists of four stimulus cards—one red triangle, two green stars, three yellow crosses, and four blue circles. The subject is presented with a deck of cards printed with one of four symbols in one of four colors and instructed to match these cards to the stimulus cards according to an unstated rule (either by color, shape, or number). Subjects are not told what the rule is, only whether each response is correct or incorrect. After 10 consecutive correct responses, the previously correct rule is changed and a new rule must be derived. Therefore, to successfully complete the WCST, subjects must deduce the abstract rules, apply these rules to sort the cards, maintain these response patterns as long as appropriate, and flexibly change the rules when the old response rules are no longer adequate—all examples of "executive" functioning.

Some studies of executive functioning in OCD have demonstrated an increase in perseverative responses on the WCST.[2,19,20] Perseverative responses are those in which subjects show difficulty shifting to a new rule when the old one is changed. Problems also have been noted in OCD groups on the Trail Making Test, Part B,[7] the Category Test,[8,9] visual attention tests,[18,21] and organizational measures on the RCFT.[6,11] Martin, et al[22] also found that OCD patients were slower on self-paced measures of working memory, but it was unclear whether this represented an impairment or a secondary "epiphenomenon" of OCD (e.g., indecisiveness). Executive problems, particularly on the WCST and Trail Making Test, have been most frequently interpreted to reflect difficulty "shifting mental set." This refers to the characteristic trouble some patients have when thinking about something one way and then having to "shift" and think about it in another way.

Areas of Normal Function in Obsessive-Compulsive Disorder

An important point to be made here is that OCD patients are by no means impaired across all cognitive skill areas. In fact, the vast majority of individuals with OCD are high functioning and strikingly able to cope on a daily basis given the severity of their disorder. Patients with OCD consistently demonstrate normal general intelligence and language abilities. In addition, studies have shown normal verbal memory abilities in patients with OCD. Thus, although OCD patients tend to have problems on measures of nonverbal memory, verbal memory appears to be preserved. This finding is intriguing, and some investigators have hypothesized that this is consistent with predominantly right hemisphere dysfunction.[3,10,17] Another possibility, and the one which is favored here, is that cognitive problems in patients with OCD reflect frontal-striatal system dysfunction. This hypothesis will be discussed in detail later in the chapter. The main point to be emphasized here is that neither brain dysfunction nor the resulting cognitive problems appear to be global; rather, very specific brain systems and cognitive functions have been implicated in OCD.

Some Caveats

Lest the reader get the impression of more consistency in the literature than is actually the case, it should be noted that results from these studies reflect group data and there is considerable individual variability. Not all OCD patients are identical cognitively and not all individual patients are equally impaired. In fact, some patients demonstrate normal performance across all measurable cognitive domains. It is not clear why this is the case. Many of these inconsistencies occurred in early studies and might have been related to variability in the patient populations studied, such as the inclusion of patients on psychotropic medications or with comorbid major depression. Perhaps there are also different forms of OCD, some more directly associated with dysfunction in brain systems leading to cognitive impairments. For example, Malloy[19] found a tendency to perseverate on the WCST only in one subgroup of his OCD sample, whereas the other group performed normally. This "impaired" subgroup was also described as more "psychotic" and had lower general intelligence scores. Results also differ between studies in that some report impairment on one test, whereas others do not. For example, some studies have not shown a significant tendency for OCD groups to perseverate on the WCST,[3] and at least one study found no statistically significant abnormalities in neuropsychologic functioning in an OCD group.[23] Of course, some of these negative findings may reflect inadequate statistical power to detect the generally subtle disturbances of cognitive functioning found in OCD.

Another caveat is that most neuropsychologic domains are interrelated, so there is really no such thing as a "pure" measure of visuospatial skill, nonverbal memory, or executive functioning. Dividing tests into "domains" of function is simply a means of organizing patterns of results; aspects of all these functions are tapped by individual tests to some degree, and the assignment of a test into one domain usually reflects dominance of that function rather than unimodality. Finally, it should be noted that terms such as "dysfunction" and "impairment" have little intrinsic meaning. The presence or absence of dysfunction in a group is usually determined by the performance in comparison with another group, rather than passage beyond some absolute criterion. It is not always clear where function ends and dysfunction begins.

NEUROBIOLOGY OF OBSESSIVE-COMPULSIVE DISORDER

A brief review of the neurobiology of OCD is necessary to understand how neuropsychologic deficits might relate to disturbances in brain function (for more detail on the neurobiology of OCD, see Chapter 12). Much of what is known about brain function in OCD comes from functional neuroimaging studies using positron emission tomography (PET), which provides a measure of brain function based on quantification of regional metabolism or blood flow. A number of PET studies of OCD have indicated increased metabolism or blood flow in the orbital prefrontal cortex,[24–26] caudate nuclei,[24,25] anterior cingulate,[27] and right lateral prefrontal cortex.[27] Metabolic abnormalities in the orbital prefrontal cortex and caudate nuclei have been noted to normalize in OCD following successful treatment with serotonergic reuptake inhibitors[28–30] or behavior therapy.[29,31] A recent study by Rauch, et al[32] measured regional cerebral blood flow (rCBF) with PET during obsessional symptom provocation. During obsessional states, OCD subjects showed increased rCBF in the right caudate nucleus, bilateral orbital prefrontal cortex, and anterior cingulate. In two follow-up PET studies, Rauch, et al[33,34] demonstrated that the changes in the caudate and orbital prefrontal cortex were unique to OCD when compared with two other anxiety disorders (simple phobia and posttraumatic stress disorder), whereas the anterior cingulate activation was common to all three anxiety disorders.

Support for the importance of striatal dysfunction in OCD also comes from well-documented symptomatic and familial associations with Tourette's disorder,[35] as well as reports of OCD–like behavior in cases of postencephalitic Parkinson's disease, Huntington's disease, Sydenham's chorea, and focal striatal lesions.[36–39] Current neurobiologic theories of OCD (e.g., see Chapter 12)[40–42] emphasize the importance of corticostriatal system dysfunction in the etiology of OCD. In the prefrontal component of this system, the head of the caudate nucleus receives extensive projections from dorsolateral and orbital prefrontal cortex, as well as from visual and auditory association areas in temporal and parietal cortex. These circuits then project through the globus pallidus and substantia nigra, pars reticulata to thalamic nuclei, where the system is closed by reciprocal projections back to the dorsolateral and orbital prefrontal cortex.[43] Thus, these various structures function together as a distributed frontal-striatal system. Taken together, the weight of evidence from these studies provides significant support for the importance of frontal-striatal networks in the etiology of OCD.

NEUROPSYCHOLOGY OF FRONTAL-STRIATAL NEUROLOGIC DISORDERS

This chapter briefly changes focus from psychiatric disorders to neurologic disorders. To understand the impact of brain dysfunction on cognitive ability, it is useful to understand the patterns of cognitive function observed in patients with neurologic disorders affecting frontal-striatal function, because these disorders have been more thoroughly characterized. Examples of such disorders include Parkinson's disease (PD) and Huntington's disease (HD).[44] Symptoms of PD result from degeneration in a nucleus of the substantia nigra (pars compacta) which provides dopaminergic enervation to the striatum. HD is an autosomal dominant–transmitted disorder which causes degeneration in the caudate nucleus early in its course. Cognitive dysfunction in both disorders is believed to reflect disruption of frontal-striatal systems.[45]

Studies in PD and HD have pointed to the importance of executive dysfunction in memory and spatial deficits in these groups. For example, Pillon et al[46] found that subjects with PD and HD were impaired on memory processes requiring spontaneous organization, and that this pattern was distinct from memory problems observed in subjects with Alzheimer's disease (AD), who demonstrated an abnormal forgetting rate. Further, memory performance was significantly correlated with measures of executive functioning in subjects with PD and HD but not in subjects with AD. Pillon, et al[46] concluded that memory impairment in PD and HD reflected inefficient planning strategies resulting from frontal-striatal dysfunction. Bondi et al[47] demonstrated that visuospatial and memory impairment in PD could be explained by considering performance on executive function tests. They found that visuospatial and memory problems in PD were no longer significant when performance on executive function tests was statistically controlled. Buytenhuijs, et al[48] demonstrated that PD subjects were not able to impose an internally generated strategy during multiple verbal learning trials, whereas control subjects spontaneously relied on an internally generated strategy.

The RCFT[49] is a well-characterized measure of nonverbal learning and memory that has been studied in neurologic disorders and in OCD. This test is multidimensional, including components of visuospatial, nonverbal memory, and executive processing. Visuospatial functioning is measured by the patient's ability to accurately copy the complex figure, nonverbal memory is gauged by the ability to encode and recall the figure, and executive functioning is evaluated by the organizational approach to the figure. The term *organizational approach* describes the strategic process of breaking down the complex figure into simpler components and using these components to control the action of drawing the complex figure. Recent studies of RCFT performance in PD have pointed to the importance of the organizational approach to construction and memory performance on the RCFT. For example, Ogden, et al[50] and Grossman, et al[51] found that PD subjects were impaired in their organizational approach when they copied the figure. They concluded that the PD subjects did not have difficulty with the spatial aspects of copying the figure, but rather had difficulty with the "executive" aspects of the tasks, including planning and shifting mental set. Similarly, Grossman, et al[51] found that executive problems, such as impaired organization, accounted for most of the variance in copy and recall performance in their PD patients.

Thus, a consistent picture is emerging from this literature which is pointing to the impact of frontal-striatal system dysfunction on executive functioning and the secondary impact of executive dysfunction on other cognitive domains, such as visuospatial and memory abilities. Impaired executive functioning affects planning, organization, and set-shifting abilities, which in turn disrupt spatial skills and the ability to encode and retrieve new memories. Results from studies of neurologic disorders now can be used to generate testable hypotheses in OCD. If cognitive problems in OCD also are related to frontal-striatal dysfunction, they should demonstrate similar patterns of results.

EFFECTS OF EXECUTIVE FUNCTIONING ON NONVERBAL MEMORY IN OBSESSIVE-COMPULSIVE DISORDER

The literature reviewed thus far points to the importance of frontal-striatal system function in OCD and suggests a mechanism by which this dysfunction might lead to widespread problems in executive, visuospatial, and memory abilities. Given these findings, we recently investigated the impact of frontal-striatal, system-mediated executive dysfunction on other cognitive abilities in OCD—in this case, nonverbal memory using the RCFT.[11] Our question was how executive functioning (reflected in the organizational approach used to copy the figure) would affect patients' subsequent ability to recall the figure. We administered the RCFT and other neuropsychologic measures to 20 patients with OCD (without depression, comorbid neurologic disorders, or psychotropic medications) and 20 age-, education-, and gender-matched controls. As expected, OCD patients were impaired both in the organizational approach when copying the figure and in the ability to recall the figure after the model was removed (immediate recall). They also recalled less of the figure than control subjects after a 30-minute delay (delayed recall), but this did not represent any additional loss of information (memory storage was preserved) (Figure 13-1).

Figure 13-1 shows drawings of the RCFT taken from three representative subjects. It illustrates the general finding that patients with poor organizational strategies at copy also were the patients who had difficulty recalling the figure. Multiple regression modeling[52] indicated that statistical differences between groups in immediate recall could be explained by considering organizational scores measured when subjects first copied the figure. Therefore, our OCD patients did not have a primary memory deficit; rather, their organizational approach during figure copy determined how much they subsequently remembered. These results indicate that the cognitive dysfunction involved organizational processes, and this dysfunction had a secondary effect on the ability to encode and retrieve the RCFT figure. These findings are consistent with neurobiologic theories of frontal-striatal system dysfunction in OCD.

A strong case can be made for ways in which organizational problems might affect memory. For example, the RCFT figure can be broken into various component elements when it is drawn—this is how the organizational approach is identified. Figure 13-2 provides examples of the RCFT figure and the organizational approaches used by one control subject and one subject with OCD in the Savage, et al[11] study.

Figure 13-2 illustrates what happened in the majority of subjects in this study: most OCD subjects fixated on small details, while most control subjects focused on the overall contours and configural elements. It should be obvious how an organized drawing strategy should lead to better memory for the figure. First, there are fewer parts to remember in a well-organized drawing. Secondly, the component elements comprise features that are "meaningful" to perceptual systems (i.e., rectangle, diagonal "X," horizontal and vertical "+," triangle). Information encoded into visual memory thereby has a meaningful semantic structure which makes it easier to retrieve. This detail-oriented approach used by the OCD subjects appeared to put them at a disadvantage when they were subsequently asked to recall the figure. Therefore, the "deficit" in this study of OCD was primarily in executive functioning and only secondarily in learning and memory.

A NEUROPSYCHOLOGIC MODEL OF OBSESSIVE-COMPULSIVE DISORDER

This review has presented evidence that frontal-striatal dysfunction is etiologically implicated in OCD, and that this dysfunction results in a primary executive disturbance that secondarily affects other cognitive abilities, such as nonverbal memory. The neuropsychologic findings are still preliminary and must be independently replicated and validated. However, these findings can already be used to develop a more comprehensive neuropsychologic model of

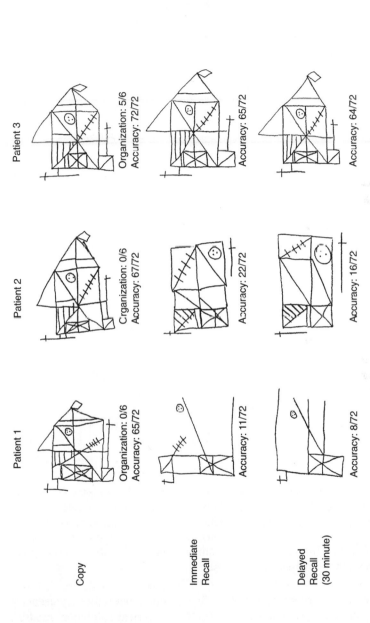

Fig. 13-1   Rey-Osterrieth Complex Figure Test drawings of three obsessive-compulsive disorder (OCD) patients, on copy, immediate recall, and delayed recall (30-minute) conditions. Organization and accuracy scores are listed under the copied figures, and accuracy scores are provided under the recalled figures. Patients 1 and 2 were chosen as examples of OCD subjects with poor organization during copy, and Patient 3 was selected as an example of an OCD subject with good organization.

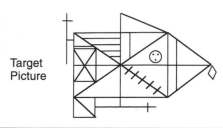

Target
Picture

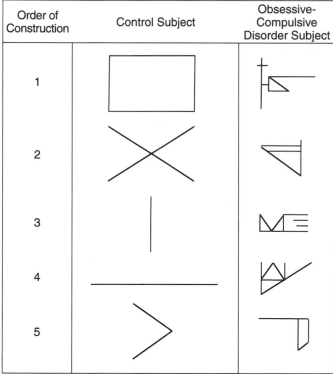

Fig. 13-2 The top of this picture shows the Rey-Osterrieth Complex Figure Test (RCFT) figure. Under this are examples of two organizational approaches—one for a control subject and the other for a patient with OCD. These summaries were prepared by taking the first five drawn units, with the order of construction running from top to bottom. This figure is meant to communicate the effects of poor organization on memory for the RCFT figure.

OCD. This model is not intended to be a final product, but rather represents a working hypothesis—one that will lend itself to empirical validation, modification, or rejection. This is not the only possible model; for instance, Otto[53] proposed a neuropsychologic model for OCD, which formed the basis for some of the ideas presented here.

The current model is founded on four general concepts: (1) the locus of primary brain dysfunction in OCD is frontal-striatal; (2) dysfunction in this brain system leads to primary executive disturbance and nonverbal memory disturbance as a secondary outcome; (3) neuropsychologic dysfunction represents an intermediate impairment, which has an impact on clinical symptoms; (4) the effects of changes in clinical symptoms feed back into brain function, creating a "vicious cycle" of brain dysfunction and cognitive and clinical symptoms.

A central aspect of this model is the effect of executive functioning on clinical symptoms. This chapter previously described executive functioning as the ability to appreciate the larger environmental context and use it to prioritize and plan behavior, to implement strategic action, and to self-monitor and flexibly change behavior as needed. These characteristics of executive dysfunction are somewhat reminiscent of the symptoms of OCD. An example is the OCD patient who worries that he will forget to turn off the stove and that some catastrophic event will take place as a result (e.g., the house will burn down). In response to this obsession, the patient compulsively checks the stove, hoping to neutralize the fear. However, no matter how many times the stove is checked, the fear continues, and he is locked into a repetitive cycle of obsessions and compulsions.

Clinical symptoms such as these may be related to executive dysfunction. For example, the obsessive fear of forgetting to turn off the stove could be linked to failure to appreciate the larger context of the environment and misappropriating attentional resources—that is, the stove is given greater importance than is objectively warranted (Otto[53] also discusses this issue). Checking the stove might also be related to difficulty planning and implementing strategic actions—the OCD sufferer engages in "automatic" repetitive behaviors rather than considering and initiating more productive alternatives. In addition, repeating compulsive behaviors in the face of their failure to reduce anxiety could be related to difficulty self-monitoring and flexibly modifying behavior. These are all examples of impaired executive functioning.

Shimamura[54] describes another key feature of patients with frontal lobe lesions which is directly relevant to this discussion. He states that a central characteristic of frontal system dysfunction is the failure of patients to inhibit irrelevant information (i.e., having difficulty controlling "inadvertent" information processing). According to this description, frontal system function is viewed as a "dynamic filtering mechanism," which, if disrupted may account for the intrusive quality of obsessions in OCD.

Anxiety also is a core feature of OCD[55] and is possibly related to frontal-striatal system dysfunction. The orbital prefrontal cortex and anterior cingulate are "paralimbic" cortical structures which are functionally and anatomically connected to the limbic system,[56] as is also the case for the most ventral regions of the caudate nucleus.[43,45] These systems likely serve to integrate cognitive and motivational information.[57] Neuroimaging data have indicated that these structures are *hyper*activated in OCD (see Chapter 15); thus, it is possible that unimportant environmental cues might be inappropriately labelled as "important" and behavior oriented toward a stimulus because of baseline hyperactivity in this system. These problems could be conceptualized as the "motivational aspects" of executive dysfunction in OCD.

Therefore, both ineffective attentional filtering and inappropriate labelling of environmental cues might be added to the beginning of the "executive" chain of dysfunction. OCD patients may feel "compelled" to process every detail in the environment because irrelevant features intrude into consciousness and are inappropriately labelled as important.

As noted previously, executive dysfunction also has secondary effects on other cognitive abilities, such as memory, which in turn further contribute to the symptoms of the disorder. One of the hallmark symptoms of OCD is a persistent and debilitating doubt regarding the adequacy of previous actions, despite their repetition. This suggests a potentially important role for memory in these symptoms of chronic doubt and repetitive behavior.[53] Although memory deficits are secondary in this model, they likely contribute to cycles of obsessions and compulsions (e.g., "Did I in fact turn off the stove? I don't know. Better check again.").

This model is rather complicated and is probably more easily understood by considering it in figure form. The proposed neuropsychologic model is illustrated in Figure 13-3.

In this model, frontal-striatal dysfunction leads to impaired executive functioning, which is manifest in a number of ways, including: (1) difficulty appreciating the larger context of the environment (possibly because irrelevant features intrude into consciousness and are inappropriately labelled as important); (2) difficulty prioritizing and planning behavior; (3) difficulty initiating strategic action to carry out the plan; and (4) difficulty monitoring behavior and "shifting" to more appropriate behavioral response patterns when the old ones are ineffective. These problems then contribute to the clinical symptoms of obsessions and compulsions. Memory impairment, secondary to executive dysfunction, also may contribute to the difficulty patients have confirming the accuracy of obsessions and the adequacy of compulsive behaviors.

In this model, neuropsychologic function is the intermediate step between brain dysfunction and clinical phenomenology. This view conceives neuropsychologic dysfunction as more than the outcome of disturbed brain function—it also is part of the problem. In addition, disrupted psychologic functioning "feeds-back" and affects brain function, contributing to the vicious cycle that maintains and compounds obsessions and compulsions. This idea of psychologic function impacting brain function is supported by PET studies showing normalization of metabolism in OCD patients following successful treatment, whether with medication or behavior therapy.[29,31] Therefore, there is evidence

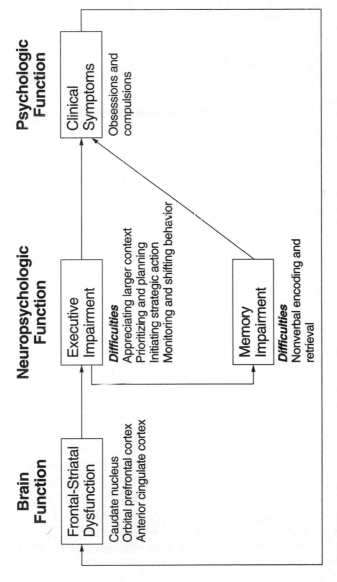

Fig. 13-3 This figure summarizes an hypothesized neuropsychologic model for obsessive-compulsive disorder.

that changes at the behavioral level (breaking obsessions and compulsions) can lead to stable alterations of function at the neural systems level.

DESIGNING NEW INTERVENTIONS

One ultimate goal of clinical research is to develop better treatments. The neuropsychologic model proposed here (Figure 13-3) suggests three potential levels of intervention: brain function, neuropsychologic function, and psychologic function. Although the etiology may initially arise at the lowest level (brain function) with dysfunction spreading upward (neuropsychologic and psychologic function), intervention can occur at any level, because changes at any level should propagate to other levels. Psychotropic medications intervene at the level of brain function, through mechanisms such as altering brain chemistry and receptor density. Behavior therapy intervenes at the level of psychologic function, by exposing patients to the trigger stimulus and preventing them from engaging in compulsive rituals (i.e., exposure and response prevention, described in Chapter 17).

One might also intervene at the intermediate level of neuropsychologic functioning, using a cognitive retraining approach to treatment (which should be distinguished from cognitive therapy approaches discussed in Chapter 10). A cognitive retraining approach has been previously proposed for other psychiatric disorders, such as schizophrenia[58] and also has been suggested by Otto[53] for OCD. Watts[59] proposed a related approach for compulsive checking (a symptom he specifically tied to deficits in information processing): he suggested using cognitive strategies to maximize the effectiveness of the first check, a so-called "one-check" approach. Watts proposed that techniques such as focusing attention during the first check and the use of memory aids to confirm the accuracy of checks might help patients stop after a single checking episode. This approach does not try to change the information-processing style, but rather to minimize the consequences afterward.

A cognitive retraining approach uses neuropsychologic theory as the basis for interventions which are designed to alter cognitive dysfunction. Based on the model proposed here, one point of intervention should be at the level of executive function; perhaps OCD patients can learn to improve executive functioning and thereby improve other cognitive abilities (e.g., memory) and ultimately reduce clinical symptoms. In contrast to the Watts approach, the goal of intervention here is to directly change cognitive processes.

At the Massachusetts General Hospital OCD Unit, we are currently studying the effectiveness of such an intervention aiming to improve organizational ability in OCD subjects and thereby improve memory (specifically, memory for the RCFT figure). As already noted, there is some evidence that OCD patients show impaired organization when copying the RCFT figure and this leads to difficulty remembering the figure. The goal of this ongoing study is to train OCD patients to use efficient configural-based organizational strategies when copying the figure (such as the one used by the control subject in Figure 13-2). In this protocol, subjects are given organizational training on another figure, which is similar but not identical to the RCFT, and the effects of training are subsequently evaluated in the patient's ability to copy and recall the RCFT figure.

What is being taught in this study is essentially a type of executive function; OCD patients tend to focus on extraneous details of the figure, rather than meaningful configural elements. They then continue to use this detail-oriented approach even after it has proven to be ineffective. Thus, one central feature of this training is to teach patients to appreciate the larger configural features, or context, of the figure. Such difficulty appreciating the larger context is described by the proverb: "He can't see the forest for the trees." This is referring to a tendency to miss the big picture—the larger context of a situation—because of a tendency to focus on minutia. In essence, the study described here is teaching patients to focus on the forest rather than the trees. This approach is only theoretic at this point, and the effectiveness has yet to be determined, but it may prove to be a productive approach to treating OCD, perhaps as an adjunct to pharmacotherapy or behavior therapy.

FUTURE DIRECTIONS FOR RESEARCH

There are, of course, many possible directions for future research in addition to the intervention approach just described. Additional research is needed to understand the apparent specificity of memory problems to visual stimuli, because verbal memory has been consistently normal in OCD.[3,15] There are several possible explanations for this dissociation between verbal and nonverbal memory performance. It has been proposed that nonverbal memory impairment, along with visuospatial impairment, might be associated with right hemisphere dysfunction.[3,10,17] It also is possible that nonverbal memory impairment is primarily the outcome of frontal-striatal dysfunction, not necessarily lateralized, because the primary deficit on the RCFT in OCD is organizational, rather than memory per se. Most verbal memory tests place less demand on organizational ability, because words are innately more familiar and have more semantic structure than novel figures. Future studies should examine memory performance in OCD patients on verbal memory tests, which place a larger emphasis on organizational capacity. It is possible that a general organizational impairment also impacts verbal memory under the right conditions. What may be important is not so much the verbal-nonverbal distinction, but rather the load placed on organizational strategies during learning.

More research also is needed to define the boundaries of executive dysfunction in OCD. Several neuropsychologic studies have not found evidence of executive impairment in OCD groups. For example, not all studies show evidence of increased perseverative tendencies on the WCST (e.g., Reference 3). One possibility, as noted previously (e.g., see Reference 19), is that there are different subgroups of OCD, only some of which have executive impairment. Another likely explanation is that OCD patients have specific deficits in executive functioning which are only consistently tapped by certain tests. "Executive functioning" is a broad and complex domain of cognitive functioning and there is significant variability in the types of deficits exhibited, depending on factors such as lesion location (e.g., see Reference 45). The current review has used the term *executive function* as a general label to describe the pattern of cognitive deficits in OCD, but the deficit may express itself only on certain measures that require patients to integrate complex information in an unstructured setting. For example, the RCFT is a complex test in which subjects are initially provided with very little external structure; they are given no guidance about the best approach, nor are they informed that they will later be asked to recall the test. It may be that the executive deficit in OCD is manifest most reliably in these complex unstructured situations. This is certainly more similar to the real-life experiences of patients, in which they are faced with a complex environment and little guidance about how to structure their actions.

Other promising areas of research include investigations into the qualitative aspects of memory in OCD. In addition to memory performance scores, research from both normal and neurologic patients has pointed to the importance of qualitative aspects of the recollective experience (e.g., see Reference 54). Critical qualitative characteristics of memory include distinctions between "remembering" and "knowing,"[60,61] "metamemory,"[62] and source memory.[13,63,64] There appear to be at least two major aspects to the recollective experience: (1) remembering; and (2) knowing (R-K). In the basic R-K paradigm, subjects are instructed to report their mental experience when remembering single items.[60,61] "Remember" responses are made to items that evoke conscious recollection of having previously encountered that specific item. "Know" responses are made to items that evoke only a sense of familiarity, without actual recollection (i.e., just a "feeling of knowing"). Previous research has indicated that the recollective process normally begins with "Remember" responses predominating, and with the passage of time "Know" responses begin to predominate. Studies using R-K paradigms have indicated that impairment of "Remember" responses is associated with frontal system impairment, and this impairment disrupts later feelings of knowing.

A closely related concept is the idea of "metamemory," referring to the ability to make accurate judgments about one's own memory ability.[54,62] In this paradigm, subjects are asked to rate their "feeling of knowing." For example, subjects might be asked to rate how likely they would be to recognize an answer in a multiple-choice situation and are later evaluated on how accurately they actually predicted their performance.

Source memory refers to the ability to recall the specific situation in which information was originally learned. Patients with frontal system dysfunction tend to have normal memory for facts but have difficulty remembering the source of recently learned information.[54,63] Although new memories are retained, these patients have difficulty remembering where or when they originally learned these things.

A central clinical feature of OCD is chronic doubt about the adequacy of previous actions and thoughts. This doubt is reminiscent of feelings of knowing, tapped by "Know" responses and the ability to accurately rate the quality of one's memory ability, measured by metamemory and source memory tests. These observations suggest that a core feature of OCD may arise from the disruption of the normal relationships between "Remembering" and "Knowing" ("I remember, but it doesn't feel right") as well as impaired ability to make accurate judgments of either memory accuracy ("Did I actually check?") or its source ("Did I check this time, or is it some other time I'm remembering?").

An information-processing study sheds light on this issue (see Chapter 18 for a review of the information processing literature): McNally and Kohlbeck[65] tested OCD patients on a reality monitoring task, which required them to distinguish memories of having actually done something from memories of having imagined doing something. OCD patients were as accurate as controls in their ability to distinguish real from imagined memories, but they expressed less confidence in their performance. The authors concluded that OCD patients had a deficit affecting memory confidence rather than memory accuracy. Future studies of such qualitative aspects of memory may advance our understanding of the cognitive neuroscience of the disorder (i.e., how brain function affects cognition), as well as its phenomenology (i.e., what it is like to have OCD).

SUMMARY

There have been a number of neuropsychologic studies of OCD reported in the literature over the past 7 years. This chapter reviewed these studies and concluded that nonverbal memory and executive functioning are most consistently affected in OCD. There have been corresponding advances in delineating the neurobiology of OCD, and this chapter discussed ways in which brain dysfunction might be tied to the cognitive problems measured by neuropsychologic techniques. The preponderance of evidence points to frontal-striatal system dysfunction in OCD, and this dysfunction is believed to underlie neuropsychologic problems—particularly the executive dysfunction characteristic of OCD. This chapter proposed a model to describe the relationships between brain function (frontal-striatal system), neuropsychologic function (executive and memory problems), and psychologic function (clinical symptoms) in OCD. It is hoped that understanding these "brain and behavior" relationships might lead to better treatments for OCD. This chapter described one ongoing study evaluating the ability to improve memory in OCD patients by training them to use more efficient strategies during learning. Finally, this review proposed some directions for future research, specifically focusing on increasing our understanding of the qualitative aspects of memory, such as how memory accuracy is tied to "feelings of knowing" in OCD. These features of memory may be tied more directly to the day-to-day experiences of OCD patients.

REFERENCES

1. Lezak MD: *Neuropsychological assessment*, ed 3, New York, 1995, Oxford University Press.
2. Head D, Bolton D, Hymas N: Deficit in cognitive shifting ability in patients with obsessive-compulsive disorders, *Biol Psychiatry* 25:929–937, 1989.
3. Christensen KJ, Kim SW, Dysken MW, Hoover KM: Neuropsychological performance in obsessive-compulsive disorder, *Biol Psychiatry* 31:4–18, 1992.
4. Hollander E, Cohen L, Richards M, et al: A pilot study of the neuropsychology of obsessive-compulsive disorder and parkinson's disease: Basal ganglia disorders, *J Neuropsychiatr Clin Neurosci* 5:104–106, 1993.
5. Hollander E, et al: Signs of central nervous system dysfunction in obsessive-compulsive disorder, *Arch Gen Psychiatry* 47:27–32, 1990.
6. Behar D, Rapoport JL, Berg CJ, et al: Computerized tomography and neuropsychological test measures in adolescents with obsessive-compulsive disorder, *Am J Psychiatry* 141:363–368, 1984.
7. Aronowitz BR, Hollander E, DeCaria C, et al: Neuropsychology of obsessive-compulsive disorder: Preliminary findings, *Neuropsychiatr Neuropsychol Behav Neurol* 7:81–86, 1994.
8. Flor-Henry, et al: Neuropsychological and power spectral EEG investigations of the obsessive-compulsive syndrome, *Biol Psychiatry* 14, 119–130, 1979.
9. Insel TR, et al: Neurological and neuropsychological studies of patients with obsessive-compulsive disorder, *Biol Psychiatry* 18:741–751, 1983.
10. Boone KB, Ananth J, Philpott L, et al: Neuropsychological characteristics of non-depressed adults with obsessive-compulsive disorder, *Neuropsychiatry Neuropsychol Behav Neurol* 4:96–109, 1991.
11. Savage CR, Baer L, Keuthen NJ, et al: Organizational strategies and nonverbal memory in obsessive-compulsive disorder, *Clin Neuropsychol* 9:293–294, 1995.
12. Squire LR: Memory and the hippocampus: A synthesis from findings with rats, monkeys, and humans, *Psychol Rev* 99:195–231, 1992.
13. Shimamura AP, Squire LR: Memory and metamemory: A study of the feeling-of-knowing phenomenon in amnesic patients, *J Exp Psychol: Learn Mem Cog* 12:452–460, 1986.
14. Wheeler MA, Stuss DT, Tulvin E: Frontal lobe damage produces episodic memory impairment, *J Int Neuropsychol Soc* 1:525–536, 1995.
15. Savage CR, Keuthen NJ, Jenike MA, et al: Recall and recognition memory in obsessive-compulsive disorder, *J Neuropsychiatr Clin Neurosci* 8:99–103, 1996.
16. Cohen LJ, et al: Specificity of neuropsychological impairment in obsessive-compulsive disorder: A comparison with social phobic and normal control subjects, *J Neuropsychiatr Clin Neurosci* 8:82–85, 1996.
17. Zielinski CM, Taylor MA, Juzwin KR: Neuropsychological deficits in obsessive-compulsive disorder, *Neuropsychiatr Neuropsychol Behav Neurol* 4:110–126, 1991.

18. Dirson S, et al: Visual memory impairment in patients with obsessive-compulsive disorder: A controlled study, *Psychother Psychosom* 63:22–31, 1995.
19. Malloy P: Frontal lobe dysfunction in obsessive-compulsive disorder. In Perecmam E, editor: *The frontal lobes revisited*, 1987, IRBN Press, pp 207–223.
20. Harvey NS: Impaired cognitive set-shifting in obsessive-compulsive neurosis, *IRCS Med Sci* 14:936–937, 1986.
21. Nelson E, Early TS, Haller JW: Visual attention in obsessive-compulsive disorder, *Psychiatr Res* 49:183–196, 1993.
22. Martin A, Pigott TA, Lalonde FM, et al: Lack of evidence for Huntington's disease-like cognitive dysfunction in obsessive-compulsive disorder, *Biol Psychiatry* 33:345–353, 1993.
23. Martin A, et al: Working memory as assessed by subject-ordered tasks in patients with obsessive-compulsive disorder, *J Clin Exp Neuropsychol* 17:786–792, 1995.
24. Baxter LR, Phelps ME, Mazziotta JC, et al: Local cerebral glucose metabolic rates in obsessive-compulsive disorder: A comparison with rates in unipolar depression and in normal controls, *Arch Gen Psychiatry* 44:211–218, 1987.
25. Baxter LR, Schwartz JM, Mazziotta JC, et al: Cerebral glucose metabolic rates in nondepressed patients with obsessive-compulsive disorder, *Am J Psychiatry* 145:1560–1563, 1988.
26. Nordahl TE, Benkelfat C, Semple WE, et al: Cerebral glucose metabolic rates in obsessive-compulsive disorder, *Neuropsychopharmacology* 2:23–28, 1989.
27. Swedo SE, Schapiro MB, Grady CL, et al: Cerebral glucose metabolism in childhood-onset obsessive-compulsive disorder, *Arch Gen Psychiatry* 46:518–523, 1989.
28. Benkelfat C, Nordahl TE, Semple WE, et al: Local cerebral glucose metabolic rates in obsessive-compulsive disorder, *Arch Gen Psychiatry* 47:840–848, 1990.
29. Baxter LR, Schwartz JM, Bergman KS, et al: Caudate glucose metabolic rate changes with both drug and behavior therapy for obsessive-compulsive disorder, *Arch Gen Psychiatry* 49:681–689, 1992.
30. Swedo SE, Pietrini P, Leonard HL, et al: Cerebral glucose metabolism in childhood-onset obsessive-compulsive disorder: Revisualization during pharmacotherapy, *Arch Gen Psychiatry* 49:690–694, 1992.
31. Baxter LR: Role of the striatal complex in ritualistic territorial behaviors—300,000 millennia of progress. Annual meeting of the American College of Neuropsychopharmacology, San Juan, 1994.
32. Rauch SL, Jenike MA, Alpert NM, et al: Regional cerebral blood flow measured during symptom provocation in obsessive-compulsive disorder using oxygen 15-labeled carbon dioxide and positron emission tomography, *Arch Gen Psychiatry* 51:62–70, 1994.
33. Rauch SL, Savage CR, Alpert NM, et al: A positron emission tomographic study of simple phobic symptom provocation, *Arch Gen Psychiatry* 52:20–28, 1995.
34. Rauch SL, van der Kolk BA, Fisler RE, et al: A symptom provocation study of posttraumatic stress disorder using positron emission tomography and script-driven imagery, *Arch Gen Psychiatry* 53:380–387, 1996.
35. Pauls DL: The genetics of obsessive compulsive disorder and Gilles de la Tourette's syndrome, *Psychiatr Clin North Am* 15:759–766, 1992.
36. Bertheir ML, et al: Obsessive-compulsive disorder associated with brain lesions:

Clinical phenomenology, cognitive function, and anatomic correlates, *Neurology* 47:353–361, 1996.

37. Cummings JL, Cunningham K: Obsessive-compulsive disorder in Huntington's disease, *Biol Psychiatry* 31:263–270, 1992.
38. Rapoport JL: Obsessive compulsive disorder and basal ganglia dysfunction, *Psychol Med* 20:465–469, 1990.
39. Weilburg JB, Mesulam MM, Weintraub S, et al: Focal striatal abnormalities in a patient with obsessive-compulsive disorder, *Arch Neurol* 46:233–235, 1989.
40. Baxter LR, Schwartz JM, Guze BH, et al: Neuroimaging in obsessive-compulsive disorder: Seeking the mediating neuroanatomy. In Jenike MA, Baer L, Minichiello WE, editors: *Obsessive-compulsive disorders: Theory and management,* Chicago, 1990, Year Book Medical Publishers, pp 167–188.
41. Rauch SL, Jenike MA: Neurobiological models of obsessive-compulsive disorder, *Psychosomatics* 34:20–32, 1993.
42. Insel TR: Toward a neuroanatomy of obsessive-compulsive disorder, *Arch Gen Psychiatry* 49:739–744, 1992.
43. Alexander GE, Crutcher MD, DeLong MR: Basal ganglia-thalamocortical circuits: Parallel substrates for motor, oculomotor, "prefrontal" and "limbic" functions, *Prog Brain Res* 85:119–146, 1990.
44. Cote L, Crutcher MD: The basal ganglia. In *Principles of neural science*, New York, 1991, Elsevier Science, pp 647–659.
45. Wise SP, Murray EA, Gerfen CR: The frontal cortex-basal ganglia system in primates, *Crit Rev Neurobiol* 10:317–356, 1996.
46. Pillon B, Deweer B, Agid Y, Dubois B: Explicit memory in Alzheimer's, Huntington's, and Parkinson's diseases, *Arch Neurol* 5:374–379, 1993.
47. Bondi MW, Kaszniak AW, Bayles KA, Vance KT: Contributions of frontal system dysfunction to memory and perceptual abilities in Parkinson's disease, *Neuropsychology* 7:89–102, 1993.
48. Buytenhuijs EL, Berger HJC, Van Spaendonck KPM, et al: Memory and learning strategies in patients with Parkinson's disease, *Neuropsychologia* 32:335–342, 1994.
49. Osterrieth PA: Le test de copie d'une figure complex: Contribution à l'étude de la perception et de la memoire, *Arch Psychologie* 30:286–350, 1944.
50. Ogden JA, Growdon JH, Corkin S: Deficits in visuospatial tests involving forward planning in high-functioning parkinsonians, *Neuropsychiatr Neuropsychol Behav Neurol* 3:125–139, 1990.
51. Grossman M, Carvell S, Peltzer L, et al: Visual construction impairments in Parkinson's disease, *Neuropsychology* 7:536–547, 1993.
52. Baron RM, Kenny DA: The moderator-mediator variable distinction in social psychological research: Conceptual, strategic, and statistical considerations, *J Personal Social Psychol* 51:1173–1182, 1986.
53. Otto MW: Normal and abnormal information processing: A neuropsychological perspective on obsessive-compulsive disorder, *Psychiatr Clin North Am* 15:825–848, 1992.
54. Shimamura AP: Memory and frontal lobe function. In *The cognitive neurosciences,* Cambridge, 1995, MIT Press.
55. American Psychiatric Association: *Diagnostic and statistical manual of mental disorders*, ed 4, Washington, 1994, American Psychiatric Association.

56. Mesulam M-M: Patterns in behavioral neuroanatomy: Association areas, the limbic system, and hemispheric specialization. In Mesulam M-M, editor: *Principles of behavioral neurology*, Philadelphia, 1985, FA Davis.
57. Weinberger DR: A connectionist approach to the prefrontal cortex, *J Neuropsychiatr Clin Neurosci* 5:241–253, 1993.
58. Green MF: Cognitive remediation in schizophrenia: Is it time yet? *Am J Psychiatry* 150:178–187, 1993.
59. Watts FN: An information-processing approach to compulsive checking, *Clin Psychol Psychother* 2:69–77, 1995.
60. Gardiner JM, Java RI: Recognising and remembering. In Collins, Gathercole, Conway, Morris, editors: *Theories of memory*, Manhwah, NJ, 1993, Lawrence Erlbaum, pp 163–188.
61. Knowlton BJ, Squire LR: Remembering and knowing: Two different expressions of declarative memory, *J Exp Psychol: Learn Mem Cog* 21:699–710, 1995.
62. Janowski JS, Shimamura AP, Squire LR: Memory and metamemory: Comparisons between patients with frontal lobe lesions and amnesic patients, *Psychobiology* 17:3–11, 1989.
63. Janowski JS, Shimamura AP, Squire LR: Source memory impairment in patients with frontal lobe lesions, *Neuropsychologia* 27: 1043–1056, 1989.
64. Schacter DL, Harbluk J, McLachlin D: Retrieval without recollection: An experimental analysis of source amnesia, *J Ver Learn Ver Behav* 23: 593–611, 1984.
65. McNally RJ, Kohlbeck P: Reality monitoring in obsessive-compulsive disorder, *Behav Res Ther* 31:249–253, 1993.

14

The Genetics of Obsessive-Compulsive Disorder

John P. Alsobrook II, Ph.D., David L. Pauls, Ph.D.

Although the psychiatric literature has long recognized the symptoms of obsessive-compulsive disorder (OCD), this disorder has been viewed in varying ways: (1) In Westphal's[1] neurologic framework, it was devoid of any underlying emotive basis; (2) in Freud's[2] psychodynamic terms, OCD was a manifestation of internal libidinal conflict; and (3) to Janet,[3,4] OCD was a psychasthenia arising from nonsexual psychologic tensions.

Obsessive-compulsive disorder was traditionally believed to be "apparently rare in the general population."[5] In 1988, Karno, et al[6] reported a lifetime prevalence rate of OCD of 1.9% to 3.3%, determined from the National Institute of Mental Health (NIMH)–sponsored Epidemiologic Catchment Area (ECA) survey.[7] These rates were obtained from data collected using the Diagnostic Interview Schedule (DIS),[8] a structured interview that elicits information to establish *Diagnostic and Statistical Manual of Mental Disorders* (DSM-III) diagnoses. The DIS was specifically designed to be administered by lay interviewers in the ECA project.

The epidemiology of OCD was further investigated in a cross-national study that surveyed populations in six countries other than the United States.[9] Data from Edmonton, Alberta, Canada; Puerto Rico; Munich, Germany; Taiwan; Seoul, Korea; and Christchurch, New Zealand, showed lifetime prevalence rates of OCD that were comparable with those seen in the United States, ranging from 1.1% in Korea to 1.8% in New Zealand. The mean age of onset of OCD was also consistent across the international sites, ranging from 22 years in Edmonton to 35 years in Puerto Rico.

Evidence for genetic influences in the manifestation of OCD has come primarily from family and twin studies. Neurobiologic investigations, including drug-treatment and functional neuroimaging studies, add strength by emphasizing the biochemical nature of the disorder.

FAMILY STUDIES

Although a number of family studies of OCD and obsessional neurosis have been completed over the past 60 years, the evidence for the familiarity of OCD remains controversial. Familial aggregation of a disorder is necessary, but not sufficient, for the inference of genetic transmission, because the family transmits not only genes but also sociocultural factors that contribute to human phenotypes. Environmental variables can have a large influence on phenotypic development and outcome, especially in family units in which aspects of the environment may be shared by all members. This caveat is critical to the investigation of traits with complex etiologies, such as psychiatric disorders. For this reason, genetics alone may not explain familial aggregation of a disorder. The demonstration of aggregation is, however, an important first step.

Family study paradigms begin with the ascertainment of index cases (probands) that are affected with the disorder under investigation.[10,11] The prevalence of the disorder among the biologic relatives of probands is then determined, and this rate is compared with that seen in separately ascertained control groups, or with general population prevalences. Control groups may be ascertained as relatives of unaffected cases, or relatives of cases affected with a different, unrelated disorder. Population prevalence estimates, if obtained using the same assessment methodology, also are appropriate. However, these studies are very expensive and difficult to undertake. Thus, accurate estimates of a disorder in the general population may be unavailable.

Two general methods are used to determine prevalence in relatives: (1) the family-history method; and (2) the direct-interview or family-study method. Both methods endeavor to collect accurate symptom information on relatives that will allow the assignment of a best-estimate diagnosis.[12] The family-history method relies on the proband to report diagnostic information on all first-degree relatives. The direct-interview method relies on directly interviewing the first-degree relatives to obtain diagnostic information. The most robust studies combine information of both types to assign diagnoses. Because some subjects fail to report symptoms in a direct interview, the family-history method can provide information that would otherwise be unavailable. In a similar fashion, some probands may be unaware of specific symptoms in their first-degree relatives, in which case the direct interview is a source of otherwise unattainable information.

Family History Method

As early as the 1930s, OCD was observed to be a familial disorder.[13–16] In 1936, Lewis[13] reported that 37 parents and 63 siblings of 306 first-degree relatives of obsessive-compulsive patients displayed pronounced obsessional traits, yielding a rate of 32.7%. In 1942, Brown[14] found obsessional neuroses in 3 of 40 parents and 4 of 56 siblings of obsessive-compulsive neurotics—a rate of 7.3% among first-degree relatives. Further, in 1965, Kringlen[15] reported that half of all fathers and mothers of 91 patients ascertained at the time of first admission for obsessional neurosis were "nervous," and 18 of the parents qualified as obsessional neurotics. In 1967, Rosenberg[16] studied 547 first-degree relatives of 144 obsessional neurotics and found an increased rate of psychiatric illness among first-degree relatives of obsessional neurotics, but no significant increase of OCD specifically among those relatives. Insel, et al[17] in 1983 studied the parents of 27 OCD patients using the family-history method and found no OCD in any of the parents. However, when 20 parents were administered the Leyton Obsessional Inventory (LOI), three were found to have obsessive thoughts about contamination that were not recognized as problematic by their offspring proband. No information on siblings was provided. In 1986, Rasmussen, et al[18] described a sample of 44 patients who met DSM-III criteria for OCD; data concerning the parents of these patients were obtained by the family-history method. Four of the 88 (4.5%) parents met full criteria for OCD, and another 10 (11.4%) had significant obsessive-compulsive traits that were not ego dystonic; thus, 15.9% of the parents of OCD patients were affected to some degree. In contrast, McKeon and Murray[19] studied first-degree relatives of 50 obsessive-compulsive patients and those of matched controls and did not find evidence that OCD was familial. All individuals completed the LOI and relatives identified as "possible cases" by high LOI scores were interviewed. Although these relatives have a significantly higher rate of mental illness in general, only one met criteria for obsessive-compulsive neurosis. A possible shortcoming of this study is the fact that individuals can have low scores on the LOI but still have a few obsessions or compulsions that cause significant distress. Thus, it is possible that some affected relatives may have been missed in the ascertainment scheme employed.

Direct-Interview Method

Seven recent studies of OCD[20–26] directly interviewed all available relatives using standard diagnostic criteria. Findings from these studies provide further support for a familial component for the expression of some forms of OCD. Three of the studies focused on families of children with OCD;[20–22] the other four investigated families of adult probands.[23–26]

Lenane and colleagues[20] studied 145 first-degree relatives (89 parents and 56 siblings) of 46 children and adolescents with severe primary OCD. The probands were consecutive admissions to an NIMH study of severe primary childhood OCD. No control group was examined. All parents and relatives were personally interviewed using structured psychiatric interviews, and diagnoses were based on DSM-III criteria. This study used an additional diagnostic category of "subclinical OCD" for subjects who met all DSM-III criteria for OCD except one of the following: their obsessions/compulsions consumed less than 1 hour per day, or they lacked insight into the unreasonable nature of their obsessions and compulsions. Twenty-five percent of fathers and 9% of mothers had OCD. When subthreshold OCD was included, the age-corrected morbid risk for all first-degree relatives was 35%.

Lenane, et al[20] also looked for any relationship between the probands' primary OCD symptoms and those of their respective relatives. They found no consistent pattern between parents and children, nor between older and younger siblings. Hence, a simple modeling hypothesis whereby obsessive-compulsive symptoms are observed and learned by susceptible younger relatives was not supported by the data.

A second family study of childhood-onset OCD probands[21] interviewed the parents of 21 clinically referred children and adolescents with OCD; DSM-III-R diagnostic criteria were used. Interviewers and raters were never blind to the status of the proband. Fifteen of forty-two (35.7%) parents (1 parent from each of 15 families) received a diagnosis of clinical (N = 4) or subclinical (N = 11) OCD. No information concerning siblings or rates of diagnosis in siblings was given. The high rate of OCD among parents may be partly the result of the early age of onset in these children, because early onset is often considered indicative of a more severe form of a disorder. On the other hand, these rates may reflect an ascertainment bias, in that parents who themselves were affected might be more likely to bring in their children than unaffected parents. Because this study was intended primarily as a description of the phenomenology seen in childhood OCD, no control group was ascertained.

Finally, a third family study of childhood-onset OCD probands[22] examined 171 first-degree relatives of 54 childhood probands who had previously been consecutively admitted into a drug treatment trial (46 of these probands and their families were reported previously by Lenane[20]). This study was a slightly expanded 2- to 7-year follow-up evaluation of those probands and their families. Using DSM-III-R criteria, 13% (age-corrected rate) of all first-degree relatives met criteria for OCD.

Bellodi, et al[23] studied the families of 92 adult patients with OCD. These patients were consecutive admissions for primary OCD at a specialty Anxiety Disorders Clinic in Milan, Italy. All first-degree relatives were evaluated by either direct interview or family history, and the rate of OCD among parents and siblings was only 3.4%. However, when probands were separated on an age-of-onset basis, and early onset was defined as 14 years of age or younger, the rates were significantly higher among the relatives of early-onset probands. The morbid risk for OCD among relatives of the 21 early-onset probands was 8.8% compared with 3.4% among the relatives of 71 later-onset probands. The number of relatives in each proband-onset category was not given. Here again, this study did not ascertain or assess a comparison sample.

Nicolini, et al[24] studied the families of 27 OCD probands ascertained through the Instituto Mexicano de Psiquiatria in Mexico City. Probands and all available first- and second-degree relatives were evaluated by direct interview, and unavailable relatives were evaluated by the family-history method. All diagnoses used DSM-III-R criteria. A total of 268 first-degree relatives and 187 second-degree relatives were evaluated; 13 first-degree relatives received an OCD diagnosis, giving a raw rate of 4.9%. This rate was significantly different at the $p < 0.05$ level from the comparison rate of 1.8% population prevalence of OCD reported in the U.S. ECA study.[6] Use of a separate sociocultural population for a control comparison is problematic, because there is no reason to expect rates of OCD in the Mexican population to be the same as in the U.S. population (although Mexican-Americans constituted approximately 10% of the ECA sample primarily the result of the Los Angeles site).

A significant methodologic weakness of the five family studies just described was the lack of a comparison sample. Thus, the investigators could not determine whether the rates observed among the family members for OCD or subthreshold OCD were significantly higher than would be observed by these same investigators employing the same diagnostic methods in an independent sample of comparison subjects. In addition, no population studies have been performed using similar methods to allow for an appropriate prevalence comparison for subthreshold OCD.

A study by Black, et al[25] did use an appropriate control group. The study sample included 120 first-degree relatives of 32 OCD probands and 129 relatives of 33 psychiatrically normal controls. Assessments of relatives were made using direct structured interviews with the interviewer blind to the proband's status, and diagnoses of relatives were made using DSM-III criteria. The age-corrected rate of OCD was 2.5% in relatives of OCD probands compared with 2.3% in relatives of controls; both values agree with the ECA lifetime prevalence for OCD and thus provided no evidence that OCD was familial. However, the risk of a more broadly defined OCD (i.e., including subclinical OCD) was increased among the parents of OCD probands (15.6%) when compared with parents of normal individuals (2.9%).

Finally, Pauls, et al[26] reported results from a family study in which all available first-degree relatives were interviewed directly, and best-estimate diagnoses were assigned using DSM-III-R criteria. One hundred OCD probands, their 466 biologic first-degree relatives, and 113 comparison subjects were included in the study. The 113 control individuals were first-degree relatives of 33 psychiatrically unaffected subjects. Rates of OCD and subthreshold OCD were significantly higher among relatives of OCD probands compared with control subjects (OCD: 10.3% vs. 1.9%, $p < 0.005$; subthreshold OCD: 7.9% vs. 2.0%, $p < 0.05$; total: 18.2% vs. 4.0%, $p < 0.0001$). Of note in this study was that approximately half of the probands did not have any relative with OCD; that is, they were isolated cases in their families. Thus, OCD appears to be a heterogeneous condition, with some cases being familial and others having no family history of either OCD or related conditions.

These studies of OCD probands and their relatives cumulatively provide strong evidence that some forms of OCD are familial. Although these findings are consistent with a genetic etiology of OCD, family studies by themselves cannot demonstrate that genetic factors are necessary for the manifestation of the illness. Twin studies are an important adjunct that can provide additional evidence that genetic factors are important.

TWIN STUDIES

Twin studies have provided some evidence for the role of genetic factors in the manifestation of OCD. The degree of phenotypic similarity among twins is generally characterized by concordance (defined as the morbid risk of disease to the co-twin of an affected twin). The twin method consists of comparing the number of monozygotic (MZ) twins in which both members are affected (i.e., concordant) with the number of dizygotic (DZ) twin pairs concordant for the trait of interest. If the concordance of MZ twins is significantly higher than the concordance of DZ twins, it is taken as evidence for the contribution of genetic factors to the expression of the disorder under study. More recently, the similarity between twins has been expressed by heritability, defined as the proportion of phenotypic or observable variance caused by additive genetic factors. This statistic describes the variance in a particular population at a particular time and is descriptive rather than predictive. Large heritability does not preclude substantial influences by environmental factors within the population,[27,28] but does indicate a potentially significant biologic component in a disorder's etiology.

In an early twin study of OCD, Inouye[29] reported 80% concordance for "obsessional neurosis" among 10 pairs of MZ twins compared with 50% concordance among four pairs of DZ twins. The small sample size in this study precludes any conclusions, but the data are suggestive of some genetic involvement. Of note is that this twin sample was ascertained in Japan, making this paper one of the earliest modern reports of non-Western obsessionality.

More recently, Rasmussen and Tsuang[18] reviewed the OCD literature on twins and found reports of 32 of 51 (63%) MZ twins being concordant for OCD. Even when those twins in whom zygosity was in doubt were eliminated from the sample, 65% (13 of 20) were concordant for OCD. These MZ concordance rates are similar to those reported for affective and anxiety disorders.[30,31] However, because no data from DZ twins were available for comparison, it is not possible from these twin data to determine the extent to which they support the hypothesis that genetic factors contribute to the expression of OCD.

Two recent twin studies included data from DZ twins. Carey and Gottesman[31] used a diagnosis of "obsessive symptoms and features" in reporting 87% concordance between MZ twins and 47% concordance between DZ twins. The subjects for this study were ascertained from the Maudsley Twin Register and represent consecutive series of 15 MZ and 15 DZ twins. The index twin in each pair had received a psychiatric diagnosis of obsessional neurosis, obsessional personality, or "phobic neurosis" at local hospitals during a 32-year interval (1948 to 1979). Along with hospital notes on the index cases and family members, each twin pair was followed-up by personal interview and assessment of psychiatric status unblinded to the index twin's diagnosis.

Two methodologic weaknesses of these studies critically limit their usefulness. The first weakness is the lack of standardized diagnostic criteria across studies. To compare rates among different studies, it is essential to show that the same disorder is being diagnosed. Additionally, without standardization, the diagnostic criteria may tend to be "loose," increasing the chance for type II errors (false positives) and thereby inflating the concordance rates. The second weakness is the lack of any procedural blind for obtaining diagnostic information or for making the actual diagnoses (i.e., knowledge of an index case's status when evaluating the co-twin [or vice versa] is an unacceptable source of bias). All studies also were constrained by small sample sizes—a common disadvantage in twin studies.

Clifford[32] and Clifford, et al[33] performed genetic analyses on data collected from 419 pairs of unselected twins who had been given the 42-item version of the LOI. Multivariate analyses provided heritability estimates of 44% for obsessional traits (as defined by the 10-item "Trait Scale" of the LOI) and 47% for obsessional symptoms (as defined by the 32-item "Symptom Scale" of the LOI). These results support earlier findings that genetic factors are important for the expression of some symptoms of clinical or subclinical OCD and obsessive-compulsive personality traits. These results also suggest that the genetic factors important for obsessional symptoms and traits are partly independent of each other.

ASSOCIATION WITH TOURETTE'S DISORDER

Additional support for the hypothesis that genetic factors are important in the transmission and expression of some forms of OCD comes from the finding of high rates of OCD and obsessive-compulsive symptoms among Tourette's disorder patients and families.[37–40] Tourette's disorder (TD) is characterized by a changing course of chronic involuntary motor and phonic tics and is a familial condition that appears to have a significant genetic basis[41] (see Chapter 8). An association with obsessions was noted by Gilles de la Tourette in his initial report of the syndrome in 1885. Since that time, many studies have reported increased OCD–related behaviors in both TD probands and their relatives, suggesting that some forms of OCD might be etiologically (and perhaps genetically) related to TD.

The family-genetic studies of TD provide the strongest evidence for a genetic basis of some form of OCD. The rate of OCD is similar in families regardless of the OCD diagnosis of the TD proband. Pauls, et al[42] studied 86 TD probands and 338 of the probands' biologic relatives and found a rate of OCD of 11.5%. Among relatives of TD probands who lacked sufficient symptoms for a concomitant diagnosis of OCD (TD – OCD probands), the age-corrected morbid risk of OCD was 10.4% (19 of 223), whereas among relatives of TD probands with a concomitant diagnosis of OCD (TD + OCD probands), the morbid risk was 13.6% (13 of 115) (the three rates were not significantly different). If the two disorders were unrelated, one would expect that OCD in the relatives would depend on the presence or absence of OCD in the proband; this was not the case, because OCD occurred with equal frequency among relatives of TD probands with or without OCD. These findings suggest a spectrum of TD expressivity, ranging from TD to OCD with a middle ground between the two occupied by chronic tic disorder. Interestingly, in the previously mentioned study by Leonard, et al[22] of OCD probands, TD was an exclusionary criterion for participation in the study, yet at 2 to 7 years' follow-up, 12% of probands were diagnosed with TD.

SEGREGATION ANALYSES

Once familial aggregation of a disorder is established, a logical next step is to determine if the patterns of aggregation can be explained by Mendelian genetic models. Segregation analysis accomplishes this by examining the goodness-of-fit of the observed data to various genetic and nongenetic models. Although segregation studies cannot prove the existence of genes, a finding of patterns within families consistent with simple modes of inheritance can be taken as evidence for the importance of genes in the etiology of the disorder. Only two segregation analysis studies of nuclear families of probands with OCD have been reported.

Nicolini and colleagues[43] performed segregation analyses on data collected from 24 families of OCD probands to test whether transmission patterns were consistent with simple Mendelian models of inheritance. The probands were ascertained through the UCLA Child Psychiatry Clinic and had a mean age of onset of 9.1 years. Eleven of the 24 probands had a positive family history of OCD; no further characterization of the sample is given. All available first-degree relatives were directly interviewed, with family history information used for unavailable relatives. Segregation analysis was performed using the SEGRAN program, assigning affected status to all individuals with a diagnosis of OCD, chronic motor tics, or TD. Because of the small sample size, these investigators were unable to statistically reject either an autosomal dominant or autosomal recessive model.

More recent segregation analyses have been consistent with these results.[44] Using more comprehensive analytic methods, Cavalini and colleagues found evidence for a major gene effect in a sample of 92 families ascertained through an OCD proband. Although the most parsimonious result was an autosomal dominant model, other major gene solutions (i.e., additive) could not be statistically rejected.

FUTURE WORK

Because many published reports suggest that some forms of OCD have a genetic basis, genetic-linkage studies are warranted as the next step in our understanding of the inheritance of the disorder. Genetic-linkage studies provide a powerful method for confirming the hypotheses of genetic involvement, because linkage results can demonstrate the existence of a genetic locus and help clarify the pattern of inheritance.

The localization of a gene or genes responsible for the expression of OCD would be a major step forward in our understanding of the genetic and biologic risk factors for the expression of this disorder. The identification of a linked marker would permit more precise studies of the physiologic and biochemical etiology of OCD, by examination of the gene product and its impact on the manifestation of the disorder. In addition, by controlling for genetic factors, it would be possible to document more carefully the nongenetic environmental factors important for the expression of obsessions and compulsions.

Once the location of a gene or genes was verified, it would be possible to test the unaffected children in high-risk families to determine those carrying a susceptibility gene, making it possible to study the interaction between genotype and environment in OCD. Linked genetic markers also can help define an appropriate control group for a "genetic case-control" design;[57] such closely linked genetic markers can accurately identify children who are genetically identical to their affected siblings or parents at the relevant loci.* Comparing probands with their respective genetically identical siblings or children provides the basis of a genetic case-control paradigm. This particular control provides optimal power for identifying major nongenetic risk factors for the TD spectrum.

The ability to use genetic linkage and other aspects of genetic studies to design and carry out a study of nongenetic etiologic factors of a psychiatric illness is a significant methodologic advancement that has not been possible heretofore. Data from prospective studies of at-risk children will make it possible to examine individuals with specific genotypes to determine which factors protect some from manifesting the syndrome. It is important to begin collecting data on potential environmental risk factors now, before genes

---

* Genetically identical individuals constitute an ideal control group for the identification of environmental factors relevant to the onset of psychiatric disorders. Genetically identical but unaffected siblings have the genetic susceptibility but have presumably not been exposed to necessary environmental agents or stimuli. Alternatively, the unaffected siblings may have been exposed to those agents or stimuli at different times in development or may have encountered factors that protected them from manifesting the disorder. In contrast, siblings who are not genetically identical at the relevant loci might very well have experienced the same environmental risks but be unaffected because they lack the necessary genetic susceptibility.

are localized. After the genes are localized, it will be ethically unacceptable to withhold a test for identification of carriers from at-risk individuals. Knowledge of carrier status may change the at-risk individual's caregiving and developmental environment, invalidating the genetic case-control design.

SUMMARY

Twin and family genetic studies provide some support for the hypothesis that genetic factors play a role in the manifestation of OCD. However, that evidence is somewhat controversial, because in some studies, there is no evidence for the specific inheritance of OCD. It is possible that OCD is part of a larger spectrum of "anxiety disorders," and that genetic factors may be important for the expression of a broader category of anxiety disorders. More work is needed to further understand this potential relationship. None of the extant studies provides conclusive evidence that specific genes are involved in the manifestation of OCD, but rather each serves as an indicator of a potentially significant biologic component in the etiology of OCD. As discussed elsewhere in this volume, both neuroanatomic and pharmacologic data also suggest that biologic factors are important in the expression of OCD. At the present time, the underlying genetic mechanisms are not understood. It is expected that with the application of recently developed methods in molecular genetics, genes important for OCD will eventually be identified.

ACKNOWLEDGMENTS

This work was supported in part by grants NS-16648, MH-49351, and MH-00508 (an NIMH Research Scientist Award to Dr. Pauls). Portions of this chapter have appeared in other publications authored by Dr. Pauls.

REFERENCES

1. Westphal C: Uber Zwangsvorstellungen, *Archive für Psychiatrie und Nervenkrankheiten* 8:734–750, 1878.
2. Freud S: The predisposition to obsessional neurosis, *Collected papers* 2:122–132, London, 1913/1924, Hogarth Press.
3. Janet P: *Les obsessions et la psychasthenie,* vol 1, Paris, 1903/1976, Alcan. (Reprinted in New York, 1976, Arno.)
4. Pitman RK: Janet's obsessions and psychasthenia: a synopsis, *Psychiatr Q* 56: 291–314, 1984.
5. American Psychiatric Association Committee on Nomenclature and Statistics: *Diagnostic and statistical manual of mental disorders,* ed 3, Washington, 1980, American Psychiatric Association.
6. Karno M, Golding JM, Sorenson SB, Burnam MA: The epidemiology of obsessive-compulsive disorder in five U.S. communities, *Arch Gen Psychiatry* 45:1084–1099, 1988.
7. Eaton WW, Kessler LG, editors: *Epidemiologic field methods in psychiatry: The NIMH epidemiologic catchment area program,* Orlando, Fla, 1985, Academic Press.

8. Robins LN, Helzer JE, Croughan J, Ratcliff KS: National Institute of Mental Health Diagnostic Interview Schedule: its history, characteristics, and validity, *Arch Gen Psychiatry* 38:381–389, 1981.

9. Weissman MM, Bland RC, Canino GJ, et al: The cross national epidemiology of obsessive compulsive disorder, *J Clin Psychiatry* 55(3,suppl):5–10, 1994.

10. Khoury MJ, Beaty TH, Cohen BH: *Fundamentals of genetic epidemiology. Monographs in epidemiology and biostatistics,* vol 19, New York, 1993, Oxford University Press.

11. Weissman MM, Merikangas KR, John K, et al: Family-genetic studies of psychiatric disorders, *Arch Gen Psychiatry* 43:1104–1116, 1986.

12. Leckman JF, Sholomskas D, Thompson WD, et al: Best estimate of lifetime psychiatric diagnosis: a methodologic study, *Arch Gen Psychiatry* 39:879–883, 1982.

13. Lewis A: Problems of obsessional illness, *Proc R Soc Med* 29:325–336, 1935.

14. Brown FW: Heredity in the psychoneuroses, *Proc R Soc Med* 35:785–790, 1942.

15. Kringlen E: Obsessional neurotics: a long term follow-up, *Br J Psychiatry* 111:709–722, 1965.

16. Rosenberg CM: Familial aspects of obsessional neurosis, *Br J Psychiatry* 113:405–413, 1967.

17. Insel T, Hoover C, Murphy DL: Parents of patients with obsessive compulsive disorder, *Psychol Med* 13:807–811, 1983.

18. Rasmussen SA, Tsuang MT: Clinical characteristics and family history in DSM-III obsessive-compulsive disorder, *Am J Psychiatry* 143:317–322, 1986.

19. McKeon P, Murray R: Familial aspects of obsessive-compulsive neurosis, *Br J Psychiatry* 151:528–534, 1987.

20. Lenane MC, Swedo SE, Leonard H, et al: Psychiatric disorders in first degree relatives of children and adolescents with obsessive-compulsive disorder, *J Am Acad Child Adolesc Psychiatry* 29:407–412, 1990.

21. Riddle MA, Scahill L, King R, et al: Obsessive compulsive disorder in children and adolescents: Phenomenology and family history, *J Am Acad Child Adolesc Psychiatry* 29:766–772, 1990.

22. Leonard HL, Lenane MC, Swedo SE, et al: Tics and Tourette's disorder: a 2- to 7-year follow-up of 54 obsessive-compulsive children, *Am J Psychiatry* 149:1244–1251, 1992.

23. Bellodi L, Sciuto G, Diaferia G, et al: Psychiatric disorders in the families of patients with obsessive-compulsive disorder, *Psychiatr Res* 42:111–120, 1992.

24. Nicolini H, Weissbecker K, Mejia JM, Sanchez de Carmona M: Family study of obsessive-compulsive disorder in a Mexican population, *Arch Med Res* 24(2):193–198, 1993.

25. Black DW, Noyes R Jr, Goldstein RB, et al: A family study of obsessive-compulsive disorder, *Arch Gen Psychiatry* 49:362–368, 1992.

26. Pauls DL, Alsobrook JP II, Goodman W, et al: A family study of obsessive compulsive disorder, *Am J Psychiatry* 152:76–84, 1995.

27. Vogel F, Motulsky AG: *Human genetics,* ed 2, New York, 1986, Springer-Verlag.

28. Lewontin R: Comment on an erroneous conception of the meaning of heritability, *Behav Gene* 6:373–374, 1976.

29. Inouye E: Similar and dissimilar manifestations of obsessive-compulsive neurosis in monozygotic twins, *Am J Psychiatry* 121:1171–1175, 1965.

30. Bertelsen A: A Danish twin study of manic-depressive disorders. In Schou M, Stromgren E, editors: *Origin, prevention and treatment of affective disorders,* London, 1978, Academic Press.
31. Carey G, Gottesman II: Twin and family studies of anxiety, phobic and obsessive disorders. In Klien DF, Rabkin J, editors: *Anxiety: new research and changing concepts,* New York, 1981, Raven Press.
32. Clifford CA: Twin studies of drinking behavior and obsessionality. Doctoral dissertation, London, 1983, Institute of Psychiatry.
33. Clifford CA, Murray RM, Fulker DW: Genetic and environmental influences on obsessional traits and symptoms, *Psychol Med* 14:791–800, 1984.
34. Torgersen S: Genetic factors in anxiety disorder, *Arch Gen Psychiatry* 40: 1085–1089, 1983.
35. Andrews G, Stewart G, Allen R, et al: The genetics of six neurotic disorders: a twin study, *J Affect Dis* 19:23–29, 1990.
36. Andrews G, Stewart G, Morris-Yates A, et al: Evidence for a general neurotic syndrome, *Br J Psychiatry* 157:6–12, 1990.
37. Pauls DL, Towbin KE, Leckman JF, et al: Gilles de la Tourette syndrome and obsessive compulsive disorder: evidence supporting an etiological relationship, *Arch Gen Psychiatry* 43:1180–1182, 1986.
38. Robertson MM, Trimble MR, Lees AJ: The psychopathology of the Gilles de la Tourette: a phenomenological analysis, *Br J Psychiatry* 152:383–390, 1988.
39. Pauls DL, Leckman JF: The inheritance of Gilles de la Tourette's syndrome and associated behaviors: evidence for autosomal dominant transmission, *N Engl J Med* 315:993–997, 1986.
40. Eapen V, Pauls DL, Robertson MM: Evidence for autosomal dominant transmission in Tourette's Syndrome—United Kingdom Cohort Study, *Br J Psychiatry* 162:593–596, 1993.
41. Pauls DL: The inheritance pattern. In Kurlan R, editor: *Handbook of Tourette's syndrome and related tic and behavioral disorders,* New York, 1992, Marcel Dekker.
42. Pauls DL, Raymond CL, Stevenson JM, et al: A family study of Gilles de la Tourette's syndrome, *Am J Hum Genet* 48:154–163, 1991.
43. Nicolini H, Hanna G, Baxter L, et al: Segregation analysis of obsessive compulsive and associated disorders. Preliminary results, *Ursus Medicus* 1:25–28, 1991.
44. Cavalini MC, Macciardi F, Pasquale L, et al: Complex segregation analysis of obsessive compulsive and spectrum related disorders, *Psychiatr Genet* 5(suppl 1): 31, 1995.
45. Insel T: A neuropeptide for affiliation: evidence from behavioral, receptor, autoradiographic and comparative studies, *Psychoneuroendocrinology* 17:3–35, 1992.
46. Zohar J, Insel TR: Obsessive-compulsive disorder: psychobiological approaches to diagnosis, treatment and pathophysiology, *Biol Psychiatry* 2:667–687, 1987.
47. Goodman WK, McDougle CJ, Price LH, et al: Beyond the serotonin hypothesis: a role for dopamine in some forms of obsessive compulsive disorder? *J Clin Psychiatry* 51(suppl):36–43, 1990.
48. Hanna GL, McCracken JT, Cantwell DP: Prolactin in childhood obsessive-compulsive disorder: clinical correlates and response to clomipramine, *J Am Acad Child Adolesc Psychiatry* 30:173–178, 1991.

49. McDougle CJ, Goodman WK, Leckman JF, et al: The efficacy of fluvoxamine in obsessive compulsive disorder: effects of comorbid chronic tic disorder, *J Clin Psychopharmacol* 13:354–358, 1993.
50. McDougle CJ, Goodman WK, Leckman JF, et al: Haloperidol addition in fluvoxamine-refractory obsessive compulsive disorder: a double blind placebo-controlled study in patients with and without tics, *Arch Gen Psychiatry* 51:302–308, 1994.
51. Altemus M, Pigott T, Kalogeras KT, et al: Abnormalities in the regulation of vasopressin and corticotropin releasing factor secretion in obsessive-compulsive disorder, *Arch Gen Psychiatry* 49:9–20, 1992.
52. de Boer JA, Westenberg HGM: Oxytocin in obsessive compulsive disorder, *Peptides* 13:1083–1085, 1992.
53. Leckman JF, Goodman WK, North WG, et al: Elevated levels of CSF oxytocin in obsessive compulsive disorder: comparison with Tourette's syndrome and healthy controls, *Arch Gen Psychiatry* 51:782–792, 1994.
54. Marazziti D, Hollander E, Lensi P, et al: Peripheral markers of serotonin and dopamine function in obsessive-compulsive disorder, *Psychiatr Res* 42:41–51, 1992.
55. Weizman A, Mandel A, Barber Y, et al: Decreased platelet imipramine binding in Tourette syndrome children with obsessive-compulsive disorder, *Biol Psychiatry* 31:705–711, 1992.
56. Stahl SM: The human platelet: a diagnostic and research tool for the study of biogenic amines in psychiatric and neurological disorders, *Arch Gen Psychiatry* 34:509–516, 1977.
57. Kidd KK: New genetic strategies for studying psychiatric disorders. In Sakai T, Tsuboi T, editors: *Genetic aspects of human behavior,* Tokyo, 1984, Igaku-Shoin.

15

Neuroimaging in Obsessive-Compulsive Disorder and Related Disorders

Scott L. Rauch, M.D., Lewis R. Baxter, Jr., M.D.

Neuroimaging technologies and their applications have advanced to become the most powerful tools available for assessing human brain structure and function *in vivo*. This chapter emphasizes neuroimaging research findings that have influenced current neurobiologic models of obsessive-compulsive disorder (OCD) and related disorders. Contemporary neuroimaging techniques are described briefly, and their role in the clinical assessment of OCD is discussed.

CONTEMPORARY NEUROIMAGING TECHNIQUES

For didactic purposes, neuroimaging technologies can be divided into methods that assess structure and methods that assess function. Structural neuroimaging techniques yield images that reflect the size, shape, and composition of brain components, whereas functional techniques yield images that reflect indices of brain activity (e.g., cerebral blood flow or glucose metabolism), neuroreceptor binding characteristics, or other neurochemical parameters (e.g., brain concentrations of endogenous or exogenous compounds). A comprehensive review of neuroimaging techniques is beyond the scope of this chapter, but can be found elsewhere.[1-5] This section is intended as a primer for readers otherwise unfamiliar with these technologies; readers already knowledgeable about neuroimaging may want to proceed to the next section (i.e., "Contemporary Neuroimaging Research Strategies").

Structural Methods

X-ray computed axial tomography (CT) uses the same principles as plain radiographs to produce images that reflect x-ray blocking capacity (i.e., attenuation values) at each location in space. The rotating ring-shaped CT

289

scanner allows x-ray beams to be directed through the head while detectors on the opposite side determine how much of the energy is transmitted versus how much is blocked. By gathering such data from multiple angles within each horizontal slice, an attenuation value can be calculated for each volume element (i.e., "voxel"). Data are gathered and subsequently displayed in a slice-wise fashion (i.e., tomographically), one horizontal slice at a time. With current conventional CT scanners, each slice is approximately 1 cm thick and requires approximately 1 minute to obtain. The patient lies on a mechanical bed, which is advanced through the bore of the scanner, such that the entire brain can be imaged in approximately 10 minutes. Attenuation values obtained provide ample contrast between gas, fluid, brain substance, and bone, but provide limited capability for distinguishing among different soft tissues (e.g., white versus gray matter, or old blood clots versus brain tissue). CT remains the imaging modality of choice in acute trauma, for instance, where rapid imaging of sometimes uncooperative or agitated patients must be performed to assess possible fractures or acute internal bleeding. Additional limitations of CT include those of slice geometry (i.e., typically acquired as relatively thick slices in the transaxial plane) and exposure to ionizing radiation (e.g., CT is contraindicated in pregnancy).

Magnetic resonance imaging (MRI) exploits the intrinsic magnetic properties of tissue to produce exquisite pictures of brain anatomy and pathology. For MRI, the patient is placed within a strong magnetic field, which induces alignment (or "coherence") of a subpopulation of hydrogen atoms within the brain. A series of radiofrequency pulses are then used to perturb this steady state. Following each perturbation, the scanner "listens" to detect the energy released as the perturbed hydrogen dipoles "relax" back into alignment within the constant magnetic field. Because subtle differences in the concentration of, or immediate surroundings near, these hydrogen atoms influence the way in which they are perturbed and relax, these differences can be captured and computer processed as sources of contrast in the images. The radiofrequency pulse sequences can be varied to accentuate different aspects of anatomy or pathology (i.e., so-called "T1-weighted" or "T2-weighted" images).

MRI is superior to CT in that it provides excellent soft-tissue contrast, particularly with regard to the definition of white versus gray matter. Moreover, MRI provides greater flexibility in terms of slice orientation and slice thickness, so that imaging data can be gathered to optimally visualize specific structures of interest. Limitations of MRI include exposure to the high magnetic field environment (e.g., MRI is contraindicated for patients with paramagnetic prostheses, such as pacemakers), and the greater imaging time and sense of confinement engendered by the narrow bore of the magnet (although claustrophobia can be prevented by pretreatment with low-dose benzodiazepines). CT is also superior for visualizing bone or calcifications and acute bleeding (i.e., < 48 to 72 hours old).

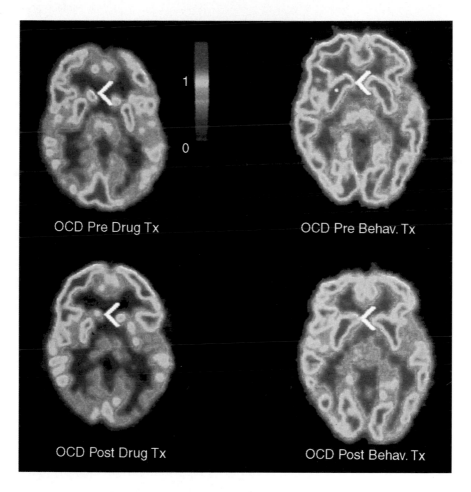

OCD Pre Drug Tx

OCD Pre Behav. Tx

OCD Post Drug Tx

OCD Post Behav. Tx

Fig. 15-1 Examples illustrating the results of Baxter and colleagues' positron-emission tomography pretreatment and posttreatment study of obsessive-compulsive disorder,[12] using F-18-fluorodeoxyglucose. Data are presented from representative patients in a horizontal plane at the level of the caudate nucleus, before (top panels) and after (bottom panels) successful treatment with medication (left panels) or behavior therapy (right panels). The inset color bar reflects the scale for normalized glucose metabolic rates. The arrows highlight the reduction in metabolism within the right caudate nucleus from the pretreatment to the posttreatment time point (note that the images are displayed according to radiologic convention; the left side of the image represents the right side of the brain). (From Baxter et al: *Arch Gen Psychiatry* 49:681-689, 1992. Copyright 1992-1994 by the American Medical Association.)

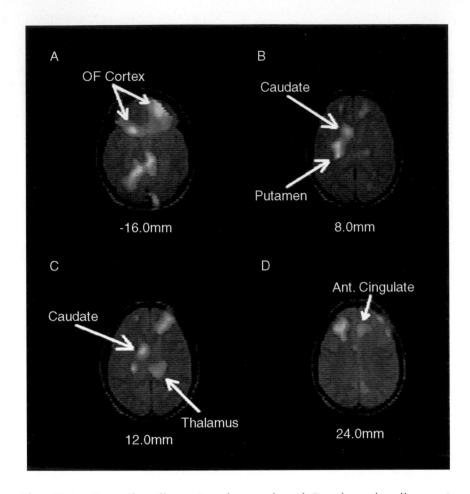

Fig. 15-2 Examples illustrating the results of Rauch and colleagues' positron-emission tomography symptom provocation study of obsessive-compulsive disorder,[57] using O-15-labelled-CO_2. Statistical parametric maps reflecting composite results from the provoked minus control contrast across the group of patients studied are depicted in "hot iron scale," superimposed over gray-scale structural magnetic resonance images for anatomic reference. The four horizontal slices shown are from different levels of the brain (corresponding z coordinates are given beneath each image; positive values are superior to the intercomissural plane), displayed according to radiologic convention (i.e., the left side of the image represents the right side of the brain). Arrows highlight key areas of interest. Regions of significant activation associated with the provoked state were the bilateral orbitofrontal cortex, right caudate nucleus, and the anterior cingulate cortex. Activation within the left anterior orbitofrontal locus correlated with subjective ratings of obsessionality. (From Rauch et al: *Arch Gen Psychiatry* 51:62-70, 1994. Copyright 1992-1994 by the American Medical Association.)

Functional Methods

Positron emission tomography (PET) uses radioactive tracers that emit positrons (the antimatter counterpart to electrons) to produce images reflective of brain function or chemistry. Although a variety of such tracers are employed, the basic principles are the same in every case. Namely, the radioactive substance is introduced into the body (via injection, inhalation, or ingestion) and gains access to the vasculature, travels to the brain, redistributes according to particular rules governed by the nature of the tracer, and then the PET camera detects the signal emitted by the radioactive label, allowing maps to be made that reflect regional tracer concentrations. More specifically, as positrons are emitted, they travel a short distance before meeting up with an electron, which results in annihilation producing two high-energy photons sent in opposite directions. The PET camera actually detects photons that arrive on opposite sides of the scanner at the same time. It is this dual-photon production allowing for coincidence detection that underlies the high spatial resolution of PET.

For example, the PET tracer F-18-fluorodeoxyglucose (FDG)—a radiolabelled sugar analog—is injected intravenously and is actively taken up by brain cells over a 20- to 40-minute period. Following injection, patients are typically instructed to rest quietly during the uptake period and then are placed in the PET scanner for image acquisition. The resulting images reflect glucose metabolism and hence gross brain activity, integrated over the 20- to 40-minute uptake period.

Alternatively, oxygen-15 (O-15)–labelled tracers are injected (i.e., O-15-water or O-15-butanol) or inhaled (i.e., O-15-carbon dioxide in air) when patients are actively being scanned. Because these substances are freely diffusible, they redistribute in brain proportionally to cerebral blood flow (CBF). CBF is known to be coupled with neuronal activity, and CBF maps are likewise inferred to reflect gross brain activity. In contrast to PET-FDG, PET-CBF studies produce images that are snapshots of brain activity integrated over approximately 1 minute. Because the half-life of O-15 is only 2 minutes in duration, a washout period of 10 minutes (i.e., 2-minute half-life x 5 half-lives) allows for dissipation of radioactivity such that O-15 PET scans can be repeated several times in the same scanning session.

Thirdly, a variety of positron-emitting radionuclides can be used to label drugs or other ligands of interest. Such radioligands then can be used to perform *in vivo* receptor-binding studies; the redistribution of the labelled compound is inferred to reflect binding characteristics and receptor concentrations in brain. Complex mathematical models are typically necessary, however, to tease apart specific versus nonspecific binding, and the influences of endogenous ligands pose daunting problems for image interpretation.

It is noteworthy that positron-emitting nuclides must be produced via a cyclotron. Because most positron-emitting nuclides are short-lived, the cyclotron should be in close proximity to the PET scanner. Consequently, PET scanning is of limited availability and relatively high cost.

Single photon emission computed tomography (SPECT) involves principles and procedures similar to those of PET, but, as the name indicates, employs single photon–emitting nuclides. Like PET, SPECT allows for CBF and receptor characterization studies. SPECT-CBF studies are performed using injected tracers (99m-Technetium hexamethyl-propylene amine oxime [Tc-HMPAO] or ethyl cysteine dimer [ECD]). The tracers are injected and uptake occurs over approximately 1 to 3 minutes; however, because of the long half-life of single photon emitters (e.g., the half-life of 99m-Technetium = 6 hours), patients may be injected outside the scanning environment, and then may be transported and scanned minutes or hours later. Within this time scale, regardless of when the scan is performed, the image will reflect brain activity during the few minutes of uptake following the injection. Conversely, this long half-life necessitates that serial studies on the same patient be separated by hours to days.

Older xenon-133-inhalation methods also rely on single photon emission and yield images reflective of CBF. However, the low-energy characteristics of this nuclide only allow for visualization of superficial cortical structures. Consequently, xenon-inhalation images are typically displayed as two-dimensional projections, rather than tomographically.

Receptor characterization studies analogous to those performed with PET can be conducted via SPECT. In general, radiochemical factors make it more challenging to synthesize radioligands for SPECT than for PET, because positron-emitting nuclides (i.e., O-15, N-13, C-11, F-18) can be attached more easily to a parent compound without altering its pharmacologic activity than can single photon emitters (e.g., 99m-Tc or I-123).

Limitations of SPECT include more modest spatial resolution that is not uniform throughout the brain (i.e., resolution is poorer for deep structures) and has no capacity for performing metabolic imaging or absolute quantitation of brain activity. However, one advantage of SPECT is that single photon emitters can be synthesized at relatively low cost in a conventional radiochemistry laboratory. Therefore, although PET has been the gold standard modality for functional imaging, SPECT is more widely available and usually is less costly.

Functional MRI (fMRI) is a term that may be used generically to encompass a broad range of MRI–based techniques that yield images reflective of brain function or chemistry. Here, however, we will use the term fMRI more restrictively, referring to the revolutionary discovery of blood-oxygen-level–dependent (BOLD) imaging with MRI.[6,7] This technique exploits the intrinsic magnetic properties of hemoglobin to image subtle changes in brain blood flow and blood volume. Because oxygenated and deoxygenated hemoglobin have different magnetic characteristics, special MRI pulse sequences and hardware modifications allow for images to be made that reflect brain activation patterns akin to PET and SPECT-CBF images. The great advantage of fMRI, however, is that it promises unparalleled spatial and temporal resolution, without exposure to ionizing radiation. Consequently, serial fMRI studies can be performed on the same subject, unlimited by cumulative exposure considerations. Further, in one visit to the scanner, high-quality structural and functional data can be obtained and coregistered. At this juncture, the main limitations of fMRI are related to its sensitivity or "contrast-to-noise ratio." This is a new technology, but one that is evolving rapidly.

Magnetic resonance spectroscopy (MRS) likewise represents an adaptation of fundamental MR principles and hardware. MRS allows investigators to measure the relative concentration of particular chemicals in brain volumes of interest. Specific MRS visible nuclei (e.g., H-1, Li-7, C-13, F-19, P-31) can be assayed to produce spectra specific to those elements; by measuring the area under designated peaks from such a spectrum, the relative regional concentration of the specific compound can be calculated. This technology can be used to measure in vivo brain concentrations of endogenous compounds (e.g., N acetyl aspartate or choline) or exogenous compounds (e.g., lithium or fluoxetine). The main limitation of this technique is its modest spatial resolution.

Neuroimaging Applications in Psychiatry

Clinical applications of neuroimaging in psychiatry are limited. CT and MRI are principally used to "rule in" or "rule out" structural brain lesions as causes of disturbed mental status. Functional neuroimaging techniques, such as PET and SPECT, occasionally may be useful as adjunctive diagnostic tests in neuropsychiatric conditions such as dementia or seizures. Presently, MRS and fMRI remain research tools.

CONTEMPORARY NEUROIMAGING RESEARCH STRATEGIES

Neuroimaging research paradigms have grown increasingly sophisticated in parallel with the development of new and progressively more powerful imaging tools. A historic perspective reveals that neuroimaging studies have gradually advanced from naturalistic to hypothesis-driven modes of inquiry. It is now clear that in addition to replication, convergence of findings across complementary studies using a variety of different modalities has provided the most convincing results.

Structural Imaging Studies

Morphometric studies have used high-resolution structural images from cohorts of patients and matched controls. Then, by performing careful "segmentation" (which entails tracing the outline of specified structures in each slice of the image), volumetric indices can be calculated and compared between groups. Regional volumetric differences between groups may indicate structural abnormalities, which may reflect maldevelopment, degeneration, and/or fundamental dysfunction. Morphometric MRI (mMRI) now represents the gold standard. Early studies with CT should be viewed with caution owing to poor soft-tissue contrast, thick slices (often of suboptimal orientation), and less well-refined segmentation.

Functional Imaging Studies

Neutral-state paradigms refer to single-session studies in which subjects are imaged during a nominal resting state, or during performance of some non-specific standardized task. Neutral-state studies involve between-group comparisons of gross brain activity, and are intended to determine whether specific regions exhibit abnormally high or low levels of activity in patients with OCD or related disorders. The term *resting state* is problematic in the sense that the brain is never truly at rest. Contemporary brain mapping research underscores the sensitivity of functional imaging techniques to state-dependent differences in brain activity. Therefore, studies that employ a nominal resting condition yield results that can be influenced by state as well as trait differences. Studies that employ a standardized task are intended to better control mental state at the time of scanning, thereby reducing variability. Depending on the task, however, such paradigms may serve to accentuate or obscure between-group differences. Neutral-state studies have been performed in conjunction with PET-FDG or SPECT-CBF imaging.

Pre/posttreatment studies typically involve imaging parameters identical to those of neutral-state paradigms; however, data are gathered from a patient group before and after some particular treatment intervention. Then, a within-subject, by-group comparison enables investigators to determine regional brain activity changes that accompany symptomatic improvement as a consequence of treatment. The premise here is that brain areas showing changes in activity associated with symptom reduction might be involved in mediating the symptoms of the disease. Again, pre/posttreatment studies are usually performed in conjunction with PET-FDG or SPECT-CBF imaging.

Symptom provocation paradigms represent one of several approaches that seek to capitalize on the sensitivity of imaging tools for capturing transient state-dependent changes in brain activity. By using CBF or fMRI techniques, investigators can acquire one set of images during a control state and another set of images during a provoked (i.e., more symptomatic) state, both from the same group of patients. Then, in the context of a within-subject, by-group design, the brain activity values from the control state can be compared with those from the symptomatic state, yielding a map that graphically illustrates which brain areas are differentially active during the provoked state. Hence, the activated brain system is implicated in mediating the state changes in question. For example, symptoms can be actively provoked behaviorally (via *in vivo* exposure or imagery, in OCD) or pharmacologically.

Cognitive activation paradigms also exploit the power of CBF or fMRI techniques to perform within-subject, by-group comparisons of state-dependent brain activity profiles. However, in this case, rather than inducing symptoms, refined cognitive tasks are employed to selectively recruit brain systems of interest.[8] In this way, investigators can establish normal brain activity patterns in response to standardized tasks and then test patients with diseases of interest to determine whether or not they activate or deactivate particular brain systems in a normal manner. Failure to exhibit such normal recruitment patterns implies abnormal brain function, as does aberrant recruitment of collateral systems. Such results are further informed by the analysis of behavioral measures to determine whether or not task performance is impaired.

Data analytic methods also have developed considerably over the past decade. Although a detailed discussion of these various techniques is beyond the scope of this chapter, a few general concepts will be introduced.

In the case of PET studies, it is possible to calculate absolute values of CBF or glucose metabolism. To accomplish this, however, a line for blood access is required so that an "input function" can be determined by taking frequent blood samples to measure the amount of radioactivity in them. Although for glucose metabolic rates there are many advantages to absolute quantitation (e.g., if the major differences between groups involve global brain increases or decreases), the method also has inherent inaccuracies that may propogate error. Moreover, absolute quantitation requires a number of mathematical corrections (e.g., for pCO_2) that may introduce error as well as variability, thereby diminishing essential statistical power. Consequently, many PET studies, as is the case for all SPECT studies, report "relative values" that reflect "normalization" to some reference—that is, taking the ratio of the value obtained in one region to that of another. Although there is fair debate as to the optimal reference area, most often values are calculated relative to global brain or ipsilateral hemisphere. Even in cases in which PET is performed to yield absolute values, relative values are typically reported. Therefore, for consistency, findings reviewed here will reflect relative rather than absolute values unless specified otherwise.

Another critical aspect of data analysis relates to anatomic definition and demarcation of regions to be measured. Originally, so-called region-of-interest (ROI)–based approaches were most popular. These approaches entail the outlining of various ROIs and calculating the mean value within each ROI, so that conventional statistics can be used to contrast values obtained from these ROIs between different groups or conditions. Varying levels of sophistication can be seen in methods of ROI definition—from using standard templates, to user-modified or user-repositioned standard templates, or the contemporary practice of coregistration with MRI structural scans, which allows for morphometric quality ROI definition. Even with the most sophisticated ROI–based methods, however, the areas defined are often large and constrained by gross anatomic landmarks. Given that functional subterritories may not adhere to such structural landmarks, a voxel-by-voxel method of brain map analysis has been developed. In this manner, parametric (or nonparametric) statistics can be applied within or across subjects to yield a statistical value at each position in space for the entire brain volume. For such methods to be applied across cohorts of subjects, brain size and shape must be standardized via a structural warping procedure. Although these highly complex maneuvers greatly enhance statistical power and provide a common coordinate system for expressing the location of each finding, they are imperfect and necessarily contribute another source of potential error. Methods that rely on transformation to a common brain shape may be particularly problematic in studies of neuropsychiatric disorders for which structural abnormalities exist. Nonetheless, the voxel-by-voxel approach represents the current gold standard method for human brain mapping research in individual subjects and provides an important additional method for group comparisons. The resulting statistical maps can provide a graphic illustration of brain activity differences between conditions or groups by condition.

NEUROIMAGING RESEARCH: NEUROBIOLOGIC MODELS OF OBSESSIVE-COMPULSIVE DISORDER

Before reviewing the vast body of imaging research data that has accrued regarding OCD and related disorders, it is useful to construct a scheme for organizing the findings. Contemporary neurobiologic models of OCD and related disorders have been shaped to a large degree by neuroimaging results, but also by information from other modes of inquiry. Such models are comprehensively reviewed elsewhere in this text (see Chapter 12). During the 1980s, several groups theorized that the basal ganglia and their relationships with frontal cortical structures might mediate the pathophysiologic processes that underlie OCD.[9,10] Neuroanatomic models of OCD[9,11–16] were progressively influenced by contemporaneous research delineating the nature of corticostriatal anatomy and physiology.[17,18] An emerging appreciation of parallel segregated corticostriatal circuits and their potential role in psychiatric disorders provides a useful heuristic (Table 15-1).[17–19] These parallel circuits each project from a specific group of cortical territories, to a corresponding subterritory of striatum, then ultimately to a specific territory of thalamus, and complete the loop via reciprocal projections to the very same cortical territories in frontal cortex. Most importantly, each of these circuits normally subserves a distinct type of function. Hence, dysfunction in any one of these circuits could be responsible for a specific brand of psychopathology. To elaborate, focusing on the corticostriatal elements, the sensorimotor circuit involves sensorimotor cortex projecting to the putamen; the affective/motivational circuit involves paralimbic cortex (e.g., anterior cingulate and posteromedial orbitofrontal cortex; see Mesulam 1985[20] for a description and comprehensive discussion of the "paralimbic belt") projecting to the ventral striatum (i.e., the nucleus

Table 15-1   Anatomy and Function of Relevant Segregated Cortico-striatothalamocortical Circuits

Circuits	Functions	Structural Elements		
		Cortex	Striatum	Thalamus
Sensorimotor	Sensorimotor	Sensorimotor	Putamen	Ventral tier nuclei
Dorsal cognitive	Cognitive/ Executive	Lateral prefrontal	Caudate (dorsolateral)	Medial dorsal and anterior nuclei
Ventral cognitive	Socioemotional/ Contextual	Anterior and lateral orbito-frontal cortex	Caudate (ventromedial)	Medial dorsal and anterior nuclei
Limbic	Affective/ Motivational	Paralimbic	Nucleus accumbens	Medial dorsal nucleus

accumbens); and there are two cognitive circuits: (1) the dorsal cognitive circuit involves dorsolateral prefrontal cortex projecting to the dorsolateral portion of caudate nucleus; and (2) the ventral cognitive circuit involves anteromedial and posterolateral orbitofrontal cortex projecting to the ventromedial portion of the caudate nucleus. This ventral cognitive circuit represents the interface, both conceptually and anatomically, between the dorsal cognitive and affective systems and is the one primarily implicated in OCD. There is not an absolute dissociation between the different cognitive functions subserved by the two cognitive circuits. However, although both mediate executive functions, the dorsal cognitive system has been more strongly implicated in working memory, planning, and organization, whereas the ventral system is typically associated with response inhibition, especially in relation to context or socially relevant cues.[21] One also should appreciate that, in general, all of these corticostriatal systems are purported to mediate automatic, rule-based, or nonconscious aspects of the designated functions. Thus, each corticostriatal circuit also has a counterpart descending pathway from the very same prefrontal territories via thalamus, which involves analogous functions, but, unlike the corticostriatal systems, is under volitional control and consciously accessible.

With the above functional anatomy in mind, Baxter and colleagues[11,13] suggested what others have termed "the striatal topography model" of obsessive-compulsive spectrum disorders,[15,16] the notion being that these disorders fundamentally involve corticostriatal dysfunction; however, they differ with respect to the specific systems involved. Thus, the clinical presentation reflects and is governed by the topography of dysfunction within the striatum. In other words, whereas putamen dysfunction leads to the sensorimotor symptoms of Tourette's disorder (TD), ventromedial caudate dysfunction leads to the obsessions and compulsions of OCD.

STRUCTURAL STUDIES IN OBSESSIVE-COMPULSIVE DISORDER AND RELATED DISORDERS

Early Studies

Early structural imaging studies, employing CT or MRI with more limited acquisition or segmentation methods, have yielded mixed results. Insel et al[22] used CT to study 10 patients with OCD and an equal number of healthy controls, and found no structural differences. Behar, et al[23] used CT to study 17 patients with OCD and 16 healthy controls, and found increased ventricular-to-brain volumetric ratios in OCD. Behar and colleagues' findings are consistent with reduced caudate volume (because the caudate defines one of the medial boundaries of the ventricle). Yet, interpretations of this study are complicated by both the indirect nature of the measurement and the fact that many of the OCD subjects suffered from comorbid depression. Luxenberg, et al[24] used CT to study 10 male OCD patients and an equal number of male controls, and found reduced caudate volume in OCD. Kellner, et al[25] used MRI to study 12 OCD patients and an equal number of matched controls and found no difference in caudate cross-sectional area. Taken together, these initial studies suggested that there might be some subtle caudate structural abnormality associated with OCD. If present, however, the methods of the era were insufficient to detect the abnormality reliably.

Contemporary Morphometric Magnetic Resonance Imaging Studies of Obsessive-Compulsive Disorder

More recently, four independent mMRI studies of OCD have been conducted using contemporary image acquisition and segmentation methods (Table 15-2).[26–29] Three of these four investigations found volumetric abnormalities involving the caudate nucleus. Nonetheless, perhaps owing to methodologic differences, the nature of the caudate abnormalities described differed among the three positive studies (Table 15-3).[26–28]

Scarone, et al[29] used mMRI to study a mixed-gender cohort of 20 patients with OCD versus 16 matched controls and found increased right caudate volume in the OCD group. Robinson, et al[28] studied a mixed-gender cohort of 26 patients with OCD versus 26 matched controls and found bilaterally decreased caudate volumes in the OCD group. Jenike, et al[27] studied an all-female cohort of 10 patients with OCD versus matched controls and found a rightward shift in caudate volume (p = 0.06), as well as a trend toward overall reduced caudate volume (p = 0.10) in the OCD group. Aylward, et al[26] studied a mixed-gender cohort of 24 patients with OCD versus 21 matched controls and found no differences in striatal volumes. The likelihood that three of four studies would yield type I error with regard to caudate volumetric differences seems low; therefore, these findings also argue for a subtle structural abnormality of the caudate nucleus in at least some OCD patients.

Table 15-2 Striatal Findings in Structural Neuroimaging Studies of Obsessive-Compulsive Disorder and Related Disorders

Early Studies of OCD[22–25]	Modality	Findings
Insel, et al (1983)	CT	No difference in caudate volume
Behar, et al (1984)	CT	Increased ventricle:brain ratio
Luxenberg, et al (1988)	CT	Decreased caudate volume
Kellner, et al (1991)	MRI	No difference in striatal areas

Contemporary Studies of OCD[26–29]	Modality	Findings
Scarone, et al (1992)	MRI	Increased right caudate volume
Robinson, ct al (1995)	MRI	Decreased caudate volume
Jenike, et al (1996)	MRI	Rightward shift in caudate asymmetry
Aylward, et al (1996)	MRI	No difference in caudate volume

Contemporary Studies of Related Disorders[35–38]	Study Groups	Modality	Findings
Peterson, et al (1993)	TD vs controls	MRI	Rightward shift in lenticulate volume
Singer, et al (1993)	TD vs controls	MRI	Rightward shift in lenticulate volume
Hyde, et al (1995)	TD twin pairs	MRI	Decreased caudate volume
O'Sullivan, et al (1997)	TTM vs controls	MRI	Rightward shift in putamen volume

CT, computed axial tomography; MRI, magnetic resonance imaging; OCD, obsessive-compulsive disorder; TD, Tourctte's disorder; TTM, trichotillomania.

Several methodologic differences among the studies may explain the disparity in findings. First, there are several obvious differences in study populations and possible differences that are not as readily apparent. Gender compositions differed among the studies both in terms of the male-to-female ratios and with respect to the closeness of gender matching between comparison groups within each study. This factor is critical, because morphometric characteristics of the basal ganglia show significant gender dimorphism.[30,31] Medication status at the time of scanning might explain the disparate findings by Scarone, et al,[29] although the brain volumetric effects of ongoing therapy with serotonin reuptake inhibitors (SRIs) are not known. However, documented reversible effects of neuroleptics on striatal volume[32,33] underscore the relevance of medication status at the time of imaging, but also raise questions as to possible effects of past treatments, which were incompletely characterized for this collection of studies. Finally, other potentially important factors related to the heterogeneity of OCD might have systematically differed among

Table 15-3 Comparison among Contemporary Morphometric Magnetic Resonance Imaging Studies of Obsessive-Compulsive Disorder (OCD)

Study	Scarone, et al[29]	Robinson, et al[28]	Jenike, et al[27]	Aylward, et al[26]
Total N (OCD:Normal controls)	20:16	26:26	10:10	24:21
Gender mix (OCD:Normal controls)				
Males	8:10	14:16	0:0	17:14
Females	12:6	12:10	10:10	7:7
Age at study (mean±SD)				
OCD	32.5 ± 10.1	32.2 ± 8.3	31.6 ± 8.7	34.4 ± 9.8
Normal controls	31.1 ± 6.5	29.8 ± 6.3	28.5 ± 11.4	31.1 ± 10.4
OCD Y-BOCS (mean±SD)	24.3 ± 6.7	22.3 ± 6.4	17.6 ± 5.6	25.8 ± 5.0
Medication status (N)	SRI (20)	None	SRI (1)	None
Slice thickness	5 mm	3 mm	3 mm	5 mm
Slice orientation	Axial	Coronal	Coronal	Axial
Segmentation techniques	Manual	Semiautomated	Semiautomated	Semiautomated
Caudate segmentation				
Number of slices	3	13	21	N/A
Subterritories included	Head	Head + part of body	Total caudate + accumbens	Head
Findings:				
Caudate volume in OCD	Right increase	Bilateral decrease	Rightward shift	No difference

Y-BOCS, Yale-Brown Obsessive-Compulsive Scale; SRI, serotonin reuptake inhibitor; N/A, not available.

these study populations; for instance, probands' psychiatric comorbidities, OCD symptom types, duration of illness, and family histories (e.g., regarding tic disorders and/or OCD) were incompletely characterized across these studies.

Secondly, and probably more importantly, there were substantial differences in the image acquisition and segmentation schemes employed across the four studies. Technically, the semiautomated tools for segmentation used in the three more recent reports are likely superior, as is the practice of acquiring thinner slices and segmenting the striatum in the coronal plane. Much more striking, however, is the gross disparity in the actual territories studied under the rubric of "caudate." Here, it is critical to appreciate that no universally accepted procedures have been established for defining the subterritories of the caudate (i.e., head vs. body vs. tail) or for demarcating the boundary between caudate nucleus and nucleus accumbens in a valid and reliable manner.

Although each of these studies awaits true replication, there seems to be some convergence that suggests a volumetric abnormality of the caudate nucleus in OCD. Moreover, Jenike, et al[27] provide data that are consistent with an overall reduction in caudate volume as observed by Robinson, et al,[28] as well as a rightward shift in caudate volume as suggested by Scarone, et al[29] in OCD, which are analogous to replicated findings in related disorders.

Further, beyond the striatum, it should be noted that white matter reductions in OCD were reported in a preliminary retrocallosal analysis.[34] This finding was subsequently replicated and extended to include multiple white matter territories.[27] These results are in keeping with the notion that, in some cases, OCD is fundamentally a disorder of brain development and decreased white matter volume may be closely related to abnormal caudate morphology.

Related Disorders

Several analogous mMRI studies have now been performed in Tourette's disorder (TD) and one preliminary study in trichotillomania (TTM) (Table 15-2); both TD and TTM are believed to be related to OCD (see Chapters 7 through 9, 12, and 14). In accordance with the striatal topography model of OCDs, the studies of TD and TTM also show volumetric abnormalities involving the striatum. In particular, two studies comparing patients with TD to normal controls have shown a rightward shift in lenticulate (which is the name of a region inclusive of putamen plus globus pallidus) or putamen volume.[35,36] In fact, it was this replicated result that prompted Jenike, et al[27] to specifically look for caudate laterality differences in OCD. Likewise, the phenomenologic similarity between TTM and TD inspired O'Sullivan and colleagues[37] to test these same *a priori* hypotheses; their study of 10 women with TTM versus an equal number of matched controls yielded identical results of rightward shift in putamen volumetric asymmetry. Hyde and colleagues[38] have taken a different approach, using mMRI to study volumetric differences between 10 monozygotic twin pairs concordant for TD but discordant for TD severity. Complementing the previously reported results, Hyde, et al[38] found that the twins with more severe TD had smaller caudate volumes. This suggests that, in the case of TD, more severe disease does not reflect a greater volumetric difference in the putamen, but instead a greater breadth of pan-striatal involvement. In fact, although this twin study focused on tic severity, no data are reported that speak to the relative severity of obsessive-compulsive symptoms or attentional deficits which are hypothesized to be more directly mediated via the caudate. It is most parsimonious to hypothesize that those twins with the most severe TD had not only the most severe tics, but also the most severe disease overall (i.e., including prominent obsessive-compulsive or perhaps attentional manifestations). Of course, this is an empirical question that awaits an answer.

Taken together, mMRI findings in OCD and related disorders provide strong preliminary support for the striatal topography model. Striatal abnormalities have been detected in the preponderance of studies, and caudate involvement is primarily implicated in OCD, whereas putamen involvement is implicated in TD and TTM. Morphologic studies, however, do not provide direct information regarding the functional consequences of these apparent differences. Therefore, these mMRI data are best understood in conjunction with functional imaging data. Conversely, this information regarding apparent structural abnormalities should guide and must be incorporated into any models of pathophysiology and etiology.

FUNCTIONAL STUDIES IN OBSESSIVE-COMPULSIVE DISORDER AND RELATED DISORDERS

Neutral-State Paradigms

Neutral-state studies in OCD are summarized in Table 15-4. Although reviewed comprehensively elsewhere,[13,39] we have chosen to deemphasize some early investigations, because study populations confounded by comorbidities,[40] ongoing medication use,[41] or problematic methods[42] yield data that are difficult to interpret.

To date, all neutral-state studies of OCD have employed ROI–based methods. Three PET studies employed a nominal resting state. Baxter, et al[43] used PET-FDG to study 10 patients with OCD versus 10 matched controls and found relative hypermetabolism in orbitofrontal cortex bilaterally. Swedo, et al[44] used PET-FDG to study 18 patients with childhood-onset OCD versus an equal number of matched controls, and found relative hypermetabolism in left anterior cingulate and right prefrontal cortex. Of note, they also found numerous regions of absolute hypermetabolism, including left orbitofrontal, bilateral anterior cingulate, and bilateral prefrontal cortex. Perani, et al[45] used PET-FDG to study 11 patients with OCD versus 15 healthy controls, and found relative hypermetabolism in cingulate cortex, lenticulate, and thalamus. Two PET studies employed a continuous performance task condition in an effort to better control the neutral state. Nordahl, et al[46] used PET-FDG to study eight patients

Table 15-4   PET-FDG and SPECT-HMPAO Studies in Obsessive-Compulsive Disorder Versus Normal Control Subjects: Neutral-State Paradigms

Study[43–49]	Modality	Findings: Indices of Brain Activity
Baxter, et al (1988)	PET-FDG	Increased in orbitofrontal cortex
Swedo, et al (1989)	PET-FDG	Increased in anterior cingulate cortex
Nordahl, et al (1989)	PET-FDG	Increased in orbitofrontal cortex
Benkelfat, et al (1990)	PET-FDG	Increased in frontal cortex, caudate and putamen
Perani, et al (1995)	PET-FDG	Increased in cingulate cortex, lenticulate, and thalamus
Machlin, et al (1991)	SPECT-HMPAO	Increased in medial frontal cortex
Rubin, et al (1992)	SPECT-HMPAO	Increased in orbitofrontal cortex; decreased in caudate

with OCD versus 30 controls, and found relative hypermetabolism in bilateral anterior orbitofrontal cortex and in right lateral and medial orbitofrontal cortex. Other areas of relative hypermetabolism were noted in bilateral parietal cortex. Benkelfat, et al[47] used PET-FDG to study eight patients with OCD versus 30 controls in the context of a continuous performance task condition, and found relative hypermetabolism in inferomedial, right anterior, and right posterior frontal cortex, as well as caudate and putamen. Two SPECT studies employed a nominal resting state. Machlin, et al[48] used SPECT-HMPAO to study 10 patients with OCD versus eight controls, and found relative hyperactivity in medial frontal cortex. Rubin, et al[49] used SPECT-HMPAO to study 10 patients with OCD versus an equal number of controls, and found relative hyperactivity in bilateral orbitofrontal cortex, left posterior frontal cortex, and bilateral parietal cortex, as well as relative hypoactivity in bilateral caudate.

Taken together, these neutral-state studies of OCD most consistently implicate hyperactivity in prefrontal cortex. The combination of ROI–based methods with ROIs that are inclusive of multiple functional areas (particularly in SPECT) and are not standardized between laboratories makes it difficult to specify which frontal subterritories are involved. Nonetheless, to the degree that such interpretations are possible, orbitofrontal cortical hyperactivity appears most prominent across studies. Striatal and cingulate involvement has been found inconsistently. This implies that either cingulate and striatal dysfunctions are not reliably present or that these techniques, in the context of a neutral state, are insufficiently sensitive to demonstrate them. The poorly controlled nature of the neutral state (and especially the nominal resting state), together with the intrinsic lesser power of between-subject analyses, may well underlie variable or negative results. Further, neutral-state paradigms do not allow us to distinguish between state and trait abnormalities. Thus, for state-dependent phenomena, such as brain activity associated with specific obsessive-compulsive symptoms, one should expect great intersubject variability that would mitigate against consistent findings from neutral-state studies. Finally, in the case of the striatum, the convolution of volume and activity, where subtle volume reductions in small structures cause underestimates and greater variability in activity values, probably serves to further obscure functional abnormalities in that region. Thus, more powerful approaches described in the subsequent sections help to elaborate on these initial findings.

Neutral-state studies in related disorders have thus far been few in number: one such study in TD[50] used PET-FDG and a resting state to study 18 patients versus 16 matched controls. They found relative *hypo*metabolism in orbitofrontal, striatal, and paralimbic territories, and relative *hyper*metabolism in sensorimotor cortex associated with TD. In addition, a secondary analysis was employed in which interregion correlations in activity were emphasized. The investigators found an abnormal (inverse) correlation between activity in the sensorimotor cortex and striatum associated with TD. George, et al[51] used SPECT-HMPAO and a resting state to study 10 patients with TD plus OCD versus 10 patients with TD alone versus 10 controls. They found relative hyperactivity in the right frontal cortex for the TD versus control group and no other differences. The only neutral-state study in TTM to date[52] used PET-FDG and a resting state to study 10 patients versus an equal number of matched controls. In an exploratory manner, comparing numerous ROIs without correction for multiple comparisons, they found relative hypermetabolism in the right parietal cortex and bilateral cerebellum.

These initial neutral-state imaging data from disorders purportedly related to OCD do not yet yield a cohesive picture regarding pathophysiology. Only the results of Stoetter, et al,[50] which suggest an abnormal interaction between sensorimotor cortex and the striatum in TD, can be viewed as supportive of the striatal topography model.

Pre/Posttreatment Paradigms

Pre/posttreatment studies of OCD are summarized in Table 15-5. One SPECT study and four PET studies assessed the effects of medication treatment in the context of resting-state paradigms. Hoehn-Saric, et al[53] used SPECT-HMPAO to study six patients with OCD before and after 12 weeks or more of fluoxetine therapy and found decreased activity in medial frontal cortex. Benkelfat, et al[47] used PET-FDG to study eight patients with OCD before and after 16 weeks of clomipramine therapy and found decreased activity in left caudate nucleus and right orbitofrontal cortex. Treatment response was correlated with reduced activity in left caudate; a similar but nonsignificant trend was found for the right caudate. Swedo, et al[54] used PET-FDG to study 13 patients with childhood-onset OCD before and after 1 year of clomipramine or fluoxetine therapy. They found decreased activity in the bilateral orbito-

Table 15-5   PET-FDG and SPECT-HMPAO Studies in Obsessive-Compulsive Disorder: Pretreatment and Posttreatment Paradigms

Study[12,45,47,53–55]	Modality	Sites of Reduced Activity with Treatment	Type of Treatment
Benkelfat, et al (1990)	PET-FDG	Orbitofrontal cortex and caudate	Medication
Hoehn-Saric, et al (1991)	SPECT-HMPAO	Medial frontal cortex	Medication
Baxter, et al (1992)	PET-FDG	Caudate	Medication or behavior therapy
Swedo, et al (1992)	PET-FDG	Orbitofrontal cortex	Medication
Perani, et al (1995)	PET-FDG	Cingulate cortex	Medication
Schwartz, et al (1996)	PET-FDG	Caudate	Behavior therapy

frontal cortex; treatment response was correlated with activity in the right frontal cortex. Perani, et al[45] used PET-FDG to study nine patients with OCD before and after 3 months of medication therapy (various SRIs) and found decreased activity in cingulate cortex. Baxter, et al[12] used PET-FDG to study nine patients with OCD before and after 10 weeks of fluoxetine therapy, as well as nine different patients with OCD before and after 10 weeks of behavior therapy. They found decreased right caudate activity in both groups (Figure 15-1, see insert); additional areas showing decreases for the medication group were right cingulate cortex and left thalamus. Only activity at the right caudate locus correlated with treatment response. Moreover, a secondary analysis pooling patients from both treatment groups revealed that abnormally high inter-region correlations between orbitofrontal cortex and right caudate in OCD were decoupled with effective treatment. The UCLA group has gone on to replicate these caudate findings in a second study of behavior therapy in OCD.[55] A subsequent study suggests that the "linkage" between orbitofrontal cortex and caudate may be an important prognostic indicator in OCD; robust treatment responders showed significant positive correlations between orbito-frontal and caudate activity pretreatment that disappeared posttreatment (for both medication and behavior therapy treatment) and was nonsignificant at the pretreatment time point in a group of nonresponders.[13]

To our knowledge, no such pre/posttreatment studies of obsessive-compulsive–related disorders have been performed.

Although replication across laboratories has been imperfect, the pre/post-treatment findings in OCD are more consistent than those from between-group, neutral-state paradigms. A picture begins to emerge whereby orbitofrontal cortex, caudate nucleus, or cingulate cortex show reduced activity with effective treatment, regardless of the treatment modality. It is tempting to interpret these results in terms of a common mechanism of action for these various treatments. However, an alternative, and perhaps more prudent, explanation suggests that these brain differences may be state-dependent, reflecting the profile of the OCD symptomatic brain versus that of the relatively symptom-free brain. Thus, regardless of the circumstances that bring about symptom reduction, one might expect to see attenuation of hyperactivity in these brain systems. In this context, the greater reliability seen among pre/posttreatment studies may be understood as a direct consequence of accentuating the contrast between severity of symptoms while using a within-subject design that minimizes other sources of variability. Symptom provocation studies were designed to test this hypothesis more directly, by using the converse approach of inducing (thereby momentarily exacerbating) symptom severity in the context of a within-subject design.

Symptom Provocation Paradigms

The first symptom provocation study of OCD used the xenon-inhalation technique, which did not allow visualization of the very structures subsequently implicated in the mediating anatomy of OCD.[56] Nonetheless, this work by Zohar and colleagues[56] was a landmark contribution that spurred subsequent studies employing this same paradigmatic approach. Zohar, et al[56] studied 10 patients with OCD during relaxation versus imaginal flooding versus *in vivo* exposure. They found increased CBF in temporal cortex during flooding; *in vivo* exposure was associated with widespread decreases in cortical CBF. In retrospect, these widespread decreases in dorsal and superficial territories may have been an indication of CBF shunting to more ventral or deeper structures, including orbitofrontal cortex, anterior cingulate cortex, and the basal ganglia.

Positron emission tomographic and fMRI symptom provocation studies of OCD, as well as selected analogous studies of other anxiety states, are summarized in Table 15-6. These symptom provocation studies used statistical mapping techniques. Rauch, et al[57] used PET-CBF methods to study eight patients with OCD during exposures to provocative or control stimuli (e.g., patients with contamination obsessions were touched with a "contaminated" versus a "clean" version of the same object). During the symptomatic versus the control state, statistically significant increases in activity were found in the left anterior and right posterior orbitofrontal cortex, right caudate, and left anterior cingulate cortex; a trend toward significant activation was found in the left thalamus (p = 0.07) (Figure 15-2, see insert). Further, the magnitude of subjective obsessional symptom severity was correlated with the magnitude of activation at the left anterior orbitofrontal locus. McGuire, et al[58] used PET-CBF methods to study four patients with OCD during exposure to a hierarchy of 12 potentially provocative stimuli. This approach allowed the investigators to perform within-subject analyses to determine brain loci for which CBF correlated with symptom severity in individuals as well as across the cohort. Although

Table 15-6   Select PET and fMRI Studies of Obsessive-Compulsive Disorder and Other Anxiety States: Symptom Provocation Paradigms

Study[57-62]	Diagnosis	Modality	Regions Activated During Symptomatic State		
			Caudate	A/LOFC	Paralimbic
Rauch, et al (1994)	OCD	PET	Yes	Yes	Yes
McGuire, et al (1994)	OCD	PET	Yes	Yes	Yes
Breiter, et al (1996)	OCD	fMRI	Yes	Yes	Yes
Rauch, et al (1995)	Simple phobia	PET	No	No	Yes
Rauch, et al (1996)	PTSD	PET	No	No	Yes
Benkelfat, et al (1995)	Normal	PET	No	No	Yes

fMRI, functional magnetic resonance imaging; A/LOFC, anterior or lateral orbitofrontal cortex; PET, positron emission tomography; PTSD, posttraumatic stress disorder

some intersubject variability was evident, areas of significant positive correlation for the group included right inferior frontal cortex (lateral orbitofrontal cortex), left cingulate, right striatum, right thalamus, left hippocampus, and secondary visual cortex. The Massachusetts General Hospital (MGH) group sought to replicate and extend their own PET findings[57] using new fMRI techniques.[59] Studying 10 patients with OCD and a comparison group of healthy controls, they sought to detect sites of significant activation associated with exposure to provocative versus control stimuli. Healthy control subjects underwent an identical paradigm to determine whether or not similar activation patterns would be produced as a consequence of differential stimulus exposure in the absence of bonafide OCD symptoms. Toward that end, more provocative stimuli were used in this study, such that healthy controls experienced mild levels of disgust. Breiter and colleagues[59] replicated findings in OCD of orbitofrontal activation (greatest in left anterior and right posterior quadrants), caudate activation (most pronounced on the right), and anterior cingulate activation. Of note, additional areas of significant activation were present in the multiple frontal cortical territories and in the lenticulate, paralimbic cortices, and amygdala. No significant activations were found in healthy controls.

One important confound in symptom provocation studies of OCD is the induction of anxiety as a nonspecific element of the symptomatic state. Therefore, additional studies were necessary to tease out which of the brain activations seen in OCD might be specific to that disorder versus elements of some system that might mediate anxiety or arousal nonspecifically (Table 15-6). The group at MGH has performed a series of symptom provocation studies involving other anxiety disorders, including patients with simple phobia of small animals and patients with posttraumatic stress disorder.[60,61] Briefly, in both of these studies, analysis of the provoked versus control state yielded activation patterns that comprised paralimbic territories, including the posterior orbitofrontal cortex and anterior cingulate cortex; however, in neither case was anterior/lateral orbitofrontal cortex nor caudate activation observed. Similarly, Benkelfat, et al[62] studied an anxiety state induced by injection of cholecystokinin tetrapeptide in healthy control subjects and found activation in paralimbic territories but not in the anterior orbitofrontal cortex nor caudate nucleus.

Taken together, the data from symptom provocation studies in OCD and other anxiety states suggest that the symptomatic state in OCD is mediated by one system involving the anterior/lateral orbitofrontal cortex and caudate nucleus, as well as another system involving structures of the paralimbic belt. The former circuit, composed of the anterior/lateral orbitofrontal cortex and caudate, we call the *ventral cognitive corticostriatal system*; the latter paralimbic system now is implicated across a variety of anxiety states and presumably mediates anxiety—or perhaps more broadly, adverse emotion or arousal—nonspecifically.

Although no symptom provocation studies have yet been published regarding obsessive-compulsive–related disorders, two ongoing projects should be mentioned. First, Stern, et al[63] have used innovative PET techniques to "capture" the mediating anatomy of transient tic phenomena in TD. Preliminary data from these investigators suggest that sensorimotor cortices, putamen and thalamus, as well as paralimbic and language areas, play a role in mediating the tics of TD. Second, the MGH group has completed data acquisition for an fMRI symptom provocation study of TTM, although analysis of those data is currently pending.

Cognitive Activation Paradigms

Convergent data from the previously mentioned imaging studies implicate orbitofrontal cortex and caudate nucleus in the pathophysiology of OCD, sensorimotor cortex and putamen in TD, and paralimbic or limbic structures across various anxiety and/or affective disorders. Therefore, obvious targets for cognitive activation probes include subterritories of striatum, orbitofrontal cortex, anterior cingulate cortex, and perhaps the amygdala (which has been implicated in fear conditioning and the assessment of threat). Based on the findings of striatal structural abnormalities and the striatal topography model of OCDs, the development of a reliable and sensitive probe of striatal function seemed a rational first step. With this goal in mind, the MGH group conducted a series of studies validating neuroimaging paradigms involving a modified version of the serial reaction time (SRT) task.[64] This implicit sequence learning task was selected both because its performance was believed to rely on intact corticostriatal function and because implicit learning represents a kind of unconscious information processing that we and others hypothesized might be dysfunctional in OCD and related disorders. Rauch, et al[65] first validated this probe in normal subjects for use with PET-CBF methods; similar findings in normal subjects have been reported by several research groups,[66,67] documenting the reliability of striatal activation with this type of paradigm. A very similar probe now also has been validated in normal subjects for use with fMRI.[68] The next step was to employ this probe and study patients with OCD and related disorders versus control subjects. In an initial study, nine women with OCD and an equal number of healthy controls, matched for age, gender, and years of education, were studied using the PET-SRT.[69] Behaviorally, patients with OCD showed no decrement in performance on the task; in other words, they were able to process the information and learn effectively. However, whereas healthy controls showed normal striatal activation, patients with OCD failed to display activation in inferior or right-sided striatal territories. Moreover, patients with OCD instead activated medial-temporal regions (bilateral hippocampal/parahippocampal areas) not previously observed in normal subjects on this task. Therefore, this initial PET cognitive activation study of OCD supports the hypothesis that patients with OCD fail to activate the striatum normally when confronted with an automatic information-processing task that typically relies on intact striatal function. Further, and perhaps most intriguingly, these patients with OCD instead activated brain regions, which are typically involved in conscious information processing or affect. These data suggest a new heuristic model of OCD: because of striatal dysfunction, patients with OCD process information via different brain systems, which may confer preferential access to consciousness and affect. Consequently, patients with OCD might suffer intrusions into consciousness of information that healthy individuals are able to "put to rest" automatically and outside the conscious domain.[13,69,70] Analogous studies of OCD and TD now are ongoing, using the fMRI-SRT. Other candidate probes of anterior cingulate, orbitofrontal, and amygdalar function are likewise the subject of ongoing research.[71,72]

Receptor Characterization Studies

To our knowledge, no neuroimaging receptor characterization studies have yet been completed in OCD. Given the efficacy of serotonergic medications in OCD, future studies might seek to target the serotonergic system. Several neuroimaging studies of the dopaminergic system already have been conducted in patients with TD. Malison, et al[73] used SPECT and I-123-β-CIT to measure binding capacity of the dopamine transporter in striatum. They studied five patients with TD and an equal number of matched healthy control subjects, and found a significant increase in binding capacity within the striatum in the TD group. These results suggest dysregulation of presynaptic dopamine function in TD. Most recently, Wolf, et al[74] reported the results of another TD study, in which twin pairs concordant for TD but discordant for TD severity were compared. The investigators used SPECT and I-123-iodobenzamide to measure D2 receptor-binding capacity, and found increases in the caudate nucleus associated with more severe TD. These findings further suggest dysregulation of the striatal dopaminergic system in TD.

FUTURE DIRECTIONS IN NEUROIMAGING RESEARCH

First, it is important to replicate and expand on research findings to date. Morphometric mMRI studies should focus on a clearer delineation of striatal subterritories, with special attention to the distinction between dorsolateral and ventromedial anterior striatum. In addition, investigators will undoubtedly follow-up on leads regarding white matter abnormalities in OCD. Emergent availability of higher field strength MRI devices will provide superior resolution for all MRI–based techniques.

Within the functional imaging domain, studies might emphasize the cognitive activation approach. Validating paradigms to probe the functional integrity of the various corticostriatal systems, as well as key limbic and paralimbic structures, remains a high priority. Although study of OCD, TD, and other related disorders with versions of the SRT represents one rational line of inquiry, a broad battery of other cognitive-behavioral probes is needed.[75] Receptor characterization studies of OCD will likely initially focus on the serotonergic system. Although techniques are already available for assaying 5-HT$_2$ receptor-binding capacity,[76] the development of radioligands specifically targeting additional serotonergic receptor subtypes will be essential to advancement on this front. Despite this focus on serotonin, investigation of other neurotransmitter systems also is indicated; dopaminergic, noradrenergic, and peptidergic receptors may likewise yield important insights. Beyond conventional receptor characterization studies, Morris, et al[77,78] have developed a theoretic basis for performing receptor-based activation studies. In fact, the approach they propose may allow investigators to graphically demonstrate regional endogenous serotonergic or dopaminergic release associated with various repetitive behaviors. MRS also offers many as yet unexploited strategies for exploring the pathophysiology of OCDs. For instance, MRS measurement of N-acetyl aspartate (a neuronal marker) might provide complementary evidence for abnormal cellular integrity within striatum. Further, whereas most imaging studies to date have compared patients with OCD or related disorders to healthy control subjects, future studies should incorporate psychiatric control groups to assess the specificity of all key findings.

Aside from these scientific questions, investigators will no doubt begin to address clinical applications. As our understanding of pathophysiology increases and more refined imaging probes are identified, diagnostic and prognostic tests can be explored.[79] For instance, findings from cognitive activation, receptor characterization, or other studies might provide a neurobiologic basis for OCD subtyping or prediction of treatment response.[13]

NEUROIMAGING IN THE CLINICAL ASSESSMENT OF OBSESSIVE-COMPULSIVE DISORDER

Case series suggest that OCD is not generally associated with gross abnormalities of brain structure detectable by conventional clinical imaging tests.[80] Certainly, there are anecdotal reports in the literature of cases in which the clinical presentation was indistinguishable from OCD, and a structural lesion was found on routine CT or MRI, implicating a general medical etiology.[81–83] Consequently, structural imaging may be indicated in OCD to help rule out an underlying general medical process. Guidelines that have been developed for structural imaging use in psychiatry suggest that, in the clinical setting, patients with OCD–like presentations should receive a structural brain imaging test if: (1) onset of OCD occurs later than 50 years of age, (2) focal neurologic signs are present; (3) there is a history of significant head trauma (especially if it is temporally related to onset of symptoms); or (4) the OCD proves treatment refractory.[3,15] Generally, MRI is the modality of choice; CT is preferred only in cases of acute head trauma (i.e., within 48 hours), or if MRI is contraindicated because of paramagnetic prostheses or intolerance of the confined scanning environment.

At present, there are no compelling data to support indications for functional neuroimaging in the clinical assessment of OCD. Recommendations regarding functional imaging assessments of OCD in the clinical setting are tentative, because no large-scale studies have been performed to determine the sensitivity or specificity of this diagnostic tool. Anecdotally, functional imaging tests in patients with OCD can reveal hyperactivity in orbitofrontal cortex, striatum, or anterior cingulate cortex; thus, they may provide helpful adjunctive information, although the cost effectiveness of these tests remains unproven.

SUMMARY

Although neuroimaging has a limited role in the diagnostic assessment of OCD, neuroimaging research has been critical to the evolution of neurobiologic models of OCD and related disorders. Neuroimaging data provide the strongest evidence in support of the "striatal topography model." Structural neuroimaging studies of OCD have indicated subtle volumetric abnormalities in the caudate nucleus. Functional imaging studies of OCD have shown increased activity in the corticostriatal pathway involving anterior/lateral orbitofrontal cortex and the caudate nucleus, which is accentuated during symptom provocation and attenuated following effective treatment. An abnormal linkage between orbitofrontal and caudate activity may distinguish a subgroup of patients with OCD that is particularly treatment responsive. Preliminary findings from cognitive activation studies suggest that patients with OCD fail to exhibit normal striatal recruitment during performance of an implicit learning task and instead rely on systems typically associated with conscious information processing. Paralimbic elements, such as the anterior cingulate and posterior orbitofrontal cortex, appear to play a nonspecific role in mediating anxiety or arousal. Future research will include analogous studies of other purported obsessive-compulsive spectrum disorders to establish whether or not these conditions share a common pathophysiology. In parallel, new research strategies—including receptor characterization studies, MRS, and various cognitive activation paradigms—will be exploited to advance our understanding of corticostriatal physiology and dysfunction in OCD and related disorders.

ACKNOWLEDGMENTS

Dr. Rauch is supported in part via the National Institute of Mental Health (grant MH01215) and a Young Investigator Award from the National Alliance for Research on Schizophrenia and Depression. Dr. Baxter is supported by grant RO1-MH53565 and The Kathy Ireland Chair for Psychiatry Research.

REFERENCES

1. Andreasen NC, editor: Brain imaging. In Oldham JM, Riba MB, Tasman A, editors: *Review of psychiatry*, Washington, 1993, American Psychiatric Press.
2. Mazziotta JC, Gilman S, editors: *Clinical brain imaging: principles and applications*, Philadelphia, 1992, FA Davis.
3. Rauch SL, Renshaw PF: Clinical neuroimaging in psychiatry, *Harv Rev Psychiatry* 2:297–312, 1995.
4. Roland PE: *Brain activation*, New York, 1993, Wiley-Liss.
5. Toga AW, Mazziotta JC: *Brain mapping: The methods*, San Diego, 1996, Academic Press.
6. Kwong KK, Belliveau JW, Chesler DA, et al: Dynamic magnetic resonance imaging of human brain activity during primary sensory stimulation, *Proc Natl Acad Sci U S A* 89:5675–5679, 1992.
7. Ogawa S, Lee TM, Kay AR, et al: Brain magnetic resonance imaging with contrast dependent on blood oxygenation, *Proc Natl Acad Sci U S A* 87:9868–9872, 1990.
8. Weinberger DR, Berman KF, Zec RF: Physiologic dysfunction of dorsolateral prefrontal cortex in schizophrenia I. Regional cerebral blood flow evidence, *Arch Gen Psychiatry* 43:114–124, 1986.
9. Modell J, Mountz J, Curtis G, et al: Neurophysiologic dysfunction in basal ganglia/limbic striatal and thalamocortical circuits as a pathogenetic mechanism of obsessive-compulsive disorder, *J Neuropsychiatry* 1:27–36, 1989.
10. Rapoport JL, Wise SP: Obsessive-compulsive disorder: is it a basal ganglia dysfunction, *Psychopharmacol Bull* 24:380–384, 1988.
11. Baxter LR, Schwartz JM, Guze BH, et al: Neuroimaging in obsessive-compulsive disorder: seeking the mediating neuroanatomy. In Jenike MA, Baer L, Minichiello WE, editors: *Obsessive compulsive disorder: theory and management*, ed 2, Chicago, 1990, Mosby.

12. Baxter LR Jr, Schwartz JM, Bergman KS, et al: Caudate glucose metabolic rate changes with both drug and behavior therapy for obsessive-compulsive disorder, *Arch Gen Psychiatry* 49:681–689, 1992.
13. Baxter LR, Ackermann RF, Swerdlow NR, et al: Specific brain system mediation of OCD responsive to either medication or behavior therapy. In Goodman WK, Rudorfer MV, Maser JD, editors: *Treatment resistant obsessive-compulsive disorder*, (in press).
14. Insel TR: Toward a neuroanatomy of obsessive-compulsive disorder, *Arch Gen Psychiatry* 49:739–744, 1992.
15. Rauch SL, Bates JF, Grachev ID: Obsessive compulsive disorder. In Peterson BF, editor: *Neuroimaging. Child and Adolescent Psychiatric Clinics of North America*, Philadelphia, 1997, WB Saunders.
16. Rauch SL, Jenike MA: Neural mechanisms of obsessive-compulsive disorder, *Curr Rev Mood Anx Dis* 1:84–94, 1997.
17. Alexander GE, DeLong MR, Strick PL: Parallel organization of functionally segregated circuits linking basal ganglia and cortex, *Ann Rev Neurosci* 9:357–381, 1986.
18. Alexander GE, Crutcher MD, DeLong MR: Basal ganglia-thalamocortical circuits: parallel substrates for motor, oculomotor, "prefrontal" and "limbic" functions, *Prog Brain Res* 85:119–146, 1990.
19. Cummings JL: Frontal-subcortical circuits and human behavior, *Arch Neurol* 50:873–880, 1993.
20. Mesulam M-M: Patterns in behavioral neuroanatomy: association areas, the limbic system, and hemispheric specialization. In Mesulam M-M, editor: *Principles of behavioral neurology*, Philadelphia, 1985, FA Davis.
21. Zald DH, Kim SW: Anatomy and function of the orbital frontal cortex II: function and relevance to obsessive-compulsive disorder, *J Neuropsychiatry* 8:249–261, 1996.
22. Insel TR, Donnely EF, Lalakea ML, et al: Neurological and neuropsychological studies of patients with obsessive-compulsive disorder, *Biol Psychiatry* 18:741–751, 1983.
23. Behar K, Rapoport JL, Berg CJ, et al: Computerized tomography and neuropsychological test measures in adolescents with obsessive-compulsive disorder, *Am J Psychiatry* 141:363–368, 1984.
24. Luxenberg JS, Swedo SE, Flament MF, et al: Neuroanatomical abnormalities in obsessive-compulsive disorder detected with quantitative X-ray computed tomography, *Am J Psychiatry* 145:1089–1093, 1988.
25. Kellner CH, Jolley RR, Holgate RC, et al: Brain MRI in obsessive-compulsive disorder, *Psychiatry Res* 36:45–49, 1991.
26. Aylward EH, Harris GJ, Hoehn-Saric R, et al: Normal caudate nucleus in obsessive-compulsive disorder assessed by quantitative neuroimaging, *Arch Gen Psychiatry* 53:577–584, 1996.
27. Jenike MA, Breiter HC, Baer L, et al: Cerebral structural abnormalities in obsessive-compulsive disorder: a quantitative morphometric magnetic resonance imaging study, *Arch Gen Psychiatry* 53:625–632, 1996.
28. Robinson D, Wu H, Munne RA, et al: Reduced caudate nucleus volume in obsessive-compulsive disorder, *Arch Gen Psychiatry* 52:393–398, 1995.

29. Scarone S, Colombo C, Livian S, et al: Increased right caudate nucleus size in obsessive compulsive disorder: detection with magnetic resonance imaging, *Psychiatry Res Neuroimaging* 45:115–121, 1992.

30. Filipek PA, Kennedy DN, Caviness VS: Neuroimaging in child neuropsychology. In Rapin I, Sagalowitz SJ, Boller F, et al, editors: *Handbook of neuropsychology*, vol 6, *Child neuropsychology*, New York, 1992, Elsevier Science Publishers.

31. Filipek PA, Richelme C, Kennedy DN, et al: The young adult human brain: an MRI-based morphometric analysis, *Cereb Cort* 4:344–360, 1994.

32. Frazier JA, Giedd JN, Kaysen D, et al: Childhood-onset schizophrenia: brain MRI rescan after 2 years of clozapine maintenance treatment, *Am J Psychiatry* 153: 564–566, 1996.

33. Keshavan MS, Bagwell WW, Haas GL, et al: Changes in caudate volume with neuroleptic treatment (letter), *Lancet* 344:1434, 1994.

34. Breiter HCR, Filipek PA, Kennedy DN, et al: Retrocallosal white matter abnormalities in patients with obsessive compulsive disorder, *Arch Gen Psychiatry* 51:663–664, 1994.

35. Peterson B, Riddle MA, Cohen DJ, et al: Reduced basal ganglia volumes in Tourette's syndrome using three-dimensional reconstruction techniques from magnetic resonance images, *Neurology* 43:941–949, 1993.

36. Singer HS, Reiss AL, Brown JE, et al: Volumetric MRI changes in basal ganglia of children with Tourette's syndrome, *Neurology* 43:950–956, 1993.

37. O'Sullivan R, Rauch SL, Breiter HC, et al: Reduced basal ganglia volumes in trichotillomania by morphometric MRI, *Biol Psychiatry* 42:39–45, 1997.

38. Hyde TM, Stacey ME, Coppola R, et al: Cerebral morphometric abnormalities in Tourette's syndrome: a quantitative MRI study of monozygotic twins, *Neurology* 45:1176–1182, 1995.

39. Hoehn-Saric R, Benkelfat C: Structural and functional brain imaging in obsessive compulsive disorder. In Hollander E, Zohar J, Marazziti D, et al, editors: *Current insights in obsessive compulsive disorder*, New York, 1994, John Wiley and Sons.

40. Baxter LR, Phelps ME, Mazziotta JC, et al: Local cerebral glucose metabolic rates in obsessive compulsive disorder: a comparison with rates in unipolar depression and in normal controls, *Arch Gen Psychiatry* 44:211–218, 1987.

41. Martinot JL, Allilaire JF, Mazoyer BM, et al: Obsessive-compulsive disorder: a clinical neuropsychological and positron emission tomography study, *Acta Psychiatr Scand* 82:233–242, 1991.

42. Mindus P, Ericson K, Greitz T, et al: Regional cerebral glucose metabolism in anxiety disorders studied with positron emission tomography before and after psychosurgical interventions, *Act Radiol* 369(suppl):444–448, 1986.

43. Baxter L, Schwartz J, Mazziotta J, et al: Cerebral glucose metabolic rates in nondepressed patients with obsessive-compulsive disorder, *Am J Psychiatry* 145: 1560–1563, 1988.

44. Swedo SE, Shapiro MB, Grady CL, et al: Cerebral glucose metabolism in childhood-onset obsessive-compulsive disorder, *Arch Gen Psychiatry* 46:518–523, 1989.

45. Perani D, Colombo C, Bressi S, et al: FDG PET study in obsessive-compulsive disorder: a clinical metabolic correlation study after treatment, *Br J Psychiatry* 166: 244–250, 1995.

46. Nordahl TE, Benkelfat C, Semple W, et al: Cerebral glucose metabolic rates in obsessive-compulsive disorder, *Neuropsychopharmacology* 2:23–28, 1989.
47. Benkelfat C, Nordahl TE, Semple WE, et al: Local cerebral glucose metabolic rates in obsessive-compulsive disorder: patients treated with clomipramine, *Arch Gen Psychiatry* 47:840–848, 1990.
48. Machlin SR, Harris GJ, Pearlson GD, et al: Elevated medial-frontal cerebral blood flow in obsessive-compulsive patients: a SPECT study, *Am J Psychiatry* 148: 1240–1242, 1991.
49. Rubin RT, Villaneuva-Myer J, Ananth J, et al: Regional xenon-133 cerebral blood flow and cerebral Technetium 99m HMPAO uptake in unmedicated patients with obsessive-compulsive disorder and matched normal control subjects, *Arch Gen Psychiatry* 49:695–702, 1992.
50. Stoetter B, Braun AR, Randolph C, et al: Functional neuroanatomy of Tourette syndrome: limbic-motor interactions studied with PET FDG, *Adv Neurol* 58:213–226, 1992.
51. George MS, Trimble MR, Costa DC, et al: Elevated frontal cerebral blood flow in Gilles de la Tourette syndrome: a 99Tm-HMPAO SPECT study, *Psychiatr Res Neuroimag* 45:143–151, 1992.
52. Swedo SE, Rapoport JL, Leonard IIL, et al: Regional cerebral glucose metabolism of women with trichotillomania, *Arch Gen Psychiatry* 48:828–833, 1991.
53. Hoehn-Saric R, Pearlson GD, Harris GJ, et al: Effects of fluoxetine on regional cerebral blood flow in obsessive-compulsive patients, *Am J Psychiatry* 148:1243–1245, 1991.
54. Swedo SE, Pietrini P, Leonard HL, et al: Cerebral glucose metabolism in childhood-onset obsessive-compulsive disorder: revisualization during pharmacotherapy, *Arch Gen Psychiatry* 49:690–694, 1992.
55. Schwartz JM, Stoessel PW, Baxter LR, et al: Systematic changes in cerebral glucose metabolic rate after successful behavior modification, *Arch Gen Psychiatry* 53:109–113, 1996.
56. Zohar J, Insel T, Berman K, et al: Anxiety and cerebral blood flow during behavioral challenge: dissociation of central from peripheral and subjective measures, *Arch Gen Psychiatry* 46:505–510, 1989.
57. Rauch SL, Jenike MA, Alpert NM, et al: Regional cerebral blood flow measured during symptom provocation in obsessive-compulsive disorder using ^{15}O-labeled CO_2 and positron emission tomography, *Arch Gen Psychiatry* 51:62–70, 1994.
58. McGuire PK, Bench CJ, Frith CD, et al: Functional anatomy of obsessive-compulsive phenomena, *Br J Psychiatry* 164:459–468, 1994.
59. Breiter HC, Rauch SL, Kwong KK, et al: Functional magnetic resonance imaging of symptom provocation in obsessive-compulsive disorder, *Arch Gen Psychiatry* 53:595–606, 1996.
60. Rauch SL, Savage CR, Alpert NM, et al: A positron emission tomographic study of simple phobic symptom provocation, *Arch Gen Psychiatry* 52:20–28, 1995.
61. Rauch SL, van der Kolk BA, Fisler RE, et al: A symptom provocation study of posttraumatic stress disorder using positron emission tomography and script-driven imagery, *Arch Gen Psychiatry* 53:380–387, 1996.
62. Benkelfat C, Bradwejn J, Meyer E, et al: Functional neuroanatomy of CCK4-

induced anxiety in normal healthy volunteers, *Am J Psychiatry* 152:1180–1184, 1995.

63. Stern E, Silbersweig DA, Chee K-Y, et al: A functional neuroanatomy of involuntary action in Tourette's syndrome (abstract). Second International Conference on Functional Mapping of the Human Brain, *Neuroimage* 3(suppl):S600, 1996.
64. Nissen MJ, Bullemer P: Attentional requirements of learning: evidence from performance measures, *Cog Psychol* 19:1–32, 1987.
65. Rauch SL, Savage CR, Brown HD, et al: A PET investigation of implicit and explicit sequence learning, *Hum Brain Map* 3:271–286, 1995.
66. Doyon J, Owen AM, Petrides M, et al: Functional anatomy of visuomotor skill learning in human subjects examined with positron emission tomography, *Eur J Neurosci* 8:637–648, 1996.
67. Grafton ST, Hazeltine E, Ivry R: Functional mapping of sequence learning in normal humans, *J Cog Neurosci* 7:497–510, 1995.
68. Rauch SL, Whalen PJ, Savage CR, et al: Striatal recruitment during an implicit sequence learning task as measured by functional magnetic resonance imaging, *Hum Brain Map* 5:124–132, 1997.
69. Rauch SL, Savage CR, Alpert NM, et al: Probing striatal function in obsessive compulsive disorder: A PET study of implicit sequence learning, *J Neuropsychiatry* 9:568–573, 1997.
70. Rauch SL, Savage CR: Investigating cortico-striatal pathophysiology in obsessive compulsive disorders: procedural learning and imaging probes. In Goodman WK, Rudorfer MV, Maser JD, editors: *Treatment resistant obsessive-compulsive disorder,* (in press).
71. Whalen PJ, Bush G, McNally R, et al: The Digital Emotional Stroop activates anterior cingulate cortex: An fMRI study ([abstract]). Third International Conference on Functional Mapping of the Human Brain, (in press).
72. Whalen PJ, Rauch SL, Etcoff NL, et al: Masked presentation of emotional facial expressions modulate amygdala activity without explicit knowledge, *J Neurosci* 18(1):411–418, 1998.
73. Malison RT, McDougle CJ, van Dyck CH, et al: I-123-β-CIT SPECT imaging of striatal dopamine transporter binding in Tourette's disorder, *Am J Psychiatry* 152:1359–1361, 1995.
74. Wolf SS, Jones DW, Knable MB, et al: Tourette syndrome: prediction of phenotypic variation in monozygotic twins by caudate nucleus D2 receptor binding, *Science* 273:1225–1227, 1996.
75. Breiter HC, Rauch SL: Functional MRI and the study of OCD: from symptom provocation to cognitive-behavioral probes of cortico-striatal systems and the amygdala, *Neuroimage* 4:S127–S128, 1996.
76. Fischman AJ, Bonab AA, Babich JW, et al: Positron emission tomographic analysis of central $5HT_2$ receptor occupancy in normal humans treated with the atypical neuroleptic ziprasidone, *J Pharmacol Exp Ther* 279:939–947, 1996.
77. Morris ED, Fisher RE, Alpert NM, et al: In vivo imaging of neuromodulation using positron emission tomography: optimal ligand characteristics and task length for detection of activation, *Hum Brain Map* 3:35–55, 1995.
78. Morris ED, Fisher RE, Rauch SL, et al: PET imaging of neuromodulation: designing experiments to detect endogeneous transmitter release. In Myers R, Cunningham

V, Bailey D, Jones T, editors: *Quantification of brain function using PET,* San Diego, 1996, Academic Press.

79. Rauch SL: Advances in neuroimaging research: how might they influence our diagnostic classification scheme? *Harv Rev Psychiatry* 4:159–162, 1996.
80. Garber HJ, Ananth JV, Chiu LC, et al: Nuclear magnetic resonance study of obsessive-compulsive disorder, *Am J Psychiatry* 146:1001–1005, 1989.
81. Rauch SL, Jenike MA: Neurobiological models of obsessive-compulsive disorder, *Psychosomatics* 34:20–32, 1993.
82. Weilburg JB, Mesulam MM, Weintraub S, et al: Focal striatal abnormalities in a patient with obsessive-compulsive disorder, *Arch Neurol* 46:233–235, 1989.
83. Williams AC, Owen C, Heath DA: A compulsive movement disorder with cavitation of caudate nucleus, *J Neurol Neurosurg Psychiatry* 51:447–448, 1988.

16

Veterinary Models of Obsessive-Compulsive Disorder

Nicholas H. Dodman, B.V.M.S., M.R.C.V.S., D.A.C.V.B.

People believe it must be difficult for veterinarians to diagnose and treat medical problems when their patients cannot tell them how they feel. On the contrary, I believe that, in some situations, the lack of communication can be a great advantage. To illustrate this point, when 250 human patients were asked about obsessions that included fear of some disastrous consequence, 13% were certain that their feared consequence would *not* occur, 27% were mostly certain, 30% were uncertain, 25% were mostly certain that the consequence *would* occur, and 4% were completely certain that it would occur.[1] Veterinarians do not have to contend with such subjective matters, relying exclusively on objective *signs* to reach their conclusions. Because of this, it has been easy for us to embrace the concept of obsessive-compulsive disorder (OCD) in animals, as many of the repetitive behavior conditions we see look like obsessive-compulsive spectrum disorders, fit the *Diagnostic and Statistical Manual of Mental Disorders* (DSM) definition of a compulsive behavior, and respond to the same types of drugs used to treat human OCD. Some of these conditions also have construct validity as biologically equivalent conditions.

In a recent review of animal models of OCD, Insel, et al[2] posed "the fundamental question" of whether OCD is a disorder of aberrant thoughts or a primary disturbance of primitive motor circuits. In other words, is OCD a uniquely human disorder, stemming from spontaneous worry, doubt, or guilt? Or, is it a consequence of inappropriate, repetitive activation of phylogenetically ancient neural pathways? The former anthropocentric interpretation makes it difficult to explain why compulsions sometimes occur without accompanying obsessions. On the other hand, obsessions without compulsions are not easy to account for by motor circuit dysregulation theories. The acceptance of striatum-dependent emotional and cognitive processes goes some way toward addressing this latter concern.[3,4] One explanation that would address both aspects of

318

the fundamental question is that obsessions and compulsions may be different manifestations of the same underlying neurophysiologic dysregulation. Such dysregulation could result from impairment of the gating and screening functions of the ventral striatum[5,6] or might be related to deficiencies in the intrinsic reward mechanism.[7] Behavioral functions and information processing are discharged jointly by the limbic system and the basal ganglia, with recognition of goals and evaluation of outcomes dealt with by the limbic system.[8] If limbic/basal ganglia dysregulation were fundamental in OCD, activation of the orbitofrontal or prefrontal areas of the cortex would be secondary to the underlying process of OCD rather than driving it (Figure 16-1). It has been suggested that overactivation of orbitofrontal areas may be a result of attempts to suppress adventitious thoughts or behaviors.[4] Alternatively, this activation may be a more direct sequel stemming from the massive input orbitofrontal areas receive from limbic structures.[9]

Some human OCD sufferers with insight into their behavior would be anticipated to have concerns about the appropriateness of their behavior (depending on the behavior), adding a secondary ego dystonic component to the syndrome. Such ego dystonia appears to be an exclusively human sequel to OCD—a consequence of (greater) self-awareness. Although it is unlikely that animals feel guilt or embarrassment over the performance of compulsive behaviors, a discrepancy such as this does not preclude animals exhibiting ritualistic behaviors from serving as useful models of human OCD. Both ego dystonic and ego syntonic compulsive behaviors can furnish the common endpoint of releasing inner tension.

If OCD and obsessive-compulsive spectrum disorders involve dysregulation of primitive drives *and* emotions, a new "fundamental" question becomes: What is the cause of this dysregulation? Is it an anomaly in the 5-HT$_2$ gene or an environmentally induced change resulting in activation of the Papez circuit or the striatum? Is it a genetic or acquired trait or some combination of both? Valid animal models would help provide answers to these questions.

In the discussion that follows, I will assume that the neuroethologic/dysfunctional gating theory of OCD explains what we see in animals, and will allow the reader to decide how well the observed facts fit this paradigm. If the reward deficiency theory were validated, it would simply provide a different explanation for unchecked ("freewheeling") basal ganglia function and would not substantively change the paradigm. As the number of OCD-like conditions and information pertaining to them have burgeoned, it has become increasingly difficult to do justice to them all in one chapter. Accordingly, I will confine my remarks to some of the more interesting veterinary models and will make only passing reference to the already well-documented laboratory models of OCD.[2] Veterinary conditions with OCD-like phenomenology that are not detailed in the text are presented in Table 16-1 and, for completeness, the reader is directed to other recent reviews of the subject.[10–13]

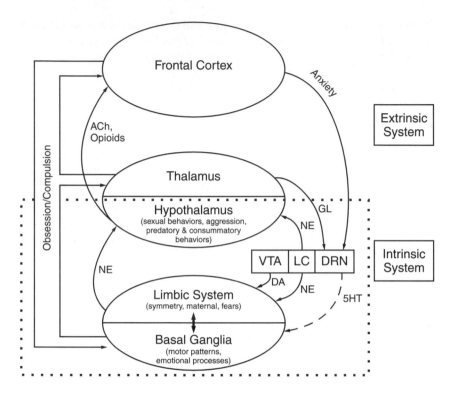

Fig. 16-1   A schematic drawing showing the punitive interaction of various brain regions and neurotransmitters in the propagation of obsessive-compulsive disorder. NE, norepinephrine; DA, dopamine; 5HT, serotonin; ACh, acetylcholine; GL, glutamate.

BACKGROUND

The neuroethologic theory of OCD derives from the concept of the fixed-action pattern. The early ethologists' view was that certain behaviors necessary for survival are encoded in the brain as motor programs to be liberated when necessary by specific environmental cues (i.e., "sign stimuli" or "releasers"). If the stimulus was removed midresponse, the behavioral program would still run to conclusion, being driven by an indivisible motor program unit. Under certain circumstances, it was believed that the motor program might discharge spontaneously, resulting in the release of a fixed-action pattern in the absence of an appropriate releaser (so-called "vacuum activity"). The basal ganglia are the best-known repositories for such "hard-wired" behavior programs (which are in fact, not purely innate, as was previously believed, but modifiable by learning[14]). Imprinting and other types of species- or breed-specific learning are necessary for the establishment of these programs.

Table 16-1 Species-Typical Compulsive Behaviors

Animal	Grooming	Predatory	Locomotor	Consummatory	Sexual	Aggressive	Fear and Avoidance
CANINE	Acral lick dermatitis	Tail chasing; object compulsion; light chasing	Pacing; circling	Air licking; aerophagia; flank sucking	Compulsive mounting	Compulsive aggression	Checking; global fear
FELINE	Paw licking; psychogenic alopecia; lip and nose licking	Tail chasing; hoarding	Circling	Wool sucking	Compulsive masturbation	Compulsive aggression	Excessive marking
EQUINE	Trichotillomania	NA	Weaving; stall walking	Lip flapping/tonguing; cribbing	Flank biting*; masturbation	Flank biting*	NR
AVIAN (psittacine)	Feather pulling	NA	Route tracing	Spot picking	Masturbation; regurgitation	NR	NR
PORCINE	NR	NA	NR	Bar biting; vacuum chewing; chain chewing	NR	Tail biting	NR
BOVINE/ OVINE	Hair licking	NA	Weaving	Tonguing; compulsive sucking	Masturbation	NR	NR
URSINE	NR	NA	Pacing	NR	NR	NR	NR
PRIMATES	Skin picking; hair pulling	NA	Bouncing in place; somersaulting	Self sucking; licking/chewing	Masturbation; rectal probing	Self-directed aggression	NR
HUMAN	Skin/nose picking; trichotillomania	Gambling; hoarding	Whirling; tics; compulsive exercising	Binge eating	Paraphilias	Self-directed aggression; pyromania	Checking; contamination

* Motor tics associated
NA, not applicable; NR, not recognized
(Table reproduced from CNS Spectrums with permission of MBL publications.)

The programming of basic circuits may not be confined to motor programs, because the basal ganglia also participate in cognitive aspects of behavior.[15] Basic emotional affiliations and interpretation of environmental cues may be imbued in the process inscribing the fundamental biologic repertoire. Although the neostriatum (caudate nucleus and putamen) is essential for the gradual, incremental learning of associations that is characteristic of habit learning,[16] limbic structures also appear to be involved in hard-wired learning. For example, the hippocampus plays a role in spatial learning in voles,[14] the anterior cingulate is important in affective valence/intensity, and the amygdaloid complex plays a role in appetitive and fear/emotional reactivity.[17] Imaging studies have indicated that limbic structures, including cingulum, septum, hippocampus, and temporal cortex, are among the prime candidates for dysfunctional sites in OCD.[18]

If the neural circuit theory of OCD is accepted, the feature common to all forms of OCD in man and animals is the inappropriate release of encrypted motor programs or emotional/cognitive programming from the basal ganglia and limbic regions of the brain, perhaps resulting from gating failure or lack of feedback about satisfactory completion of the task or thought process. Motor tics or stereotypies originating from the caudate region would be the most uncomplicated form of this dysregulation. Cognitive sequelae (obsessions), alone or in association with motor (compulsive) events, would represent either a different origin of the impulses or an extension of the same disturbance. From this standpoint, the occurrence of obsessions is immaterial to understanding the fundamental disturbance. Also, according to this interpretation, we would anticipate obsessions and compulsions relating to a spectrum of hard-wired behaviors or emotional states, not just relating to grooming or concerns over personal safety. In animals and people, hunting (predatory), grooming (maintenance), sexual (procreative), and spatial (nest building/symmetry/precision) behaviors should all be involved in the syndrome. Obsessions might represent the dysregulation of mechanisms governing intrinsic emotions, for example, fear (in humans, including concerns over personal safety) and anger. Which behavioral or emotional state is released would depend on the species and breed, as well as individual learning history. In predatory and aggressive breeds of dogs, compulsive behaviors would be expected to reflect these tendencies, as indeed they do. Because horses spend 60% of their time grazing in the wild, oral/ingestive compulsions would be anticipated; once again, this is the case. In birds, where preening is vital for feather maintenance, compulsions related to this activity would be predicted; feather picking is the most common compulsive behavior problem in captive psittacine birds. There are many other examples of species-typical compulsive behaviors, all of which represent survival behaviors gone awry (Table 16-1). Humans, who are historically a hunter/gatherer species and who are required to blend risk taking and gathering with caution to survive, are no exception, developing compulsive behaviors of gambling, hoarding, and personal-safety concerns. With this in mind, I will discuss selected animal models of OCD that may shed further light on the syndrome as a whole, viewed from an ethologic perspective.

CANINE MODELS

Several potential canine models of OCD are listed in Table 16-1. Of these, acral lick dermatitis (ALD), which affects primarily large breeds of dog, and object obsession/tail-chasing syndrome of Bull Terriers have received the most attention.[10-13]

Acral Lick Dermatitis

True ALD is a psychologic disorder of excess grooming in which affected dogs repetitively lick the lower extremities of their limbs. Various medical conditions, particularly allergies, can mimic ALD, and these must be ruled out to confirm the diagnosis.[19] The biologic function of self-grooming is to keep the body surface clear of debris, although self-grooming also appears to serve as a self-comforting behavior. ALD is most common in Labrador Retrievers, Golden Retrievers, German Shepherds, Doberman Pinschers, and Great Danes. Genetic factors predisposing individual dogs to the condition have been suggested,[20] although our attempts to locate relatives of probands have been unsuccessful. Temperamentally, affected dogs often appear anxious and high-strung; we have found 70% comorbidity of ALD with other anxiety-related conditions, such as separation anxiety and noise phobia.[11] (Similar comorbidity has been found in humans with OCD.[21]) In one survey of 15 dogs with ALD from our clinic, the average age of onset was 3.8 years (range, 0.5 to 7.5 years), equivalent to an age of approximately 25 years in humans.

Presumed stressful circumstances, such as boredom and confinement, are often associated with the onset of ALD, which may be gradual or precipitous. One dog with ALD began grooming compulsively the day his master, to whom he was closely bonded, became estranged from the family; the dog stopped the compulsive grooming a few weeks later, corresponding precisely with his master's return to the family. This case suggests that compulsive grooming can begin as a displacement behavior as a result of conflict (perhaps in the form of an unresolvable dilemma) and, at least, in the early stages, is reversible if the stressful circumstances are eliminated. Later in the course of the condition, the behavior seems to become more ingrained and is then unlikely to respond to stress-reducing measures alone. A change in liability of stereotypies over time has been noted in bank voles and pigs, in which responsiveness to pharmacologic intervention differs according to the duration of the condition.[22,23]

Working from first principles, it would be anticipated that ALD would respond to treatment with opioid antagonists, dopamine antagonists, and serotonergic drugs. A schematic illustrating the putative interaction of these neurotransmitters and the brain centers and functions/processes affected is depicted in Figure 16-1. In support of this proposed mechanism, opioid antagonists and selective serotonin reuptake inhibitors (SSRIs) have been found effective in ALD,[20,24,25] although there is currently no published information on the efficacy of dopamine antagonists for treatment of this condition. Imaging and postmortem studies of the brains of affected dogs are needed to clarify the pathophysiology of ALD. From what is known of the neurophysiology of grooming, it seems likely that the basal ganglia, specifically the caudate nucleus, would be affected in some way.[26]

Object Obsession/Tail-Chasing Syndrome

Most dogs pay attention to tennis balls, rope toys, and sticks and occasionally chase moving objects, including their own tails. This behavior probably derives from their innate predatory drive.[27] Because predatory behavior is hard-wired, it would be predicted from the motor circuit theory of OCD that some dogs would express this behavior compulsively (especially breeds selectively bred for enhancement of these predatory tendencies). Terriers and herding or retrieving breeds would be prime candidates for problems of this nature. Terriers, selectively bred for ratting (among other things), do exhibit predatory compulsions at a higher rate than other breeds, including light and shadow chasing (especially Wire-Haired Fox Terriers), compulsive fly biting (when there are no flies present), and tail chasing (particularly Bull Terriers and Bull Terrier crosses).[28] Compulsive chasing of cars, joggers, and tennis balls may be another form of predatory behavior gone awry. (In an ironic switch, one man began to chase cars compulsively as the result of manganese intoxication–induced damage to the globus pallidus![29])

Herding/retrieving breeds show a range of predatory compulsions similar to Bull Terriers but, in addition, these breeds also may herd things compulsively: one Retriever reported to us collected a shoe every 15 minutes when its owner was away and stored the shoes under a bed. If the closet in which the shoes were kept was closed, the dog would destroy the door to get at the shoes. Another dog collected pieces of dry kibble and arranged them on a couch, one piece in each depression on the couch and one beside the couch, as if spatial/symmetry also was a concern; if the dog's kibble arrangement was disturbed, it would immediately replace missing pieces to restore the symmetry.

The breed we have studied most extensively regarding predatory compulsions is the Bull Terrier: these dogs show a number of perseverant behaviors, including compulsive carrying of objects, compulsive tail chasing, fly biting, and iterative ingestion of inedible material. It is not so much *what* they do that is abnormal but rather the extent to which they do it. Some breeds cannot go anywhere without a tennis ball in their mouths, which they chew or chase almost incessantly. The mouthing often causes excessive wear of the teeth, and some dogs even wear their teeth down to the gum line. If the tennis ball is taken away from a predatory compulsive dog, the dog may displace into another compulsion, such as spinning frantically, sometimes for hours, apparently trying to catch or bite its own tail. I believe that object obsession, like tail chasing, is related to predatory drive. One Bull Terrier admitted to Boston's Angell Memorial Animal Hospital spun in circles the entire time it was not eating or sleeping, eventually wearing its rear digital pads to the bone. The only way to describe the behavior of such severely affected dogs is compulsive, and owners themselves often use such terms to describe their dog's behavior.

In one study of compulsive tail chasing in Bull Terriers and related breeds, the mean age of onset was 16 months,[27] corresponding to an age of approximately 10 years in humans. The earlier onset of tail-chasing (between 3 and 12 months of age) in unneutered dogs in this study suggests that hormones influence the development of the behavior. (It is worth noting that the processes that control the development of the basal ganglia are believed to be influenced by sex hormones.[30]) Eight of the 18 dogs in the tail chasing study showed other compulsive behaviors in addition to tail chasing: in four dogs, the ancillary compulsion was object obsession, two of the dogs were fly biters, and two were "flank suckers" (possibly derived from nursing behavior). Tail chasing breeds responded well to treatment with clomipramine, 12 of 18 dogs showing greater than 75% reduction in the behavior as determined by owner rating, although the response of the ancillary compulsive behaviors was more variable.

Tail chasing has been variously described as an opioid-mediated stereotypy,[31] a partial seizure–linked condition,[32] and a compulsive behavior.[27] The similarities between tail-chasing syndrome and human OCD are compelling, but this does not rule out an organic cause of the dysregulation. All six tail-chasing Bull Terriers in one study were found to have abnormal (epileptiform) electroencephalogram (EEG) patterns.[32] There have been several reports of temporal lobe EEG abnormalities coinciding with OCD in humans,[33–36] and EEG abnormalities consistent with frontal epileptic foci have been found in some OCD patients.[37]

FELINE MODELS

There are several potential models of OCD in cats, including psychogenic alopecia, wool sucking/pica, feline hyperesthesia, hoarding, compulsive paw-licking, and compulsive hair playing.[12] Of these conditions, feline psychogenic alopecia is best documented and appears to provide an excellent model of trichotillomania (TTM), having face validity, predictive validity (of response to modification), and construct validity of this obsessive-compulsive spectrum condition.

Feline Psychogenic Alopecia

Cats with feline psychogenic alopecia lick themselves compulsively, stripping hair from their abdomen, flanks, back, and limbs. Some cats groom themselves almost continuously, or for several hours per day; others groom for just a few minutes at a time. The frequency with which bouts occur ranges from daily to once a week.[38] As with ALD, the diagnosis is confirmed by ruling out medical conditions, such as allergy and fungal infections of the skin, that can produce similar signs. Lack of response to systemically administered steroids also is evidence supporting a psychogenic origin for the condition.[39]

Psychogenic alopecia is most common in oriental breeds of cat (Oriental Shorthair, Siamese, Abyssinian), although domestic Shorthair cats also are affected. The age of onset of psychogenic alopecia ranges from 6 months to 12 years (equivalent human age range is approximately 12 to 15 years), with a significantly higher percentage developing the condition for the first time in the first year of life (around or shortly after puberty).[38] Temperament seems to be an important factor in the initiation of the condition, with several authorities indicating that high-strung, timid, or fearful cats are at most risk.[40-42] The onset of the condition is often associated with a stressful event, such as the addition of a new cat to the family or confining a previously indoor/outdoor cat to the house.[38] The predictive value of psychogenic alopecia as a model of TTM is supported by preliminary reports of a positive response to clomipramine,[38] although more comprehensive studies are necessary.

Feline Hyperesthesia

Feline hyperesthesia, so called because affected cats have an apparent hypersensitivity to touch (which can trigger the syndrome), is a pleiomorphic compulsive behavior involving several component behaviors in various combinations. Some cases involve a syndrome of frenetic self-grooming not unlike psychogenic alopecia, but in other cases, mania and aggression are the primary signs, sometimes progressing to frank seizures.[43] Siamese or Siamese-crosses are most often affected.[44] Again, environmental pressures seem to have some bearing on the condition, which tends to occur in cats with already "unstable personalities."[45] It seems likely that there is an organic cause for this compulsive behavior akin to the seizure-related OCD sometimes reported in humans.[46] Opioid antagonists, anticonvulsants, and SSRIs have found a place in the pharmacologic management of this unusual condition.[47-49]

Wool Sucking/Pica

Not much has been written about wool sucking, an oral compulsion in which affected cats mouth/suck their own hair, a neighboring cat's hair, or woolly fabrics. This condition usually arises in juveniles prior to 6 months of age (equivalent human age 12 years) and, in some cats, appears to be related to early weaning.[38] The condition seems to originate as displaced nursing behavior, subsequently evolving into a compulsive behavior. In many cats, the condition transmutes over time into pica, involving the selective ingestion of foreign material, particularly wool-like fabrics and plastic. This switch may represent a preprogrammed ontogenic change in the orientation of feeding behavior. Oriental breeds are more commonly affected, suggesting genetic susceptibility. A genealogy of one family of Burmese cats, some of which exhibited the condition, is illustrated in Figure 16-2. Preliminary reports of open-label clinical trials suggest that the condition responds to treatment with SSRIs.[38]

AVIAN MODELS
Feather Picking

The most promising avian model of OCD is chronic (compulsive) feather-picking. This condition has been compellingly described in the literature as a model of TTM.[12,50] When feather picking is compared with TTM, there are striking similarities in phenomenology, response to pharmacologic agents, and in the basic construct of these two conditions.

Affected birds typically are of anxious breed and temperament and often have comorbid separation anxiety. A genetic predisposition for the development of feather picking is widely acknowledged, but this remains to be conclusively established. The circumstances leading to the development of feather picking (e.g., loneliness, boredom, and captivity itself) are easily interpretable as stressful for the bird. Affected birds often choose newly grown feathers to pluck with their beaks; once they have removed a feather, they will inspect it, sometimes chew and shred it, and finally discard it, before repeating the process. Feather picking, like TTM, responds to some extent, at least transiently, to treatment with dopamine antagonists and SSRIs.[51–55]

EQUINE MODELS

There are a number of conditions, including cribbing, wind sucking, stall walking, and digging, that have been known to horsemen for years as "stall vices." The etiology of these conditions is unclear (other than that they result from confinement), and a multiplicity of "traditional" treatments—some surgical and some mechanical—reflect this dilemma. Even if these conditions were not well known, their existence could be predicted from the neuroethologic (motor circuit) theory of compulsive behaviors: horses in the wild are social animals whose natural life involves much grazing and locomotion. When prevented from these activities by confinement in an unnatural environment, it would be anticipated that they would develop compulsions related to their primary drives of grazing and locomotion.

Cribbing

When horses suffer from cribbing, they repeatedly anchor their upper incisor teeth on a ledge or surface, lean back, tense their large neck muscles, and grunt as they swallow a bolus of air into their pharynx/esophagus. This compulsive behavior is related to the hard-wired behavior of grazing and to ingestive behavior. The suggestion has been made that cribbing is, to some extent, genetically determined.[56] Our observations suggest that cribbing horses

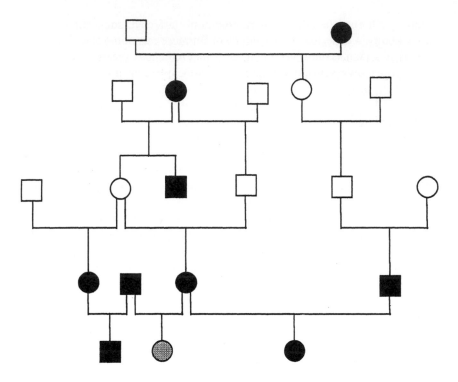

Fig. 16-2   Pedigree showing the inheritance of wool sucking/pica in a family of Burmese cats. *Open circles,* unaffected females; *Closed circles,* affected females; *Open squares,* unaffected males; *Closed squares,* affected males; *Cross-hatched circle,* compulsive paper-shredding female (Courtesy of Dr. A. Moon-Fanelli).

are more active than their noncribbing stable mates and are usually highly strung. Cribbing responds to treatment with opioid antagonists,[57] an observation that would be predicted from the significant role that opioids play in feeding behaviors.[58] Recently, serotonin reuptake blockers have been found effective for the treatment of stall vices[59] (a finding that could be predicted from the neuromodulatory role of serotonin in eating behavior).

Self-Mutilation Syndrome

Self-mutilation syndrome is a compulsive disorder that involves hyperactivity and impulsive self-directed aggressive behavior. This condition, also known as flank biting and self-directed aggression, has many features in common with human Tourette's disorder (TD), including the presence of a gross head or neck motor tic, hemiballismus, bizzare vocalizations, primarily male gender distribution, early onset, temporary suppression by absorbing activities, and an apparent genetic basis.[60] Affected horses are often preoccupied with the periphery of their stalls, and may lick or kick stall walls. Some also seem to have trouble negotiating doorways, hesitating nervously before barrelling through (a feature of some human sufferers of TD, most famously Samuel Johnson). Bearing in mind the good face validity of this condition as a model of TD and the overlapping neurobiology of TD and OCD, equine self-mutilation would appear to be a model deserving further study. Unfortunately, there are logistical problems associated with research on animals the size of horses, so many potentially interesting studies, such as attempting to correlate D2 receptor binding with the severity of symptoms,[61] would be practically out of the question.

Pharmacologically, equine self-mutilation responds to treatment with opioid antagonists, dopamine blockers, and SRIs.[60,62] Castration also may reduce the severity of the condition in stallions,[60] so it appears that androgens play a facilitatory role. There are no direct human analogies to make here, but opioid-gonadotropin interactions have been suggested in TD[63] and antiandrogen therapy of TD has met with limited success in some cases.[64]

PORCINE MODELS

Because one of the primary activities of pigs in the wild is rooting around with their snouts, compulsive behavior related to this activity would be expected in an impoverished environment in which species-typical behaviors are inhibited. Not surprisingly then, compulsive oral behaviors in the form of chain chewing, bar biting, and tail biting are seen in piggeries around the world.

Chain Chewing and Bar Biting

Chain chewing and bar biting are the best documented porcine compulsive behaviors. Approximately 20% of pigs in impoverished environments develop such behavior, suggesting genetic susceptibility to the condition.[65] The easiest way to reduce compulsive chewing and biting is to increase roughage in the diet (probably because it increases the time pigs spend feeding, causing a more natural time budget for feeding behavior and providing an alternative substrate for hard-wired oral behaviors). Houben-Gelissen, et al[65] found that pigs exhibiting oral compulsions responded to fluvoxamine in a manner and time course virtually identical to those shown by humans with OCD who are treated with SSRIs.[6] This compulsive behavior could be the most promising animal model of OCD to date, though research involving animals of this size would be price-preclusive as a pharmaceutical research model.

OTHER MODELS

There are several other veterinary models of OCD, some of which are listed in Table 16-1. Rodent models have been well described elsewhere[2] and are not addressed here. Models such as adjunctive behavior, spontaneous alternation, and delayed-response paradigms (DRL 18s) may contribute significantly toward understanding species-typical responses to conflict.[12]

SUMMARY

Fifteen years ago, OCD was believed to be a rare, narrowly defined condition of humans. By the late 1980s, it had become apparent that OCD was not rare, affecting an estimated 1% to 3% of the human population. At approximately this time, the first suggestions of spontaneous equivalents of OCD were being made, leading to a rekindling of interest in veterinary models.[20,55,66] A neuroethologic approach toward understanding OCD gradually emerged. Animal stereotypies had been known for years prior to this, but because of their pleiotropic and, in some cases, entirely different phenotypic expression, it was not immediately apparent how far the stereotypy–compulsive behavior analogy could be taken.

ALD was first recognized as a veterinary equivalent of OCD by dog owners and veterinarians who, in response to the publicity surrounding Rapoport's popular book, *The Boy Who Couldn't Stop Washing*, noticed the striking similarity between their dogs' and cats' behavior and the subject of the book.[67] Other animal "stereotypies" then began to be described as compulsive behaviors.[68,69] At this time, however, the interpretation of stereotypies as compulsive behaviors was somewhat ambivalent, with the terms *stereotypy* and *compulsive disorder* appearing interchangeably to describe various repetitive behaviors.[68] The different phenotypic expression of animal stereotypies, the infeasibility of confirming an obsessional component, and the different pharmacologic responsiveness of some animal conditions[24,57] threw many off the trail, and it was not until the concept of an obsessive-compulsive spectrum emerged[70] that the integrity of the syndrome across the species finally began to make sense. This unifying theory of OCD has led away from a narrow anthropocentric definition of OCD to a broader biologic explanation for a syndrome of dysregulation of fundamental mental processes at the level of the basal ganglia/limbic system. From this perspective, the different forms of compulsive behavior in animals (including humans) can be viewed as species-typical expressions of survival-oriented behaviors. Although animal models are inappropriate for investigations into uniquely human aspects of OCD research (e.g., ego dystonicity or cognitive therapy), they seem more than adequate for the purpose of understanding OCD from a biologic perspective.

In summary, animal models of OCD offer advantages for study of human OCD because: (1) they are ubiquitous and easily accessible; (2) they provide unique opportunities to study the inheritance and genetics of compulsive behavior; (3) animal generation times are short relative to those of humans; (4) controlled studies in animals are easier to implement; and (5) animal models give biologic insight into the obsessive-compulsive spectrum.

REFERENCES

1. Foa EB, Kozak MJ: DSM-IV field trial: Obsessive-compulsive disorder, *Am J Psychiatry* 152:90–96, 1995.
2. Insel TR, Mos J, Olivier B: Animal models of obsessive compulsive disorder: a review. In Hollander E, Zohar J, Marazziti B, Olivier B, editors: *Current insights in obsessive compulsive disorder*, New York, 1994, John Wiley and Sons.
3. Dubois B, et al: Cognitive and behavioral changes in patients with focal lesions of the basal ganglia. In Weiner WJ, Lang AE, editors: *Behavioral neurology of movement disorders, advances in neurology*, vol 65, New York, 1995, Raven Press.
4. Saint-Cyr JA, Taylor AE, Nicholson K: Behavior and the basal ganglia. In Weiner WJ, Lang AE, editors: *Behavioral neurology of movement disorders, advances in neurology*, vol 65, New York, 1995, Raven Press.
5. Baxter LR, Schwartz JM, Guze BH: Brain imaging: toward a neuroanatomy of OCD. In Zohar J, Insel TR, Rasmussen SA, editors: *The psychobiology of obsessive-compulsive disorder*, New York, 1991, Springer.
6. Baxter LR, et al: Caudate glucose metabolic rate changes with drug and behavior therapy for obsessive-compulsive disorder, *Arch Gen Psychiatry* 49:681–690, 1992.
7. Blum K, et al: Dopamine D2 receptor gene variants: Association and linkage studies in impulsive-addictive-compulsive behavior, *Pharmacogenetics* 5(3):121–142, June 1995.
8. Gray JA: A general model of the limbic system and basal ganglia: applications to schizophrenia and compulsive behavior of the obsessive type, *Revue eurologique* 150(8–9):605–613, 1994.
9. Gross-Isseroff R, et al: Alternation learning in obsessive-compulsive disorder, *Biol Psychiatry* 39:733–738, 1996.
10. Dodman NH, Moon-Fanelli A, Mertens PA: Veterinary models of OCD. In Hollander E, Stein DJ, editors: *Obsessive compulsive disorders*, New York, 1997, Marcel Dekker.
11. Moon-Fanelli A, Dodman NH, O'Sullivan RL: Veterinary models of compulsive self-grooming: parallels with trichotillomania. In Christenson GA, Stein DJ, editors: *Trichotillomania*, American Psychiatric Press, in press.
12. Dodman NH, Olivier B: In search of animal models for obsessive-compulsive disorder, *CNS Spectrums* 1(2):10–15, 1996.
13. Hewson CJ, Luescher UA: Compulsive disorder in dogs. In Voith VL, Borchelt PL, editors: *Readings in companion animal behavior*, Trenton, NJ, 1996, Veterinary Learning Systems.
14. Alcock J: The diversity of behavior. In Alcock J, editor: *Animal behavior: An evolutionary approach*, Sunderland, Mass, 1993, Sinauer Associates.
15. Cote L, Crutcher MD: Motor functions of the basal ganglia and diseases of transmitter metabolism. In Kandel ER, editor: *Principles of neural science*, ed 2, New York, 1985, Elsevier North-Holland.
16. Knowlton BJ, Mangels JA, Squire LR: A neostriatal habit learning system in humans, *Science* 273:1399–1402, 1996.
17. Saint-Cyr JA, Taylor AE, Nicholson K: Behavior and the basal ganglia. In Weiner WJ, Lang AE, editors: *Behavioral neurology of movement disorders, advances in neurology*, New York, 1995, Raven Press.

18. Rauch SL, Jenike MA: Neurobiological models of obsessive-compulsive disorder, *Psychosomatics* 34:20–32, 1993.
19. White S: Naltrexone for treatment of acral lick dermatitis in dogs, *J Am Vet Med Assoc* 196:1073–1076, 1990.
20. Rapoport JL, Ryland DH, Kriete M: Drug treatment of canine acral lick: an animal model of obsessive-compulsive disorder, *Arch Gen Psychiatry* 49:517–521, July 1992.
21. Ramussen SA, Eisen JL: The epidemiology and differential diagnosis of obsessive compulsive disorder, *J Clin Psychiatry* 55(5–10):1–14, 1994.
22. Kennes D, et al: Changes in naloxone and haloperidol effects during the development of captivity-induced jumping stereotypy in bank voles, *Eur J Pharmacol* 153:19–24, 1988.
23. Cronin GM, Wiepkema PR, VanRee JM: Evidence for a relationship between endorphins and the performance of abnormal stereotyped behaviors in tethered sows. In Cronin GM, editor: *The development and significance of stereotyped behaviors in tethered sows*, PhD Thesis, 1985, Wageringen Netherlands.
24. Dodman NH, et al: The use of narcotic antagonists as therapeutic agents to modify stereotypic self-licking, self-chewing and scratching behavior in dogs, *J Am Vet Med Assoc* 193:815–819, 1988.
25. White SD: Naltrexone treatment of acral lick dermatitis in dogs, *J Am Vet Med Assoc* 196:1073–1076, 1990.
26. Hartgraves SL, Randall PK: Dopamine agonist-induced stereotypic grooming and self mutilation following striatal dopamine depletion, *Psychopharmacology* 90:358–363, 1986.
27. Moon-Fanelli A, Dodman NH: Phenomenology, development and pharmacotherapy of compulsive tail chasing behavior in Bull Terriers and related breeds: an open trial of clomipramine, *J Am Vet Med Assoc,* in press.
28. Blackshaw JK, Sutton RH, Boyhan MA: Tail chasing or circling behavior in dogs, *Canine Pract* 19:7–11, 1994.
29. Mena I, et al: Chronic manganese poisoning, *Neurology* 33:128–136, 1967.
30. Kurlan R: Hypothesis 2: Tourette's syndrome is part of a clinical spectrum that includes normal brain development, *Arch Neurol* 51:1145–1150, 1994.
31. Brown SA, et al: Naloxone-responsive compulsive tail chasing in a dog, *J Am Vet Med Assoc* 190:884–886, 1987.
32. Dodman NH, et al: Behavioral changes associated with suspected complex partial seizures in Bull Terriers, *J Am Vet Med Assoc* 208:688–691, 1996.
33. Jenike MA, Brotman AW: The EEG in obsessive-compulsive disorder, *J Clin Psych* 45:122–124, 1984.
34. Jenike MA, Brandon AD: Obsessive-compulsive disorder and head trauma: a rare association, *J Anx Dis* 2:353–359, 1988.
35. Kettl PA, Marks IM: Neurological factors in obsessive-compulsive disorder: two case reports and a review of the literature, *Br J Psychiatry* 149:315–319, 1986.
36. Levin B, Duchowny M: Childhood obsessive-compulsive disorder and cingulate epilepsy, *Biol Psychiatry* 30:1049–1055, 1991.
37. Ward CD: Transient feelings of compulsion caused by hemispheric lesions: three cases, *J Neurosurg Psychiatry* 51:266–268, 1988.
38. Sawyer L, Moon-Fanelli AA, Dodman NH: Phenotype establishment of feline

compulsive behaviors, Data on file, Tufts University of Veterinary Medicine, Grafton, Mass.

39. Stewart L: Veterinary Dermatology of New England, Acton, Mass, personal communication, 1996.

40. Young MS, Manning TO: Psychogenic dermatoses, *Dermatol Rep* 3(2):1–8, 1984.

41. Muller GH, Kirk RW, Scott DW: *Small animal dermatology*, Philadelphia, 1989, WB Saunders.

42. Scott DW: Feline dermatology 1900–1978: a monograph, *J Am Anim Hosp Assoc* 16:331–562, 1980.

43. Shell LG: Feline hyperesthesia syndrome, *Feline Pract* 22:10, 1994.

44. Scott DW: The skin. In Holzworth J, editor: *Diseases of the cat: medicine and surgery*, Philadelphia, 1987, WB Saunders.

45. Parker AJ, O'Brien DP, Sawchuk SA: The nervous system. In Pratt PW, editor: *Feline medicine*, Santa Barbara, Calif, 1983, American Veterinary Publications.

46. Caplan R, et al: Intractable seizures, compulsions, and coprolalia: a pediatric case study, *J Neuropsychiatry Clin Neurosci* 4(3):315–319, 1992.

47. Dodman NH: Pharmacological treatment of behavioural problems in cats, *Vet International* 6(4):13–20, 1994.

48. Shell LG: Feline hyperesthesia syndrome, *Feline Pract* 22.10, 1994.

49. Dodman NH: *The cat who cried for help,* New York, 1997, Bantam.

50. Bordnick PS, Thyer BA, Ritchie BW: Feather picking disorder and trichotillomania: an avian model of human psychopathology, *J Behav Ther Exp Psychiatry* 25(3):189–196, 1994.

51. Iglauer F, Rasim R: Treatment of psychogenic feather picking in psittacine birds with a dopamine antagonist, *J Sm Anim Pract* 34:564–566, 1993.

52. Mertens PA, Dodman NH: Data on file, University of Munich, Germany.

53. Stein DJ, Hollander E: Low dose pimozide augmentation of serotonin reuptake blockers in the treatment of trichotillomania, *J Clin Psychiatry* 53:123–126, 1992.

54. VanAmerigen M, Mancini C: Treatment of trichotillomania with haloperidol, Abstract: Anxiety Disorders Association of America Annual Meeting, Orlando, Fla, 1996.

55. Swedo SE, et al: A double-blind comparison of clomipramine and desipramine in the treatment of trichotillomania (hair pulling), *N Engl J Med* 321:497–501, 1989.

56. Vechiotti GG, Galanti R: Evidence of heredity of cribbing, weaving, and stall-walking in thorough-bred horses, *Livestock Prod Sci* 14:91–95, 1986.

57. Dodman NH, Shuster L, Court MH: Investigation into the use of narcotic antagonists in the treatment of a stereotypic behavior pattern (crib-biting) in the horse, *Am J Vet Res* 48:311–319, 1987.

58. Grandison L, Guidotti A: Stimulation of food intake by muscimol and beta endorphin, *Neuropharmacology* 16:533–536, 1977.

59. McDonald S: University of Pennsylvania, personal communication.

60. Dodman NH, et al: Equine self-mutilation syndrome (57 cases), *J Am Vet Med Assoc* 204(8):1219–1223, 1994.

61. Wolf SS, et al: Tourette syndrome: prediction of phenotypic variation in monozygotic twins by caudate nucleus D2 receptor binding, *Science* 273:1225–1227, 1996.

62. Dodman NH, Shuster L: Data on file, Tufts University of Veterinary Medicine, Grafton, Mass.
63. Sandyk R, et al: Deranged modulatory midbrain opioid and gonadotrophin functions: relevance to Tourette's syndrome, *Med Hypoth* 36:95–97, 1991.
64. Peterson BS, et al: Steroid hormones and Tourette's syndrome: Early experience with antiandrogen therapy, *J Clin Psychopharmacol* 14(2):131–135, 1994.
65. Houben-Gelissen M, Moss J, Olivier B: Animal models for obsessive-compulsive disorder: new perspectives. In Olivier B, Manceaux A, editors: *Destructive drives and impulse controls—preclinical considerations*, Denhaag, 1991, CIP.
66. Rapoport JL, Wise SP: Obsessive-compulsive disorder: evidence for basal ganglia dysfunction, *Psychopharmacol Bull* 24:380–384, 1988.
67. Rapoport J: Quoted by R Jerome: *The sciences*, Sept/Oct 1992, pp 5–6.
68. Luescher UA, MCKeown DB, Halip JH: Stereotypic or obsessive compulsive disorders in dogs and cats. In Marder AR, Voith V, editors: *Veterinary clinics of North America, small animal practice,* Philadelphia, 1991, WB Saunders.
69. Overall KL: Recognition, diagnosis, and management of obsessive compulsive disorders, *Canine Pract* 17:39–42, 1992.
70. Stein DJ, Hollander E: Dermatology and conditions related to obsessive-compulsive disorder, *J Am Acad Dermatol* 26:237–242, 1992.

Part IV

Treatment

17

Behavior Therapy for Obsessive-Compulsive Disorder

Lee Baer, Ph.D., William E. Minichiello, Fd.D.

The apparent simplicity of behavior therapy for obsessive-compulsive disorder (OCD) can be misleading, as the following two examples indicate: two recent neuroimaging studies at UCLA[1,2] have proven this seemingly simple treatment to be the first nonsomatic intervention to result in neurophysiologic changes that mirror observable clinical improvements. In a similar vein, Professor Isaac Marks lectured on the vital importance of spreading comparatively simple medical information. He notes that, despite all the money spent on high technology medical and imaging equipment, the following simple instructions from the World Health Organization (WHO) to mothers in Third World countries have saved many more lives: "The instruction is for the mother to boil a cup of water, put into it a pinch of salt lifted with three (not 2 or 4) fingers, stir it, taste it, and if it's no saltier than tears and not too hot, to spoon it to her baby, who is likely to absorb it without vomiting. Behind that simple instruction are 200 years of Western scientific endeavor concerning the nature of dehydration and blood osmolarity and how to correct it. With that instruction one can do away with the need for intravenous fluid and all the paraphernalia it entails. Mums can treat their babies in the bush."[3] The simple rules of behavior therapy are similar to the WHO instructions in that both are behavioral instructions, and both rely on the individual accepting the advice as worthwhile, nondangerous, and effective.

This chapter begins with a brief history of behavioral treatments for OCD and critically reviews outcome studies that illustrate the effective components of treatment, with particular attention to the kinds of OCD symptoms they benefit. Next a summary of our clinical management of patients is provided. The final section considers the theoretic bases of behavior therapy for OCD. The present chapter considers only behavioral treatment for adult OCD; behavioral treatment for children and adolescents with OCD is covered in detail elsewhere in this text (see Chapter 19). The next chapter (see Chapter 18) gives detailed treatment descriptions of patients to assist the reader in understanding and implementing these effective techniques.

BACKGROUND

The behavioral techniques of exposure and response prevention (i.e., extended exposure to the stimuli that trigger OCD symptoms along with prevention of rituals during this exposure and afterward) consistently yield 60% to 70% of patients "much improved" after brief treatment.[4] Further, behavior therapy is free of the side effects of drug treatment, and improvements are generally maintained at follow-up after several years.[5]

Behavior therapy produces the largest changes in behavioral rituals, such as compulsive cleaning or checking.[4] This is in contrast to traditional psychotherapy, in which changes are produced mainly in obsessional thoughts, whereas little effect is seen in behavioral rituals.[6] This difference reflects the specific effects of behavioral treatment, in which the behaviors themselves are the targets of treatment.

The use of behavioral techniques to treat obsessions and compulsions is not new. A century ago, French neurologist Pierre Janet gave a remarkably accurate description of what is now termed *exposure therapy,* including the name itself:

> The guide, the therapist, will specify to the patient the action as precisely as possible. He will analyze it into its elements if it should be necessary to give the patient's mind an immediate and proximate aim. By continually repeating the order to perform the action, that is, exposure, he will help the patient greatly by words of encouragement at every sign of success, however insignificant, for encouragement will make the patient realize these little successes and will stimulate him with the hopes aroused by glimpses of greater successes in the future.

Other patients need strictures and even threats and one patient told (Janet), "Unless I am continually being forced to do things that need a great deal of effort I shall never get better. You must keep a strict hand over me."[4]

This early description of the behavioral treatment of OCD remains concise and accurate today, and exposure therapy as described by Janet remains the major behavioral treatment of OCD nearly a century later.

Besides describing clinical treatment for this disorder, Janet was ahead of his time in noting improvements produced by societal pressures to engage in informal exposure and response prevention: he reported 14 cases of "accidental" cure of OCD symptoms when patients served in the French military.[4] Later, Marks[4] noted that many obsessive-compulsive women remained well when living in convents, and Lewis[4] reported that many patients had severe obsessions, which disappeared during service in the war, but later returned after the war ended. Thus, it appears that patients suffering from obsessions and compulsions require an outside agent to assist them in keeping their habits under control. This agent may take the varied forms of social institution, family member, or behavior therapist. Regardless of the agent, when an OCD sufferer is in some way forced to engage in the feared practices without ritualizing, therapeutic improvement usually results.

A natural question then is, if behavioral techniques were successfully employed almost a century ago, why then was it not until the late 1960s that these techniques were widely and effectively employed in the treatment of this disorder? A major reason lies with the impact of psychoanalytic theory, which was gaining popularity at the turn of the century. Soon after Janet gave his description of exposure therapy, Freud published his analysis of semantic conditioning in the formation of obsessions and compulsions in the patient known as the Rat Man,[7] and interest turned toward the meaning of obsessions and compulsions, and away from considering the compulsive behaviors as treatment targets in and of themselves.

Any clinician familiar with OCD patients can attest that the presentation of many of these cases coincides with psychodynamic themes; that is, the majority of patients with cleaning compulsions are inordinately concerned with contamination from dirt, feces, urine, and sexually related objects, whereas those patients with checking compulsions tend to be preoccupied with fears of hurting others, saying or writing obscene or blasphemous things, and handling money. However, although psychodynamic formulations do have descriptive value, they have not yielded any reliable techniques for modifying obsessions and compulsions. That patients can have OCD symptoms that fit a dynamic theme yet still improve with behavior therapy is demonstrated by the following case.

Case 1

The patient, a 42-year-old married woman, presented with obsessive thoughts and ritualistic behaviors including washing her hands up to 100 times per day and using approximately seven rolls of paper towels per week. In addition, she avoided touching any object that might have been touched by a person who was now dead for fear of becoming contaminated by "germs or death." She was also unable to touch dozens of objects in her home including objects associated with sex, money, doorknobs, light switches, shoes, and kitchen utensils. She could not sit on furniture that she believed a person now deceased might have sat on at some time in the past. The patient had members of her family touch these objects for her and use them for her. She was depressed because of the constriction in her activities produced by the rituals.

Eight years earlier, her father died from a stroke when on a business trip. The patient had been in the habit of abstaining from certain sexual activities when her father was away, for fear that God would punish her by hurting her father. When he was away on this particular business trip, she did not abstain, and he in fact did die, and the patient experienced greatly increased guilt.

Two years later, she developed systemic lupus erythematosus and accepted this as punishment for what she had done to her father. Two years after that, and 4 years before treatment, she began hand-washing rituals because she "decided not to follow in her father's footsteps" and because she felt "like I had to wash something off my hands." The rituals and obsessions began with objects that had belonged to her father and then spread to other objects. Her father's belongings still produced the strongest sensations of anxiety. At initial interview, the patient reported that she did not truly believe that her actions in fact had killed her father. She acknowledged guilt over his death and briefly described her close relationship with him.

The process of exposure therapy was explained, and the patient agreed that she would be willing to experience moderate levels of anxiety to overcome the problem. She agreed to have her husband attend the second session and to ask him to bring along a "contaminated" object belonging to her father so that exposure and response prevention could be demonstrated.

The patient's husband attended the second session, in which the principles of exposure and response prevention were explained to him. With the therapist's encouragement, the patient was able to hold the "contaminated" object for 30 minutes and refrained from washing her hands for 1 hour afterward. A homework assignment was agreed upon whereby she would touch six kitchen objects and engage in response prevention with her husband's help.

At the third session, she stated that she had been able to touch kitchen utensils and shoes that she had not touched for months. The exposure practice of 30 minutes was done three times per week and produced minimal discomfort. The patient brought the most "contaminated" object, her father's wristwatch, to the session in a plastic bag. With the therapist's urging, she was able to hold the watch during the final 30 minutes of the session. It was pointed out to the patient that her anxiety ratings decreased over the time she had been holding the watch, and this was presented as a model for the remainder of the treatment. Several more target behaviors were agreed upon as homework assignments.

When the couple returned for the fourth session 1 month later, they reported that almost all of the patient's rituals had been eliminated and that she was feeling better and more confident. Family tensions had decreased as the patient made fewer demands.

The couple was seen for a fifth session 1 month later; the patient had maintained her gains and the few remaining rituals—touching shoes and placing her hands in her mouth—were not interfering with her functioning. Because the couple lived a great distance from the hospital, it was agreed that they would continue to work on the rituals in home practice sessions.

The patient was seen for a follow-up session after 1 year. At this time, she had maintained her goals. However, she requested additional behavioral treatment for a ritual that she had not presented as a target behavior at the initial

> sessions. Following instructions provided at this session, the patient controlled the remaining ritual through exposure and response prevention carried out at home with the aid of her husband. She was most recently seen at 5-year follow-up and had maintained her goals; although some mild rituals remained, they did not interfere with her life.

The need for direct behavioral treatment, even in cases such as this that can also be explained in psychodynamic terms, finds support in an unexpected observation by Freud in discussing the psychoanalytic treatment of agoraphobia[8] (pp 399–400):

> Our technique grew up in the treatment of hysteria and is still directed principally to the cure of this affliction. But the phobias have made it necessary for us to go beyond our former limits. One can hardly master a phobia if one waits till the patient lets the analysis influence him to give it up . . . take the example of agoraphobia. It succeeds only when one can induce them through the influence of the analysis to behave like the first class, that is, to go out alone and to struggle with their anxiety while they are making the attempt. One first achieves therefore, a considerable moderation of the phobia and it is only when this has been attained by the physician's recommendation that the associations and memories come into the patient's mind, enabling the phobia to be solved.

MISCONCEPTIONS ABOUT BEHAVIOR THERAPY

Before considering the theory and clinical management of obsessions and compulsions, we address some misconceptions we have encountered in case conferences and lectures.

• *Substitute Symptoms Will Result from Behavioral Change* A frequent criticism of behavior therapy is that although target behaviors may be modified, other insidious substitute symptoms may arise. This idea is a result of the Freudian hydraulic theory, which predicts that an unconscious conflict will express itself in some form until that conflict is resolved. In fact, research on behavior therapy in general, and on behavior therapy for OCD in particular, has found no evidence for substitute symptoms.[9] When anxiety, depression, or adjustment in job, marital, or family relationships is examined, the results of follow-up studies show improvements in these areas. It is true, however, that unless a careful behavioral analysis is performed at the outset of treatment, a controlling variable, can be overlooked, such as excessive guilt, which might result in a large number of apparently shifting checking rituals. The issue of substitute symptoms was addressed by Foa and Steketee[10] who found that 3 of 21 patients experienced emergent fears during behavioral treatment for OCD. The emergent fears were from the same hierarchy as the initially treated fears and were hypothesized to have resulted from a reduction in conditioned inhibition; these fears were reduced with direct behavioral treatment.

Given the recent realization of the overlap of OCD symptoms and the symptoms of Tourette's and other tic disorders—many of which change over time—it is possible that some symptoms believed to be compulsive rituals may be complex tics (especially those not involving subjective experience of fear) and may therefore change in form over time.

• *It Is Dangerous to Interrupt Rituals* The fear that it is dangerous to interrupt a person who is actively engaged in ritualistic behavior[11] may result from viewing the ritual as a defense against breakthrough into consciousness of an unconscious impulse with its associated anxiety. Thus, it is feared that ritual interruption may produce overwhelming anxiety, which may reach psychotic proportions.

Rachman and associates[11] have found that interruption of rituals in OCD patients does not ultimately result in any increase in self-reports of anxiety, in psychophysiologic measures of anxiety, or in subjective reports of discomfort. Further, follow-up studies pursued up to 7 years of more than 150 OCD patients have revealed no lasting problems caused by the response prevention procedure. At worst, the patient may find the process temporarily distressing, and in some cases may refuse the treatment, but there are no long-range dire consequences.

On the other hand, Foa and Chambless[12] did find that, on average, OCD sufferers experienced stronger anxiety during behavioral treatment than did agoraphobics, and these high levels of anxiety lasted approximately twice as long as those in the OCD sufferers. However, this study found that after six or seven exposure sessions, strong anxiety was experienced only briefly by either group.

• *Thoughts Are Ignored in Behavior Therapy* Behavior therapy is sometimes accused of being overly simplistic by not dealing with the patient's thoughts or unconscious motivations. In fact, a thorough behavioral analysis examines all variables that can be empirically demonstrated to have an effect on behavior.[13] The trend in behavioral analysis is to evaluate the motoric, affective, physiologic, and cognitive spheres of behavior. Rachman[14] has proposed a three-system approach to fears. In brief, this theory is derived from work by Lang;[15] instead of the old concept of fear as a unitary or "lumped" concept, there are in fact three systems of behavior (i.e., motoric, physiologic, and verbal), which are at best loosely correlated. The lump model of fear implicitly assumes a perfect correlation among these systems, an assumption proved untenable by much behavioral research indicating the often low correlation among these systems. As an example, an OCD patient may report strong fears of a situation, yet may force himself to confront it and show only slight increases in physiologic measures of arousal. This low correlation is termed "desynchrony" by Rachman, and when this desynchrony persists after treatment, it may predict treatment failures.

A clinical example of conditioning along a symbolic or semantic dimension was provided by Wolpe,[16,17] a pioneer in the application of classical conditioning theory to the neuroses. A woman presented complaining of a fear of cockroaches. She was then treated with the standard behavior therapy technique of systematic desensitization, a deconditioning procedure. To Wolpe's surprise, the fear of cockroaches remained after this treatment. In further discussion with the patient, it was discovered that she had been undergoing severe marital problems for some time. Further, it happened that her pet name for her husband was "cockroach." When it was determined that the generalization to real cockroaches was symbolic, the treatment was switched to focus on the marital relationship, after which the phobia of cockroaches disappeared. As a result of such cases, Wolpe estimated that approximately one third of all phobias are not the result of direct autonomic conditioning, but rather are the result of misinformation or of semantic generalization. He has found that such cases do not respond to direct systematic desensitization. Instead, these cases require either the correction of misinformation or an understanding of the lines along which the symbolic or semantic conditioning has occurred.[16,17]

The current state-of-the-art of cognitive therapy approaches to OCD is described in detail elsewhere in this text (see Chapter 18).

• *Behavior Therapy Assumes That All Maladaptive Behavior Is Learned Through Simple Processes* As behavior therapy has moved from the laboratory to clinical populations, it has been forced to take into account factors other than its major learning principles: operant and respondent conditioning. Among these additional factors have been individual differences in personality, genetic factors preparing individuals for ease of learning certain associations, and the concomitant presence of psychiatric diseases, such as bipolar disorder and schizophrenia, which require pharmacologic treatment. For example, the concept of biologic preparedness for learning particular fears[18] has gained acceptance and will be considered later in this chapter. In addition, behaviors are often seen to fluctuate with the patient's mood, as when the frequency of checking compulsions increases or decreases depending on the level of depressed mood.[19]

• *The Use of Drugs Is Incompatible with Behavior Therapy* There are many occasions in which psychopharmacology and behavior therapy complement one another. For example, the presence of concomitant depression poses several problems. For one, agitated depressive patients may not habituate normally to stimuli.[19,20] Thus, behavioral treatments based on habituation, such as exposure therapy, may be useless until the mood disorder is treated. In addition, a mood disorder can make it difficult or impossible for patients to comply with behavioral programs such as response prevention. In these cases, adjunctive pharmacologic interventions can smooth the way for increased compliance with the treatment protocol and increased success. This was noted by Marks, et al[5] in a study of behavior therapy and clomipramine in the treatment of OCD. Further, we have noted in our clinic that the use of antidepressants has helped improve compliance with behavioral treatment in patients who previously had difficulty complying with these techniques.

The decision to treat a patient with behavior therapy or medication should not be an "either-or" decision. In our OCD clinic, patients may be treated either with medications alone, behavior therapy alone, or a combination of the two. A recent long-term follow-up of patients treated in our clinic found that this approach has resulted in marked improvements in OCD symptoms, which have been maintained over time.[21]

Current literature provides little or conflicting data describing the efficacy of combined drug and behavioral treatment versus behavioral treatment alone; a federally funded study is ongoing in Philadelphia and New York that will help to resolve this issue.

• *All Patients Respond Equally Well to Behavior Therapy* As will be seen in the sections on outcome research and clinical management, predictors of poor outcome with behavioral treatments in OCD include: (1) schizotypal personality disorder; (2) fears that the patient feels are realistic; (3) severe depression or mania; (4) poor compliance; and (5) severe family problems. Whereas the early behavior therapy literature claimed extremely high success rates with a variety of disorders, more recent research has focused on both the strengths and limitations of this form of treatment.[22] In addition, the strongest evidence for the efficacy of exposure and response prevention has been noted in patients with cleaning and circumscribed checking rituals.[23]

OUTCOME RESEARCH
Exposure and Response Prevention

Initial attempts at behavioral treatment of OCD typically involved the technique of systematic desensitization, which had been successfully applied to the treatment of phobias. This technique produced unpredictable and unstable results when applied to OCD.[11,24]

The modern era of behavioral treatment of OCD began with Meyer and his associates,[24] who developed a method of completely preventing 15 inpatients with OCD from engaging in their rituals. Of these patients, 10 had cleaning compulsions, two had checking compulsions, and the rest had either a combination of these or repeating compulsions. After treatment, 10 of these patients were reported to be markedly improved or asymptomatic, and the other five were "improved;" of 12 patients followed-up at 6 months to 6 years, only four patients showed varying degrees of relapse. This inpatient method involved constant daily supervision during waking hours by nurses (response prevention), along with elements of exposure, therapist modeling, and social reinforcement (these techniques are described later in this chapter). Despite the high cost of staff involvement, these case reports demonstrated that a psychologic treatment could have a dramatic and lasting effect on OCD symptoms.

Drawing on this pioneering work of Meyer and associates,[11] a group at the Maudsley Hospital in London, including Rachman, Hodgson, Marks, and Mawson, embarked on a series of partially controlled trials of Meyer's response prevention method combined with exposure to feared stimuli as well as modeling by the therapist. This group provided evidence in a series of crossover trials that the combination of these treatments was superior to a relaxation control.[11]

These findings have been extended and refined by research teams led by Foa (USA),[25] Emmelkamp (The Netherlands),[26] and Boulougouris (Greece).[27] The successful replication of cross-cultural results has strengthened confidence in the efficacy of behavior therapy for this disorder.

There have been more than 10 outcome studies (with varying degrees of control) of behavior therapy for OCD over the past 15 years, involving more than 200 patients in various countries (reviews[4,11,28,29]). The treatment protocol nearly always involves exposure to the feared situation and response prevention, a procedure in which the patient is prevented from carrying out the ritualistic behavior. These studies have examined only OCD patients exhibiting ritualistic behavior, usually of the checking or cleaning variety.[23] Patients with only obsessive thoughts without ritualistic activity have been studied separately, with unpredictable results.[4]

In general, these studies have found that 60% to 70% of patients with ritualistic behaviors were much improved after behavioral treatment. Approximately 20% to 30% of the patients were found to be resistant to the treatment, whereas the dropout rate averaged 20%.[11] Treatment was carried out over a relatively short period averaging 3 to 7 weeks, with a 10-session treatment program most common. At follow-ups of 2 years or more, improvements in rituals were maintained in nearly all patients.[4]

Early studies were performed with hospitalized patients,[30] whereas more recent studies were performed with outpatients. The outpatient studies frequently involved home treatment, which appeared to be necessary for adequate generalization of treatment gains.[11]

Although obsessive and compulsive symptoms are usually significantly reduced with behavioral treatment, and interference with occupational and social functioning is reduced, the ritualistic behavior is rarely totally eliminated. Marks[4] has observed:

> Although most patients who are cooperative (and those are the great majority) improve with exposure in vivo, few of them are totally cured. Patients are generally told that they need to acquire a coping set to deal with tendencies to ritualize that might recur after discharge. Occasionally brief booster treatment is needed, but this is minimal apart from explicit advice about regular homework, which may be needed for many months after discharge.

Outcome studies have differed in their relative emphases on the various components of the treatment. For example, Meyer and associates[24] stressed the importance of strictly enforced response prevention, whereas Rachman and associates[11] have emphasized exposure and the addition of participant modeling (i.e., the therapist modeling, or demonstrating, the desired behavior along with the patient). The optimal length of exposure to the feared situation also has been studied; in general, results indicate that the effects of the treatment combination of exposure and response prevention are quite robust across studies, producing comparable results despite various modifications in the procedures.

Commenting on the many studies comparing the importance of various components of the treatment package, Rachman and Hodgson[11] noted: "The most striking outcome of these comparison studies is that so few significant differences have emerged" (p 341).

Several early studies by Rachman and associates[30] controlled for the effects of exposure therapy by also requiring patients to undergo a relaxation training group as a control for therapist exposure and nonspecific factors. Results indicated that relaxation reduced the anxiety and depression ratings of the OCD patients but did nothing to reduce rituals, thus providing evidence for the specific effects of exposure therapy.

Foa, et al[31] shed some light on the relative contributions of the components of the treatment package. These authors found that the exposure and response prevention components produced differential effects in the treatment of compulsive washers. Exposure therapy was found to help mainly in reducing anxiety, whereas response prevention had its greatest effect in reducing ritualistic washing. Further, it was found that the combined treatment was more effective than either component alone. These authors also provided evidence that in the treatment of checking rituals, a combination of imaginal exposure (i.e., having the patient vividly imagine the most feared consequences of not ritualizing) and response prevention led to better treatment outcome than response prevention alone. This response may occur because the catastrophic consequences many checkers fear will never actually occur in real life, so that habituation must be carried out in the patients' imagination.[31]

Metaanalysis Results

Although a controversial technique,[31a] metaanalysis nonetheless provides a summary of the efficacy of various treatments for a particular disorder in the absence of controlled comparison studies and can be more objective than a narrative review. A recent metaanalysis by investigators with the Quality Assurance Project of Australia and New Zealand[32,33] studied 71 papers published between 1961 and 1984, 38 of which included enough information to calculate effect sizes between pretreatments and posttreatments. The effect size statistic is calculated as (posttest mean − pretest mean)/pretest standard deviation. Only eight studies provided double-blind trials versus placebo treatments, and no two of these studies tested the same treatment versus placebo.[32]

The most effective treatment, with an effect size of 1.8 at the end of treatment and 1.7 at a mean 80-week follow-up, was the behavior therapy combination of exposure and response prevention. Treatment with clomipramine produced an effect size of 1.7, with no studies including follow-up after discontinuation of treatment. Treatment with psychosurgery (cingulate and other regions) produced an effect size of 1.4, which fell to 1.0 at 60 weeks' follow-up. Thus, behavior therapy was found to produce the highest mean effect size, which also was best maintained on discontinuation of treatment.

This metaanalysis also examined effect sizes for relaxation treatments and waiting list controls, which are not believed to directly reduce either obsessions or compulsions. The average effect size of these conditions was 0.20, and for those studies of these methods that involved a follow-up score, the effect size at follow-up fell to –0.18, indicating that patients were worse at follow-up than at baseline. These findings indicated that few OCD patients improve without treatment, and there was little lasting placebo response.

More recently, Van Balkom and associates in The Netherlands[34] replicated and updated this metaanalysis through the early 1990s, and again concluded that behavior therapy (only that involving exposure and response prevention) and treatment with a number of serotonin reuptake inhibitor (SRI) drugs then available produced highly significant and approximately equal improvements in OCD symptoms, as measured by the same within-subject effect size statistic described above. However, improvement with SRI drugs tended to be rated by assessors as greater than improvement with behavior therapy, even though patients rated this SRI improvement as lesser.

Conclusions from metaanalyses are limited by any biases inherent in the treatment literature on which they are based. As noted above, three quarters of patients in past behavioral treatment studies have had primarily cleaning rituals (47.6%) or circumscribed checking rituals (27.0%).[23] On the other hand, only 13.5% have been reported as having obsessions without motor rituals, and only 4.0% have been reported as having hoarding, slowness, exactness, or other less common types of rituals.[23] Therefore, the results of these metaanalyses regarding behavioral treatments are generalizable mainly to patients with cleaning or circumscribed checking rituals. In addition, modern cognitive therapy treatments for OCD (as described in detail in Chapter 18) were not available at the time of these metaanalyses and are not represented.

Maintenance of Gains

Marks[4] reviewed eight studies with follow-up data collected at least 1 year after completion of behavioral treatment. In these studies, improvements at the end of treatment were maintained or strengthened at follow-ups of 1 to 5 years.

In many of these studies, follow-up periods were not free of continued and confounding treatments. For example, Foa and Goldstein[25] followed 21 patients, of whom 12 had a mean of 16 additional behavioral sessions. Similarly, Marks, et al[35] followed 11 patients, who had a mean of 7.7 additional sessions, including a mean of three home visits. Nine of the patients required antidepressant medication during the follow-up period, two required marital therapy, and one required assertiveness training.

Hiss and associates[36] in Philadelphia recently reported encouraging results of a relapse-prevention program following intensive behavioral treatment of OCD. Eighteen patients (17 with cleaning or checking rituals) were treated with 3 weeks of intensive imaginal and *in vivo* exposure for their cleaning and checking symptoms, including home practice and two home visits by the therapist. Patients were then randomly assigned to either a relapse-prevention condition (consisting of four 90-minute sessions over 1 week) or a control condition (consisting of relaxation training and associative therapy). Using a 50% improvement on the Yale-Brown Obsessive-Compulsive Scale (Y-BOCS) as the criterion for treatment response, 75% of patients assigned to the relapse prevention condition were "responders" after initial treatment, and 75% were responders at 6-month follow-up. On the other hand, 70% of patients assigned to the control condition were "responders" after initial treatment, but only 33% were responders at 6-month follow-up. Although there were few statistically significant results because of the small sample size, this study suggested that a brief relapse-prevention program, including brief telephone contacts, may help prevent relapse, at least in patients with cleaning and checking rituals.

Generalizability of Gains

One aspect of generalizability involves the improvement of rituals other than those directly treated with exposure and response prevention. Although no studies have yet been designed to examine the specificity of treatment response, it appears that only those specific rituals that are effectively prevented (e.g., by response prevention) are reduced. The cases of partial compliance with associated partial improvement suggest that reduction of rituals is specific and does not generalize to responses that are not prevented. Such specificity of treatment effects is also found in primary obsessional slowness.[11]

As an example, Rachman, et al[30] described a patient with both cleaning and hoarding rituals: ". . . she cooperated moderately well in flooding, and her washing was reduced. The hoarding, which was not treated, did not change."

These same authors[37] also noted that the "results of the behavioral treatment were specific. The compulsive behavior changed as predicted and was not accompanied by alterations in other aspects of the person's problems."

Predicting Treatment Failures

As noted previously, despite advances in the behavioral treatment of OCD, many patients remain refractory to treatment, and the dropout rate is 20%.[11]

Outcome studies have proven that poor compliance with the treatment program is the most common reason for treatment failure with behavioral therapy for OCD. Beyond this, until recently we only had anecdotal reports of either positive or negative predictors of treatment outcome with exposure and response prevention for OCD. These are summarized in the following paragraphs.

Pervasive Checking Rituals

Rachman, et al[30] commented that: "most failures resulting from inability to comply with response prevention come from compulsive checkers. These are patients in whom response prevention may be the most important element in treatment,"[11 p. 350] and: "Our view is, however, that the most difficult patients in this group were those who complained of repetitive, pervasive checking rituals, often involving more than 100 checks per day. The patients with the best prognosis, based on our clinical impression, appear to be those with contamination fears and cleaning rituals that are focused on a restricted number of stimulus situations. To put it another way, patients whose disorders might be classified, in our terms, as 'phobic-compulsive' respond best to this kind of treatment."[11 p. 319.]

Overvalued Ideation

Foa and Goldstein[25] reported that "The three patients who relapsed at follow-up were all washers characterized by a strong belief that their fears were realistic . . . An additional washer had a slight relapse . . . three checkers who were mildly or moderately symptomatic at the end of treatment continued to improve after therapy and became asymptomatic at follow-up." This same group later reported that patients with checking rituals who were treated with *in vivo* exposure but without imaginal exposure tended to relapse at follow-up.[38]

Obsessional Slowness

Rachman and Hodgson[11] provided two case histories of patients who required many hours to complete daily activities. These authors noted: "Our feeling that flooding had little to contribute to the treatment of these patients was confirmed in clinical practice." Instead, they developed an outpatient method of "prompting, shaping, and pacing," which produced lasting improvements at 4- and 6-year follow-up in the two patients studied. Commenting on the lack of generalization of improvements in these patients, these authors remarked: "It is interesting to notice the specificity of the treatment effects; each problem required separate, direct management, and that is reflected in the stepwise sequence of the improvements."

Schizotypal Personality Disorder

Minichiello, et al[39] found that OCD patients meeting criteria for schizotypal personality disorder (SPD) do not respond well to behavioral treatment of OCD. After treating 29 patients with standard behavior therapy techniques and others with concomitant antidepressant medication, the authors independently noted that a certain proportion of patients were not responding to the standard behavioral treatment. It did not appear that these patients were merely resistant to treatment, but some seemed to "defy the laws of learning," as one of us phrased it. Ten (35%) of these 29 OCD patients also met the *Diagnostic and Statistical Manual of Mental Disorders* (DSM-III) criteria for SPD and for OCD. These patients did not meet the criteria for schizophrenia, although many of them had been diagnosed as such in the past and had been treated ineffectively with neuroleptics.[40] A retrospective review of treatment outcome of patients receiving behavior therapy (either alone or in combination with medication) revealed that 84% of OCD patients without SPD, but only 10% of those with SPD, achieved at least moderate improvement in their OCD symptoms.[39] Some of the OCD patients with concomitant SPD who did not make progress with behavior therapy later showed reductions in rituals when treated in behavioral family or couples therapy and placed in structured environments such as halfway houses or day treatment programs. The concept of SPD as a poor prognostic indicator in OCD appears to have validity in light of the literature on treatment failure. This personality disorder encompasses several of the poor predictive factors reviewed earlier. Most noticeably, these patients strongly believe that their rituals are necessary or some terrible event will occur. Also, these patients frequently have difficulty complying with the prescribed treatment and with assigned record-keeping tasks. In addition, Rachman and Hodgson[11] have similarly found that the presence of an "abnormal personality" is a negative-outcome predictor of behavior therapy for OCD, and Solyom, et al[41] recently identified a similar subgroup—"obsessive psychosis"—as having a less favorable outcome. Our clinical impression is that the poor outcome of these patients is not solely the result of resistance to the treatment. Instead, it appears that the overvalued ideas of these patients make it difficult for them to comply with treatment. In addition, although support by family members is helpful in overcoming this disorder, patients with SPD often have poor social relations and chaotic family situations.

Quantitative Analysis of Outcome Prediction

In recent years, two studies have attempted to quantify predictors of response to behavioral treatment for OCD.

Keijsers and associates[42] in The Netherlands treated 40 OCD sufferers (34 had checking and/or washing rituals and six had obsessions only) with 18 sessions of *in vivo* exposure and response prevention. The authors then categorized patients as "responders" separately for compulsive behaviors and for obsessive fear improvement, based on a greater than 30% reduction on a variety of combined outcome measures. Sixteen patients (40%) were "responders" on compulsive behaviors, and 23 patients (57.5%) were "responders" on obsessive fear improvement (Y-BOCS scores were not obtained). Greater initial severity of symptoms and greater depression significantly predicted poorer outcome on compulsive behavior. These two variables, along with longer problem duration, poorer motivation for treatment, and dissatisfaction with the therapeutic relationship, significantly predicted poorer outcome for obsessive fears.[42]

Buchanan and associates[43] in London reviewed the records of 127 OCD patients admitted to their inpatient behavioral unit between 1988 and 1991. Fifty-seven percent of the patients presented with contamination fears, and 28% had fears of harming others. The mean percentage of symptom improvement on their scale (Y-BOCS was not used) was 44% for all patients, 18% for those patients leaving the unit during the first 3 months of treatment, and between 60% and 62% for those patients remaining in treatment at least 3 months. Compliance with treatment was significantly predicted by the patient's being employed during treatment and by the patient living with his or her family. Clinical improvement was predicted by these two variables, along with no history of previous treatment; absence of depression; presence of observable rituals; and the presence of contamination fears.

CLINICAL MANAGEMENT

As noted elsewhere in this chapter, several controlled studies of behavior therapy for OCD have been conducted in inpatient settings, with greater control over the patient's environment. In actual practice, this is not possible for most clinicians. The following techniques are used with OCD patients who are seen in outpatient settings.

Behavioral Analysis

The first step in any behavioral treatment is to perform a careful behavioral analysis. Such an analysis differs from a traditional psychiatric or psychologic assessment in that the aims are to isolate the target behaviors and to determine the functional relationship between the target behaviors and environmental events. Little or no time is spent assessing theoretic constructs, such as unconscious conflicts or early life history, except for details directly relevant to the maintenance of the problem behavior.

The first step in the behavioral analysis is to identify ritualistic behaviors, which may include one or more of the following: (1) obsessive thoughts; (2) cognitive rituals (e.g., safe numbers, prayers, formulae); (3) washing and cleaning; (4) checking or seeking reassurance for an action; (5) repeating an action; (6) ordering objects; and (7) obsessive slowness (use of the Y-BOCS Symptom Checklist is particularly useful for this purpose). Questioning is directed toward determining whether the behavior occurs in the home, away from the home, or in both environments. Rachman and Hodgson[11] have found that many rituals or obsessions are triggered only in the home. This appears to be especially true among patients with checking rituals, because patients feel greatest responsibility for their actions at home.

Other assessment questions include: (1) Are there times when the patient is completely free of rituals or obsessions? (2) Are there times when rituals are reduced in intensity or frequency? and (3) Does the presence or absence of other people have an effect on the frequency or intensity of the rituals?

In addition to identifying the target rituals, the therapist must inquire about all objects or situations that the patient avoids to prevent himself or herself from engaging in rituals. As an example, a patient may avoid using public toilets to avoid extensive washing of body or clothes.

Once specific rituals and avoidance patterns are identified, the focus of questioning moves to the identification of all objects or situations that trigger anxiety, panic, or discomfort and that are reduced by engaging in rituals. Examples include: (1) objects such as dirt, urine, feces, or pesticides, which trigger washing rituals; and (2) the actions of switching off a light, checking a door, or viewing a plug in a socket, which trigger checking rituals.

When all external objects or situations that trigger rituals are identified, the focus of the interview moves to the identification of all thoughts, images, or impulses that trigger anxiety, panic, or discomfort and lead to ritualistic behavior to alleviate these feelings. Examples include "bad" numbers, sacrilegious images, and catastrophic thoughts. It is important at this point that the interviewer extract information about (1) what the patient believes will happen if he or she comes in contact with the external objects or situations that trigger the rituals; and (2) what the patient believes will happen if he or she recites "bad" numbers or experiences sacrilegious images.

We next assess the strength of the patient's belief that catastrophic events will actually happen if he or she fails to engage in ritualistic behaviors. The presence of overvalued ideation could be an indication for referral for cognitive therapy for OCD and/or an SRI drug if the patient either refuses to comply with exposure and response prevention or if this treatment is ineffective. An assessment of the patient's level of depression and anxiety also is important.

Finally, we determine whether the patient satisfies criteria for schizotypal or other personality disorders. Severe depression, overvalued ideation,[20] and SPD[39] have been identified as poor predictors of response to behavioral treatment.

If the patient is severely depressed or suffering from bipolar disorder, he or she is given a trial of antidepressant medication. Patients with severe depression respond well to behavior therapy procedures after their depression is controlled. In addition, we have reported on two patients with concomitant bipolar disorder and OCD who did not respond to behavioral treatment until their affective disorder was controlled with medication.[19]

If the patient meets criteria for SPD and is living in a stressful home environment, we attempt to arrange for a structured environment such as a day treatment center or halfway house during and after behavioral treatment. For these patients, we have found exposure and response prevention to work very slowly, if indeed at all.[44]

During the behavioral analysis, we determine whether the patient's rituals are reinforced by other members of the family (e.g., are there secondary gains?). If this is the case, then the family must be instructed that they will help the patient to overcome the OCD behaviors only if they will refrain from engaging in vicarious checking or providing reassurance in response to the patient's frequent requests. As an illustration, the family members of one ritualistic washer had agreed to enter their home through a cellar entrance, strip off all "contaminated" clothing, and dress in uncontaminated clothes provided by the patient, before being allowed to enter the living quarters.

Explanation of Exposure and Response Prevention

As described previously, the behavioral techniques consistently found effective in reducing compulsive behaviors and related obsessive thoughts are *exposure* to the feared situation and *response prevention,* in which the patient is helped to resist the urge to engage in compulsions to reduce discomfort. Exposure is often alternately termed "flooding," although this technically refers only to exposure to highly anxiety-producing situations or images.

The procedure of exposure and response prevention is straightforward in the case of a patient with compulsive handwashing and showering related to contamination fears of cancer "germs." In this case, exposure consists of gradually bringing the patient into contact with objects believed to be contaminated, such as a magazine or chair in the waiting area of an outpatient cancer clinic. The patient is then encouraged to remain in contact with the "contaminated" object for as long as possible (exposure), and then to refrain from handwashing or showering for at least 2 to 3 hours afterward (response prevention).

Although less obvious, the same principles of exposure and response prevention apply to patients with other types of compulsive rituals. For example, a patient who retraces a path when driving to ensure that he or she has not struck a pedestrian is accompanied for a ride by the therapist or family member; when driving, the patient is encouraged to engage in the feared behaviors, such as driving on a bumpy road, or passing pedestrians in the road (exposure), while resisting the urge to turn the car around to check that no one has been injured (response prevention).

Treatment Planning

It important to explain in detail to the patient the rationale and procedure of exposure and response prevention. By definition, these treatments cause discomfort. The patient must understand and be willing to accept this discomfort before treatment can commence.

It also is helpful to explain to patients that the rituals, thoughts, and emotions may respond to treatment at different rates. We explain that the easiest and most rapid changes usually come in the rituals themselves; as patients engage in response prevention, the rituals are stopped very rapidly. However, it is explained that thoughts and emotional arousal will take longer to change or "wear out;" this is a fact of learning and not something to become discouraged about. It also is explained that individuals vary in the time required for diminution of their obsessive thoughts, impulses, and feelings. This explanation appears to increase the patient's motivation.

If the patient's behaviors occur only at home, it is often necessary that a family member or a friend assist with treatment to ensure compliance (although some patients are able to engage in exposure and response prevention on their own). A therapist may make a home visit if the patient's home is near the hospital. The important point is that if the target behavior occurs only at home, then exposure therapy and response prevention carried out in the clinic will be useless.

After we determine the specific situations that are avoided or provoke rituals, these situations are ranked from least troublesome to most troublesome, forming a hierarchy of target situations, which will form the goals of the behavioral treatment. The situations are ranked on the degree of anxiety or discomfort they produce using the 100-point Subjective Units of Distress scale (SUDS)[45] (Figure 17-1). The patient is asked to rate each target situation based on the amount of anxiety it produces; after the situations are ranked from lowest to highest SUDS ratings, exposure therapy proceeds upward on the scale, beginning with the lower-rated items to maximize compliance.

Treatment of Obsessions Without Compulsions

The process of treatment will differ depending on the type of target behaviors. For example, for a patient with obsessive thoughts but without rituals, the target behaviors are the thoughts themselves. In some cases, the therapist may find that the thoughts are reliably and exclusively triggered by specific situations, such as taking public transportation, going to a beach, or shopping in a particular store. In these cases, *in vivo* exposure is often effective, supplemented by imaginal exposure often with the use of a tape-recorded description of the feared situation.

In some cases, obsessive thoughts are reliably triggered by specific mood states such as anger, anxiety, or guilt. In these cases, procedures designed to decrease these drive states, such as assertiveness training or relaxation training, can be useful. In assertiveness training, the patient is taught to express both negative and positive emotions in a socially appropriate way. This technique typically includes instruction, therapist modeling, role playing, and feedback of the patient's performance.

Emmelkamp[26] in a review of the behavioral treatment of obsessions concluded that ". . . it does seem that prolonged exposure in imagination has beneficial effects, while the results of thought-stopping are more variable. Further, assertiveness training was found to be quite effective in the treatment of harming obsessions."

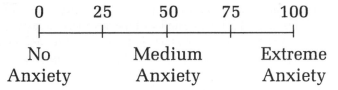

Fig. 17-1   Subjective Units of Distress Scale (SUDS) for rating anxiety.

Our clinic procedure with patients who present with obsessive thoughts with no discernible triggers has been to refer these patients for a trial of medication. Several of our patients with severe obsessive thoughts have responded to antidepressants.

When using imaginal flooding, we have found that it is important to rule out the presence of SPD in OCD patients before attempting to employ imaginal flooding. A man who sought treatment in our OCD clinic was found to meet criteria for both OCD and SPD, and had multiple obsessions and checking rituals. This patient had been treated elsewhere in the past with several sessions of imaginal flooding, which resulted in severe exacerbation of his anxiety. The patient explained that when he was asked to imagine the activities he most feared (e.g., stabbing nurses, beating people), he was later unsure as to whether he had only imagined the situations or had actually committed the actions. Although we have only evidence from this one case, it is possible that imaginal flooding may be contraindicated in patients with concomitant SPD and OCD, because of the frequent presence of magical thinking.

Treatment of Cleaning Rituals

For patients with washing or cleaning rituals but with none of the aforementioned negative predictors, the treatment is relatively straightforward. In many respects, the treatment is similar to the behavioral treatment of simple phobics with exposure and prevention of escape. Rachman and Hodgson[11] have noted the strong similarity between washers and phobics in their physiologic reaction to the feared situation and in their passive avoidance of the objects. Both types of patients attempt to avoid the feared situations at all costs.

Treatment sessions are generally 1 hour in length and involve persuading the patient to touch the feared objects. This session can often be performed in ← the clinic, as when the targets are public restrooms or common objects such as shoes or chairs. In addition, when the feared objects are in the home, but are nonetheless movable, the patient or a family member can bring objects from home into the session. We have had patients bring in objects such as mothballs, dirty clothing, and trash to facilitate *in vivo* exposure during the session.

Typically, the therapist first touches the object to demonstrate the procedure. This process is termed "participant modeling" and has been shown to enhance the effects of exposure and response prevention, probably by increasing the patient's motivation.[11] After the person touches the object, he is told not to wipe or wash his hands for the remainder of the session. No physical force is necessary. In our experience, despite fears to the contrary, all patients are able to refrain from performing cleaning rituals during the therapy session. During the time of response prevention, the patient is reminded that it is natural for urges to wash and feelings of contamination to continue for a while, but that these feelings will slowly decrease over time.

The patient is given a "homework assignment" to engage in the same types of activities daily until the next session and to refrain from engaging in cleaning rituals for at least 1 hour after the exposure. With the cooperation of the patient, a relative or friend is often asked to attend one of the early sessions and is explained the theory and procedures of exposure and response prevention. The relative or friend is then asked to act as the proxy of the therapist during the exposure and response prevention sessions at home. It is explained to the patient that if he or she feels angry during the exposure or response prevention, this anger should not be taken out on the other person, because that person is only supervising the home assignment previously agreed on by the patient and therapist.

If cleaning rituals occur only in the home, therapy should begin in the home, with either the therapist, friend, or family member carrying out the assignments. If a relative or friend participates, the assignments to be performed are determined during a session with the therapist, the patient, and the relative or friend present.

For patients with a combination of cleaning and checking rituals, we often begin behavior therapy focusing on cleaning rituals, which have a greater likelihood of rapid improvement. When cleaning rituals are controlled, behavioral treatment is shifted to other rituals.

Treatment of Checking Rituals

For patients with checking rituals, the procedure is different in several respects. First, response prevention must often be self-administered, because checkers frequently check only when they are alone. In arguing for the use of self-administered response prevention, Emmelkamp and Kraanen[46] found that therapist-controlled exposure *in vivo* may not be as effective with checkers because "several checkers in the present study were easily able to resist their urges to check when the therapist was present but were unable to do so in the periods between the treatment sessions").

The presence of another person can decrease the need to check because the patient assumes that the other person would take responsibility and notice if he or she did anything wrong or dangerous.[11] Secondly, checking occurs largely in the home, presumably because this is a place of greatest responsibility. Therefore, the response prevention assignments that can be carried out in the office or clinic are often limited. Thirdly, generalization is often poor from the office session to the home. For example, the patient may be able to shut off the light switch in the treatment office without checking, but he or she may continue to check light switches, electrical outlets, and door locks when alone at home. In some cases, the patient may engage in hundreds of checking activities per day; in these cases, the patient is often unable to enforce response prevention.[11]

We attempt to carry out any exposure and response prevention that is possible to perform in the office. For example, if the person has a fear of throwing away objects, he or she is asked to bring in trash from home and throw it away during the session without checking. If the person is afraid to enter stores for fear of closing the door on someone or afraid of handling objects in the store for fear of dropping them, the patient is accompanied into stores during the treatment hour and is requested to handle merchandise without checking afterward. If the person is afraid of walking past cars for fear of unknowingly damaging them, he or she is asked to accompany the therapist on a walk in which the patient walks approximately 3 feet away from parked cars. As soon as the patient is able to handle this, he or she may be asked to hold a set of keys in the hand closest to the cars. For those who are afraid of driving for fear that they will unknowingly run over a pedestrian, patients are asked to drive the therapist in their car during the session. Patients are frequently reminded not to check the rearview mirror or to turn the car around to check. Throughout all these activities, the patient is reminded during the session that it is natural to have urges to check, but that the thoughts about checking will decrease over time, because they are misleading signals from the body and should not be responded to.

The patient and an assistant if possible are told to practice similar activities between sessions, to keep a log of these activities, and to report back to the therapist at the next session. The patient is reminded that the rate that rituals and urges decrease is mainly a function of the number of repetitions without checking.

The treatment of checkers is complicated by the fact that they repeatedly request reassurance, as if they had an attention deficit. It is very common for a checker to report that he will continue to perform an action until "something clicks in my head and I am sure that it is right." Our practice is to tell patients that a feeling of confidence takes many practice sessions to acquire. They are also told that each time they have given in to the urge to check over the years, they have in fact decreased the feeling of confidence that is normally learned in childhood. Despite the difficulties in the treatment of checkers, this assertion is borne out for patients motivated to continue this treatment: they report that after many experiences of response prevention (sometimes hundreds), they begin to get a feeling of confidence in their actions.

In difficult patients who either do not respond to behavior therapy alone or are unable to comply fully with the treatment, a medication trial may be helpful. One patient who was unable to refrain from extensive checking rituals and who was too fearful to engage in exposure activities, found that after treatment with phenelzine she was able to engage in both the exposure and response prevention, because she felt braver and more sure of herself. This patient was able to eliminate approximately 50% of her checking rituals with this combined approach, with corresponding improvement in her social functioning.

Treatment of Primary Obsessional Slowness

This rare type of OCD is characterized by the patient's inability to complete routine tasks without getting "stuck." The patient is often unable to initiate tasks and may require many hours to complete a simple task such as dressing, walking from room to room, using a bathroom, eating, or taking medication. These patients are extremely difficult to treat without the cooperation of family members. A great deal of patience and firmness is required of both the therapist and family members when interacting with the patient.

As described in the treatment outcome section of this chapter, behavioral treatment of obsessional slowness consists of shaping procedures, in which the patient is given a specified time limit to initiate or complete a particular task. The patient must engage in the task within the allotted time, even if this means that the therapist or family member forces him to do so. If the allotted time is exceeded, treatment is likely to fail. Improvement of obsessional slowness with behavioral treatment is generally time consuming and progress is slow.

Summary of Clinical Management

The number of sessions required for treatment varies. We have found that some patients with cleaning rituals have responded in as few as three to five sessions, with appropriate home practice. On the other hand, we have treated patients with pervasive repeating and checking rituals who have been seen for years and still have rituals remaining.

The office sessions are of 1- to 1.5-hour duration and patients are instructed to engage in exposure and response prevention at home for 1 hour per day. At the outset of treatment, many patients are unable to tolerate 1 full hour in homework assignments.

Clinically, we will use any technique within reason that will help the patient to engage in the "active treatment" of exposure and response prevention. Almost all patients are willing to undergo the exposure treatment when adjunctive techniques such as thought stopping, cognitive restructuring, or medication are included. It appears that the addition of these techniques can reduce the percentage of patients who refuse to participate in exposure therapy—a figure typically found to be 20% to 30% in research trials.

At the very least, any trial of behavior therapy for OCD should include a minimum of 10 to 20 hours of actual *in vivo* or imaginal exposure to the feared situations along with good response prevention. Exposure can be carried out alone, with the therapist, or with a family member or friend; good compliance is the key. Some improvement should be noticeable by the end of this trial, although continued treatment will probably be necessary.

THEORETIC CONSIDERATIONS
Learning and Maintenance of Compulsions

Marks[4] has cogently argued that it is not necessary to assume that compulsive rituals are learned or conditioned, because this is ultimately an untestable hypothesis. Instead he suggests that we not call the environmental event that precedes the ritual a "conditioned stimulus," but rather call it an "evoking stimulus." Further, he suggests that instead of referring to the ritual as the "conditioned response," we operationally identify it as the "evoked response." As Marks[4] points out, these definitions not only possess the advantage of parsimony, but they further suggest the effective treatment procedure: break the connection between the evoking stimulus and the evoked response.

Nevertheless, a general anxiety-reduction theory of OCD has developed, and it has implicitly or explicitly influenced most behavioral treatments. The following discussion includes only those theoretic considerations that have clear clinical applications. A complete review of theories of obsessions and compulsions can be found in Rachman and Hodgson.[11]

The predominant behavioral explanation of the factors that maintain obsessive and compulsive behavior has been the two-stage learning theory of Mowrer.[47] According to this theory, anxiety is classically conditioned to a specific environmental event, such as the OCD patient who feels anxious after touching a contaminated object (stage 1—classical conditioning). The person then engages in compulsive or ritualistic behavior to decrease anxiety. If the compulsion succeeds in reducing anxiety, the compulsive behavior is reinforced and is more likely to occur again in the future, such as the OCD patient who washes to reduce anxiety (stage 2—operant conditioning). Ritualistic behavior preserves the fear response, because the person does not remain in contact with the eliciting stimulus long enough for the conditioned anxiety to habituate. In turn, the anxiety reduction preserves the compulsive behavior, producing a cycle that is difficult to break.

Wolpe[45] proposed a modification of the anxiety-reduction hypothesis, suggesting instead that there are two classes of obsessional behavior: one anxiety-increasing and the other anxiety-decreasing. Anxiety-increasing obsessions occur automatically in response to anxiety-provoking stimulation, whereas anxiety-reducing compulsions occur as a reaction to the anxiety and their performance temporarily decreases anxiety.

Although the anxiety-reduction theory has been the most-accepted behavioral theory of obsessive and compulsive behavior, others have been presented,[48] partly based on the clinical experience that some rituals actually increase anxiety. However, these are a small minority of all rituals.[11] In addition, compulsive behaviors have been conceptualized as stereotyped behaviors.[6] However, most compulsions appear to be purposeful behaviors, rather than analogs of stereotyped behaviors as seen in animals or brain-damaged humans.

The anxiety-reduction theory was tested by Rachman and Hodgson.[11] They recorded subjective measures of anxiety and physiologic measures of autonomic arousal when subjects were exposed to situations that evoked compulsive rituals. As predicted by the two-stage theory, exposure to the stimulus resulted in an increase in both physiologic and subjective measures of anxiety. Also, in accord with this theory, when patients were allowed to engage in ritualistic behavior, there were decreases in both measures of anxiety. However, interruption of the compulsive ritual by the experiments did not result in the predicted increase in anxiety. These patterns held strongest for patients with washing or cleaning rituals. On the other hand, patients with predominantly checking rituals showed smaller increases in anxiety when presented with the evoking situation. Further, engaging in the compulsive rituals produced less reduction in the elicited anxiety, and in fact, in 7 of 36 trials, it was found that engaging in checking rituals actually increased anxiety—a phenomenon not seen in any of the cleaners. In checkers, changes in anxiety were reflected only in subjective reports, but no significant changes were noted in pulse rate variability—a measure of autonomic arousal.[11]

Rachman and Hodgson[11] summarized their revised theory of obsessions and compulsions and their effects on anxiety:

> Obsessions and compulsions can (1) reduce anxiety or discomfort; (2) increase anxiety or discomfort; or (3) leave anxiety or discomfort unchanged. Compulsive cleaning rituals most often follow the type (1) pattern (i.e., they are discomfort reducing). Obsessions follow the second pattern (i.e., they increase discomfort), and checking rituals follow either the first or the second pattern.

Patients suffering with obsessions but with no compulsive behaviors have been largely ignored in behavioral theory. It is typically assumed that the obsessive thoughts, images, and urges are subject to operant and classical conditioning just as motoric responses, and they are treated in similar ways. As we will see, the literature is unclear concerning the usefulness of behavioral techniques for such patients.

Biologic Preparedness for Fears

How can learning theory account for the fact that obsessions and compulsions tend to cluster around certain themes, usually those that have been emphasized by psychoanalytic theory? Rachman and Hodgson[11] found that among their patients, 55% of obsessive thoughts involved contamination through dirt or disease, 35% involved orderliness themes, 19% involved aggressive themes, 13% involved sexual themes, and 10% involved religious themes. These proportions appear to be relatively consistent across cultures.

Seligman[18] has proposed a theory of biologic preparedness in the formation of fears. He rejects the belief that fear is determined by random factors. Instead, he proposes that we are highly prepared to acquire certain fears with speed and ease. These "prepared phobias" are said to be of particular biologic significance and are survivors from earlier periods of human history.

DeSilva, et al[49] studied 69 phobic and 82 obsessive patients to determine the relative prevalence of prepared versus unprepared fears according to Seligman's criteria. It was found that the great majority of phobias and obsessions met the criteria for biologically prepared fears.

Rachman and Hodgson[11] have hypothesized that preparedness for specific fears, mood disturbances, and family learning histories interact to produce exaggerated obsessive and compulsive behaviors. They believe that biologic preparedness may play a larger role in cleaning compulsions than in checking rituals. On the other hand, family learning history may be more significant in the etiology of checking rituals.

Stimulus Generalization of Obsessions and Compulsions

Although obsessions and compulsions may initially be evoked by circumscribed situations, they soon begin to spread to other situations. This process can be conceptualized as stimulus generalization of a classically conditioned response. Here, other situations, which are in some respect similar to the original conditioned situation, come to evoke anxiety or discomfort. The generalization may occur along various characteristics of the original situation, including size, shape, color, facial pattern, or symbolic meaning.

In OCD, it is common to see generalization along symbolic dimensions. For example, in many Western cultures, sexual or aggressive thoughts are "dirty." In general, we are able to wash off "dirt" from ourselves, and so we frequently see patients engaging in washing rituals when feelings of guilt, aggression, or sexuality are reported. A classic example of the inadvertent generalization of compulsions along symbolic lines was provided by Meyer.[9] A woman suffering from 36 years of intrusive blasphemous thoughts regarding sexual intercourse reduced guilt and anxiety by repeating ritualistic behavior a certain number of times. According to the patient, it was not until she underwent 11 years of psychoanalysis and additional stimuli were interpreted as being sexual symbols, that she began to avoid new situations including eating oblong objects and performing any activity that could conceivably have sexual connotations (e.g., shutting drawers, putting in plugs, wiping receptacles, entering underground trains). As each situation was interpreted as a sexual symbol, it came to evoke ritualistic behaviors. This patient was successfully treated by Meyer with exposure to the feared activities (e.g., eating sausages, imagining sexual intercourse with the Holy Spirit) and by preventing the patient from engaging in the rituals. This is another example of successful behavioral treatment of symptoms that conform to psychodynamic concepts.

Functional Autonomy of Rituals

In the early stages of their development, compulsive rituals may clearly serve the anxiety-reduction function as theorized by Mowrer.[47] However, in long-standing compulsive rituals, these behaviors can come under the control of other environmental stimuli.[50] In the early stages of OCD, compulsive rituals can sometimes be treated through elimination of the underlying drive states of anxiety or aggression. Walton and Mather[50] cite as evidence the case of a man with severe OCD of recent origin whose hand-washing ritual was assumed to be evoked by anxiety and guilt over violently aggressive fantasies. The handwashing disappeared after the passive client received training in assertiveness.[50] On the other hand, these authors contend that in problems of long duration, other cues besides the original conditioning ones come to elicit the rituals. In this way, the compulsive rituals become functionally autonomous or independent of the original stimulus. These authors noted only partial improvement in compulsive rituals when therapy was restricted to the original conditioned stimulus or to avoidance responses themselves. Walton and Mather's[50] explanation was partly supported by Foa, et al,[31] who found that exposure therapy was necessary to reduce anxiety, whereas response prevention was required to reduce compulsive rituals. In clinical practice, careful behavioral analysis will determine the extent of generalization and will indicate the most appropriate treatment.

Difficulties in Elimination of Compulsive Rituals

Because compulsive behavior usually prevents or reduces anxiety or discomfort, it is functionally an escape or avoidance behavior. As a clinical example, whenever the patient is exposed to the evoking situation (e.g., a can of gasoline), he engages in the ritual escape behavior of handwashing, which reduces the unpleasant feelings, thereby paradoxically strengthening the compulsion with the cycle continuing unbroken.

It is known from animal learning studies[47] that when the unpleasant stimulus to be avoided is extraordinarily intense (e.g., strong electric shock), the avoidance response will persist for hundreds of trials and is nonextinguishable unless "therapeutic" procedures, which are essentially methods of response prevention, are used. An example would be erecting a glass barrier to prevent the animal from carrying out the avoidance behaviors. This finding has been replicated in humans by Turner and Solomon;[51] the strong resistance of avoidance responses to extinction may account for the necessity of response prevention techniques in OCD patients to rid them of their symptoms.[6]

An additional difficulty in helping humans to unlearn maladaptive behaviors is that, unlike research animals, we modify our actions based on instructions about the situation and based on our expectations and predictions of future occurrences.[52] This phenomenon is especially important in OCD. Here, although the therapist or relative tells the patient that no terrible event will befall them if they do not engage in the ritual, the patient often does not fully believe this. As a result, patients repeatedly ask, "Are you sure nothing will happen if?. . . ." This is especially true in patients with checking rituals, who have little confidence in their judgment. Such patients may be unsure whether they actually heard the therapist's assurance or merely imagined it, or whether written reassurance is in the therapist's handwriting or forged by the patient to mislead himself.

Complications in Reducing Anxiety or Discomfort

The majority of desensitization procedures are based on the principle of habituation of an emotional response; that is, with repeated exposure to a feared situation, the emotional response will dissipate. Here, the patient is gradually exposed to situations that are increasingly similar to the central feared situation. With extended exposure, the evoking situations gradually lose their ability to elicit anxiety or discomfort. The behavior therapy technique of exposure as used in treating OCD is based on this principle. Several factors influence the speed of habituation of the emotional response, and in some cases determine whether it will occur at all. These factors must be taken into account in planning behavioral treatments:

1. The speed of habituation of emotional responses varies from person to person. That is, some people require 30 minutes of exposure to the stimulus, whereas others may require repeated 2-hour sessions of exposure before any diminution in the emotional response occurs. Also, some patients experience further reductions in the fear between exposure sessions, whereas others do not.[20]

2. Patients who are severely depressed may never habituate to the situation regardless of how long they are exposed to it.[19]

3. If the OCD patient truly believes that the object or situation is in fact dangerous, he/she often does not habituate, regardless of the length of exposure.[20]

4. Different types of classically conditioned responses have different habituation times. Some autonomic responses, such as animal phobias, can be deconditioned relatively rapidly, but others, such as food aversions, may require extremely long times to extinguish. Classically conditioned responses in which both the stimulus and response are internal (i.e., interoceptive) are notoriously difficult to unlearn. This may explain why associations between emotional states, such as sexual arousal and guilt, are often resistant to treatment. Further, the time required for thoughts to habituate (if in fact they do habituate) is not known, because they remain elusive dependent variables to study. As a result, a patient undergoing behavior therapy usually finds that thoughts, rituals, and emotional reactions habituate at different speeds.

5. We now know that some OCD symptoms do not involve anxiety at all, especially those that are also found as part of Tourette's disorder and other tic disorders.[53] In these cases (symptoms that may more closely resemble

complex motor tics than compulsive rituals), the anxiety habituation model of exposure and response prevention may not be applicable at all.

These complicating factors, not the least of which is that many OCD patients have concomitant affective illness and often require medication,[19] may explain why few OCD patients can overcome the problem on their own. Other fears, such as height, water, and occasionally agoraphobia, can be overcome without recourse to a therapist. If by chance a patient musters the courage to fight his obsessive fears and confront the feared situation without ritualizing, feelings of fear and discomfort are likely to remain strong for some time. Unless some form of external support is available (e.g., therapist, friend, social institution), the patient is likely to revert to ritualizing before the anxiety can be totally diminished.

SUMMARY

We have known how to successfully treat the most common obsessions and compulsions for more than a quarter of a century. However, new methods for treating less common (and less phobic-like) symptoms are needed and should be tested "off-line" when we strive to make our first-line treatment of exposure and response prevention more widely available.

REFERENCES

1. Baxter LR Jr, Schwartz JM, Bergman KS, et al: Caudate glucose metabolic rate changes with both drug and behavior therapy for obsessive-compulsive disorder, *Arch Gen Psychiatry* 49:681–689, 1992.
2. Schwartz JM, Stoessel PW, Baxter LR Jr, et al: Systematic changes in cerebral glucose metabolic rate after successful behavior modification treatment of obsessive-compulsive disorder, *Arch Gen Psychiatry* 53:109–113, 1996.
3. Marks IM, Personal communication, 1995.
4. Marks IM: Review of behavioral psychotherapy. I: Obsessive-compulsive disorders, *Am J Psychiatry* 138:584–592, 1981.
5. Marks IM, Stern RS, Mawson D, et al: Clomipramine and exposure for obsessive-compulsive rituals, *Br J Psychiatry* 136:1–25, 1980.
6. Sturgis ET, Meyer V: Obsessive-compulsive disorders. In Turner SM, Calhoun KC, Adams HE, editors: *Handbook of clinical behavior therapy,* New York, 1980, John Wiley and Sons.
7. Freud S: *Three case histories,* New York, 1973, Macmillan, (Translated by P. Rieff; Originally published in 1909.)
8. Freud S: Turnings in the ways of psychoanalytic therapy. In *Collected papers,* vol 2, London, 1924, Hogarth Press. (Originally published in 1919.)
9. Bandura A: *Principles of behavior modification,* New York, 1969, Holt, Rinehart and Winston.
10. Foa EB, Steketee G: Emergent fears during treatment of three obsessive compulsives: symptom substitution or deconditioning? *J Behav Ther Exp Psychiatry* 8:353–358, 1977.

11. Rachman SJ, Hodgson RJ: *Obsessions and compulsions,* Englewood Cliffs, NJ, 1980, Prentice Hall.
12. Foa EB, Chambless DL: Habituation of subjective anxiety during flooding in imagery, *Behav Res Ther* 16:391–399, 1978.
13. Latimer PR, Sweet AA: Cognitive versus behavioral procedures in cognitive-behavior therapy: a critical review of the evidence, *J Behav Ther Exp Psychiatry* 15:9–22, 1984.
14. Rachman SJ: *Fear and courage,* San Francisco, 1978, WH Freeman and Co.
15. Lang PJ: Fear reduction and fear behavior: problems in treating a construct. In Schlien JM, editor: *Research in psychotherapy,* vol 3, Washington, 1968, American Psychological Association.
16. Wolpe J: The two modes of conditioning of neurotic anxiety. Presented at Seventh World Congress of Psychiatry, Vienna, July 14, 1983.
17. Wolpe J, Lande SD, McNally RJ, et al: Differentiation between classically conditioned and cognitively based neurotic fears: two pilot studies. *J Behav Ther Exp Psychiatry* 16:287–293, 1985.
18. Seligman MEP: Phobias and preparedness, *Behav Res Ther* 2:307–320, 1971.
19. Lader M, Wing L: Physiological measures in agitated and retarded depressed patients, *J Psychiatr Res* 7:89–100, 1969.
19a. Baer L, Minichiello WE, Jenike MJ: Behavioral treatment in two cases of obsessive-compulsive disorder with concomitant bipolar affective disorder, *Am J Psychiatry* 142:358–360, 1985.
20. Foa EB: Failures in treating obsessive-compulsives, *Behav Res Ther* 17:169–176, 1979.
21. Orloff LM, Battle MA, Baer L, et al: Long-term follow-up of 88 patients with obsessive-compulsive disorder, *Am J Psychiatry* 151:441–442, 1994.
22. Foa EB, Grayson JB, Steketee G, et al: Success and failure in the behavioral treatment of obsessive-compulsives, *J Consult Clin Psychol* 51:287–297, 1983.
23. Ball SG, Baer L, Otto MW: Symptom subtypes of obsessive-compulsive disorder in behavioral treatment studies: a quantitative review, *Behav Res Ther* 34:47–51, 1996.
24. Meyer V, Levy R, Schnurer A: The behavioural treatment of obsessive-compulsive disorders. In Beech HR, editor: *Obsessional states,* London, 1974, Methuen.
25. Foa EB, Goldstein A: Continuous exposure and complete response prevention in the treatment of obsessive-compulsive neurosis, *Behav Res Ther* 9:821–829, 1978.
26. Emmelkamp PMG: *Phobic and obsessive-compulsive disorders: theory, research, and practice,* New York, 1982, Plenum.
27. Boulougouris JC: Variables affecting the behavior modification of obsessive-compulsive patients treated by flooding. In Boulougouris JC, Rabavilas AD, editors: *The treatment of phobic and obsessive compulsive disorders,* Oxford, 1977, Pergamon Press.
28. Rasmussen SA, Tsuang MT: The epidemiology of obsessive compulsive disorder, *J Clin Psychiatry* 45:450–457, 1984.
29. Baer L, Minichiello WE: Behavior therapy for obsessive compulsive disorder. In Burrows GD, Noyes R, Roth M, editors: *Handbook of anxiety,* vol 4, Amsterdam, 1990, Elsevier Science.
30. Rachman SJ, Hodgson RJ, Marks IM: The treatment of chronic obsessional neurosis, *Behav Res Ther* 9:237–247, 1971.

31. Foa EB, Steketee G, Milby JB: Differential effects of exposure and response prevention in obsessive-compulsive washers, *J Clin Consult Psychol* 48(1):71–79, 1980.

31a. Fonagy P, Higgitt AC: A note on statistical inference in meta-analysis, *Behav Res Ther* 21(1):87–88, 1983.

32. Christensen H, Hadzi-Pavlovic D, Andrews G, et al: Behavior therapy and tricyclic medication in the treatment of obsessive-compulsive disorder: a quantitative review, *J Consult Clin Psychol* 55(5):701–711, 1987.

33. Quality Assurance Project: Treatment outlines for the management of obsessive-compulsive disorders, *Austr NZ J Psychiatry* 19:240–253, 1985.

34. Van Balkom AJ, Van Oppen P, Vermeulen AWA, et al: A meta-analysis on the treatment of obsessive-compulsive disorder: a comparison of antidepressants, behavior therapy, and cognitive therapy. *Clin Psychol Rev* 14:359–381, 1994.

35. Marks IM, Hodgson R, Rachman S: Treatment of chronic obsessive-compulsive neurosis by in-vivo exposure: a two-year follow-up and issues in treatment, *Br J Psychiatry* 127:349–364, 1975.

36. Hiss H, Foa EB, Kozak MJ: Relapse prevention program for treatment of obsessive-compulsive disorder, *J Consult Clin Psychol* 62:801–808, 1994.

37. Rachman S, Cobb J, Grey S, et al: The behavioural treatment of obsessional-compulsive disorders, with and without clomipramine, *Behav Res Ther* 17:467–478, 1979.

38. Steketee G, Foa E, Grayson JB: Recent advances in the behavioral treatment of obsessive-compulsives, *Arch Gen Psychiatry* 39:1365–1371, 1982.

39. Minichiello WE, Baer L, Jenike MA: Schizotypal personality disorder: a poor prognostic indicator for behavior therapy in the treatment of obsessive-compulsive disorder, *J Anx Dis.* 1:273–276, 1987.

40. Carey R, Baer L, Minichiello WE, et al: MMPI correlates of obsessive-compulsive disorder, *J Clin Psychiatry* 47:371–372, 1986.

41. Solyom L, DiNicola VF, Phil M, et al: Is there an obsessive psychosis? Aetiological and prognostic factors of an atypical form of obsessive compulsive neurosis, *Can J Psychiatry* 30:372–380, 1985.

42. Keijsers GPJ, Hoogduin CAL, Schaap CPDR: Predictors of treatment outcome in the behavioral treatment of obsessive-compulsive disorder, *Br J Psychiatry* 165:781–786, 1994.

43. Buchanan AW, Meng KS, Marks IM: What predicts improvement and compliance during the behavioral treatment of obsessive-compulsive disorder? *Anxiety* 2:22–27, 1996.

44. Jenike et al: Concomitant obsessive-compulsive disorder and schizotypal personality disorder, *Am J Psychiatry* 143:530–533, 1986.

45. Wolpe J: *Psychotherapy by reciprocal inhibition,* Stanford, Calif, 1958, Stanford University Press.

46. Emmelkamp PMG, Kraanen J: Therapist-controlled exposure in vivo versus self-controlled exposure in vivo: a comparison with obsessive-compulsive patients, *Behav Res Ther* 15:491–495, 1977.

47. Deese J, Hulse SH: *The psychology of learning,* New York, 1967, McGraw Hill.

48. Beech HR, editor: *Obsessional states,* London, 1974, Methuen.

49. DeSilva P, Rachman S, Seligman M: Prepared phobias and obsessions: therapeutic outcome, *Behav Res Ther* 15:54–77, 1977.

50. Walton D, Mather MD: The application of learning principles to the treatment of obsessive compulsive states in the acute and chronic phases of illness, *Behav Res Ther* 1:163–174, 1963.
51. Turner LH, Solomon RL: Human traumatic avoidance learning: theory and experiments on the operant-respondent distinction, *Psychol Mongr* 1962.
52. Lindley RH, Moyer KE: Effects of instructions on the extinction of a conditioned finger-withdrawal response, *J Exp Psychol* 61:82–88, 1961.
53. Miguel EC, Coffey BJ, Baer L, et al: Phenomenology of intentional repetitive behaviors in obsessive-compulsive disorder and Tourette's disorder, *J Clin Psychiatry* 56:246–255, 1995.

18

Cognitive Theory and Treatment of Obsessive-Compulsive Disorder

*Gail S. Steketee, Ph.D, Randy O. Frost, Ph.D,
Josée Rhéaume, Ph.D, Sabine Wilhelm, Ph.D*

Several theorists have proposed that people with obsessive-compulsive disorder (OCD) exhibit mental phenomena (e.g., irrational beliefs and attitudes, inaccurate reasoning) that may contribute to the development of the disorder and interfere with treatment. In this chapter, we briefly present some general cognitive models proposed for OCD and follow this with a more extended discussion of several cognitive domains or areas that appear to contain most of the dysfunctional beliefs and attitudes exhibited by patients with OCD. These domains include threat estimation, control over thoughts, perfectionism, tolerance for ambiguity, excessive responsibility, and overimportance of thoughts. In this context, we describe theoretic ideas pertinent to these domains, along with empirical evidence of their importance. A discussion of recent strategies for assessing cognition in OCD follows, with recommendations for clinically useful strategies. Finally, clinical cognitive therapy procedures are reviewed, both as stand-alone treatments and as adjuncts to exposure and medication treatment.

COGNITIVE APPRAISAL MODELS FOR OBSESSIVE-COMPULSIVE DISORDER

Two major cognitive models have been proposed for OCD: one emphasizing threat appraisal, the other emphasizing cognitive processes. The latter model hypothesizes deficits in basic processes like attention, memory, and the structuring of information[1] and is discussed later in this chapter. The former hypothesizes concerns faulty appraisals or interpretations of intrusive thoughts based on beliefs and assumptions about the world that in turn lead to faulty attempts at coping. Although specific beliefs may be too idiosyncratic to be useful in understanding OCD, research has suggested certain general cognitive or belief domains that are characteristic of OCD patients.

Most contemporary cognitive theories grow out of an appraisal model of the development and maintenance of stress and anxiety.[2] In this model, an appraisal of threat (primary appraisal) is followed by an appraisal of one's ability to cope (secondary appraisal). In the context of OCD, primary appraisal occurs in conjunction with the intrusive thought, whereas secondary appraisal leads to faulty coping (compulsions, avoidance). With regard to primary appraisal in OCD, Carr[3,4] first suggested that sufferers make unusually high estimates of the probability of unfavorable outcomes. Hence, they anticipate danger or negative outcomes more frequently, thus presuming threat more readily. Compulsive behaviors are seen as attempts to reduce the threat based on this erroneous judgment. McFall and Wollersheim[5] hypothesized that this inaccurate primary appraisal process is produced by four types of beliefs or assumptions: (1) one must be perfectly competent to feel worthwhile and avoid criticism; (2) making mistakes or failing to meet one's goals should result in punishment or condemnation; (3) magical rituals can prevent disastrous outcomes; and (4) certain thoughts and feelings are unacceptable, potentially catastrophic, and worthy of punishment. These authors also hypothesized that secondary appraisals underestimating coping capacity lead to uncertainty, fears of loss of control, and anxiety, resulting in rituals and ruminations to cope with discomfort.

Guidano and Liotti[6] suggested that several irrational beliefs described by Ellis[7] as a target of rational-emotive therapy (RET) are relevant to OCD. Several are similar to beliefs discussed by McFall and Wollersheim[5] that were described previously (competence, certainty, and the need to avoid criticism). Other such beliefs are "I should be very concerned with potential danger," and "there are perfect solutions to problems and I must achieve them." Warren and Zgourides[8] also emphasized the importance of beliefs about perfection, certainty, and the unacceptability of certain types of thoughts and impulses. They suggested that biologic vulnerability and learning experiences shape the development of these irrational thoughts. As these beliefs develop in response to intrusive thoughts, attentional focus narrows, exacerbating hypervigilance for the intrusions.

Salkovskis[9,10] has formulated a cognitive model of OCD that draws heavily on Beck's cognitive theory of emotional disorders.[11] Salkovskis argued that intrusive cognitions are normal phenomena that are universally experienced. In fact, research has shown that approximately 90% of the population have intrusive cognitions whose content is difficult to distinguish from that of obsessions.[12-14] According to Salkovskis' model, what distinguishes people with OCD is not that they experience intrusive thoughts, but how they appraise them. Whereas most people simply ignore these phenomena, people with OCD pay attention to them and believe them to be important. The nature and extent of the attention given to these intrusive thoughts depend on a set of underlying beliefs and assumptions about them. For people with OCD, these beliefs are characterized by an exaggerated sense of responsibility for causing or failing to prevent harm to oneself or others.

Normally, people judge themselves to be responsible when their actions bring about an unpleasant outcome, and they do not judge themselves to be responsible (or do so to a much lesser extent) if their lack of action brings about a negative outcome.[15] Spranka, et al[15] called this the "omission bias." Salkovskis, Richards, and Forrester[16] suggested that OCD patients do not show this omission bias. Further, by paying attention to intrusive thoughts about negative outcomes, the person with OCD considers the possibility of a catastrophe that can be prevented. Not acting to prevent such a catastrophe is experienced as an "omission" that could bring about a tragedy. The person then feels responsible for "failing to act."

OCD patients experience guilt and seek ways to reduce discomfort, perceived responsibility, and feared consequences of having the thought.[9,10,16] Such attempts to neutralize possible harm take the form of overt compulsions (washing, checking, etc.), mental rituals, attempts to put things right, thought suppression, and reassurance seeking.

With respect to the appraisal process described previously, the person first appraises the intrusive thought as an indication that he is in some way responsible for harm or its prevention. Secondary appraisal involves an assessment of how to respond to the situation. Because the initial effort to complete rituals is minimal compared with the effort to tolerate the discomfort, the cost:benefit ratio favors this mode of coping. Paradoxically, such neutralizing efforts actually maintain the obsessive thoughts via negative reinforcement of anxiety reduction.

This model has generated a great deal of research, which has supported the hypothesis that beliefs about responsibility are important features of OCD. In an anecdotal report, Rachman[24a] suggested that perceived responsibility for harm was central to OCD. Some studies have found significant correlations between responsibility and OCD symptoms,[17,18] and manipulation of responsibility has led to temporary changes in symptom severity.[19,20] This model has also generated treatment strategies designed to reduce excessive responsibility which are described later in this chapter (e.g., see References 23 and 136).

Several revisions and extensions of this cognitive model have also been proposed. Clark and Purdon[21] suggested that dysfunctional beliefs about the need and ability to control thoughts and the consequences of not doing so should be emphasized. They proposed that neutralization may be prompted only when efforts at thought control fail, and that depressed mood interferes with efforts at thought control. Freeston, et al[22] broadened earlier cognitive models of OCD to include five domains: (1) the tendency to attribute excessive importance to the occurrence of a thought; (2) an excessive sense of responsibility for harm coming to oneself or someone else as a result of one's actions (or inaction); (3) the need for perfection, especially with regard to certainty and control; (4) the overestimation of the probability and severity of negative outcomes;[4] and (5) the belief that the experience of anxiety caused by intrusive thoughts is dangerous. Freeston, et al[23] also postulated a role for negative mood in this process: negative mood increases the frequency and duration of intrusive thoughts, thus decreasing the efficacy of neutralization strategies. Further, mood may activate distorted appraisals and increase attention to obsessional cues.

COGNITIVE DOMAINS IN OBSESSIVE-COMPULSIVE DISORDER

An international group of researchers recently attempted to determine the most relevant domains of OCD–related beliefs and appraisals.[24] This group identified six general domains of belief relevant to OCD; these are described in the following paragraphs.

Responsibility

Salkovskis' cognitive model of OCD[9] (described previously) focused mainly on distorted beliefs about responsibility, proposing that these are both central and specific to OCD. Rachman[24a] concurred that excessive responsibility often characterizes this disorder. Responsibility has been defined as, "the belief that one possesses pivotal power to provoke or prevent subjectively crucial outcomes that may be real or occur at a moral level."[25] Following Rachman's and Salkovskis' views, responsibility is the cognitive variable that has received the most attention from recent research. Findings related to various components of responsibility are discussed in the following paragraphs.

1. Beliefs about responsibility and perceived responsibility. Self-report data have provided some support for the responsibility model. In a recent study with nonclinical subjects, perceived pivotal influence predicted perceived responsibility better than overestimation of threat, giving empirical support for this model.[26] Other studies of nonclinical samples have found a significant link between responsibility and OCD symptoms. For example, perceived responsibility has been found to be significantly related to self-reports of obsessive-compulsive symptoms and thought suppression[27] and compulsive activities.[28] However, Rachman, Thordarson, Shafran, and Woody[29] reported that participants who scored high on obsessive-compulsive symptoms did not differ from low obsessive-compulsive scorers on several aspects of responsibility, including responsibility for harm.

Several studies have experimentally manipulated responsibility. For example, when Lopatka and Rachman[19] had experimenters assume full responsibility for any consequence resulting from not checking compulsively, patients reported significant decreases in both subjective discomfort and urges to check. However, these results were not replicated for patients with compulsive washing, perhaps because this group included people who feared contaminating themselves as well as people who felt responsible for contaminating others.

According to Ladouceur and colleagues,[25] nonclinical subjects in a high-responsibility condition checked significantly more during a classification task and reported being more preoccupied with errors and more anxious during the task, compared with those who performed the task under the low-responsibility condition. These results were recently replicated and expanded by this same group.[30] Overall, the results suggest that responsibility is related to checking, but it is not yet clear whether this can be generalized to other compulsive behaviors.

2. Omission and commission. It has been suggested that normal subjects have an omission bias, meaning that they place more weight on deliberately causing an adverse outcome (commission) and less emphasis on failing to prevent a negative event from happening (omission).[15] Although the social psychologists have extensively studied the evaluation of responsibility through omission or commission,[15,31,32] no studies have directly addressed this question in OCD patients. Salkovskis and colleagues[16] suggested that OCD patients are equally concerned about failing to prevent an outcome as about directly causing that outcome. Our clinical observations point to the presence of such fears of being responsible for omission among OCD symptoms, but direct empirical evidence for this hypothesis is lacking.

3. Guilt. Although guilt is considered a negative mood, it is often associated with the cognitive evaluation of responsibility. Perceived responsibility for threat would be expected to lead to guilt that could be alleviated by taking restorative action in the form of neutralizing.[33] Consistent with this hypothesis, obsessional subjects have reported significantly more guilt than nonobsessional subjects.[29,33] Shafran, et al[33] also found trait guilt to be a significant predictor of obsessionality. Studying college students, Niler and Beck[34] reported that guilt was the strongest predictor of the content of obsessive thoughts and compulsive rituals, whereas Freeston, et al[12] observed that guilt (as well as sadness and worry) was more commonly associated with escaping or avoiding intrusions than not responding to them. However, guilt does not appear to be specific to OCD. In a study using clinical subjects, Manchanda, Sethi and Gupta[35] failed to distinguish OCD patients from depressed patients on a measure of guilt, and Steketee, Quay and White[36] noted that guilt scores were not higher in OCD subjects compared to anxious controls. Taken together, the results provide good support for the existence of a link among responsibility, guilt, and obsessive-compulsive symptoms, but further study of these cognitive aspects is clearly needed.

Threat Estimation

Several writers have suggested that OCD results from the overestimation of the probability (risk) and severity of harm, as well as the underestimation of one's coping abilities.[3,5] McFall and Wollersheim[5] also proposed that individuals with OCD overestimate the likelihood of making mistakes. Consistent with these theorists, other writers have pointed out that many individuals with OCD overestimate the risk of negative consequences for a variety of actions,[37-39] and presume worse outcomes.[37] The overprediction of probability and severity of subjective risk may be an important clinical feature of OCD that must be addressed in treatment.

The mechanism underlying the overestimation of threat has been the subject of some speculation. Kozak, Foa, and McCarthy[40] hypothesized that people with OCD have difficulty with epistemologic reasoning related to their excessive fear of harm. Although most people assume that a situation is safe unless it has been determined to be dangerous, most OCD sufferers seem to view situations as dangerous unless proven safe. They appear to base their beliefs about danger in the absence of evidence that guarantees safety. Further, they fail to assume general safety in spite of specific experiences of exposure to feared situations in which no harm occurred. Consequently, although rituals are performed to reduce the likelihood of harm, they can never really guarantee safety and therefore must be repeated over and over. Frost and Hartl[41] have hypothesized a related phenomenon among compulsive hoarders: The possessions of hoarders seem to serve as signals of safety and comfort in a world that is perceived as threatening (see Chapter 23).

Barlow[42] has suggested that biologic vulnerabilities lead to false-alarm reactions to thoughts perceived as threatening. Attention narrows onto these thoughts, followed by unsuccessful attempts to avoid them and subsequent efforts (compulsions) to prevent the unfortunate perceived consequences. Other cognitive processes may contribute to the overprediction of threat as well. Butler and Mathews[43] have proposed that available heuristics (e.g., recency, frequency, saliency, and selective exposure effects) influence probability estimates for particular events. For example, having recently read an account of an automobile accident increases the subjective estimate of the probability of having an automobile accident. Consistent with this notion, the increased frequency and saliency of obsessional thoughts about harm may lead individuals to overestimate the likelihood of such events.

A limited amount of research supports the hypothesis that obsessive-compulsives overestimate threat. In one study, people who scored high on obsessive symptoms, as well as those people diagnosed with OCD, preferred to avoid taking even ordinary risks like leaving their car unlocked very briefly or drinking out of a friend's cup.[44] In another laboratory, overestimation of harm was identified as a feature of volunteer subjects who complained of obsessive-compulsive symptoms.[28] Also, Rhéaume, Ladouceur and Freeston[45] found that measures of perceived danger correlated with OCD severity among nonclinical subjects. Working with clinical samples, Steiner[39] found obsessional patients more cautious than other groups in self-reported questionnaire responses about risk taking in real situations. However, an earlier study that used a behavioral task failed to substantiate reluctance to take risks.[46] These findings suggest that

OCD is associated with less risk taking, but they do not clearly demonstrate that people with OCD overestimate the probability or severity of unpleasant outcomes. More detailed research is needed on these topics among OCD patients.

The overprediction of danger has been observed in other forms of anxiety besides OCD.[43,47] However, it may be a salient characteristic of OCD and essential to the formulation of a comprehensive cognitive theory of OCD. For example, Freeston, et al[22] suggest that overestimating threat is a necessary precursor to overestimating responsibility.

Perfectionism

Various theories of OCD have emphasized the role of perfectionistic thinking. Janet[48] described perfectionism as central to the first two stages of his OCD theory. Psychoanalytic writers have described perfectionism as one way an OCD patient maintains control to reduce the risk of harm.[49,50] As noted earlier, cognitive theorists also have suggested the importance of perfectionism in the development and maintenance of OCD. McFall and Wollersheim[5] suggested that perfectionistic beliefs or assumptions contribute to increased appraisal of threat. Likewise, Guidano and Liotti[6] proposed that OCD patients consider perfect performance both possible and necessary to avoid criticism and risk.[8] Consistent with these writings, Freeston, et al[22] hypothesized several forms of perfectionism in OCD, including the need (1) to know something perfectly; (2) for things to be "just right;" and (3) for perfect symmetry, certainty, and control over thoughts.

Evidence linking perfectionism and OCD comes from anecdotal reports, studies of nonclinical populations, and a few studies of OCD patients compared with other patient and nonpatient groups. Anecdotal reports have identified excessive levels of perfectionism among OCD patients, among the parents of OCD patients, and among children who later develop OCD.[38,51,52] Unfortunately, these findings are based on unsystematic observations with unvalidated measures of perfectionism.

A number of studies of perfectionism and obsessive-compulsive characteristics have now been conducted on nonclinical populations using a validated measure of perfectionism, the Frost Multidimensional Perfectionism Scale (FMPS). Frost and colleagues[53,54] found perfectionism, concern over mistakes, and doubt about actions to be associated with OCD symptoms in multiple samples. Likewise, Gershuny and Sher[55] reported that nonclinical compulsive checkers had higher perfectionism scores than noncheckers, and that perfectionism partially mediated the relationship between obsessive-compulsive symptoms and both perceived and actual task performance. Rhéaume and colleagues[17] also found significant correlations between concern over mistakes and doubts about actions and obsessive-compulsive symptoms. Further, they found that perfectionism accounted for a significant portion of the variance in obsessive-compulsive symptom severity, even when level of responsibility was controlled. Perfectionism also was correlated with specific obsessive-compulsive symptoms, including compulsive hoarding.[56]

Only two studies reported using validated perfectionism measures with diagnosed OCD patient samples. Using a different perfectionism measure, Ferrari[57] reported significant correlations between perfectionism and obsessive-compulsive symptom severity. In a study comparing OCD, agoraphobic, and nonpatient samples, Frost and Steketee[58] found that the OCD group scored higher than nonpatient controls on concern over mistakes, doubts about actions, and total perfectionism. However, the OCD patients did not report more frequently on concern over mistakes than agoraphobic patients, although they did have more doubts about actions. These latter findings raise some questions about the extent to which perfectionism is specific to OCD.

In addition to the finding that panic disorder patients had higher levels of perfectionism than controls, other research has found higher levels of perfectionism among social phobics,[59] eating disorder patients,[60] and depressed individuals.[61] Thus, perfectionism may be a background variable associated with a wide variety of psychopathologies. Although probably not specific to OCD, it may still be an important determiner of the shape and course of this disorder. For this reason, it was included as one of the primary cognitive domains of OCD by the Obsessive-Compulsive Cognition Working Group (OCCWG).

Overimportance of Thoughts

Some OCD patients appear to attach too much importance to the content or the presence of their thoughts. Here, the most important feature may not necessarily be the fear of being responsible for harm, but the meaning associated with the occurrence of these thoughts. For example, if having these terrible thoughts is taken to mean, "I am a bad, abnormal person," considerably more anxiety and effort at suppression or removal are likely to follow than if the thoughts are viewed as unimportant. Another feature associated with OCD is thought-action fusion, the idea that having a thought will lead the patient to act on this thought. Although some authors[9,29] consider thought-action fusion to be a component of responsibility, others have suggested that these types of beliefs may be better conceptualized separately.[22]

Although these types of beliefs are commonly seen in patients, so far only a few studies have examined how people attach importance to their intrusive thoughts. Purdon and Clark[62] found that students who believed that they could act on intrusive thoughts experienced more persistent intrusions, and highly obsessional students rated their intrusive ideas as more believable than low obsessive students. Consistent with this report, Rachman and colleagues[29] found that a measure of thought-action fusion correlated positively with obsessionality. Freeston and colleagues recently developed a measure of overimportance given to thoughts, thought-action fusion, and consequences of having intrusive thoughts. In OCD subjects, they found that this measure was significantly associated with more obsessive-compulsive symptoms, obsessional thoughts, and efforts to suppress thoughts.[63] In a related vein, Freeston and Bouchard[64] demonstrated that a decrease in obsessions during the treatment of a patient suffering from harming obsessions was immediately followed by a decrease in thought-action fusion. That is, the patient reduced his belief that, "I'm dangerous; I'm not normal." These findings, then, support the notion that intrusions become obsessions when they are imbued with special importance and beliefs about acting on the thoughts.

Control

Researchers have long speculated that a need to exert control over all aspects of their lives is central to OCD. Psychoanalytic theorists[49,50] have suggested that OCD patients attempt to control their environment to reduce the risk of harm by doing everything perfectly. Cognitive theorists have similarly suggested that establishing perfect control over the environment is one way to limit risk and criticism.[6,8] A hypothesized link between perfectionism and control is evident in these writings.

More recently, investigators have focused on the importance of beliefs about control over thoughts in OCD. Clark and Purdon[21] asserted that mistaken beliefs about the need to control thoughts are determinants in the development and maintenance of OCD. They hypothesized that obsessions result from a breakdown in the usually effective mental system that controls distractor thoughts. As a result, the individual becomes more sensitive and vigilant to all kinds of cues reminiscent of the unwanted thoughts. Supporting these hypotheses are findings that perceived uncontrollability of intrusive thoughts was associated with increased frequency and persistence of intrusions in nonclinical samples.[62]

In the same vein, Wegner[65] suggested that obsessive thinking may arise because initial efforts to control thoughts fail, leading to escalated efforts at suppression, which further highlight the unpleasant thoughts. The person exercises even greater vigilance and enhanced efforts to control thoughts, and the cycle escalates still further. Self-distraction efforts work only temporarily and interfere with habituation of negative reactions to unwanted thoughts. Such habituation is needed to actually reduce obsessive thinking, although Wegner notes that this may not be all that is needed.

A series of studies by Wegner[65] on nonclinical samples indicated that efforts to control particular thoughts usually resulted in a rebound effect; suppressed thoughts actually recurred more frequently after subjects tried to block them. According to analog studies, conditioning may play a role in this process: trying not to think about something in a particular situation may become associated with that context, which then serves as a reminder of the unwanted thought. Mood state may also influence this process. Depressed individuals are less successful at suppressing negative thoughts than positive thoughts, and the more negative the tone of the distractor thoughts, the more effective they are in suppressing negative thoughts. These findings imply that obsessive thoughts, which are invariably unpleasant, will be more easily suppressed by using other unpleasant distractor thoughts, which perhaps can in turn become obsessions. The cycle of attention to intrusions followed by attempts at suppression is hypothesized to escalate to an obsessional pattern.[65,66]

Recently, an international group of researchers on cognition in OCD[24] identified beliefs about the need to control thoughts as an important belief domain relevant to OCD. This domain was defined to include (1) hypervigilance for mental events; (2) moralistic beliefs that controlling thoughts is a virtue; (3) beliefs that failure to control results in negative psychologic and behavioral consequences (e.g., insanity, decreased functioning); and (4) beliefs about immediate efficiency and future success of control efforts. Further study of the effect of beliefs about control on OCD patient groups is needed.

Tolerance for Ambiguity

Although not a diagnostic criterion for OCD, doubting the veracity of one's experience and the quality of one's actions is a hallmark of this disorder.[1] Doubts about the validity of sensory experience can lead to uncertainty about whether one's actions are effective in warding off danger. Beech and Liddell[67] proposed that ritualistic behaviors are maintained not only to reduce immediate discomfort, but also to address the obsessive-compulsive patient's need for certainty before terminating an activity. According to Makhlouf-Norris and colleagues,[68] they create "islands of certainty" amidst confusion, in an effort to control and predict events. The need for certainty, or intolerance of uncertainty, is a commonly noted feature of OCD.[38,40] Reed[1] emphasized the importance of doubts among OCD patients. Several laboratory studies support the need for certainty in OCD and corresponding difficulties with decision making (the reader is referred to our discussion of decision making in the section of this chapter entitled, "Cognitive Processing"). We note, however, that Tallis[69] has recently identified methodologic limitations to these studies.

Several investigators have tied intolerance for uncertainty to perfectionism and perceptions of risk. For example, Guidano and Liotti[6] suggested that OCD patients believe that patients feel uncertain about the quality of their efforts to minimize risk when perfect solutions cannot be identified. Frost, et al[53] considered doubting the quality of actions to be a central domain of perfectionism, and this dimension of perfectionism was the only one that distinguished OCD patients from panic disorder patients.[58] Further studies with better methodologic controls are needed to verify the relevance of tolerance for uncertainty to OCD and to other features of this disorder such as overestimation of threat and perfectionism. A working definition for use in such research has been provided by the OCCWG. They proposed that intolerance of ambiguity includes "beliefs about the necessity of being certain, about the capacity to cope with unpredictable change, and about adequate functioning in situations which are inherently ambiguous."

Other Cognitive Domains

Beliefs About Coping

Beliefs about coping among OCD patients have been given some attention in theorizing about OCD. Guidano and Liotti[6] and Carr[3,4] observed that OCD patients devalue or underestimate their ability to deal adequately with threatening situations, resulting in pervasive uncertainty and discomfort. As a result, OCD patients view rituals and avoidance as the only available coping strategy. McFall and Wollersheim[5] suggested that negative beliefs about coping capacity derive from a sense of perfectionistic ideals that lead these patients to believe that they must be perfectly competent or punished for their failures. Thus, coping is either perfect or a failure deserving of punishment. There is very limited empirical evidence for these ideas. One study by Steketee, et al[18] demonstrated that OCD patients endorsed more negative beliefs about coping than nonpatients, but not more than other anxious patients. Beliefs about coping, then, may not be specific to OCD.

Beliefs About Emotional Discomfort

Some patients who experience frequent high levels of discomfort report irrational beliefs in their tolerance for anxiety. Such beliefs about emotional discomfort may play a predominant role in the development and maintenance of obsessive-compulsive symptoms for some patients.[23] When asked to predict their anxiety level before the first exposure sessions, OCD patients often anticipate higher levels than they actually experience. Some patients who refuse exposure provide irrational explanations that reflect their beliefs about the negative effects of experiencing a high anxiety level such as losing control, doing something unwanted, or experiencing sickness, craziness, or death. Empirical evidence that these beliefs are specific to OCD is lacking, but if they predict poorer outcome following therapy, they may be clinically important targets of cognitive restructuring.

Summary

Six general belief domains listed in Table 18-1 have been identified as central to OCD by an international group of researchers.[24] These domains were established and defined by expert consensus and form a framework for the study of cognition in OCD. First, the overperception of responsibility appears to be consistently associated with OCD symptoms and behavior. Other domains of importance include threat estimation, perfectionism, overimportance of thoughts, control over thoughts, and tolerance for ambiguity. More research on these features is clearly needed to clarify their meaning, interconnection, and role in maintaining OCD.

Table 18-1   Belief Domains in Obsessive-Compulsive Disorder

1. Responsibility
2. Threat estimation
3. Perfectionism
4. Overimportance of thoughts
5. Control over thoughts
6. Tolerance for ambiguity

Finally, the variety of OCD beliefs and the postulated cognitive schemas of several models suggest that different levels of cognitive content may exist. For example, for some patients, an excessive sense of responsibility, as well as deeper moralistic values, may influence their interpretation of intrusive thoughts. It may be relatively easy to assess the presence and intensity of beliefs about responsibility, estimation of threat, and so forth, whereas determining deeper "schema" or basic assumptions may require priming in an OCD-relevant context. Strategies for assessment of cognitions are discussed below.

ASSESSMENT OF COGNITION IN OBSESSIVE-COMPULSIVE DISORDER

Freeston[24] has drawn a distinction between several levels of cognition measurement in OCD. The first level concerns the assessment of intrusive thoughts themselves—that is, the obsessions. The nature and measurement of these OCD symptom phenomena can be studied idiographically through self-report or laboratory tasks. The second level of measurement focuses on interpretations or appraisals of the intrusive thoughts. These appraisals include judgments about an intrusive thought, its content, and its perceived consequences. The next levels consist of basic beliefs or assumptions that are relevant to OCD. Some of these beliefs may be OCD specific, and some may be found in other clinical populations. Such beliefs are thought to influence appraisals or interpretations of intrusive thoughts. We comment on each of these levels in the following paragraphs.

Assessment of Intrusive Thoughts

Several studies have demonstrated that unwanted intrusive thoughts, images, or impulses appear in approximately 90% of the general population.[13] However, such intrusions only are considered obsessions if they cause marked anxiety or distress.[70] The possibility that clinical obsessions have their origins in normally occurring unwanted intrusive thoughts has prompted much research into the nature of normally occurring unwanted intrusive thoughts. Within this context a number of idiographic, self-report, and laboratory measures of intrusive thoughts have emerged.[71] Idiographic measures of intrusive cognitions might include open-ended interviews in which subjects identify and rate their emotional reactions to unwanted intrusions. Another idiographic method consists of daily journal recordings of specific intrusive thoughts and ratings of these on pertinent dimensions.[72] Although these methods can more precisely pinpoint subjects' responses to their own individual intrusions, as yet there is little evidence that these techniques are more useful than self-report measures.

Self-report questionnaires are more structured, but limit subjects' responses to predetermined content. Several such instruments have been developed to measure intrusive thoughts. The Distressing Thoughts Questionnaire (DTQ)[73] asks subjects to rate six anxious and six depressing thoughts on five dimensions (frequency, sadness, worry, removal, and disapproval). However, questions have arisen regarding the extent to which these thoughts are separate and relevant to OCD.[71] Consequently, derivatives of this questionnaire have been developed in an attempt to create a questionnaire more relevant to OCD. The Cognitive Intrusions Questionnaire (CIQ)[12] expanded the number of thoughts and dimensions on which the thoughts were appraised. Although more research has been completed on this questionnaire, Clark and Purdon[71] suggest that it may be measuring general anxiety or worry more than OCD–specific cognitions. These authors developed the Obsessional Intrusions Inventory (OII) in an attempt to assess intrusive cognitions occurring during obsessional thinking.[74] Like the CIQ, the OII has limited data supporting its validity of the scale. Still other self-report attempts have been made to measure specific aspects of intrusive thoughts, including the tendency to suppress unwanted thoughts.[75]

Laboratory assessment of intrusive thoughts has taken the form mainly of examining attempts to suppress selected thoughts. In the original studies, subjects were asked not to think about a neutral stimulus.[76] After the suppression period, these subjects showed a tendency to think more about the suppressed stimulus. Subsequent work has indicated that attempts to suppress personally relevant negative thoughts may increase thought frequency, and that monitoring of thoughts to be suppressed enhances this effect.[66] Other data have suggested that preexisting mood state (e.g., depression) may mediate this effect.[66]

Interpretations of Intrusive Thoughts

Appraisal models of OCD are based on the assumption that people with OCD interpret intrusive cognitions in peculiar ways, and that the interpretation rather than the presence of intrusive thoughts determines the development of obsessive symptoms. Although few attempts have been made to generate measures of interpretation about intrusive thoughts, idiographic, self-report, and laboratory tasks could be used for assessing these interpretations. The OCCWG[24] identified three domains considered relevant to the interpretation or appraisal of intrusive thoughts: responsibility, control over thoughts, and overimportance of thoughts. A self-report measure including each of these "interpretations" has been developed by this group and is undergoing validation.

General Beliefs Common in OCD

Individuals with OCD may have beliefs that are specific to this disorder or beliefs that are general in the sense that they also are associated with other forms of anxiety or depression. For example, there is a general belief that there is only one perfect solution that will avoid criticism, which is likely to be held by patients with various types of anxiety disorders. Several researchers have attempted to measure these beliefs. The OCCWG identified 16 different scales designed to measure such OCD–related beliefs.[24] Although investigators have used slightly different definitions for similar constructs, most of these measures have overlapping content. At least four multidimensional scales have been developed for this purpose.

Freeston, et al[77] developed a 20-item Inventory of Beliefs Related to Obsessions (IBRO), which identifies problematic thoughts and beliefs. Findings from both clinical and nonclinical samples suggest that this is a reliable and valid instrument. The IBRO generates a single obsessive-compulsive belief score, although the items reflect most of the domains reviewed earlier. The Obsessive Compulsive Cognitive Schemata Scale (CSS)[78] is a 206-item measure containing 12 dimensions or subscales. These subscales overlap substantially with the OCCWG-recommended domains. Sookman, et al[79] reported good evidence for the reliability and convergent and discriminate validity of most of their subscales. They also reported that OCD patients scored higher on many of their subscales than other psychiatric groups. The 90-item Obsessive-Compulsive Beliefs Questionnaire (OCBQ)[18] also has subscales that significantly overlap with the domains reviewed previously, including responsibility, control, tolerance of risk or threat, and tolerance for uncertainty. Likewise, this scale showed good reliability and validity, with OCD patients scoring higher on each subscale than other psychiatric groups. Finally, Clark and Purdon's[80] Meta-Cognitive Beliefs Questionnaire also has multiple subscales, including the importance of thought control, responsibility and guilt, and behavioral consequences. These subscales were related to the frequency of unwanted intrusive thoughts in nonclinical populations and to appraisals of intrusive thoughts consistent with OCD.

In addition to these self-report measures covering multiple domains, a number of scales have been designed to tap individual domains regarding OCD beliefs. These measures assess responsibility alone.[26,81,82] Shafran, et al[33] have developed a self-report measure of thought-action fusion, and others have created measures to assess perfectionism.[53]

Each of the measures described previously has some evidence supporting its reliability and validity, yet none has been sufficiently studied, nor have domains been adequately defined for widespread adoption. Such a large number of measures of related phenomena create difficulties in comparing findings across studies, and in generating enough suitable subjects for validation studies. For this reason, a large group of international researchers have begun a collaborative effort to develop and validate a consensually generated cognitive measure for general OCD beliefs.[24]

Six identified domains described previously of general obsessive-compulsive beliefs (responsibility, threat estimation, perfectionism, overimportance of thoughts, tolerance for ambiguity, and control) have been defined. A self-report measure containing these domains has been generated and is now being validated. The OCCWG[24] also recommended the development of idiographic and laboratory assessments. Idiographic measures might include ratings of subjective probability or cost with stimuli for these ratings kept specific for each person. Another strategy might be a "self-debate" in which the subject is asked to present arguments for and against a proposition, then to rate the degree of conviction he has for each side in the debate. Laboratory tasks have not yet been well studied, but recently several attempts have been made to develop laboratory manipulations of belief domains considered important for OCD. For instance, several investigations have attempted to manipulate feelings of responsibility,[19,25,30] and these studies show some promise for methods of assessment and study of OCD–related beliefs.

In addition to the presence of these beliefs in OCD, another important variable is the strength or fixity of obsessions and beliefs. Overvalued ideation of obsessional material has been hypothesized to influence the outcome of behavioral treatment[83] and to be critical in the maintenance of OCD.[84] Several measures of this construct have been developed such as the Fixity of Beliefs Scale;[85] the Brown Assessment of Beliefs Scale (BABS)[86]; and the Overvalued Ideation Scale.[87] These scales have been multifaceted, examining dimensions such as the strength and bizarreness of the belief, insight about the belief, and so on. These scales assess the form or structure of beliefs rather than the content. Such advances in the assessment of fixity of obsessions and associated beliefs are essential to determining their role in the onset and persistence of OCD symptoms.

COGNITIVE PROCESSES IN OBSESSIVE-COMPULSIVE DISORDER

Traditionally, cognition was considered equivalent to conscious thought, and psychopathologists used self-report measures to investigate cognitive aspects of emotional disorders. But self-report data describing internal processes, such as thoughts or beliefs, have methodologic limitations. Therefore, researchers began to use concepts and methods of cognitive psychology to better understand information-processing difficulties and biases that might play important roles in the etiology and maintenance of psychologic disorders.[88] In recent information-processing studies, OCD patients have shown biases and deficits with respect to decision making, attention, and memory.

Decision Making

Indecision has been considered a core cognitive feature of OCD.[40] OCD patients might have difficulty making decisions because they want to be certain that they always find the "correct" solution.[6] The need for certainty and the inability to make decisions may account for the difficulties that patients with OCD and obsessive-compulsive personality disorder (OCPD) display in category formation. For example, Reed[89,90] presented OCPD and control subjects with a concept word (e.g., table) and five other words (e.g., cloth, vase, legs, drawer, top). They were asked to choose which of the five words were essential to the concept word. Reed found that individuals with OCPD were more likely to overdefine categories (i.e., they selected fewer choices) than control subjects. In a similar experiment, he observed that OCPD subjects produced more classes in a category-formation task than did controls.

Consistent with these results, Persons and Foa[91] found that clinical OCD patients needed more categories and more time to sort items in a category-formation task than did clinical controls. Although Frost and colleagues did not replicate these findings of underinclusion in nonclinical checkers, they observed that individuals with high scores on obsessive-compulsive symptoms took more time to sort items into categories compared with individuals with low obsessive-compulsive symptom scores.[92]

A recent study by Frost and Shows[93] on college students revealed that indecisiveness was related to perfectionism, hoarding, compulsivity, and procrastination—features that are associated with either OCD or OCPD. Moreover, the subjects who scored high on indecisiveness took longer to make decisions than subjects who scored low on the scale. Similar experiments have shown that, compared with other psychiatric patients, OCD subjects requested more repetition of information[94] and required more evidence[96] before they could make a decision. There also is evidence that OCD patients demonstrate more uncertainty and doubt about decisions already made compared with phobic and nonpsychiatric controls.[95,96] Tallis[69] has recently identified various methodologic limitations of the studies cited previously. Specifically, he emphasized that elevated levels of anxiety or depression might have produced the underinclusive levels of responding in the category-formation tasks. Moreover, he stressed that asking for repetition is not necessarily related to indecision; it might instead be an expression of caution. Thus, further and better controlled studies are needed to substantiate the findings on indecisiveness, and such studies should clarify the observed effects in OCD and OCPD.

Attention

Thus far, attempts to measure attention directly in obsessional patients have been rare. Two types of studies have predominated. Some studies examined attention regardless of emotional content. Here, subjects were asked to process information that varied in complexity but not in emotional valence. In other studies, subjects were asked to process information that varied in emotional valence or was relevant to their fears.

An important content-independent study of nonclinical subjects with high obsessionality scores measuring obsessional personality has been conducted by Broadbent and colleagues.[97] The authors asked their subjects to perform two tasks that required a reaction to the presentation of certain stimuli. In the filtering task, the subjects were told the spatial location of the stimulus in advance, whereas in the selective set task, the subjects did not know where the stimulus would appear. Obsessional subjects tended to perform relatively worse on the selective set task than on the filtering task. The authors concluded that the obsessional individuals appeared "blind to relevant events that are happening outside the focus of attention."[97] However, similar studies have failed to show a correlation between attentional tasks and obsessionality.[98]

Inhibition of Attention

The process of selecting specific material should require reduced attention to less relevant stimuli.[99] This general inhibition effect has been demonstrated in nonclinical samples.[100,101] Recently, researchers[102–105] have hypothesized that OCD sufferers may fail to inhibit their attention to irrelevant material, thereby interfering with the patients' control over intrusive thinking. Pitman noted that obsessive-compulsive individuals may not be able to effectively distract themselves from intrusive ideas and images.[21] In fact, Enright and Beech[104,105] demonstrated that OCD patients (but not patients with other anxiety disorders) experienced difficulty inhibiting the processing of irrelevant, emotionally neutral material. The authors suggested that this failure in preconscious inhibition may lead OCD patients to use more voluntary strategies, such as thought suppression, which could then paradoxically increase the frequency of intrusive thoughts.[65,106] In one study of nonclinical checkers, however, no evidence for deficient inhibitory control of attention was found.[107]

Information-Processing Research

Most of the research on attention in OCD has involved the processing of emotionally significant information. This research suggests that OCD patients might be characterized by an attentional bias for processing fear-relevant stimuli (e.g., material about contamination). Investigators have used various experimental paradigms to examine attention in OCD, including dichotic listening and modified visual paradigms.[108] Various studies employing these paradigms have provided support for the contention that attentional resources are drawn toward threat-related cues.

The dichotic listening paradigm involves the presentation of two different prose passages, one to each ear. Subjects are asked to repeat aloud one passage and to ignore the other. Moreover, they are asked to detect occasional presentations of fear-related words or neutral words that occur in either passage. Employing a dichotic listening task, Foa and McNally[109] showed that threat words were detected more readily than neutral words in the unattended passage. Moreover, they showed greater skin conductance responses to fear-related words than to neutral words. These effects disappeared after successful behavior therapy, suggesting that the attentional biases resulted from fear and not from the patient's familiarity with the words.

In modified Stroop[108] experiments, subjects are presented words of varying emotional significance and are asked to name the color in which the word is printed while ignoring the word meaning. Delays in the naming of the color occur whenever subjects focus on the meaning of the word, despite their effort to focus on its color. Therefore, if an attentional bias for threat-related information (e.g., contamination words) exists in OCD patients, these patients should take longer to color-name threat words than to color-name words that are neutral. Foa and colleagues[110] compared compulsive washers with obsessive-compulsive subjects without washing rituals and normal subjects in a modified Stroop task. They found that washers had longer response latencies for contamination words than for neutral words. Moreover, these patients had longer latencies for contamination words than did healthy control subjects.

One might argue that the attentional biases found in the studies described are not the result of threat-relatedness of the cues but that any emotional cue, regardless of its valence, might produce Stroop interference.[111] Alternatively, anxious subjects might show an attentional bias only for material that is related to their concerns and not for emotional cues in general. Lavy and colleagues[112] investigated these conflicting hypotheses with a modified Stroop task and found evidence only for the threat-relatedness hypothesis. The OCD subjects selectively attended to threat-related OCD words (e.g., "disease") but not to positive OCD words (e.g., "clean").[112]

Only a few studies have investigated attention and attentional biases in OCD. Taken together, these studies suggest that OCD subjects may have difficulties with the allocation of attention and the inhibition of attention to irrelevant material. Moreover, OCD patients appear to display an enhanced sensitivity to attend to threat-related cues.

Memory

Relatively few studies have explored memory in OCD, despite evidence of distortions in other areas of information processing in this disorder. OCD patients have been frequently reported to display recall that is unusually accurate and detailed. On the other hand, however, the uncertainty of these patients is often considered to signal memory deficits.[1] OCD patients are believed to repeat actions compulsively because they are unsure that they performed the behavior accurately. They may have difficulty recalling a previous act, which Otto[113] has related to deficits in the decision-making process in stressful and ambiguous circumstances. He proposed that OCD patients may have difficulty separating subsequent compulsions from previous ones.

Memory for Previous Action

Several investigations examined memory in subclinical OCD populations or in non–OCD psychiatric patients who have obsessive-compulsive–like symptoms but with less debilitating rituals. For example, Sher and colleagues[114,115] found that checkers had a worse recall of their own actions performed during the course of an experimental session relative to subjects with low obsessive-compulsive checking scores. A similar study was conducted by Sheffler-Rubenstein and colleagues.[116] These authors asked subclinical checkers and noncheckers to participate in various memory tests. In one of the tasks, checkers were confused more often than noncheckers about whether they had read or generated certain words. Moreover, checkers more frequently believed that they had studied words that actually had not been on the study list. Thus, several studies with subjects showing excessive checking rituals demonstrated that these individuals might have an action-memory deficit. However, this hypothesis requires further investigation with clinical OCD patients.

Reality Monitoring and Confidence in Memory

Researchers have hypothesized that individuals with OCD might have a deficit in their ability to distinguish memories of previous experiences from memories of experiences that were only imagined. This reality monitoring deficit hypothesis is based on the OCD patient's uncertainty about whether he has actually performed a check or whether he only imagined performing it. To test for such a deficit, McNally and Kohlbeck[117] instructed their patients to either trace or to imagine tracing line drawings and words. The authors predicted that if OCD patients' reality monitoring is defective, they would have difficulty distinguishing memories of actual tracing from memories of imagined tracing. The OCD patients did not differ from the control subjects in their reality monitoring abilities, but they expressed less confidence in their memories. A similar study with subclinical checkers also showed that they were less confident in their memories than noncheckers.[115]

Consistent with the results reported previously, Brown and colleagues[118] found no differences between OCD patients and control subjects in their ability to distinguish words presented through visual or auditory channels. In another recent study, subjects were asked to engage in real and imagined actions.[119] Some of these actions were emotionally neutral, but others were anxiety provoking. Investigators failed to find support for either a memory impairment for actions or a reality monitoring deficit. In fact, the patients' recall of actions was superior to that of controls for distressing situations. However, OCD patients, in contrast to control subjects, reported that they desired more vivid images than they were able to produce. Thus, the authors concluded that the patients' dissatisfaction with recall—rather than an actual memory deficit—may trigger repeated checking behavior.

Finally, employing a directed forgetting paradigm, Wilhelm and associates[120] presented OCD patients and healthy controls with negative, positive, and neutral words, and instructed them to either remember or forget each word after it was presented. Subjects were given a free recall and a recognition test for all words, regardless of the original instructions. OCD patients had more difficulty forgetting negative material compared with positive and neutral material, whereas control subjects did not. In an investigation by Maki and colleagues,[107] no differences were found in directed forgetting performance between college students with high and low obsessive-compulsive symptom scores. However, these findings are not necessarily inconsistent with those of Wilhelm et al[120] because Maki and associates did not include words of negative valence and did not test OCD patients.

Many recent investigations have focused on neuropsychologic aspects of memory in OCD.[121] A review of these studies is provided in Chapter 13 of this book. The reader may also be interested in Watts'[122] treatment strategy for checking rituals derived from an information-processing approach.

In summary, investigations of memory in OCD have provided mixed results. Many studies on OCD patients suggest no memory dysfunction, whereas several studies on subclinical groups indicate memory problems. Specifically, research with non–OCD checkers suggests a deficit for action memory, but these results have not yet been replicated in clinical OCD patients. There also is evidence for a memory bias favoring threatening information in OCD patients. Moreover, although several studies failed to find a reality monitoring deficit in OCD, most suggested a lack of confidence or dissatisfaction with the OCD sufferers' recall of their own actions. This suggests that some cognitions about memory performance may play a role in OCD symptomatology. Indeed, beliefs about memory have been hypothesized to influence memory processes.[123] Thus, a better understanding of OCD might be achieved through the integration of research on beliefs and the information-processing approach.

COGNITIVE TREATMENT FOR OBSESSIVE-COMPULSIVE DISORDER

Several writers have observed that exposure-based therapies often modify thoughts and beliefs merely by requiring patients to remain in anxiety-provoking situations until their fear has subsided. Thoughts or beliefs about the danger of the situation are often reduced following such an experience. Foa and Steketee[124] suggested that treatment by exposure and response prevention (ERP) does not correct cognitive deficits, but rather reduces threat estimation as patients reclassify some situations as nondangerous based on their experience during exposure. Whether exposure also modifies other types of cognitions common in OCD, as discussed earlier, has been studied indirectly using general belief measures; modest reductions in general irrational beliefs following ERP have been reported, with significantly more gains evident following cognitive therapy.[125,126]

Although few studies of cognitive therapies for OCD had been reported until recently, intense interest in this topic has spawned several ongoing studies. The earliest cognitive therapy studies tested Rational-Emotive Therapy (RET),[7] with more recent trials testing Beck's cognitive therapy and related methods. These outcome trials have been conducted almost exclusively in the Netherlands, and thus replication in other centers is essential before effectiveness is clearly established.

Rational-Emotive Therapy

This form of therapy requires patients to become aware of patterns of illogical assumptions and to challenge these on rational grounds. Ellis[7] has proposed a series of typical assumptions that are explored, and Warren and Zgourides[8] proposed special concerns to be addressed using RET with OCD patients. These include responsibility, reassurance seeking, overvalued ideas, epistemologic reasoning, overestimating harm, depression, criticism and guilt, promoting self-acceptance, and relapse prevention.

In a case series, Neziroglu and Neuman[127] reported good outcomes for three of six patients who received RET alone before or after thought-stopping and exposure treatment. In the first group trial, Emmelkamp and colleagues[128] assigned 18 OCD patients to either RET or self-controlled exposure *in vivo*. Both treatments produced significant changes in most OCD symptom scores (average improvement 78%), with continued gains 6 months later (average improvement, 94%). However, follow-up data should be interpreted conservatively, because several clients received additional treatment as needed. Subjective ratings of anxiety and depression also improved with both methods, although RET demonstrated significant superiority over the exposure method in the treatment of depression.

In a second study of RET, Emmelkamp and Beens[125] replicated these findings in 21 clients randomly assigned to cognitive therapy or to self-controlled exposure and response prevention, followed by the addition of exposure treatment for both groups. In the cognitive intervention group, therapists used Ellis' ABC framework (A = activating event, B = beliefs, C = emotional and/or behavioral consequence) to assist clients in observing and recording their irrational beliefs and discriminating these beliefs from actual events. Therapists then taught clients to dispute their beliefs using Socratic dialogue. Homework involved practice in disputing OCD beliefs. Subsequent sessions focused on review of situations encountered during homework, with particular emphasis on analyzing irrational beliefs associated with the primary and secondary appraisal process. In the first phase of the study, both ERP and RET groups improved significantly from pretest to posttest, but these groups did not differ significantly from each other. In the second phase of the study, both groups received ERP and again improvement in pretest was seen in both groups, but there was no evidence that the addition of cognitive therapy produced any additional benefit. General irrational beliefs declined more following RET, but this difference was not significant until 4 weeks after the end of the treatment period, suggesting that change in beliefs may require more time than change in obsessions and compulsions. These studies, both conducted in the Netherlands, were the first to show that cognitive treatment alone was clinically beneficial for OCD.

Beck's Cognitive Therapy

Several recent studies have tested cognitive therapy (CT) using Beck's model,[11] in which faulty idiosyncratic beliefs and underlying assumptions are identified, examined, and challenged using several types of techniques that include Socratic questioning, identification of dysfunctional thinking, generation of alternative thoughts, testing these thoughts through behavioral experiments, and several other techniques intended to challenge the patients' usual thinking processes. Both single case studies and reports of a series of cases have shown positive effects. Among case studies, Kearney and Silverman[129] reported that alternating between CT and response prevention was effective in treating a suicidal adolescent with OCD who found *in vivo* exposure too distressing to tolerate. Salkovskis and Warwick[130] used CT to alter unrealistic beliefs when exposure therapy failed to resolve the contamination fears of a patient who believed she could develop skin cancer. Although CT has been disputed as the cause of the successful outcome,[131] the addition of CT appeared to enable the patient to benefit from exposure treatment. This case study may offer treatment possibilities for OCD patients who lack insight into the irrationality of their fears.

Ladouceur and colleagues[132] also reported positive outcomes using CT without ERP to correct thoughts of inflated responsibility in four patients with checking rituals. In this case series, a detailed behavioral analysis was used to provide the patients with the following therapy rationale: "Environmental or internal stimuli lead to mental intrusions that are then evaluated in such a way that the patient inflates his or her own degree of responsibility. This increases the perception of danger and provokes efforts to neutralize the fear (rituals, avoidance, reassurance) and adversely influences mood." During CT, therapists helped patients identify thoughts of inflated responsibility and to correct unreasonable beliefs. Techniques for correction of negative automatic thoughts included Socratic dialogue, pie chart techniques* for reevaluating actual versus presumed responsibility, and playing devil's advocate. Patients were encouraged to generate adequate explanations for their anxious, overresponsible reactions.

Recently, Ladouceur,[133] reported positive results for three patients with checking symptoms using CT alone focusing on overestimation of danger,

---

* The pie chart technique involves asking patients how much responsibility all relevant persons including themselves *might have* on a particular outcome, and drawing each proportion in the shape of a pie. Usually, on considering others' responsibilities, the proportion assigned to their own responsibility reduces.

responsibility, and perfectionism. For these patients, reduced checking was correlated with a decrease in specific beliefs about these domains. Freeston and colleagues[22] reported on six OCD patients treated with CT, three of whom showed marked benefit, two were much improved, and one improved minimally. At the 6-month follow-up, only one patient relapsed, and one improved further.

In the first controlled trial, Van Oppen, et al[126] randomly assigned 28 OCD patients to CT and 29 patients to self-exposure. Patients in the CT group experienced exposure only in the context of homework assignments designed to test assumptions and correct faulty thinking. Treatment was similar to that described previously[133]: Intrusions were viewed as stimuli; negative automatic thoughts were identified, challenged, and corrected; and underlying dysfunctional assumptions were sought and challenged in the office and during homework assignments. CT appeared to produce slightly more benefit, but differences were not statistically significant. However, more of the patients in the CT group were recovered to a clinically significant degree (50%) than in the behaviorally treated sample (28%). This finding appeared to hold true at 1-year follow-up.[134] However, the relatively high average Yale-Brown Obsessive-Compulsive Scale (Y-BOCS) scores of the exposure group after treatment suggest that the self-controlled exposure procedure may not have been as successful as in some other studies. It is reasonable to conclude that ERP and CT did not differ in the effects on obsessive-compulsive symptoms (Figure 18-1).

Freeston, et al[135] treated 29 ruminators with exposure and CT and compared them with a wait list control condition. Cognitive intervention addressed patients' overestimation of the importance of thoughts, probability and severity of feared consequences, personal responsibility, and perfectionism. The combined treatment produced an 84% success rate and therapeutic gains were maintained at 1-year follow-up. This study, conducted in Canada, offers some evidence of generalization of the benefits of CT outside of the Netherlands.

Evidence of the benefits of CT for severe OCD is provided by Sookman, et al,[136] who described successful outcomes for three patients receiving lengthy (up to 5 years) and often intensive CT mixed with exposure or medications. This cognitive treatment was focused on several levels described earlier in this chapter, including appraisals, specific and general beliefs, and especially core beliefs. Further study is required to determine whether CT or RET will be helpful for OCD patients whose severe symptoms and comorbid disorders require inpatient treatment. Drummond[137] reported the use of CT in 10 of 49 chronic and treatment-resistant inpatient cases, of whom approximately 50% had comorbid diagnoses. The authors reported that 31 (63%) of these 49 cases were clinically improved at discharge, but unfortunately, no specific information was available about the outcome of those patients who had received CT in combination with other therapies.

In summary, based on the case studies and few controlled trials, it appears

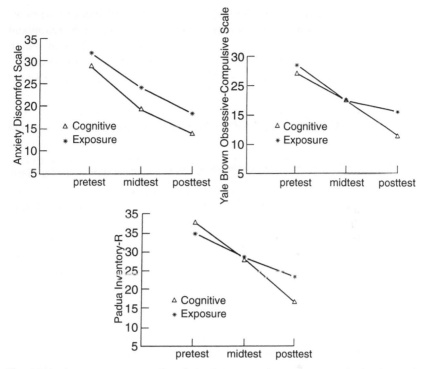

Fig. 18-1   Improvements on the obsessive-compulsive measures for both conditions. (From Van Oppen P, De Haan E, van Balkan AJLM, et al: Cognitive therapy and exposure in vivo in the treatment of obsessive-compulsive disorder, *Behav Res Ther* 33:379–390, 1995.)

that treatments tailored specifically to correct cognitive distortions in OCD patients have demonstrated positive short-term effects. These treatments have been described in detail by Van Oppen and Arntz[138] and by Freeston, et al.[22] Whether these treatments also reduce relapse is not yet clear. More study of outcomes in both outpatient and chronic treatment–refractory inpatients is needed, especially to demonstrate efficacy across centers. This research should include longer trials with large sample sizes, and treatment comparisons that include or omit specialized cognitive interventions. We are aware of at least one such ongoing trial using a group intervention at the University of British Columbia.

Comment

Reed[1] has suggested that cognitive procedures commonly used in other disorders may not be appropriate for obsessive-compulsive patients who generally recognize their obsessions to be irrational. However, the degree to which

OCD patients recognize the irrationality is variable, depending on whether they are in a feared situation when they are questioned.[84] CT involving logical discussion of the actual probability of a negative outcome or of its potential impact seems to produce little change in a patient's firmly held beliefs. Efforts to correct misconceptions may be useful in cases in which there is genuine inaccuracy in assumptions, but this is rarely the problem. Instead, OCD patients may have exaggerated the perceived danger of a potentially harmful situation. Beck's model recommends deliberate testing of the accuracy of such automatic beliefs. Such testing requires direct exposure to the stimuli, which some patients refuse; others may complete exposure assignments but explain the apparent absence of expected catastrophe by special circumstances such as luck.

Cognitive treatments may have more use for OCD patients if they are focused not only on appraisals and specific beliefs, but also focused on basic assumptions about the self, the world, and the future. Indeed, there is both anecdotal and research evidence that OCD patients often hold unrealistic assumptions in the several domains described earlier. Our clinical impression is that many failures and relapses occur among those patients who hold such unrealistic beliefs, particularly when guilt and excessive responsibility are involved.

Further study of these beliefs is needed, first to establish which cognitions are important in the development or maintenance of OCD symptoms. We can then begin to determine whether needed cognitive changes are best achieved through cognitive treatments or through behavioral or drug treatments. Because there is currently inadequate evidence of the efficacy of CT for OCD symptoms, it is not routinely included in standard behavioral treatment programs. Informally, however, many clinicians engage in dialogue with clients regarding their beliefs and assumptions when these beliefs surface during exposure sessions and are judged to interfere with habituation of anxiety or discomfort. The effect of such efforts must be more carefully examined to determine the potential benefit of CT in OCD.

SUMMARY

Cognitive models of OCD have emphasized problems with threat appraisal and cognitive processing. Research on appraisal models has generally supported hypotheses about the importance of specific belief domains (e.g., responsibility). Some consensus has developed about which domains are most important, and efforts to measure these beliefs are under way. Research on cognitive-processing models has suggested deficits and biases with respect to decision-making, attention, and memory. Only a few studies have investigated cognitive deficits and information-processing biases in OCD, and many subjects have had either obsessive-compulsive personality style or subclinical OCD, rather than clinical OCD.

To date, research on cognitive processes, cognitive content, and cognitive treatments has mainly developed independently. A cross-fertilization among researchers of various cognitive approaches might prove fruitful and may help in the design of measures of cognitive belief and cognitive processes that can be included in comparative treatment trials of OCD. One example might be repeated assessments to identify cognitive changes and their triggers during therapy. Investigating the nature and causes of beliefs and cognitive deficits and information-processing biases that underlie OCD may help clinicians to develop better treatment methods. For example, the use of mnemonic strategies to address identified memory deficits or sensory focus to alleviate perceptual processing deficits[122] might be beneficial.

Experimental information-processing paradigms might help to evaluate treatment effects because these methods may be less prone to response bias than commonly used self-report measures. Such examination of changes in information-processing measures in relation to therapeutic improvement also could shed light on the underlying mechanisms of change with drug or behavioral treatment in OCD.[69]

Although some evidence suggests that CT may be as effective as ERP in the treatment of OCD, much additional research is needed before CT is firmly established as a first-line treatment for OCD (e.g., controlled trials comparing CT with ERP and comparing the combination of CT and ERP with standard ERP).

REFERENCES

1. Reed GF: *Obsessional experience and compulsive behavior: A cognitive-structural approach*, Orlando, 1985, Academic Press.
2. Lazarus R: *Psychological stress and the coping process*, New York, 1966, McGraw-Hill.
3. Carr AT: Compulsive neurosis: Two psychological studies, *Bull Br Psychol Soc* 24:256–257, 1971.
4. Carr AT: Compulsive neurosis: A review of the literature, *Psychol Bull* 81: 311–318, 1974.
5. McFall ME, Wollersheim JP: Obsessive-compulsive neurosis: A cognitive-behavioral formulation and approach to treatment, *Cogn Ther Res* 3:333–348, 1979.
6. Guidano VF, Liotti G: *Cognitive processes and emotional disorders*, New York, 1983, Guilford.
7. Ellis A: *Reason and emotion in psychotherapy*, New York, 1962, Lyle Stuart.
8. Warren R, Zgourides G: *Anxiety disorders: A rational-emotive perspective*, New York, 1991, Pergamon.
9. Salkovskis PM: Obsessional-compulsive problems: A cognitive-behavioural analysis, *Behav Res Ther* 23:571–583, 1985.
10. Salkovskis PM: Cognitive-behavioural factors and the persistence of intrusive thoughts in obsessional problems, *Behav Res Ther* 27:677–682, 1989.
11. Beck AT, Emery G, Greenberg RL: *Anxiety disorders and phobias: A cognitive perspective*, New York, 1985, Basic Books.
12. Freeston MH, Ladouceur R, Thibodeau N, Gagnon F: Cognitive intrusions in a non-clinical population. I. Response style, subjective experience, and appraisal, *Behav Res Ther* 29:585–597, 1991.
13. Rachman SJ, de Silva P: Abnormal and normal obsessions, *Behav Res Ther* 16:233–248, 1978.

14. Salkovskis PM, Harrison J: Abnormal and normal obsessions: A replication, *Behav Res Ther* 22:549–552, 1984.
15. Spranka M, Minsk E, Baron J: Omission and commission in judgement and choice, *J Exp Soc Psychol* 27:76–105, 1991.
16. Salkovskis PM, Richards HC, Forrester E: The relationship between obsessional problems and intrusive thoughts, *Behav Cogn Psychother* 23:281–299, 1995.
17. Rhéaume J, Freeston MH, Dugas ML: Perfectionism, responsibility and obsessive-compulsive symptoms, *Behav Res Ther* 33:785–794, 1995a.
18. Steketee G, Frost RO, Cohen I: *Measuring beliefs specific to OCD*, Manuscript in preparation, 1996.
19. Lopatka C, Rachman SJ: Perceived responsibility and compulsive checking: An experimental analysis, *Behav Res Ther* 33:673–684, 1995.
20. Shafran R: *The manipulation of responsibility in obsessive-compulsive disorder.* Paper presented at the World Congress of Behavioural and Cognitive Therapies, Copenhagen, Norway, July 1995.
21. Clark DA, Purdon C: New perspectives for a cognitive theory of obsessions, *Austr Psychol* 28:161–167, 1993.
22. Freeston MH, Léger E, Rhéaume J, Ladouceur R: The treatment utility of cognitive assessment in obsessive-compulsive disorder. Poster presented at the 30th annual convention of the Association for Advancement of Behavior Therapy, New York, November 1996.
23. Freeston MH, Rhéaume J, Ladouceur R: Correcting faulty appraisals of obsessional thoughts, *Behav Res Ther* 34:433–446, 1996.
24. Obsessive Compulsive Cognitions Working Group: Cognitive assessment of obsessive compulsive disorder, *Behav Res Ther* 35:667–681, 1997.
24a. Rachman SJ: Obsessions, responsibility and guilt, *Behav Res Ther* 31:149–154, 1993.
25. Ladouceur R, Rhéaume J, Freeston MH, et al: Experimental manipulations of responsibility: An analogue test of models of obsessive-compulsive disorder, *Behav Res Ther* 33:937–946, 1995.
26. Rhéaume J, Ladonceur R, Freeston MH et al: Inflated responsibility and its role in OCD. I. Validation of a theoretical definition of responsibility, *Behav Res Ther* 33:159–169, 1995b.
27. Rhéaume J, Ladouceur R, Freeston MH, Letarte H: Inflated responsibility and its role in OCD. II. Psychometric studies of a semi-idiographic measure, *J Psychopathol Behav Assess* 16:265–276, 1995c.
28. Freeston MH, Ladouceur R, Thibodeau N, Gagnon F: Cognitive intrusions in a non-clinical population II. Associations with depressive, anxious and compulsive symptoms, *Behav Res Ther* 30:263–271, 1992.
29. Rachman SJ, Thordarson D, Shafran R, Woody SR: Perceived responsibility: Structure and significance, *Behav Res Ther* 33:779–784, 1995.
30. Ladouceur R, Rhéaume J, Aublet F: Manipulating both components of responsibility in nonclinicals: An experimental analysis, *Behav Res Ther,* in press.
31. Baron J, Hershey JC: Outcome bias in decision evaluation, *J Personal Soc Psychol* 4:569–579, 1988.
32. Landman J: Regret and elation following action and inaction: Affective responses to positive and negative outcomes, *Personal Soc Psychol Bull* 4:524–536, 1987.

33. Shafran R, Watkins E, Charman T: Guilt in obsessive-compulsive disorder, *J Anx Dis* 10:509–516, 1996.
34. Niler ER, Beck SJ: The relationship among guilt, dysphoria, anxiety, and obsessions in a normal population, *Behav Res Ther* 27:213–220, 1989.
35. Manchandi R, Sethi BB, Gupta SC: Hostility and guilt in obsessive-compulsive neurosis, *Br J Psychiatry* 135:52–54, 1979.
36. Steketee G, Quay S, White K: Religion and guilt in OCD patients, *J Anx Dis* 5:359–367, 1991.
37. Foa EB, Kozak MJ: Emotional processing of fear: Exposure to corrective information, *Psychol Bull* 99:20–35, 1986.
38. Rasmussen SA, Eisen JL: Clinical features and phenomenology of obsessive compulsive disorder, *Psychiatr Ann* 19:67–73, 1989.
39. Steiner J: A questionnaire study of risk-taking in psychiatric patients, *Br J Med Psychol* 45:365–374, 1972.
40. Kozak MJ, Foa EB, McCarthy P: Assessment of obsessive-compulsive disorder. In Last C, Hersen M, editors: *Handbook of anxiety disorders*, Elmsford, 1987, Pergamon.
41. Frost RO, Hartl T: A cognitive-behavioral model of compulsive hoarding, *Behav Res Ther* 34;341–350, 1996.
42. Barlow DH: Disorders of emotion, *Psychol Inq* 2:58–71, 1991.
43. Butler G, Mathews A: Cognitive processes in anxiety, *Adv Behav Res Ther* 5:51–62, 1983.
44. Steketee G, Frost RO: Measurement of risk-taking in obsessive compulsive disorder, *Behav Cogn Psychother* 22:269–298, 1994.
45. Rhéaume J, Ladouceur R, Freeston MH: The prediction of obsessive compulsive symptoms: New evidence for multiple cognitive vulnerability factors, Unpublished manuscript, 1996.
46. Steiner J, Jarvis M, Parrish J: Risk-taking and arousal regulation, *Br J Med Psychol* 43:333–348, 1970.
47. Salkovskis PM: The importance of behaviour in the maintenance of anxiety and panic: A cognitive account, *Behav Psychother* 19:6–19, 1991.
48. Pitman RK: Pierre Janet on obsessive-compulsive disorder (1903): Review and commentary, *Arch Gen Psychiatry* 44:226–232, 1987b.
49. Mallinger AE: The obsessive's myth of control, *J Am Acad Psychoanal* 12:147–165, 1984.
50. Salzman L: *The obsessive personality*, New York, 1968, Jason Aronson.
51. Honjo S, Hirano C, Murase S, et al: Obsessive compulsive symptoms in childhood and adolescence, *Acta Psychiatr Scand* 80:83–91, 1989.
52. Tallis F: Compulsive washing in the absence of phobic and illness anxiety, *Behav Res Ther* 34:361–362, 1996.
53. Frost RO, Marten P, Lahart C, Rosenblate R: The dimensions of perfectionism, *Cogn Ther Res* 14:449–468, 1990.
54. Frost RO, Steketee G, Cohn L, Greiss K: Personality traits in subclinical and nonobsessive compulsive volunteers and their parents, *Behav Res Ther* 32:47–56, 1994.
55. Gershuny BS, Sher KJ: Compulsive checking and anxiety in a nonclinical sample: Differences in cognition, behavior, personality, and affect, *J Psychopathol Behav Assess* 17:19–38, 1995.

56. Frost RO, Gross RC: The hoarding of possessions, *Behav Res Ther* 31:367–381, 1993.
57. Ferrari JR: Perfectionism cognitions with nonclinical and clinical samples, *J Soc Behav Person* 10:143–156, 1995.
58. Frost RO, Steketee G: Perfectionism in obsessive compulsive disorder patients, *Behav Res Ther* 35:291–296, 1997.
59. Juster HR, Heimberg RG, Frost RO, et al: Social phobia and perfectionism, *Person Indiv Diff* 21:403–410, 1996.
60. Bastiani AM, Rao R, Weltzin T, Kaye WH: Perfectionism in anorexia nervosa, *Int J Eating Dis* 17:147–152, 1995.
61. Hewitt PL, Flett GL: Perfectionism and depression: A multidimensional analysis, *J Soc Behav Person* 5:423–438, 1991.
62. Purdon C, Clark DA: Obsessive intrusive thoughts in nonclinical subjects. Part II. Cognitive appraisal, emotional response and thought control strategies, *Behav Res Ther* 32:403–410, 1994.
63. Freeston MH, Rhéaume J, Dugas KM, Ladouceur R: Surestimation de l'importance des pensées obsessionnelles. Paper presented at the 18th annual convention for the Quebec Society of Research in Psychology, Ottawa, Canada, October 1995.
64. Freeston MH, Bouchard S: Positive and negative interpretations and disturbed mood in the treatment of obsessive thoughts: A pilot study. Paper presented at the World Congress of Behavioural and Cognitive Therapies, Copenhagen, Denmark, July 1995.
65. Wegner DM: *White bears and other unwanted thoughts*, New York, 1989, Viking/Penguin.
66. Salkovskis PM, Campbell P: Thought suppression induces intrusion in naturally occurring negative intrusive thoughts, *Behav Res Ther* 32:1–8, 1994.
67. Beech HR, Liddell A: Decision-making, mood states and ritualistic behaviour among obsessional patients. In Beech HR, editor: *Obsessional states*, London, 1974, Methuen.
68. Makhlouf-Norris F, Norris H: The obsessive-compulsive syndrome as a neurotic device for the reduction of self-uncertainty, *Br J Psychiatry* 121:277–288, 1972.
69. Tallis F: The characteristics of obsessional thinking: Difficulty demonstrating the obvious? *Clin Psychol Psychother* 2:24–39, 1995.
70. American Psychiatric Association: *Diagnostic and statistical manual of mental disorders*, ed 4, Washington, 1994, American Psychiatric Association Press.
71. Clark DA, Purdon CL: The assessment of unwanted intrusive thoughts: A review and critique of the literature, *Behav Res Ther* 33:967–976, 1995.
72. Wells A, Morrison AP: Qualitative dimensions of normal worry and normal obsessions: A comparative study, *Behav Res Ther* 32:867–870, 1994.
73. Clark DA, deSilva P: The nature of depressive and anxious thoughts: Distinct or uniform phenomena? *Behav Res Ther* 23:383–393, 1985.
74. Purdon C, Clark DA: Obsessive intrusive thoughts in nonclinical subjects. Part I. Content and relation with depressive, anxious and obsessional symptoms, *Behav Res Ther* 31:713–720, 1993.
75. Wegner DM, Zanakos S: Chronic thought suppression, *J Personal* 62:615–640, 1994.
76. Wegner DM, Schneider DJ, Carter III SR, White TL: Paradoxical effects of thought suppression, *J Personal Soc Psychol* 53:5–13, 1987.

77. Freeston MH, Ladouceur R, Gagnon F, Thibodeau N: Beliefs about obsessional thoughts, *J Psychopathol Behav Assess* 15:1–21, 1993a.
78. Sookman C, Pinard G, Engelsmann F: The obsessive compulsive disorder cognitive schemata scale: Reliability and validity, Unpublished manuscript, 1997.
79. Sookman C, Pinard G, Engelsmann F: The obsessive compulsive disorder cognitive schema scale: Reliability and validity, Unpublished manuscript, 1997.
80. Clark DA, Purdon C: Meta-cognitive beliefs in obsessive-compulsive disorders. Paper presented at the World Congress of Behavioural and Cognitive Therapies, Copenhagen, Denmark, July 1995.
81. Kyrios M, Bhar SS: A measure of inflated responsibility: Its development and relationship to obsessive compulsive phenomena. Paper presented at the World Congress of Behavioral and Cognitions Therapies, Copenhagen, Denmark, July 1995.
82. Salkovskis PM: Cognitive models and therapy of obsessive compulsive disorder. Paper presented at the World Congress of Cognitive Therapy, Toronto, Ontario, Canada, 1992.
83. Foa EB: Failure in treating obsessive compulsives, *Behav Res Ther* 17:169–176, 1979.
84. Kozak MJ, Foa EB: Obsessions, overvalued ideas, and delusions in obsessive-compulsive disorder, *Behav Res Ther* 32:343–353, 1994.
85. Kozak MJ: Fixity of Beliefs Questionnaire. Unpublished scale, Philadelphia, 1996, Department of Psychiatry, Medical College of Pennsylvania.
86. Eisen JL, Phillips KA, Beer D, et al: Brown Assessment of Beliefs Scales (BABS). Unpublished manuscript, Providence, 1996, Department of Psychiatry, Brown University School of Medicine.
87. Neziroglu F, Yaryura-Tobias JA, McKay DR, et al: Overvalued Idea Scale. Unpublished scale, Great Neck, 1986, Institute of Bio-Behavioral Therapy and Research.
88. Williams JMG, Watts FN, MacLeod C, Mathews A: *Cognitive psychology and emotional disorders*, New York, 1988, Wiley.
89. Reed GF: 'Underinclusion' a characteristic of obsessional personality disorder: I. *Br J Psychiatry* 115:781–785, 1969a.
90. Reed GF: 'Underinclusion' a characteristic of obsessional personality: II. *Br J Psychiatry* 130:177–183, 1969b.
91. Persons, Foa EB: Processing of fearful and neutral information by obsessive-compulsives, *Behav Res Ther* 22:259–265, 1984.
92. Frost RO, Lahart CM, Dugas KM, Sher KJ: Information processing among non-clinical compulsives, *Behav Res Ther* 26:275–277, 1988.
93. Frost RO, Shows D: The nature and measurement of compulsive indecisiveness, *Behav Res Ther* 31:683–692, 1993.
94. Milner A, Beech R, Walker V: Decision processes and obsessional behavior, *Br J Soc Clin Psychol* 10:88–89, 1971.
95. Sartory G, Master D: Contingent negative variation in obsessional-compulsive patients, *Biol Psychol* 18:253–267, 1984.
96. Volans PJ: Styles of decision making and probability appraisal in selected obsessional and phobic patients, *Br J Soc Clin Psychol* 15:305–317, 1976.
97. Broadbent DE, Broadbent MHP, Jones JL: Performance correlates of self-reported cognitive failure and of obsessionality, *Br J Clin Psychol* 25:285–299, 1986.

98. Gordon PK: Allocation of attention in obsessional disorder, *Br J Clin Psychol* 24:101–107, 1985.
99. Treisman A: Verbal cues, language and meaning in selective attention, *Am J Psychol* 77:205–219, 1964.
100. Tipper SP: The negative priming effect: Inhibitory priming by ignored objects, *Q J Exp Psychol* 37:571–590, 1985.
101. Beech AR, McManus D, Baylis GC, et al: Individual differences in cognitive processes: Towards an explanation of schizophrenic symptomatology, *Br J Psychol* 82:417–426, 1991.
102. Pitman RK: A cybernetic model of obsessive-compulsive psychopathology, *Comprehens Psychiatry* 28:334–343, 1987a.
103. Enright SJ, Beech AR: Obsessional states: Anxiety disorders or schizotypes? An information processing and personality assessment, *Psychol Med* 20:621–627, 1990.
104. Enright SJ, Beech AR: Reduced cognitive inhibition in obsessive-compulsive disorder, *Br J Clin Psychol* 32:67–74, 1993a.
105. Enright SJ, Beech AR: Further evidence of reduced cognitive inhibition in obsessive-compulsive disorder, *Pers Individ Diff* 14:387–395, 1993b.
106. Lavy E, Van der Hout M: Thought suppression induces intrusions, *Behav Psychother* 18:251–258, 1990.
107. Maki WS, O'Neill HK, O'Neill GW: Do nonclinical checkers exhibit deficits in cognitive control? Tests of an inhibitory control hypothesis, *Behav Res Ther* 29:147–160, 1994.
108. Stroop JR: Studies of interference in serial verbal reactions, *J Exp Psychol* 18:643–661, 1935.
109. Foa EB, McNally RJ: Sensitivity of feared stimuli in obsessive compulsives: A dichotic listening analysis, *Cogn Ther Res* 10:477–485, 1986.
110. Foa EB, Ilai D, McCarthy PR, et al: Information processing in obsessive-compulsive disorder, *Cogn Ther Res* 17:173–189, 1993.
111. Martin M, Williams RM, Clark DM: Does anxiety lead to selective processing of threat-related information? *Behav Res Ther* 29:147–160, 1991.
112. Lavy E, van Oppen P, van Den Hout M: Selective processing of emotional information in obsessive-compulsive disorder, *Behav Res Ther* 32:243–246, 1994.
113. Otto MW: Normal and abnormal information processing. A neuropsychological perspective on obsessive-compulsive disorder, *Psychiatr Clin North Am* 15:825–847, 1992.
114. Sher KJ, Frost RO, Kushner M, et al: Memory deficits in compulsive checkers: Replication and extension in a clinical sample, *Behav Res Ther* 27:65–69, 1989.
115. Sher KJ, Frost RO, Otto R: Cognitive deficits in compulsive checkers: An exploratory study, *Behav Res Ther* 4:357–364, 1983.
116. Sheffler Rubenstein CS, Peynircioglu ZF, Chambless DL, Pigott TA: Memory in sub-clinical checkers, *Behav Res Ther* 31:759–765, 1993.
117. McNally RJ, Kohlbeck PA: Reality monitoring in obsessive-compulsive disorder, *Behav Res Ther* 31:249–253, 1993.
118. Brown HD, Kosslyn SM, Breiter HC, et al: Can patients with obsessive compulsive disorder discriminate between percepts and mental images? A signal detection analysis, *J Ab Psychol* 3:445–454, 1994.

119. Constans JI, Foa EB, Franklin ME, Mathews A: Memory for actual and imagined events in OC checkers, *Behav Res Ther* 33:665–671, 1995.
120. Wilhelm S, McNally RJ, Baer L, Florin I: Directed forgetting in obsessive-compulsive disorder, *Behav Res Ther* 34:633–641, 1996.
121. Christensen KL, Kim SW, Dysken MW, Hoover KM: Neuropsychological performance in obsessive-compulsive disorder, *Biol Psychiatry* 31:4–18, 1992.
122. Watts FN: An information-processing approach to compulsive checking, *Clin Psychol Psychother* 2:69–77, 1995.
123. Anderson RE: Did I do it or did I only imagine doing it? *J Exper Psychol* 113:594–613, 1984.
124. Foa EB, Steketee G: Obsessive compulsives: Conceptual issues and treatment interventions. In Hersen M, Eisler RM, Miller PM, editors: *Progress in behavior modification*, vol 8, New York, 1979, Academic Press.
125. Emmelkamp PMG, Beens I: Cognitive therapy with obsessive-compulsive disorder: A comparative evaluation, *Behav Res Ther* 29:293–300, 1991.
126. Van Oppen P, de Haan E, van Balkom AJLM, et al: Cognitive therapy and exposure in vivo in the treatment of obsessive-compulsive disorder, *Behav Res Ther* 33:379–390, 1995.
127. Neziroglu F, Neuman J: Three treatment approaches for obsessions. *J Cogn Psychother* 4:377–392, 1990.
128. Emmelkamp PMG, Visser S, Hoekstra RJ: Cognitive therapy versus exposure in vivo in the treatment of obsessive-compulsives, *Cogn Ther Res* 12:103–114, 1988.
129. Kearney CA, Silverman WK: Treatment of an adolescent with obsessive-compulsive disorder by alternating response prevention and cognitive therapy: An empirical analysis, *J Behav Ther Exp Psychiatry* 1:39–47, 1990.
130. Salkovskis PM, Warwick HMC: Morbid preoccupations, health anxiety and reassurance: A cognitive-behavioral approach to hypochondriasis, *Behav Res Ther* 24:597–602, 1986.
131. Gurnani PD, Wang M: Cognitive therapy of obsessive-compulsive disorder: Treating treatment failures, *Behav Psychother* 15:101–103, 1987.
132. Ladouceur R, Léger E, Rhéaume J, Dubé D: Correction of inflated responsibility in the treatment of obsessive-compulsive disorder, *Behav Res Ther* 34:767–774, 1996.
133. Ladouceur R, Rhéaume J, Léger F: Cognitive change during cognitive treatment and behavioral treatment of checking behaviors. Paper presented at the Association for Advancement of Behavior Therapy, New York, November 1996.
134. van Oppen P, 1995, Personal communication.
135. Freeston MH, Ladouceur R, Rhéaume J, et al: Cognitive behavioral treatment of obsessive thoughts, *J Consult Clin Psychol* 65:405–413, 1997.
136. Sookman D, Pinard G, Beauchemin N: Multidimensional schematic restructuring treatment for obsessions: Theory and practice, *J Cogn Psychother* 8:175–194, 1994.
137. Drummond LM: The treatment of severe, chronic, resistant obsessive-compulsive disorder, *Br J Psychiatry* 163:223–229, 1993.
138. Van Oppen P, Arntz A: Cognitive therapy for obsessive-compulsive disorder, *Behav Res Ther* 32:79–87, 1994.

19

Cognitive-Behavioral Psychotherapy for Pediatric Obsessive-Compulsive Disorder

John S. March, M.D., MP.H.

Over the past 10 years, cognitive-behavioral and pharmacologic treatments for young persons with obsessive-compulsive disorder (OCD) have become widely available.[1] It is unclear whether insight-oriented psychotherapy for OCD has proven as disappointing in children and adolescents[2] as it has in adults;[3] cognitive-behavioral therapy (CBT), however, has become the psychotherapeutic treatment of choice for OCD patients of all ages.[4,5] Unlike other psychotherapies that have been applied to OCD, CBT presents a logically consistent and compelling relationship among the disorder, the treatment, and the specified outcome.[4,6] Despite the previous consensus of CBT,[7] clinicians routinely report that *patients will not comply* with behavioral treatments and parents complain that *clinicians are poorly trained* in CBT; this situation results in many, if not most, patients lacking effective treatment. This unfortunate situation may be avoided with an increased understanding of CBT implementation in cases of children and adolescents with OCD.

This chapter reviews the cognitive-behavioral treatment of children and adolescents with OCD, as implemented in *How I ran OCD off my land: A guide to the treatment of obsessive-compulsive disorder in children and adolescents*.[8] We begin with a brief review of the principles that underlie the cognitive-behavioral treatment of OCD, move on to discuss our OCD protocol, summarize our results using this protocol, and conclude by discussing directions for future research in specific treatment recommendations.

Interested readers may wish to peruse a more in-depth treatment of assessment issues;[9,10] diagnosis and comorbidity;[11–14] OCD in the school setting;[15] spectrum disorders;[16–18] natural history;[19] cognitive-behavioral psychotherapy;[20–22] and pharmacotherapy.[23,24] Each of these treatment strategies is discussed as an integrated approach to the treatment of OCD across the patient's life span in the *Expert Consensus Guidelines for OCD*,[7] which also covers level of care issues, such as number of sessions and treatment setting—issues that are of critical importance in managed care.

FIRST PRINCIPLES

Flexible, empirically supported, cognitive-behavioral treatments are available now for many childhood mental illnesses aside from OCD,[25] including anxiety, aggression, depression, attention deficit–hyperactivity disorder, pain, and learning disabilities. As Kendall indicates, because these treatments are linked tightly to their targets, they often differ from each other in both theory and applications,[26] which in turn makes manualized treatment protocols essential to treatment dissemination.[27] In contrast to disruptive behavior disorders in which contingency management is the rule, and depression, in which cognitive therapy dominates, exposure-based interventions are paramount in treating anxiety disorders, including OCD.[25]

Exposure and Response Prevention

As applied to OCD, the exposure principle relies on the fact that anxiety usually attenuates after sufficient duration of contact with a feared stimulus.[6,28] Thus, a child with fear of germs must confront relevant feared situations until his or her anxiety decreases. Repeated exposure is associated with decreased anxiety across exposure trials, with anxiety reduction largely specific to the domain of exposure, until the child no longer fears contact with specifically targeted phobic stimuli.[29,30] Exposure is typically implemented in a gradual fashion (sometimes termed *graded exposure*), with exposure targets under patient or, less desirably, therapist control.[30] Adequate exposure depends on blocking rituals or avoidance behavior—a process termed *response prevention.* For example, a child with a fear of germs must not only touch "germy things," but also must refrain from ritualized washing until the anxiety diminishes substantially.

Extinction

Because blocking rituals or avoidance behaviors remove the negative reinforcement effect of the rituals or avoidance, response prevention is technically an extinction procedure. By convention, however, extinction is usually defined as the elimination of OCD–related behaviors through the removal of parental positive reinforcement for rituals. For example, for a child with reassurance-seeking rituals, the therapist may ask parents to refrain from gratifying the child's actions. Extinction frequently produces rapid effects but can be hard to implement when the child's behavior is bizarre or very frequent. In addition, nonconsensual extinction procedures often elicit unmanageable distress on the part of the child, disrupt the therapeutic alliance, miss important exposure and response prevention (ERP) targets that are not amenable to extinction procedures, and, most importantly, fail to help the child develop a strategy for resisting OCD. Hence, as with ERP, placing the extinction program under the child's control leads to increased patient compliance and improved outcomes.[21,22]

Cognitive Therapy

Many children lack the cognitive framework to succeed at ERP, although they know what to do. When actually undertaking an ERP task, children and adolescents (perhaps more than adults) tend to engage in negative self-talk that disables the child and empowers OCD. Thus, it can be helpful clinically to provide the child a cognitive strategy for "bossing-back" OCD. Similar interventions have been helpful in some adults with OCD as well.[31,32] Targets for cognitive therapy include reinforcing accurate information regarding OCD and its treatment, encouraging cognitive resistance ("bossing-back OCD"), cultivating a sense of detachment,[33] and developing self-administered positive reinforcement and encouragement.

Anxiety Management

Anxiety management training (defined here as a combination of relaxation training, breathing control training, and cognitive training directed at general anxiety rather than OCD) is an effective treatment for overanxious children and adolescents,[34] but preliminary data in younger patients suggest that relaxation is an inert and cognitive intervention, a somewhat weaker treatment for OCD than ERP.[35] Where indicated, anxiety management training may contribute to the successful cognitive-behavioral treatment of younger persons with OCD (1) by targeting comorbidities that might interfere with OCD treatment; and (2) by facilitating exposure through reducing the amplitude of exposure-related anxiety.

Operant Techniques

In clinical practice, operant procedures involve the application of rewards, punishments, and negative reinforcement for various targeted behaviors. Positive reinforcement (imposition of a positive or desirable event) does not directly alter OCD symptoms but may help encourage exposure and produce an indirect clinical benefit. We routinely use within-session prizes and between-session reward ceremonies to recognize and solidify treatment gains. In contrast, punishment (imposition of an aversive event) or response-cost (removal of a positive event) procedures have been uniformly unhelpful in the treatment of OCD.[36] The same can be said for negative-reinforcement procedures, namely the removal of an aversive event to increase a desired behavior. An example of unhelpful negative reinforcement (the child avoids an aversive situation) is a parent caving in to a child's refusal to clean his or her room. Conversely, a constructive use of negative reinforcement in parent training for disruptive behavior might be letting a child out of "time out" after a sufficient period of time. In OCD, rituals relieve dysphoric affects through negative reinforcement; blocking this effect is the job of response prevention. Conversely, the process of negative reinforcement also characterizes successful treatment for OCD in that a reduction in aversive OCD symptoms through ERP produces an increase in the child's motivation to engage in ERP, and consequently reduces additional symptoms. Thus, in the National Institute of Mental Health (NIMH) cohort, children who did well seemed to have spontaneously discovered how to successfully say "no" to OCD;[37] we explicitly rely on the negative-reinforcement value of OCD treatment to negotiate graded exposure.[29]

Modeling and Shaping

Therapist modeling—whether overt (the child understands that the therapist is demonstrating more appropriate or adaptive behavior) or covert (the therapist informally models a behavior)—helps improve compliance with in-session ERP and generalization to between-session ERP homework. Similarly, shaping involves positively reinforcing successive approximations to a desired target behavior. Modeling and shaping also reduce anticipatory anxiety and provide an opportunity for increased constructive self-talk before and during ERP.[38] Because ERP has not proved particularly helpful with obsessional slowness, modeling and shaping procedures are currently the behavioral treatment of choice for children with this OCD subtype.[39] Unfortunately, relapse often occurs when therapist-assisted shaping, limit-setting, and temporal-speeding procedures are withdrawn.[40]

SUMMARY OF OUR TREATMENT PROTOCOL

Table 19-1 summarizes the treatment protocol, which assumes that the child has already completed a thorough evaluation. Treatment takes place in four steps, usually over 12 to 20 sessions. Each session includes (1) a statement of goals; (2) a careful review of the preceding week; (3) introduction of new information; (4) therapist-assisted "nuts-and-bolts" practice; (5) selection of homework for the coming week; and (6) monitoring procedures. Information sheets describing the goals and homework for that week are given at the end of each session. Step One focuses on psychoeducation during two sessions in the first week. Step Two provides an anxiety-management "tool kit" which overlaps with Step One in the first and second weeks. Step Three, which maps OCD, is completed during the second week. These first three steps form the basis for Step Four. Step Four initiates intensive graded ERP over week 3 to 20 sessions, although many children require far fewer sessions.

Step One places OCD firmly within a neurobehavioral model by linking OCD with a specific set of behavioral treatments and a desired outcome (i.e., symptom reduction). To cement the neurobehavioral framework, the therapist makes use of analogies to medical illnesses, such as asthma or diabetes. Metaphors for obsessions also are introduced, such as "brain hiccups" or

Table 19-1 Cognitive-Behavioral Therapy Treatment Protocol

Visit Number	Goals
Session 1/Week 1	Psychoeducation
Session 2/Week 1	"Tool kit"
Session 3/Week 2	Mapping obsessive-compulsive disorder
Session 4/Week 2	"Tool kit"
Weekly sessions 5–20	Exposure and response prevention
Sessions 17–19	Relapse prevention
Weeks 1, 7, and 11	Parent sessions

"problems with the volume-control knob," which are used with younger children. This analogy is not as far-fetched as it might seem at first. Because OCD presumably has its roots in disordered information processing in the brain,[41] changes in symptoms with CBT ought to reflect changes in brain function, which is just what Lew Baxter and Jeff Schwartz discovered when they looked at images of brains at work in OCD patients before and after drug or behavior therapy. In those who responded to treatment, the positron emission tomography images changed toward normal in both patients treated with drugs and in patients treated with CBT (see Chapter 15).[33,42] Examined this way, patients with OCD can be approached in the same way as patients with diabetes—except that the target organ is the brain rather than the pancreas, and thus the symptom picture differs. Each disorder involves medications, which might be insulin in diabetes and a serotonin reuptake inhibitor in OCD. Each disorder involves psychosocial interventions that work in part by moving the somatic substrate toward more normal function. In diabetes, the psychosocial treatments of choice are diet and exercise; in OCD, treatments involve CBT. Finally, not all patients recover completely, so some interventions must target coping with residual symptoms, such as foot care in diabetes and patient and family management of residual symptoms in OCD.

In addition to providing an extensive discussion of OCD as a medical illness, Step One also presents the risks and benefits of behavioral treatment for OCD and reviews specific details of the treatment protocol. Step One also begins the process of externalizing OCD—younger children may give OCD a nasty nickname, and older children often simply calling the problem OCD. In this way, the child and his or her family can ally with the therapist against OCD to "boss-back" the obsessions and compulsions. Adolescents and parents ordinarily appreciate a more detailed discussion of OCD as a neurobehavioral disorder.

Step two introduces a cognitive training "tool kit" consisting of training in cognitive tactics for resisting OCD as distinct from response prevention for mental rituals. Goals of cognitive therapy include increasing a sense of personal efficacy, predictability, controllability, and self-attributed likelihood of a positive outcome for ERP tasks. Targets for cognitive therapy include reinforcing accurate information regarding OCD and its treatment, encouraging cognitive resistance ("bossing-back OCD"), and developinig self-administered positive reinforcement and encouragement. To increase the patient's sense of predictability and controllability, we explicitly frame ERP as the strategy, and the therapist and parents (and sometimes teachers or friends) as the allies in the child's "battle" against OCD. To further emphasize the child's responsibility for resisting OCD without inviting further "blaming" by family members, teachers, and friends, we ask the child to give OCD a nasty nickname. By always using a disparaging name to refer to OCD, the therapist "externalizes" OCD,[43] so that the disorder becomes a discrete "enemy" and not a "bad habit" that may have been associated with previous punishment. Adolescents frequently find this procedure silly and prefer to refer to OCD by its medical appellation, but the principle of externalizing the disorder remains the same. Approaching OCD in this way allows everyone to ally with the child to "boss-back" OCD and thereby provides a narrative scaffolding on which to hang family interventions.

We also use three cognitive techniques to help our patients monitor and skillfully control themselves under the stress of exposure-based interventions: (1) constructive self-talk;[44] (2) cognitive restructuring;[31,45] and (3) cultivation of detachment.[33] Each technique must be individualized to match the specific OCD symptoms and must mesh with the child's cognitive abilities, developmental stages, and preference among the three techniques. It also is generally best to develop a tailored "short form" that the child can use on a regular basis during ERP. Used in this fashion, cognitive therapy provides the child with a cognitive "tool kit" to use during ERP tasks, which in turn facilitates ERP compliance.

Step Three maps the child's experience with OCD, including specific obsessions and compulsions, triggers, avoidance behaviors, and consequences (Figure 19-1). In behavioral terms, these steps generate a stimulus hierarchy within a narrative context. We use cartographic metaphors, diagrammed in Figure 19-1, to understand where the child is free from OCD, where OCD and the child each "win" some of the time, and where the child feels helpless against OCD. We call the central region where the child already has some success in resisting OCD, the transition zone. Continuing the map metaphor, "standing" with the child on territory free from OCD allows the therapist to strengthen the twin beliefs that (1) he or she is on the child's side in the struggle against OCD; and (2) the therapist is interested in the child as a person who wants desperately to free himself from OCD. The therapist teaches the child to recognize and use the transition zone, thereby providing a reliable guide to selecting ERP targets throughout the treatment program. In practice, the transition zone is usually defined by the lower end of the stimulus hierarchy.

Steps Two and Three include easy trial ERP tasks to gauge the patient's tolerance of anxiety, level of understanding, and willingness or ability to com-

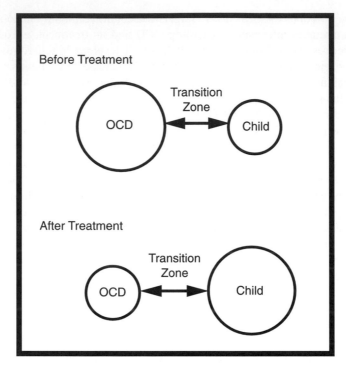

Fig. 19-1 Mapping obsessive-compulsive disorder.

ply with treatment, while instilling the idea that it is possible to successfully resist and "win" against OCD. Trial ERP tasks also demonstrate whether or not the transition zone has been accurately located, thereby avoiding disruptive "surprises" caused by mistargeted goals for ERP.

Step Four implements the core of CBT for anxiety disorders, namely, intensive, graded ERP, including therapist-assisted imaginal and *in vivo* ERP practice coupled with weekly homework assignments. Exposure occurs when the child exposes himself or herself to the feared object, action, or thought. Response prevention is the process of blocking rituals or minimizing the avoidance behaviors. Consider the child with a "contamination" fear about touching doorknobs. In this case, because doorknobs trigger the obsession, a contrived exposure task would require the child to touch the "contaminated" doorknob until his or her anxiety disappears. Response prevention takes place when the child refuses to perform the usual anxiety-driven compulsion, such as handwashing or using a tissue to grasp the doorknob.

As in a contest, OCD is framed as the adversary, and all parties remain intransigent against OCD. This framework explicitly requires that the child use his or her allies (therapist and parents or friends) and new strategies (cognitive therapy and ERP) to resist OCD, thereby preventing the therapy from becoming an excuse to avoid exposure. However, because only the child can perform the actual combat (i.e., ERP), he or she necessarily remains in charge of choosing targets from the transition zone. We update the transition zone at the beginning of each session as the child becomes more competent and successful at resisting OCD.

Beginning with Step One, which emphasizes psychoeducation, parents are an important part of the treatment process. At the end of Step One, parents receive an information booklet ("Tips for Parents," included with the manual) that includes tips for managing OCD. Parents typically attend sessions one, seven, and eleven. Parent sessions seven and eleven focus on incorporating targets for parental response prevention or extinction, with the child again selecting targets from the transition zone. Parents also may attend sessions toward the end of treatment that focus on generalization training and relapse prevention. Parents check in with the therapist at the beginning or end of each session, and we invite parents to comment on the child's progress in his or her struggle against OCD.

Homework assignments are presented each week with individualized clues to help the child successfully "boss-back" OCD. We liberally use positive reinforcers, such as within-session praise and small prizes, like pencils or gum, and between-session larger rewards, such as a trip for pizza with friends. To encourage positive reinforcement and to extinguish punishment by adults and peers, we also make a special effort to help the youngster tell other people (e.g., friends, teachers, or grandparents) how he or she has successfully reduced OCD influence over his or her life.

Treatment ends with a "graduation ceremony," followed by a booster session 6 weeks later.

Logistical Considerations

Questions about the frequency and number of sessions usually are uppermost in the minds of the child and parents. Because the first four sessions involve mostly teaching and information gathering, they can be scheduled twice weekly and are best not drawn out further than once a week. In addition to building rapport and enlisting the child's cooperation in the treatment process, these first few sessions lay the groundwork for the child to think differently about OCD. It is important early on for both child and adolescent to become well informed about the treatment process, especially the centrality of ERP. The sessions following session four can be scheduled at weekly or, less desirably, bi-weekly intervals. If bi-weekly sessions are chosen, progress-check phone calls between sessions are recommended.

A second logistical issue is a place to hold CBT sessions. The therapist need not be bound to the office, although often this is the case out of necessity. When ERP practice becomes the bulk of the session, field trips to places that will trigger OCD are especially valuable. The therapist should be creative in ways to practice ERP in the office, which may include bringing in household items, such as a chemical cleanser, to serve as a trigger for ERP practice.

A third logistical issues involves time—how much should be allotted and how to organize it (Table 19-2). Each session lasts approximately 50 minutes. Before the session begins, parents are given a handout of parent tips for the week and are encouraged to read through these as the child is meeting with the therapist and jot down any questions they may want to ask during the 10-minute parent check-in at the end of the first session. This procedure of course can be modified for adolescents who come alone, in which case parents may receive all parent tips for sessions one through four during the session. The first 10 minutes of each session are spent checking in with the child and reviewing the previous week's homework. If the child proved unable to complete the homework, this time is spent identifying what the obstacles were to completing the homework successfully. The next 20 minutes are spent presenting and completing the goals for the current session. When session goals are completed, the final 10 minutes are spent helping the child choose the week's homework task. This time includes review of the strategies identified earlier to increase homework success. A brief check-in with the parent(s) is completed at the end of the session, to answer any immediate questions or concerns. During the middle and end of treatment, as much as 30 to 40 minutes of each session may be spent in therapist-assisted exposure tasks. As a reward for participating in the hard work of ERP, time at the end of the session may be allocated to a social reward, such as playing a game or talking about something other than OCD.

Developmental Considerations

It is understood that treatment must be adjusted so that it is appropriate to the level of cognitive functioning, social maturity, and capacity for sustained attention of each patient. Additionally, developmental considerations sometimes may be confused with the diagnosis of OCD. For example, bedtime rituals, eating or dressing rituals, and collections are common in children at different ages. In a pioneering study,[46] Henrietta Leonard indicated that these developmentally normal rituals may be distinguished from OCD on the basis of frequency (common), setting (normal even across cultures), and context (adaptive rather than dysfunctional). Making these distinctions can sometimes help sharpen insight, particularly in younger patients. Younger patients also usually require more redirection and activities; adolescents are more sensitive to the effects of OCD on peer interactions, which in turn requires more discussion. Cognitive interventions especially require adjustment to the developmental level of the patient. For example, adolescents typically are less likely to appreciate the meaning of giving OCD a "nasty nickname" than are younger children.

More importantly, developmental themes involving separation (becoming

Table 19-2   What Happens at Each Session?

Session Goals	Time, min
Check-in with child and parents	5
Review homework	5
Teaching and learning tasks for week	20
Therapist-assisted practice	10
Discuss and agree on homework	10
Parent review of session and homework	10

his or her own boss) and individuation (becoming his or her own person) may affect the therapist's ability to implement treatment. For example, patients who are grappling with separation or individuation themes may find OCD tangled up in "boss battles with parents," which are inherently developmental in nature and may, as a result, cause such patients experience some difficulty engaging in CBT. Such difficulties may be more common in patients in the early elementary years and in early adolescence. In either case, helping the child and parents differentiate what is developmental, what is a symptom related to OCD, and how the two interact, will help move therapist, patient, and family toward a consensus treatment plan.

Graded Family Involvement

Because each family is different in the ways its members affect and are affected by OCD, the child's treatment must be individualized with respect to the extent of family involvement.[47] It is important to incorporate families into treatment, especially in those cases in which (1) family members are engulfed by OCD; or (2) family problems obstruct the treatment of OCD. Too little family involvement may reduce the effectiveness of CBT; too much family involvement may not only cause the therapy to stall, but also the therapy may (appropriately) anger the family. In all cases, family members are helped to ally with the affected child in the struggle with OCD and are provided with extensive information about the disorder and its treatment. To get treatment started on the best possible footing, two specific interventions—stop giving advice and differentially reinforce of other behavior—also are provided beginning with the first session.

More on Combining Cognitive-Behavioral Therapy and Pharmacotherapy

Although many childhood behaviors are in some sense problematic, not all behaviors—even symptomatic behaviors—are appropriate targets for medication management or treatment with CBT. It is crucial to clearly define the target symptoms for psychopharmacologic as compared with psychosocial interventions whenever possible. In OCD, we usually use the analogy of a "dimmer switch" for a light bulb to communicate the idea that pharmacotherapy decreases obsessions and the accompanying dysphoric effects, and, at the same time, makes it easier to resist OCD. However, because antiexposure instructions (i.e., avoid the things that make you anxious, and if you can, do your rituals as fast as possible to get them over with) completely attenuate the potential benefits of medications,[48] the combination of CBT and medication is likely more helpful than medication alone for most patients. In this context, we usually recommend beginning treatment with CBT alone whenever possible. Patients with either severe OCD or complicating conditions—such as panic disorder or depression, which may interfere with CBT—will frequently wish to start with medication, adding in CBT once the medicine has provided some symptom relief. If satisfactory progress isn't forthcoming within 6 to 8 weeks with weekly CBT, despite a strong effort by the patient to resist OCD, the addition of medication is usually a good idea.[7] For many patients, starting both treatments from the beginning will be attractive because combined treatment may offer greater benefit. We see many patients who have "failed" multiple medication trials; it is our experience that returning to standard, well-delivered pharmacotherapy, combined with CBT and academic intervention, converts nonresponders more reliably than does the introduction of polypharmacy.

Comorbidity

Not surprisingly, comorbidity complicates both the diagnosis and treatment of pediatric OCD. In some cases, the presence of a comorbid disorder (e.g., a tic or thought disorder) indicates the need for an additional treatment, such as a neuroleptic medication, that is both augmentative (for the OCD) and adjunctive (for the comorbidity).[24] In other cases, although treatments such as stimulants for attention deficit–hyperactivity disorder are multimodal, these treatments target different symptom constellations.[49,50] In a comprehensive discussion on the influence of treatment planning on comorbidity, Clarkin and Kendall[51] make the obvious but often neglected point that treatments must be matched to their targets. Likewise, we recommend parsimoniously combining treatments that are appropriate for OCD and the comorbid conditions, while carefully monitoring treatment outcomes for each intervention.[7,24] For example, comorbid depression can be conceptualized as a problem of loss in relationships, so CBT targets thoughts and behaviors designed to reconstitute relationships—be they intrapsychic, interpersonal, work, or spiritual.[52] Interestingly, CBT for depression is the least-specific treatment with respect to response (e.g., supportive, dynamic, and interpersonal psychotherapies are probably equally effective, and all are associated with large "placebo" responses). As for anxiety disorders, CBT targets cognitions and behaviors designed to promote habituation or extinction of inappropriate fears, as we have seen in the treatment of pediatric OCD with CBT.[53] Each of these technologies is supported by robust research literature, and manuals are available to guide practitioners in the use of CBT for specific problems.[26,54]

Multimodal "Team" Treatment

By now, it should be clear that successful treatment of pediatric OCD requires the clinician to wear many professional "hats," including those of supportive psychotherapist, behavior therapist, psychopharmacologist, and perhaps, family therapist. Few mental health providers are equally skilled in all these areas. For example, psychiatrists and psychologists are often poorly trained in cognitive-behavioral and medication treatments, respectively. Further, in many settings, such as large multispecialty groups or community mental health centers, child psychiatrists regularly function as diagnostic and psychopharmacologic consultants, reserving other aspects of OCD treatment for professionals from other disciplines. In this context, initiation of a multimodal treatment plan for a child with OCD requires a team approach, with different providers coordinating and carrying out different aspects of the treatment program. With each provider from a potentially different theoretic orientation or mental health discipline, every "hat" must be subsumed under a common neurobehavioral framework, such as the one outlined in this chapter. Using this approach, many children labelled treatment-resistant may become treatment-responsive. Providers should consider referring children who are nonresponsive to standard treatment or who have complex medical or psychiatric conditions to an OCD subspecialty clinic for consultation and definitive treatment.

Stylistic Considerations

As noted earlier, some therapists prefer to be nondirective, letting the child's internal processes emerge naturally; others are more directive, with much therapist activity during the session. Although the former often gravitate toward psychodynamic "play-therapy" techniques and the latter toward CBT or family therapy, it is important to note that therapists of all persuasions can be effective using this protocol if they follow the methods outlined previously. Doing so, however, may require adjusting the style of therapy to fit the treatment of OCD. Failure to do so will be frustrating to the therapist and patient. Also, the therapist should consider whether CBT is suitable to his or her expertise level. If not, then referral should be made to another provider who is experienced in CBT for OCD.

Cognitive-behavioral therapy for OCD may feel counterintuitive at first, as the therapist assists the child to "choose to be anxious" rather than providing comfort, counterarguments, or distractions against OCD–related anxiety. It is vital that the therapist ally with the child and not the OCD, even when the child may wish the opposite. Providing counter productive reassurance or trying to understand "why" the child has OCD may be tempting to the therapist, but these actions will not be helpful for the child. In addition, as the child's "coach," the therapist must emphasize that the child *practice* the techniques learned in treatment in order to get better. In this way, treatment promotes self-esteem, because the child's competence in "bossing-back OCD" is emphasized, rather than the intrusiveness of OCD or the excellence of the therapist.

A matter-of-fact stance models for the child that, although anxiety is quite uncomfortable at times, it can be tolerated and will eventually subside with implementation of ERP.

Because managing CBT is in some ways similar to coaching an athletic team (i.e., the coach instructs, models, insists on practice, and stands on the sidelines while the players play the game), it is not surprising that CBT experts do a lot of active communicating, talking as well as listening. In particular, CBT requires a molecular understanding of specific symptoms, and their triggers nature, and how the patient copes successfully or unsuccessfully. Gaining this information and working with the patient to set up an equally specific treatment intervention often requires a Socratic dialogue, in which the therapist peppers the patient with questions about his or her experiences of either "bossing-back" or being "bossed around" by OCD. As mentioned earlier, questions typically focus on and seek specific examples of greater detail about how the child successfully or unsuccessfully resisted OCD.

It is crucial for the therapist to keep the tone of the session friendly and the topic centered on OCD as the adversary so that the patient perceives both intellectually and emotionally that the therapist is an ally in seeking the end of the patient's OCD. The use of humor can greatly decrease anxiety and increase motivation; however, it is important to remember to poke fun at OCD and not the child. Examples from the therapist's experiences with other OCD patients can help calm the rough waters in treatment, such as the disclosure of aggressive or religious obsessions or fears of shaking hands with someone who has AIDS. Similarly, some degree of self-disclosure is essential to the successful conduct of treatment.

Monitoring Outcome

We monitor the course and outcome of treatment using symptom hierarchies, fear thermometer ratings to assess within-exposure anxiety to specific targets, the Yale-Brown Obsessive-Compulsive Scale (Y-BOCS), the NIMH Global Obsessive-Compulsive Scale, and Clinical Scales of Global Improvement (CGI). The most detailed instrument for assessing the outcome of treatment is the Y-BOCS, which assesses obsessions and compulsions separately on issues of time consumed, distress, interference, degree of resistance, and control.[55,56] The Y-BOCS is a clinician-rated instrument merging data from clinical observation and the parent and child report. We also use the Y-BOCS to inventory past and present OCD symptoms and their initial severity, total OCD severity, relative preponderance of obsessions and compulsions, and degree of insight. Because each session is packed with treatment goals, the Y-BOCS is generally obtained on a monthly basis, whereas the NIMH Global and the two CGIs take less than 1 minute and are completed weekly. The resulting product, when graphed, provides a valuable object lesson of the child's progress in treatment. Comorbid anxiety, depression, and disruptive behaviors can be tracked with the Multi-dimensional Anxiety Scale for Children,[57] Children's Depression Inventory,[58] and Conners' Parent and Teacher Rating Scales,[59] respectively.

TREATMENT OUTCOME STUDIES

We developed our treatment manual in response to deficiencies identified in a systematic literature review and our collective clinical experience.[20] In our first study, we used Version One of the manual to treat 15 consecutive child and adolescent patients with OCD, most of whom had been previously stabilized on medications.[22] These patients, who ranged from 6 to 18 years of age, and their families found *How I ran OCD off my land* highly acceptable, even when these patients experienced no rapid reduction in OCD symptoms. Statistical analyses showed significant benefit immediately at posttreatment and at 6-month follow-up. Nine patients showed at least a 50% reduction in symptoms on the Y-BOCS scores at posttreatment and became clinically asymptomatic on the NIMH Global Obsessive-Compulsive Scale. Of the 12 patients defined as responders—indicated by a greater than 30% improvement on the Y-BOCS—there were no relapses at follow-up intervals of as long as 18 months, although several patients experienced "hiccups" requiring additional CBT sessions. Booster behavioral treatment allowed medication discontinuation in six of the nine asymptomatic patients, again without relapse after 6 months or more of follow-up observation.

Because these 15 patients represented all patients who came to us for treatment (excluding consults, hospitalized patients, those living at extended distances, and patients treated by other therapists), we concluded that our protocol-driven implementation of CBT represented a safe, effective, and acceptable treatment program for OCD in young persons. We have since completed a series of single-subject designs with much the same results.[29] Other pediatric anxiety disorder researchers have had experiences similar to ours using our treatment protocol[60] and similarly inspired CBT programs.[47,61]

In another single-case study, we used a within-subject, multiple-baseline design plus global ratings across treatment weeks, to treat an 8-year-old OCD patient with CBT alone.[29] Eleven weeks of treatment produced complete resolution in OCD symptoms; treatment gains were maintained at 6-month follow-up. Figure 19-2 illustrates the progress of treatment at each week for each symptom baseline. Each box represents 1 treatment week. The Y (vertical) axis represents subjective units of distress scale (SUDS) (fear thermometer) scores for each symptom present at baseline on the symptom hierarchy, which are depicted as bars on the X (horizontal) axis. Symptom reduction within each baseline was specific to the ERP targets for that baseline. Characteristically, when the patient "got the idea," generalization across baselines appeared with some slowing down again as she reached the most difficult symptoms at the top of the hierarchy.

Time

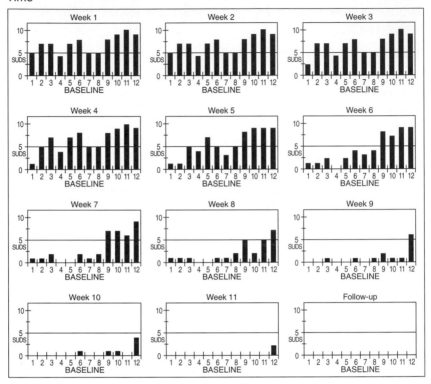

Fig. 19-2 Multiple baselines over time. Key: 1 = touching mouth; 2 = snacking after touching plants; 3 = not washing for meals; 4 = wearing turtlenecks again; 5 = touching something sticky; 6 = touching dishwashing liquid; 7 = using towel again; 8 = touching a cat; 9 = using Ajax; 10 = using Windex; 11 = using toxic paint; 12 = touching sick people.

Using similar protocols, other researchers also have shown reductions in OCD with cognitive-behavioral approaches.[47,61,62] Given the similarity between childhood-onset and adult-onset OCD in phenomenology and response to treatment, we conclude that CBT, alone or combined with pharmacotherapy, appears to be as safe, acceptable, and effective a treatment for OCD in children and adolescents as it is in adults.

FUTURE DIRECTIONS

Empirical evidence favoring CBT as a treatment for OCD in young patients remains weak, relative to the evidence favoring pharmacotherapy in these same patients[1] and CBT in adults.[63] Future research will focus on seven areas of necessity: (1) controlled trials comparing medications, behavior therapy, and combination treatment with controls that determine whether medications and behavior therapy are synergistic or additive in their effects on symptom reduction; (2) follow-up studies to evaluate relapse rates, including use of booster CBT to reduce relapse rates in patients treated with medications alone or combined with CBT; (3) component analyses, such as a comparison of ERP, anxiety management techniques, and a combination of the two, to evaluate contributions of specific treatment components to symptom reduction and treatment acceptability; (4) comparisons of individual- and family-based treatments to determine which is more effective in which children; (5) development of treatment for OCD subtypes, such as obsessional slowness, primary obsessional OCD, and tic-like OCD, that do not respond well to ERP; (6) targeting treatment innovations to factors such as family dysfunction, which constrain the application of CBT to patients with OCD; and (7) exporting research treatments to divergent clinical settings and patient populations to judge the acceptability and effectiveness of CBT as a treatment for child- and adolescent-onset OCD in real-world settings.

In this context, we are currently conducting an NIMH–funded comparative treatment outcome study to answer these questions. Using a volunteer sample of 120 (60/site) patients, ages 8 through 16, with a *Diagnostic and Statistical Manual of Mental Disorders* (DSM-IV) diagnosis of OCD, this 5-year treatment outcome study contrasts the degree and durability of improvement obtained across four treatment conditions: (1) medication with sertraline (MED); (2) OCD–specific CBT; (3) medication and CBT; and (4) two control conditions—placebo and educational support. The experimental design covers two phases. Phase I compares the outcome of medication, CBT, combination, and control conditions. In phase II, responders advance to a 16-week discontinuation study to assess treatment durability. The primary outcome measure is the Y-BOCS. Assessments blind to treatment status take place at week 0 (pretreatment); weeks 1, 4, 8, and 12 (phase I treatment); and weeks 16, 20, 24, and 28 (phase II discontinuation). In addition to addressing comparative efficacy and durability of the specified treatments, this study examines time-action effects; differential effects of treatment on specific aspects of OCD, including functional impairment; and predictors of response to treatment. Once completed, this study should advance considerably the literature on the descriptive psychopathology and treatment of OCD in young persons.

SUMMARY AND RECOMMENDATIONS FOR TREATMENT

Despite conspicuous limitations in the research literature, CBT, alone or combined with pharmacotherapy, is the psychotherapeutic treatment of choice for children and adolescents with OCD. Unlike other psychotherapies, CBT affords a logically consistent and compelling relationship between the disorder, the treatment, and the specified outcome. Moreover, as Baer[64] indicates, arguments advanced against CBT for OCD, such as symptom substitution, danger of interrupting rituals, uniformity of learned symptoms, and incompatibility with pharmacotherapy, have all proved unfounded.[64] Perhaps the most insidious myth is that CBT is a simplistic treatment that ignores "real problems." We believe that the opposite is true. Helping patients make rapid and difficult behavior changes over short time intervals requires both clinical savvy and focused treatment.

Ideally, young persons with OCD should first receive CBT that has been optimized for treating childhood-onset OCD; if the patients are not rapidly responsive, pharmacotherapy with a serotonin reuptake inhibitor should be initiated.[7] To avoid the need for medication and the side effects that may accompany pharmacotherapy, however, some experts may prefer to begin with CBT. Others will choose medication, in an attempt to avoid the time, effort, expense, and anxiety associated with behavior therapy. Because CBT, including booster treatments during medication discontinuation, may improve both short- and long-term outcome in medication-responsive patients, the majority of therapists will likely combine the two approaches, even in those patients for whom ongoing pharmacotherapy proves necessary.

For the clinician seeking to address the needs of his or her child and adolescent OCD patients, we feel confident in making the following recommendations, which are consistent with expert recommendations[7]:

- Describing OCD in a medical context (i.e., as a neurobehavioral disorder), and not as a bad habit, improves compliance with treatment.
- Giving OCD a "nickname," against which the child can do battle, keeps the focus on OCD as the identified problem.
- Graded ERP is the foundation of treatment; cognitive training and family interventions serve an important, if adjunctive, function.
- ERP and cognitive training are strategies in the child's "war" with OCD; the therapist, family, teacher, and friends then become the child's "allies."
- With the caveat that the child must make progress, the choice of ERP targets is best left to the child.
- Many if not most patients will benefit from pharmacotherapy with a serotonin reuptake inhibitor.
- Multimodality OCD treatments are more precisely delivered by a multidisciplinary team, preferably but not necessarily located in a subspecialty clinic setting.

In summary, CBT for OCD in children and adolescents is emerging from the hinterland of clinical lore to the realm of efficacy and effectiveness research. Further work is clearly necessary before the empirical database concerning CBT application to child and adolescent OCD subjects approximates that for adults. The availability of manualized, time-limited treatment programs, such as *How I ran OCD off my land*,[8] should drive this process to benefit children and adolescents with OCD.

REFERENCES

1. March J, Leonard H: Obsessive-compulsive disorder: A review of the past ten years, *J Am Acad Child Adolesc Psychiatry* 35(10):1265–1273, 1996.
2. Hollingsworth C, Tanguay P, Grossman L: Long-term outcome of obsessive compulsive disorder in childhood, *J Am Acad Child Psychiatry* 19:134–144, 1980.
3. Esman A: Psychoanalysis in general psychiatry: Obsessive-compulsive disorder as a paradigm, *J Am Psychoanal Assoc* 37:319–336, 1989.
4. Baer L: Behavior therapy for obsessive compulsive disorder in the office-based practice, *J Clin Psychiatry* 1993.
5. Foa E, Wilson R: *Stop obsessing!* New York, 1991, Bantam.
6. Foa E, Kozak M: Emotional processing of fear: Exposure to corrective information, *Psychol Bull* 90:20–35, 1985.
7. March J, Frances A, Kahn D, Carpenter D: Expert consensus guidelines: Treatment of obsessive-compulsive disorder, *J Clin Psychiatry* 58(suppl 4):1–72, 1997a.
8. March J, Mulle K: *Cognitive behavioral psychotherapy for children and adolescents, with OCD: A treatment manual,* New York, Guilford Press.
9. Goodman WK, Price LH: Assessment of severity and change in obsessive compulsive disorder (review), *Psychiatr Clin North Am* 15(4), 861–869, 1992.
10. March J, Albano A: Assessment of anxiety in children and adolescents. In Dickstein L, Riba M, Oldham M, editors: *Review of psychiatry,* vol XV, Washington, 1996, American Psychiatric Press, pp 405–427.
11. Swedo SE, Rapoport JL, Leonard H, et al: Obsessive-compulsive disorder in children and adolescents. Clinical phenomenology of 70 consecutive cases, *Arch Gen Psychiatry* 46(4):335–341, 1989.
12. Cohen DJ, Leckman JF: Developmental psychopathology and neurobiology of Tourette's syndrome (review), *J Am Acad Child Adolesc Psychiatry* 33(1):2–15, 1994.
13. Leonard H, Lenane M, Swedo S: Obsessive-compulsive disorder. In Leonard HL, editor: *Child Psychiatric Clinics of North America: Anxiety disorders,* vol 2, New York, 1993a, Saunders, pp 655–666.
14. March JS, Leonard HL, Swedo SE: Obsessive-compulsive disorder. In March J, editor: *Anxiety disorders in children and adolescents,* New York, 1995c, Guilford Press, pp 251–275.
15. Adams GB, Waas GA, March JS, Smith MC: Obsessive compulsive disorder in children and adolescents: The role of the school psychologist in identification, assessment, and treatment, *School Psychol Q* 9(4):274–294, 1994.
16. Rapoport JL: Recent advances in obsessive-compulsive disorder (see comments), *Neuropsychopharmacology* 5(1):1–10, 1991.
17. Leonard HL, Lenane MC, Swedo SE, et al: A double-blind comparison of clomipramine and desipramine treatment of severe onychophagia (nail biting), *Arch Gen Psychiatry,* 48(9):821–827, 1991.
18. Swedo S: Trichotillomania, *Psychiatr Ann* 23(7):402–407, 1993.
19. Leonard HL, Swedo SE, Lenane MC, et al: A 2- to 7-year follow-up study of 54 obsessive-compulsive children and adolescents, *Arch Gen Psychiatry* 50(6):429–439, 1993b.
20. March JS: Cognitive-behavioral psychotherapy for children and adolescents with

OCD: A review and recommendations for treatment, *J Am Acad Child Adolesc Psychiatry* 34(1):7–18, 1995b.

21. March JS: Cognitive-behavioral psychotherapy for children and adolescents with OCD: A review and recommendations for treatment, *J Am Acad Child Adolesc Psychiatry* 34(1):7–18, 1995c.

22. March J, Mulle K, Herbel B: Behavioral psychotherapy for children and adolescents with obsessive-compulsive disorder: An open trial of a new protocol driven treatment package, *J Am Acad Child Adolesc Psychiatry* 33(3):333–341, 1994a.

23. Leonard HL, Rapoport JL: Pharmacotherapy of childhood obsessive-compulsive disorder, *Psychiatr Clin North Am* 12(4):963–970, 1989.

24. March J, Leonard H, Swedo S: Pharmacotherapy of obsessive-compulsive disorder. In Riddle M, editor: *Child psychiatric clinics of north America: Pharmacotherapy*, New York, 1995a, Saunders, pp 217–236.

25. Kendall PC: Cognitive-behavioral therapies with youth: Guiding theory, current status, and emerging developments, *J Consult Clin Psychol* 61(2):235–247, 1993.

26. Kendall PC, Panichelli-Mindel SM: Cognitive-behavioral treatments, *J Abnorm Child Psychol* 23(1):107–124, 1995.

27. Clarke GN: Improving the transition from basic efficacy research to effectiveness studies: Methodological issues and procedures, *J Consult Clin Psychol* 63(5):718–725, 1995.

28. Foa E, Steketee G, Milby J: Differential effects of exposure and response prevention in obsessive-compulsive washers, *J Consult Clin Psychol* 48(1):71–79, 1980.

29. March J, Mulle K: Manualized cognitive-behavioral psychotherapy for obsessive-compulsive disorder in childhood: A preliminary single case study, *J Anx Dis* 9(2):175–184, 1995.

30. March JS, Mulle K, Herbel B: Behavioral psychotherapy for children and adolescents with obsessive-compulsive disorder: An open trial of a new protocol-driven treatment package, *J Am Acad Child Adolesc Psychiatry* 33(3):333–341, 1994b.

31. van Oppen P, Arntz A: Cognitive therapy for obsessive-compulsive disorder, *Behav Res Ther* 32(1):79–87, 1994.

32. van Oppen P, Emmelkamp P, et al: Cognitive therapy and exposure in vivo in the treatment of obsessive compulsive disorder, *Behav Res Ther* 33(4):370–390, 1995.

33. Schwartz J: *Brain lock*, New York, 1996, Harper Collins.

34. Kendall PC: Treating anxiety disorders in children: Results of a randomized clinical trial, *J Consult Clin Psychol* 62(1):100–110, 1994.

35. Kearney CA, Silverman WK: Treatment of an adolescent with obsessive-compulsive disorder by alternating response prevention and cognitive therapy: An empirical analysis, *J Behav Ther Exp Psychiatry* 21(1):39–47, 1990.

36. Harris CV, Wiebe DJ: An analysis of response prevention and flooding procedures in the treatment of adolescent obsessive compulsive disorder, *J Behav Ther Exp Psychiatry* 23(2):107–115, 1992.

37. Flament MF, Koby E, Rapoport JL, et al: Childhood obsessive-compulsive disorder: A prospective follow-up study, *J Child Psychol Psychiatry Allied Discipl* 31(3):363–380, 1990.

38. Thyer BA: Diagnosis and treatment of child and adolescent anxiety disorders, *Behav Mod* 15(3):310–325, 1991.

39. Ratnasuriya RH, Marks IM, Forshaw DM, Hymas NF: Obsessive slowness revisited, *Br J Psychiatry* 159(273):273–274, 1991.
40. Wolff R, Rapoport J: Behavioral treatment of childhood obsessive-compulsive disorder, *Behav Mod* 12(2):252–266, 1988.
41. March J, Leonard H, Swedo S: Neuropsychiatry of pediatric obsessive compulsive disorder. In Coffey E, Brumback R, editors: *Textbook of pediatric neuropsychiatry*, Washington, 1998, American Psychiatric Association Press.
42. Schwartz JM, Stoessel PW, Baxter LR Jr, et al: Systematic changes in cerebral glucose metabolic rate after successful behavior modification treatment of obsessive-compulsive disorder, *Arch Gen Psychiatry* 53(2):109–113, 1996.
43. White M, Epston D: *Narrative means to therapeutic ends*, New York, 1991, WW Norton and Company.
44. Kendall PC, Howard BL, Epps J: The anxious child. Cognitive-behavioral treatment strategies, *Behav Mod* 12(2):281–310, 1988.
45. March JS, Mulle K, Herbel B: Behavioral psychotherapy for children and adolescents with obsessive-compulsive disorder: An open trial of a new protocol-driven treatment package, *J Am Acad Child Adolesc Psychiatry* 33(3):333–341, 1994c.
46. Leonard HL, Goldberger EL, Rapoport JL, et al: Childhood rituals: Normal development or obsessive-compulsive symptoms? *J Am Acad Child Adolesc Psychiatry* 29(1):17–23, 1990.
47. Piacentini J, Gitow A, Jaffer M, Graae F: Outpatient behavioral treatment of child and adolescent obsessive compulsive disorder, *J Anx Dis* 8(3):277–289, 1994.
48. Marks IM, Lelliott P, Basoglu M, et al: Clomipramine, self-exposure and therapist-aided exposure for obsessive-compulsive rituals, *Br J Psychiatry* 152(522):522–534, 1988.
49. March J, Wells K, Conners C: Attention-deficit/hyperactivity disorder: Part I. Assessment and diagnosis, *J Pract Psychiatr Behav Health* 2:23–32, 1995b.
50. March J, Wells K, Conners C: Attention-deficit/hyperactivity disorder: Part II. Treatment, *J Pract Psychiatr Behav Health* 1:219–228, 1996.
51. Clarkin JF, Kendall PC: Comorbidity and treatment planning: Summary and future directions, *J Consult Clin Psychol* 60(6):904–908, 1992.
52. Hoberman HM, Clarke GN, Saunders SM: Psychosocial interventions for adolescent depression: Issues, evidence, and future directions, *Prog Behav Mod* 30:25–73, 1996.
53. March J: *Anxiety disorders in children and adolescents*, New York, 1995a, Guilford Press.
54. March J, Mulle K: Banishing obsessive-compulsive disorder. In Hibbs E, Jensen P, editors: *Psychosocial treatments for child and adolescent disorders*, Washington, 1996, American Psychological Association Press, pp 82–103.
55. Goodman WK, Price LH, Rasmussen SA, et al: The Yale-Brown Obsessive Compulsive Scale. II. Validity, *Arch Gen Psychiatry* 46(11):1012–1016, 1989a.
56. Goodman WK, Price LH, Rasmussen SA, et al: The Yale-Brown Obsessive Compulsive Scale. I. Development, use, and reliability, *Arch Gen Psychiatry* 46(11):1006–1111, 1989b.
57. March J, Parker J, Sullivan K, et al: The Multidimensional Anxiety Scale for Children (MASC): Factor structure, reliability and validity, *J Am Acad Child Adolesc Psychiatry* 36(4):554–565, 1997b.

58. Kovacs M: The Children's Depression Inventory (CDI):*Psychopharmacol Bull* 21:995–998, 1985.
59. Conners C: *Conners' rating scales,* Toronto, 1995, Multi-Health Systems.
60. Foa E, Last C: Personal communication.
61. Albano AM, Knox LS, Barlow DH: *Obsessive-compulsive disorder.* Jason Aronson, Inc, Northvale, NJ, US, 606:282–316.
62. Franklin M, Foa E: Personal communication.
63. Dar R, Greist J: Behavior therapy for obsessive-compulsive disorder, *Psychiatr Clin North Am* 15(4):885–894, 1992.
64. Baer L: Behavior therapy for obsessive-compulsive disorder and trichotillomania. Implications for Tourette syndrome (review):*Adv Neurol* 58(333):333–340, 1992.

20

Clinical Case Examples of Outpatient Behavioral Therapy for Obsessive-Compulsive Disorder

William E. Minichiello, Ed.D.

This chapter presents clinical examples of the treatment of both simple and complex cases of obsessive-compulsive disorder (OCD). These case examples communicate the nuances of behavioral treatment, the flexibility and creativity needed to successfully apply the straightforward principles and techniques, and the qualities of the therapist that affect outcome, particularly with difficult and complex patients.

As noted in Chapter 17, the theory and techniques involved in treating OCD are fairly simple and straightforward. The assumption that exposure and response prevention will result in *all* patients overcoming OCD has led some therapists, after attempting these treatments or instructing the patient to self-administer these techniques, to conclude that a trial of behavior therapy has failed when the anticipated results were not forthcoming. Although exposure and response prevention (ERP) constitute the most important elements necessary to successfully treat OCD, in clinical practice, where the goal is to return the patients to normal functioning and not merely to achieve clinical significance on a series of scales, much more is necessary.

THERAPEUTIC RELATIONSHIP

Contrary to popular opinion, in behavior therapy the therapeutic relationship is a key variable in successful outcome, particularly with OCD patients. Our clinical experience, supported by Alexander,[1] indicates that the therapist and client must feel comfortable with each other and the therapist must not be "mechanical" in interaction, but rather must convey warmth, empathy, and confidence[2] about his or her skills and the method of treatment. The therapist also must convey respect for the patient and not make him or her feel foolish, bizarre, weird, or crazy, no matter how strange the particular OCD symptoms may be. Sweet,[3] in his excellent review of the therapeutic relationship in behavior therapy, states: "If the therapeutic relationship is important to behavior therapy process . . . its power lies in the client's like, trust, and respect for the therapist, which increase the likelihood that the client will listen to the therapist and allow the techniques to be implemented." These factors should be kept in mind as we discuss clinical applications, because as Sweet[3] indicates: "Some therapists obtain very poor results, and some are significantly better than other therapists, regardless of the techniques employed."

Our clinical experience is that a positive patient-therapist relationship is a necessary but not sufficient element in positive treatment outcome in OCD. Certainly, an OCD patient who does not feel respect, empathy, and genuineness from the therapist may either not stay in therapy long enough for the critical ERP, or he will not follow the therapist's instruction or allow these important procedures to be implemented. But the relationship alone is not sufficient to effect change. Most OCD patients come to behavior therapy with a general knowledge of the treatment components needed for change, but they are unable to implement them alone and consequently rely on a therapist whom they can trust, who is caring, and who is respectful of the apparent bizarreness of their behavior. Thus, the behavior therapist must be both kind and firm when exposing the patient to the anxieties and discomforts that have been avoided, often for many years. Rabavilas, et al[4] assessed therapist qualities related to outcome in 36 OCD patients, and found that therapists' respect, understanding, and interest toward the client were significantly correlated with favorable outcome. They also found that the therapist's manner of conducting treatment (i.e., being encouraging, demanding, challenging, and explicit) was positively related to favorable outcome, whereas a permissive, tolerant, and neutral manner had a significant negative effect. In extrapolating the work of Matthews, et al[5] with agoraphobia, Sweet[3] concluded that "firm therapists who are demanding, explicit, directive, and challenging, while still being warm, understanding, and respectful of their clients, have a higher probability of positive treatment results when using exposure treatments."

The remainder of this chapter presents case examples of behavioral treatment for each major symptom type of OCD, as well as of some of the less frequently encountered types. We assume that the reader is knowledgeable of behavioral assessment and treatment techniques (for review, see Chapter 17).

Uncomplicated Washing/Cleaning Rituals

Case 1

A professional woman in her mid-thirties presented for treatment of compulsive handwashing that began when she was 18 years of age. During the behavioral analysis, it was ascertained that external cues to handwashing were dirt, dust, ants, insects, any item brought into the house from outdoors or any item from inside the house that had been taken outdoors and then returned to the house (e.g., children's toys), any item from the garage or cellar, and contact with the garage or cellar, chemicals, and detergents.

The patient's internal cues to handwashing were, "I'll contaminate this person in some way"; "My child will get head lice and the whole house will be contaminated"; "I'll be contaminated if my husband and child don't wash their hands when they come in from outdoors"; "It's contaminated and something bad will happen to me."

The patient avoided going to the cellar or garage and having contact with any item from the cellar or garage that had been outdoors. She changed the bedsheets, pillowcases, and blankets if an ant or other insect was found on the bed. To diminish the chance of coming in contact with contaminants, the patient required both her husband and child to wash their hands after returning from work or school. When her child came into the house after playing outdoors, the child was washed from head to toe in the bathtub. The patient's husband also had to wash his hands after coming in from outdoors or from the cellar or garage.

Although the duration of each handwashing was within normal limits, her estimated baseline frequency of handwashing was 50 times per day.

At the conclusion of the first session, the patient was asked to record daily for the next week the number of handwashings as well as the cues preceding handwashing. When the patient returned for the second session, the frequency of handwashing was reduced. The patient spontaneously reported that "Knowing I had to write down when I had the urge to wash prevented me from washing. Having to stop to think why I was washing and not being able to come up with a good reason caused me not to wash as much." In approximately 10% of patients undergoing behavior therapy, record keeping alone results in a reduction in target behaviors. Daily record keeping is an important component of behavioral intervention because it provides an objective measurement of change and assesses the effectiveness of the behavioral intervention being used.

During the second therapy session, the patient, with the therapist first modeling the behavior, touched dirt, dust, chemicals, and detergent in the therapist's office, and was instructed not to wash her hands for 2 hours. The patient also was instructed in home practice of exposure to contaminants and response prevention up to 2 hours after each exposure. The patient and therapist negotiated a schedule of three trials per day of self-administered exposure to contaminants followed by refraining from washing or using Handi-Wipes or tissues for up to 2 hours. The patient was given the form shown in Figure 20-1 to keep track of her self-administered ERP.

When the patient returned for the third session her records indicated strict compliance with the ERP homework assignment. The patient reported that her anxiety level had begun to decrease but that she was still bothered by thoughts of contamination and harm. The patient was instructed in the differences in time required to change behavior versus thoughts (see Chapter 17). During the third

DAY/DATE	TIME		SUDS (0-100)		
	Begin	End	Begin	End	Comments
Sunday, 8/3/97 Exposure	___	___	___	___	_____
Response Prevention	___	___	___	___	_____
Monday, 8/4/97 Exposure	___	___	___	___	_____
Response Prevention	___	___	___	___	_____
Tuesday, 8/5/97 Exposure	___	___	___	___	_____
Response Prevention	___	___	___	___	_____
Wednesday, 8/6/97 Exposure	___	___	___	___	_____
Response Prevention	___	___	___	___	_____
Thursday, 8/7/97 Exposure	___	___	___	___	_____
Response Prevention	___	___	___	___	_____
Friday, 8/8/97 Exposure	___	___	___	___	_____
Response Prevention	___	___	___	___	_____
Saturday, 8/9/97 Exposure	___	___	___	___	_____
Response Prevention	___	___	___	___	_____

Fig. 20-1 Exposure and response prevention homework form.

session, the patient's husband also was consulted, and an agreement was reached between patient, husband, and therapist that the patient, with the assistance of her husband, would refrain from bathing their 5-year-old child whenever she returned from outdoors. ERP continued in the therapist's office, with the patient required to touch and hold an ant and an insect when refraining from washing her hands for 2 hours. The homework assignment was negotiated, with the patient required to expose herself three times daily to all items she had been exposed to in past sessions, plus being required to touch daily at least one item from outdoors.

At the outset of the fourth session, the patient was trained in specific self-control procedures to enable her to better cope with the anxiety she reported when practicing ERP at home. In particular, the patient was trained in a self-control relaxation technique, diaphragmatic breathing,[6] thought stopping, and cognitive restructuring, to enable her to modify the frequent, catastrophic self-statements that served as internal cues for her compulsions. Although Rachman, et al[7] reported no significant difference in outcome between groups trained in relaxation plus ERP versus those with ERP alone, clinically it is often helpful to the patient who becomes increasingly anxious when self-control procedures are added. It also increases the patient's compliance with ERP. After the patient was trained in self-control procedures, ERP continued in the office along with thera- pist modeling. The homework assignment was negotiated, with the patient required to take out the trash daily and to then refrain from washing her hands for 1 hour, in addition to continued ERP of all situations previously accom- plished. The patient also was required to engage in twice-daily practices of relaxation and diaphragmatic breathing.

When the patient returned for the fifth session 2.5 weeks later, she reported that self-administered ERP was much easier to accomplish with the addition of relaxation and cognitive self-control procedures. The patient's records indicated faithful compliance on all assignments, except that she was able to refrain from washing her hands for only 15 minutes after taking out the trash. With the ther- apist first modeling the behavior, the patient was exposed to touching the trash in the therapist's office and additional trash brought from the waiting room. The patient refrained from washing her hands for 1 hour after the therapy session by remaining in the waiting room. The homework assignment was again negotiated, with the patient agreeing to daily exposure to trash when refraining from hand- washing for 30 minutes after exposure. The patient also was required to contin- ue ERP to all situations already accomplished.

Because of the patient's vacation schedule, the sixth session was scheduled for 6 weeks later. A review of the patient's record keeping indicated compliance on all assignments. Therapist and patient negotiated an extension of response prevention after daily exposure to trash, from 30 minutes to 1 hour, because the patient on her own had extended the time from 30 minutes to 45 minutes. Because the patient was still unable to touch items from the cellar or garage, or even to enter these areas, her husband was instructed to bring several objects from the cellar and garage to the therapy session. Again, with the therapist first modeling exposure to these objects, the patient was exposed to these contami- nated objects and was asked to refrain from handwashing for at least 2 hours after exposure. The patient's husband was asked to monitor compliance on the way home from the therapy session. With the patient's permission, her husband was instructed to help her carry out ERP on a daily basis for 5 minutes by accompanying her into the garage and cellar and having her touch various items, then refraining from washing for 2 hours after exposure.

When the patient returned for the seventh session 1 month later, her record- keeping not only indicated compliance with daily ERP up to 2 hours after expo- sure, but she met all goals and was able to touch all trash without washing her hands. She also was able to go into the cellar and garage and touch all items without washing for up to 2 hours.

The eighth session occurred 2 months later, with the patient maintaining all her gains and able to handle with minimal discomfort two situations that prior to treatment would have triggered severe anxiety: avoidance and significant hand- washing. She reported that a skunk had entered her garage and sprayed in a trash barrel, and a dead mouse was found in the cellar. With an appropriate application of the self-control procedures she had now mastered and a thorough under-standing of the importance of not avoiding, she continued to expose herself to the cellar and garage without maladaptive washing. At 3-month, 6-month, and 1-year telephone follow-up, the patient had maintained her gains.

This is a typical example of the application of behavioral principles and tech-niques to the treatment of uncomplicated washing compulsions. The response was rapid and straightforward and was similar in degree to the response of pho-bic patients to behavioral interventions.

Mixed Rituals

Case 2

At 23 years of age, the patient began washing her hands frequently, and noticed that she had to rewash clean laundry that had fallen on the floor even though she knew it was not dirty. She spent gradually increasing amounts of time washing and noticed that the list of cues to washing had grown, so that by 29 years of age, when she sought behavior therapy, the numerous items triggered handwashing, with the accompanying Subjective Units of Distress Scale (SUDS) score if she were prevented from washing or resisted the urge to wash (Table 20-1). The average duration of her handwashing was 5 minutes, and she often spent 30 to 45 minutes in the shower if she touched the shower curtain or dropped the soap when showering.

Over the course of the past 2 years, the patient also noted a number of counting and checking rituals. For example, she had to wash her hands an even number of times, such as four or eight. When shopping at the supermarket, she had to take the second, fourth, sixth, or eighth item from the shelf. When dressing, she had to shake each item an even number of times before putting it on. Other rituals involved checking electrical plugs, doors, tops of jars and bottles, gas jets, the radio and stereo to see if they were on or off, ashtrays to see if cigarettes were out, and retrac-ing her steps after passing certain objects. She also had a number of rituals that cen-tered around getting dressed; she would dress and then have to undress and dress again if an article of clothing or jewelry did not feel correct or "just right."

The patient's rituals had been a problem mainly in her apartment, where she lived with a roommate who was unaware of her problem. She was unwilling to discuss her symptoms with her roommate or involve her in treatment in any way. At the time of treatment, she was mildly depressed but taking no medication. During behavior therapy, she was given clomipramine (50 mg twice daily) and lorazepam (0.5 mg as necessary). Prior to entering behavior therapy, the patient had been in psychodynamic psychotherapy for 3 years without alteration in OCD symptoms.

The patient's internal cues to rituals were, "If I don't repeat or retrace, some-thing bad will happen to my mother (or sister or father)," "The house will burn down and my family will get hurt if I don't check the plugs (etc.) or end up on

Table 20-1   Case 2—Items That Trigger Patient Handwashing

Trigger	Subjective Units of Distress Scale Score
Brushing up crumbs from kitchen table	30
Seeing hair on her make up bottle	40
Touching bottle of soft soap	50
Touching papers, books circulated at work	60
Touching any item picked off floor	65
Contact with sole of her shoe	70
Touching doorknobs other than to the ladies' room	80
Touching doorknobs to the ladies' room	85
Touching shower curtain when showering	90
Touching soap dropped when showering	95

the number 2, 4, 6, or 8." In general, no negative catastrophic thoughts were associated with washing except a feeling of discomfort.

Because cleaning rituals respond most rapidly to behavioral intervention, treatment focused initially on exposure to stimuli that triggered the urge to wash. Prior to initiating ERP at the second session, a thorough explanation of the theory and rationale for the behavioral treatment of OCD was presented to the patient. This is standard procedure, and it assists with compliance of ERP because the patient understands why he or she is doing something that produces feelings of discomfort. The patient is helped to understand that the fear will be overcome and he or she will get better by contacting the feared object without reducing that fear through ritualizing. The extent of the explanation is tailored to each individual patient. After the rationale for ERP was given, the patient was explained the importance of compliance with behavioral homework assignments and the discomfort that must be experienced for successful outcome. After all questions and objections were answered, exposure with therapist modeling was begun. The patient was brought to the cafeteria, where she was required to brush up crumbs from the table and throw them away without washing. This was followed by exposure to a bottle of soft soap in the clinic lavatory of the therapist's office suite. Response prevention was required for 2 hours after the therapy session. The patient was instructed in home practice of ERP for those situations accomplished in the session. Because the patient was highly motivated, it was suggested that she attempt to expose herself to touching papers and books circulated at work and prevent herself from washing for up to 2 hours.

When the patient returned for the third session, her records indicated nearperfect compliance with the ERP homework assignment. As a result of her high motivation and compliance, treatment proceeded rapidly over the next two sessions to all external cues to washing that were accessible to the therapist. The patient was instructed in self-ERP to all washing cues that were inaccessible to the therapist.

Exposure and response prevention focused next on her inability to shop in a supermarket without repeatedly picking up and putting down as many as eight items before being able to put one of them in her shopping cart. She was accompanied to a local supermarket by the therapist and was required to shop from a list, under the therapist's supervision, and place the first item touched into the shopping cart. Initially, the patient encountered significant discomfort and difficulty with this task. With therapist modeling, prompting, and lavish reinforcement of her success, as well as continued exposure, she successfully overcame this aspect of her compulsive checking over the next two sessions. With the rationale of response prevention clearly in mind, between these two sessions she forced herself to keep walking when she passed an object on the street that in the past would make her feel uncomfortable and cause her to retrace her steps.

Inasmuch as the remainder of her checking rituals involved situations that occurred only at home, and she was unwilling to involve her roommate in treatment, the frequency of ERP homework was negotiated and she was required to keep daily records of her progress in putting tops on jars and bottles two times only; checking plugs and gas jets one time only; and putting her stockings on one time only, without putting them on and taking them off until "it feels right."

When the patient returned for the fifth session, her records indicated significant improvement on all behaviors targeted. Her frequency of putting tops on jars and bottles was reduced from 6 at baseline to 1.3, checking plugs and gas jets from a baseline of 4 checks to 1.3 checks, and dressing and undressing from a baseline of 8 to 1.4. She was requested to continue ERP on the same three behaviors, in addition to three or four additional ones added each week. At the conclusion of the tenth session, all washing and checking rituals were within normal limits. Spontaneously, the patient commented at the conclusion of the eighth weekly session on the positive effect of record-keeping on her ability to reduce checking. This was a highly motivated, intelligent woman who was willing to endure the short-term discomfort involved in resisting the urge to wash or check in return for the long-term gain of freedom from compulsive rituals. She was seen once a month for the next 3 months for maintenance therapy and for four additional sessions at 2-month intervals to help her make decisions regarding graduate school, career goals, and future therapy for personal issues. The patient maintained all OCD gains at 1-year follow-up. At that time, the patient was attending graduate school part-time and was employed full-time as a research assistant. She said, "My OCD symptoms are basically gone. Sometimes one creeps in, but I'm able to control it and not get upset over it."

Uncomplicated Checking Rituals

Case 3

A 55-year-old physician presented for behavior therapy of OCD after 6 years of psychodynamic psychotherapy. His OCD symptoms began at 8 years of age, and fluctuated over subsequent years but never interfered with his ability to function at a high level. This changed 2 years prior to treatment, when a frivolous malpractice suit was initiated against him, causing him to obsess about possible errors in past medical judgment; this subsequently resulted in his rechecking patients' symptoms, ordering unnecessary medical tests, seeking reassurance from medical colleagues, calling in medical consultants when they were not justified, and avoiding specific types of patients, in particular, patients with chest pain, prostate problems, skin moles, anemia, or questionable potassium or blood gas levels.

Behavioral analysis indicated that cues to his checking were frequent, catastrophic thoughts about malpractice suits against him. Formal thought stopping was taught. After interrupting his catastrophic thoughts, he was then taught to challenge these thoughts (i.e., cognitive restructuring) and begin to deal in probabilities rather than possibilities. He was to remind himself that technically "anything is possible, but how probable is it that I misdiagnosed this patient?" "What is the probability that X will happen if I don't repeat test Y?" He was instructed to focus on probabilities and not possibilities and to take risks by not ordering unnecessary tests or checking with medical colleagues unless there was a high probability, not just a remote possibility, of a problem. He returned in 2 weeks for a second session, and his self-report and homework data indicated a reduction in obsessions of malpractice suits and in checking with colleagues and ordering unnecessary tests or consultations. He is one of the rare patients who found that thought stopping made a significant difference by enabling him to control the obsessions that trigger his compulsions. After a discussion of the effect of avoidance (of treating patients with problems such as anemia or moles, that might trigger obsessional checking) on the maintenance of his OCD symptoms, he agreed not to avoid any patients that had the potential for triggering his symptoms and also not to check with medical colleagues unless clearly indicated. The patient returned for a third session 2 weeks later, elated at not checking once with his associates and only once avoiding contact with a patient with the potential of triggering checking behavior. Although enthusiastic about his success, he reported significant anxiety as a result of his successful ERP. Consequently, he was trained in a self-control relaxation technique and diaphragmatic breathing, with instructions in home practice and data collection.[6] When he returned 2 weeks later for a fourth session, his self-reports indicated continued reduction of checking behaviors and obsessions about malpractice suits. He reported difficulty practicing relaxation because of concentration problems, so the procedure was audiotaped to assist with concentration and increase compliance with home practice. He was also instructed in the *in vivo* use of his relaxation strategy when he found himself in medical situations that had produced high anxiety in the past and had resulted in either avoidance or checking behaviors. At a fifth session 2 weeks later, he reported himself to be 85% improved, and he was not avoiding any situation, regardless of the amount of anxiety it triggered. Two situations relating to malpractice suits occurred during this period, which, prior to therapy, would have rendered him incapable of functioning: (1) the legal subpoena of medical records of an associate's patient; and (2) a newspaper report of a $1.5 million malpractice judgment against a well-known physician in his community. He also recounted a number of difficult situations involving patients that occurred during the past 2 weeks that he would have avoided or checked prior to treatment, and attributed the "challenge of wearing out his fear by not avoiding" and the "possibility versus probability concept" as responsible for his success. He also reported a decrease in obsessions about malpractice suits and a significant reduction in the number of times he had to use thought stopping.

In light of rapid progress and good compliance, the sixth appointment was scheduled for 1 month later. At that session, the patient felt 95% better, with obsessions of malpractice so insignificant that he no longer regularly used thought stopping. He was engaging in no avoidance behavior, reported no difficulty in dealing with skin cancer or prostatic cancer, ordered only an occasional unnecessary medical test, rarely sought reassurance from a medical colleague, and no longer requested unnecessary medical consultation.

The patient maintained all gains over the next 4 months. He returned in 3 months for a ninth session, having maintained all his gains but reporting difficulty with "battling the urges to check," particularly when he had weekend duty and was responsible for his colleagues' patients. Obsessions of malpractice suits were more intense and frequent at these times. At this point, a 3-minute endless Loop Tape was made of the patient's catastrophic obsessions of being sued and losing his medical license. The patient was instructed to listen to his Loop Tape for 45 to 60 minutes daily and to keep records of his pre- and post-SUDS scores. He also requested medication to make it easier to perform the ERP. A medication consultation was arranged, and he was given clomipramine 50 mg. He returned for a follow-up session 2 months after having his dosage increased to 150 mg and reported that the medication had been helpful and that the ERP was now easier to carry out. His obsessions of malpractice suits were less frequent and it was easier to dismiss them. At the eleventh session 2 months later, he reported that he had had two checking incidents during that period, one of which was nonmedical. A final session was scheduled for 3 months later. At that session, he reported that he was 100% improved and was even handling medical emergencies without difficulty and was no longer bothered by obsessions of medical malpractice suits. Telephone follow-up at 6 months, 1 year, and 2 years indicated that the patient had maintained all gains. He discontinued clomipramine after his final behavior therapy session, with no return of symptoms.

Although the preceding three cases are typical of cleaning, checking, and mixed rituals, which respond rapidly and successfully to behavior therapy either with or without medication, not all patients who come for treatment of OCD symptoms are as motivated, intelligent, or uncomplicated as these. Many OCD patients resemble the following three patients—that is, they have very severe OCD symptoms, long psychiatric histories, and severe personality disorders; they also experience great difficulty functioning in social or work situations and live in caring but often stressful family situations. Such factors are clearly important in the maintenance or exacerbation of OCD symptoms.

Complex Checking and Repeating Rituals

Case 4

A 53-year-old woman had OCD that had controlled her life and that of her aged mother and her sister with whom she lived, since she was 15 years of age. The patient had rules for everything in her environment, and she controlled many behaviors of her mother, sister, and other relatives that she perceived as having any effect on her symptoms. Prior to behavioral treatment, she was immobilized by OCD and had been unable to complete her high school education, had never been employed, had never dated, and had not left her home for the past 10 years. Terrified and obsessed by thoughts that a family member would die if everything in her life was not done in a particular way, she had a multitude of checking and repeating rituals, with rules for checking or repeating almost everything. To avoid the necessity of checking or repeating until she could assure herself that no evil would befall a family member, she engaged in extensive avoidance behaviors. For example, she did not go into stores, drive, eat certain foods, shake hands, take off her coat, allow visitors into her home, wear any clothing other than one or two "safe outfits," use a host of words associated with illness or death, or speak the names of family members. She would not engage in any behavior whatsoever when the refrigerator was running, tap water was running, the stove was on, or doors or windows were being opened or shut, nor would she allow any family member to engage in any behavior until the refrigerator was silent.

The patient also had an extreme fear of contamination and controlled her environment to avoid possible contamination. She did not engage in cleaning or washing behavior but controlled her environment through avoidance. She had her own utensils, napkins, linens, and such, which never came in contact with those of her mother or sister. She required that such items as her dishes, spoons, forks, knives, glasses, cups, soap, and napkins be stored separately from the rest of the family's and be in perfect alignment. Nothing was allowed to be stored upside down or out of perfect symmetry. All of her food was required to be kept on shelves apart from the family's and cooked separately. Whenever family members ventured outside the home to shop, go to church, visit friends, or go to a doctor, they were required to change all clothes upon returning before coming in contact with the patient or any articles belonging to the patient.

She had been hospitalized on three different occasions over a 30-year period and had been treated with a variety of antidepressant, benzodiazepine, and neuroleptic medications over that period, without effect on her obsessions or compulsions. She had been treated as an outpatient in psychodynamic psychotherapy for decades by multiple psychiatrists and psychologists, also with no effect. When initially seen for behavioral treatment, she was taking nortriptyline 75 mg/day, with the dosage eventually raised to 125 mg/day, and perphenazine 4 mg/day.

After 6 months, the medication was switched to fluoxetine 40 mg/day, which the patient took for 10 months. The medication was discontinued because the patient could not tolerate side effects of profuse hair loss and loss of appetite. For the past 6 months, she had been without medication.

Behavioral analysis indicated almost total avoidance of all behaviors except bathing, dressing, and eating (these actions took an inordinately long time, depending on the patient's obsessions at the moment). Everything else was performed for the patient by her family. She engaged in no household chores, did not leave her apartment, and because of obsessions of contamination, her family was required to turn the pages of any magazine, newspaper, or book she was reading. The patient's limited behavioral repertoire was mediated by fearful obsessions that harm would come to her family, herself, or anybody she contacted either directly or indirectly.

Because of the severity of the OCD and the role of her family in reinforcing and maintaining most of her symptoms and avoidance behavior, treatment included the family from the outset. After the behavioral analysis was completed (which included interviewing the family as well as the patient), an explanation of the behavioral theory of OCD and the rationale for the behavioral treatment was undertaken. The discomfort such treatment would cause both family and patient was discussed. This was followed by a sensitive but thorough explanation of the family's role in the maintenance of the patient's symptoms and an explanation of how the patient's behavior had unwittingly trained the family over the years to strengthen her symptoms and avoidance by giving in to her demands, tantrums, and threats.

An agreement in the form of a written contract between the therapist, patient, and family was negotiated, in which she would allow her mother and sister to act in the name of the therapist to implement the ERP homework assignments, which would be negotiated from session to session. During each session, the therapist met with the patient alone for approximately half of the time and with the patient and her family for the remainder of the session. Because of the complexity and severity of the patient's symptoms and her almost universal avoidance, treatment required a great deal of patience, sensitivity, and firmness on the part of the therapist. The patient was seen weekly for 1 year and biweekly for the next 6 months.

The initial sessions focused on exposing the patient to simple situations that were accessible to the therapist. She was required to be contaminated by the therapist by shaking hands, taking off her coat and allowing the therapist to touch it and hang it up, and sitting in the chairs in the waiting room. These behaviors became standard practice each time she returned for a therapy session. Treatment proceeded to more anxiety-producing situations, namely, listening to the therapist speak "frightening and forbidden words," such as death, accident, sickness, die, casket, funeral home, cemetery, grave, tombstone, kill, murder, without the patient allowed to think a "good thought" about her family after each word. The patient was then required to repeat the same words without thinking good thoughts about her family after each word, and this exercise was continued until the patient could tolerate listening to the words and repeating them with low anxiety levels, without any accompanying "good thoughts." When this was accomplished, treatment proceeded to the patient speaking the names of all of her family members and relatives until she was able to do so at low anxiety levels, without waiting for a "good thought" to come into her mind. A 3-minute, endless Loop Tape was made with the list of forbidden words and the names of the 42 family members recorded on the tape, which the patient agreed to listen to for 45 to 60 minutes as a daily homework assignment until these words and names triggered low anxiety levels.

Treatment proceeded to exposing the patient to additional situations accessible to the therapist. The patient was accompanied to the hospital cafeteria, where simple foods were ordered and eaten that the patient had not eaten for 30 years because of obsessions of accompanying bodily harm, with the therapist sampling the food first (i.e., modeling). After several trips to the hospital cafeteria and accompanying homework assignments, the patient was exposed to supermarkets and other stores, where she was required to pick up various items and return them to the shelf without waiting for "good thoughts" to come into her mind. After accomplishing this, she was next required to shop from a list, picking up each item and immediately putting it in her basket without the accompanying "good thought." Her homework assignment was to accompany her family on shopping trips and help with the shopping—a task that she had avoided for 20 years. When on one of these shopping trips, she spontaneously asked her sister if she could drive part of the way home. After 20 years of avoidance, she drove and continues to do so weekly when accompanying her mother and sister on shopping trips. This first phase of treatment continued until the patient was exposed to all previously avoided situations accessible to the therapist, with the patient prevented from repeating, checking, or waiting for accompanying "good thoughts."

In the second phase of treatment, the family was instructed (1) not to change their clothing when returning from errands or visits outside the home; (2) not to keep the patient's food and utensils stored separately from the family's; (3) not to turn pages for her whenever she read; (4) to invite other family members into the home; (5) to engage in all necessary and spontaneous behaviors when the refrigerator was running, the stove was on, and the doors or windows were being opened and closed, and to ignore her pleas to remain motionless until the refrigerator stopped and all was quiet; and (6) to require the patient to choose her own shoes, socks, skirt, and blouse each day.

During this phase of treatment, progress was not as rapid and steady as in the first phase. The family required much support to remain firm during the patient's pleading, tantrums, and occasional threats, as they began to extricate themselves from their unwitting role of reinforcing her avoidance, obsessions, and rituals. They also needed assistance and education in the importance of reinforcing the desired behavior by the patient as soon as it began, as well as the importance of ignoring undesirable behavior (rather than nagging the patient about it). As with most families of OCD patients, this family became impatient with the patient's steady but slow progress and had to be instructed in the principle of shaping behaviors and in understanding how behavioral change is gradual and follows a learning curve. Although progress was slow, albeit steady, it soon became liberating for the family to once again have other family members and visitors in their home. For the first time in 20 years, they were able to have other family members gather at a table with them to celebrate Thanksgiving. Life for the patient's mother and sister became less burdensome, and they were able to engage in ordinary tasks such as turning on a light or changing the television channel without first waiting for the refrigerator motor to be silent.

Once the family was disengaged from reinforcing the patient's OCD, treatment was focused on the most difficult aspect of treatment: getting the patient to refrain from rituals when alone. Progress was slow and unsteady, as attempts were made to get the patient to engage in simple behaviors such as walking from room to room when the refrigerator was on or eating when her mother drew water from the tap or dressing herself in less than 1 hour's time. In the latter instance, the patient was able to reduce her dressing time from 1 hour to 15 minutes. With this patient (as with other OCD patients with a severe personality disorder), there was little generalization between those behaviors she was able to engage in when the environment was controlled by the therapist or surrogate therapist in the home (e.g., designated family member) and those same behaviors when she was alone in the environment.

After 1.5 years of treatment requiring a great deal of patience, caring, ingenuity, and firmness by the therapist, although the patient was not cured of OCD, the quality of her life and that of her family was improved. She was no longer a total hostage to her obsessions and was able to leave her home, visit relatives, allow visitors into her home, shop in stores, eat a variety of foods, wear a variety of clothing, dress in a reasonable length of time, drive, and engage in physical contact with other humans. The quality of life for her family was also improved, and her mother and sister were no longer hostages to the patient and her OCD symptoms.

Obsessional Slowness and Comorbid Schizotypal Personality Disorder

Case 5

At 25 years of age, after working under extremely stressful conditions as an accountant in which the workload was unbearable and his immediate supervisor was critical, cruel, and humiliating, the patient became extremely anxious, began to lose confidence in his abilities, and began to check his work. Six months later, his condition had worsened to the point that not only had his checking behavior increased, but he had become so fearful of making an error that it began to take him long periods of time to complete his projects. Because of increasing difficulty in completing his work and his perpetual state of high anxiety, he was placed on temporary disability. At that time, he sought psychiatric treatment for the first time in his life, and for the next 3 years the patient underwent twice-weekly psychodynamic psychotherapy. A number of different medications were tried, including protriptyline, clorazepate, thioridazine, thio-thixene, imipramine, and trazodone, with no significant effect on his symptoms. Unemployed and socially isolated, his depression, anxiety, and obsessive-compulsive symptoms had become so severe that he was hospitalized at the time behavioral treatment was begun.

Behavioral analysis indicated that the patient was immobilized by a rare subtype of OCD called obsessional slowness (see Chapter 15). He was unable to perform most routine tasks, such as picking up and putting down an object; washing, showering, or shaving; brushing his teeth; combing his hair; dressing; picking up utensils to eat; turning a water faucet on or off; getting in and out of a chair; walking across the room; getting ready for bed; reading beyond a first sentence; clearing the table; and opening and closing a door, without becoming immobilized. The patient often spent hours trying to perform each simple task.

The internal cues to his obsessional slowness were "somebody will die if I don't do everything perfectly"; "A disaster will occur and I'll be responsible if I don't check and get everything perfect"; "If I don't do this perfectly, I'll be labelled incompetent."

Behavioral assessment also indicated a very angry young man with major deficits in the area of assertiveness, especially regarding the expression of anger or disagreement. Behavioral analysis indicated a caring home environment, which was also stressful because of difficulties with communication and negotiation between the patient and his parents, with whom he resided.

Treatment was initiated with the therapist working directly with the patient and consulting simultaneously with the staff of this nonbehavioral inpatient unit. The patient was first exposed to performing simple tasks, such as picking up and putting down a fork, spoon, or knife within 10 seconds. When he was able to successfully complete this exercise, the time limit was gradually shortened until he could accomplish the task within 5 seconds. The therapist first modeled the desired behavior. Initially, the patient picked up and put down a utensil while the therapist counted out the seconds. When he could do this, he was required to pick up the object and put it down within the prescribed time without the therapist counting. The patient was then required to repeatedly practice until he could pick up and put down the utensil without hesitation. He was given liberal positive social reinforcement as he completed the task in the prescribed time. Once the patient demonstrated proficiency, treatment proceeded to a slightly more difficult and slightly more complex task, such as picking up a glass filled with water and drinking it, or taking medication out of a bottle. There was little generalization effect with the patient's obsessional slowness behavior. This is consistent with the findings of Rachman and Hodgson[8] (see Chapter 17). Each behavior had to be worked on separately, first with the therapist and then with the ongoing supervision of the inpatient staff. A great deal of patience and persistence was required. Consultation with staff continued, including instruction in basic principles of operant conditioning, particularly the principles of shaping, prompting, and reinforcement. Instruction in the implementation of the patient's treatment program and data collection also were necessary to allow assessment of the effectiveness of the intervention and the patient's progress. Agreement was reached between the patient and the staff that whenever he got "stuck" engaging in a task, his primary nurse would give him a count of 10 and he would begin to complete the task within the required time. Whenever he was unable to begin or complete the task, he would be assisted by his primary nurse. The patient also was required to seek assistance from the staff whenever he became "stuck."

Concomitant with measures to get him to complete tasks, the patient was taught to challenge his many obsessions of disastrous things happening if he did not do things perfectly. Because of the severity of his condition, the patient was given stimulus cards that contained statements challenging his obsession, which he would read when he was trying to engage in the prescribed behavior. For example, one stimulus card read, "I don't have the power to cause disastrous things to happen if I pick up and put down this (named object)." The ultimate goal was to get the patient to challenge his obsessions without stimulus cards, but it was necessary during the early phase of treatment to periodically give him cards with restructured statements, as for example, when he became stuck taking his medication because of his obsession that "It's the wrong time to take my Nardil, and I could cause a disaster to myself if I don't take it at the exact time."

To prepare the patient for discharge from the hospital and to ensure generalization to the home, his parents were similarly instructed in the same behavioral principles and procedures as the staff. In addition, the therapist met weekly with the patient and his parents to increase communication and negotiation skills between them. Assertiveness training was also instituted, using a structured program developed by Galassi and Galassi.[9] This became a regular part of the weekly session for the first 6 months of treatment.

When the patient was hospitalized, trazodone 400 mg was tapered and phenelzine was instituted in doses up to 90 mg/day. This medication greatly assisted the patient in his ability to tolerate and comply with behavioral treatment.

After a 2-month hospitalization, the patient's condition was significantly improved but still severely impaired. Behavioral treatment continued on a weekly outpatient basis. The patient was seen alone by the therapist for ERP and assertiveness training, then together with his parents to negotiate homework assignments and implementation of assignments. At home, his parents assisted him whenever he became "stuck" and helped him to perform behaviors within prescribed time limits. Soon after discharge, the patient began to socialize and engage in activities outside the home, sometimes with difficulty and occasional setbacks, some even humorous. One such incident occurred when the patient arranged a date with a young woman he was to meet at a nightclub in his hometown. He arrived approximately 15 minutes early and decided to go to the men's room. While there, he became "stuck" and was unable to emerge until 2 hours after the time he was to meet the woman. Thinking that she had been "stood up," she left after waiting for 1 hour, unaware he was 15 feet away from where she had been waiting, "stuck" trying to get out of the men's room. On another occasion, he went to an all-night restaurant at 1:00 a.m. and became "stuck" reading a map until 6:00 a.m. In the parking lot he became "stuck" again, until 11:00 a.m., trying to get inside his car.

Progress after discharge continued at a slow, steady rate, and the patient was able gradually to initiate more behaviors and complete them within normal time limits. Five months after initiating behavioral treatment, the patient was able to get his own clothes, dress, get his own food and drinks and consume them, get ready for bed, and read up to 50 consecutive pages, all within normal time limits.

A great deal of patience and persistence is required when treating a patient with obsessional slowness. It is doubly difficult when the patient also has schizotypal personality disorder (SPD); response to behavior therapy is often inconsistent or nonexistent.[10] Success is impossible without a parent, spouse, or close friend acting as a surrogate therapist in the patient's home environment to prompt, shape, and pace the patient's behavior. Often, a parent or spouse becomes impatient or is unable to remain detached and act in a kind, positive, yet firm manner in implementing exposure and response prevention. Such was the case with this patient's parents. As well-intentioned and caring as they were, the parents became increasingly frustrated with his slow progress and experienced greater difficulty in positively reinforcing him for desired target behaviors. He, on the other hand, became more resistant to allowing his parents to act as the surrogate therapist in the home and to letting them intervene whenever he became immobilized when initiating or completing a task. If this patient were in treatment in 1997, we would refer him to The Home Based Treatment Program, which is one of the outpatient programs of the MGH-OCD Institute. In this program, trained counselors travel to the patient's home for one to three sessions per week and perform ERP in the patient's natural environment (Chapter 25).

Although recovery continued at a slow, steady rate, there were increasing signs of conflict and stress at home. Arguments became more frequent and severe, with the patient having occasional outbursts of temper, during which he would destroy furniture or run out of the house in a blind rage. The therapist witnessed one of these outbursts during a behavioral family counseling session, and it was as if the patient had become temporarily insane. Similar incidents occur in other OCD patients with SPD. This observation is consistent with the description in the *Diagnostic and Statistical Manual of Mental Disorders* (DSM-III).[11] "During periods of extreme stress, transient psychotic symptoms may be present." And again, when discussing complications of SPD, DSM-III (p. 312)[11] notes: "Psychotic disorders such as brief reactive psychosis may occur" and "when psychotic symptoms occur in schizotypal personality disorder, they are transient and not as severe." At this point, it was suggested that the patient enter a therapeutic halfway house staffed to handle his obsessional slowness. This concept was initially resisted by both patient and parents until the situation at home became so stressful that it was unbearable. During this period, it was impossible to continue behavior therapy. Supportive therapy and behavioral family counseling, aimed at convincing the parents and the patient to accept halfway house placement, was the focus of treatment. The parents were the first to agree to placement. Several months later, the patient was able to accept the suggestion, applied, and was accepted for placement at the halfway house.

Once the patient entered the halfway house, the behavioral treatment program was reinstituted and telephone consultation was provided to the staff. The behavioral treatment program was carried out impartially, systematically, and firmly by the staff. Halfway house placement often plays a significant role in reducing stress in the home environment of OCD patients with SPD and possibly other severe personality disorders. Such reduction in stress has greatly facilitated the patient's ability to comply with behavioral treatment.

Once the behavioral program was reinstituted and the halfway house staff applied the behavioral principles on a consistent basis, the patient resumed his earlier progress. At this point, he was being seen on a monthly basis by the therapist for support and reinforcement of the behavioral work being carried out by the halfway house staff.

Six months after entry to the halfway house, the patient began to experience interpersonal difficulties with housemates and staff and once again began to have rage attacks. Eight months after admission to the halfway house, he had to be hospitalized. During this hospitalization his medication was changed from phenelzine 90 mg to a brief trial of chlorpromazine, then to fluoxetine 40 mg, lithium 1,200 mg, and clonazepam 2 mg/d, which was continued for this 1-month hospitalization. After discharge, he returned to the halfway house and his behavioral protocol was reinstituted. This time, his response to behavior therapy was rapid and enduring.

Within 6 months after inpatient discharge and change of medication, the patient was able to initiate and complete all tasks within normal time limits. Within 4 months after hospital discharge, he no longer met DSM-III criteria for SPD (see Chapter 14 for information on this personality disorder). In the words of his mother, "He's now the person he was before the onset of OCD symptoms," and in the words of the patient himself, "I keep asking myself, who was that other guy?" The patient had a complete response to the combined treatment of behavior therapy and pharmacotherapy with fluoxetine, lithium, and clonazepam. He is the second patient of a previously reported group of 10 with SPD[10] who failed to respond to behavior therapy and pharmacotherapy and who, with the addition of fluoxetine, not only had a significant reduction in OCD symptoms but also no longer met criteria for SPD. One year after discharge, the patient was working 8 hours daily in a volunteer job, was actively seeking a paying job, and was anticipating, with the advent of a salaried position, discharge from the halfway house and a move to his own apartment.

Complex Repeating, Checking, and Washing Rituals with Comorbid Schizotypal Personality Disorder

Case 6

This patient became immobilized by obsessions and compulsions at 14 years of age. As a result, the patient dropped out of school in grade 7 and had no further formal education. She had received extensive psychiatric treatment since age 14, her symptoms waxed and waned in her late teens and early twenties, and she was able to marry at 27 years of age. Two years after marrying, her symptoms began to interfere with her ability to function normally, and they progressively worsened. When brought to our outpatient clinic and research unit by her husband at age 61, she was totally immobilized. In the intervening years from age 27 until she was evaluated, she had been hospitalized five times, from periods of 6 months to 2 years each time and had undergone several courses of electroconvulsive therapy, one cingulotomy, and one bifrontal leucotomy. She was one of the most severely disabled patients treated at our clinic. Behavioral analysis in this patient indicated total avoidance of almost all activity. She was housebound and avoided all behavior, except eating food prepared by her husband and toileting. Her entire day was spent in bed, and her avoidance of almost everything prevented her from engaging in constant repeating. In the period prior to total withdrawal from all activity, she repeated every action, including multiple repetitions of behaviors such as tracing and retracing steps when walking inside or outside the home; going back and forth over every threshold she passed; going in and out of each door she passed through; going up and down stairs; opening and closing doors and cabinets; picking up and putting down utensils, cups, and glasses used in eating meals; getting in and out of the chairs, sofa, and bed; putting on and taking off every item of clothing; picking up and putting down every item to be purchased; and turning lights on and off. She also washed her hair and parts of her body repetitively, and repetitively dusted and cleaned every item in her house.

The patient denied any internal cues that triggered the rituals. She stated that she was just compelled to repeat and felt anxious and uncomfortable unless she repeated.

In addition to her own repetitive behavior, the patient required her husband to also repeat many behaviors he engaged in throughout the day. For example, before leaving for work each morning, he was required to repeat the phrase, "Have your breakfast and take your medicine, there's no problem." Prior to driving off to work, he was required to back his car into and out of the garage numerous times before he was allowed to drive off. Similarly, on returning from work he was required to back in and out of the garage before emerging and coming into the house. Whenever the patient heard her husband open the refrigerator or a cabinet door, she would shout orders from her bed to open and close it numerous times. She would also call out orders for him to repeat flushing the toilet, turning the faucets on and off numerous times, and washing and wiping his hands numerous times. She required him to put his slippers on and off, retrace his steps from the parlor to the den, go up and down the stairs from the kitchen to the garage, stand and sit when eating, and get into and out of bed and stand quietly for 30 to 60 seconds before repeating the behavior again. The only time he was not given orders to repeat an action was when he was engaging in a silent behavior such as reading and she was unaware of what he was doing.

This patient met all DSM-III[11] criteria for SPD. Her medication regimen consisted of haloperidol, carbamazepine, and tranylcypromine. After an in-depth explanation of behavioral treatment of OCD and the effort that would be required by both the patient and her husband if change was to be forthcoming, both made a commitment to proceed, with the understanding that therapy would terminate if it became clear from the weekly homework assignments that maximum effort at ERP was not forthcoming. Firmness with the patient was indicated from the onset. It was necessary to model behavior for her husband that did not reinforce her symptoms. She showed a threatening and manipulative demeanor and from the onset attempted to get the therapist to repeat or avoid certain words, subjects, or bodily movements. It was made clear from the outset that this was not acceptable and that the therapist would not engage in behavior that would contribute to the maintenance of her symptoms.

With these preliminary matters resolved, treatment began slowly, with negotiation between the therapist, the patient, and her husband that before leaving for work, the husband would remind the patient one time only that she was to eat her breakfast and take her medication; he was then to leave the house without returning. She was to get out of bed by 8:30 each morning and dress herself in blouse, pants, socks, and shoes without taking them off and on. Records were kept of daily progress.

When they returned 1 week later for their next session, the husband's record indicated that he was successful 50% of the time but succumbed to his wife's temper tantrums, screaming, and threats by repeating for her the rest of the time. However, he was able to reduce the pretreatment frequency of repetition from nine times to three times. The patient's data also indicated a 50% success rate on dressing without repeating; the rest of the time, she repeated each procedure when dressing from one to three times. This was an improvement over her pretreatment baseline of five times. She was successful 100% of the time in getting out of bed each day. The husband was told that his wife initially would continue to test him, and that her screaming, yelling, and temper tantrums would probably increase temporarily as she tested his resolve not to repeat actions at her request.

Joint therapy sessions were held weekly and centered on reviewing progress of the past week, reinforcing progress made, discussing problems encountered, and negotiating homework assignments for the coming week. These assignments aimed to eliminate the husband's reinforcement of the repetitive behavior and decrease her avoidance behavior, thus exposing her to behaviors that would trigger the urge to repeat. After she had significantly reduced her avoidance behavior and was active around the house, the focus shifted to reducing the repetitious actions she had previously avoided.

The husband was able to make steady progress in reducing the repetitive behaviors he engaged in at the patient's command, and over time he was able to eliminate 90% of these behaviors. This was not done easily, because the patient's screaming and temper tantrums lasted much longer than predicted, but they did stop eventually.

The patient's progress to significantly reduce repeating was slow and at times inconsistent, erratic, and unpredictable. After several months of treatment, the extent of this couple's marital malaise came more sharply into focus. The patient's weekly data indicated a significant increase in repetitive behavior after a dispute, disagreement, or stressful event involving her husband. There also was the indication that the patient sometimes used her OCD symptoms to control and punish her husband. At this point, behavioral marital counseling was begun, which focused on negotiation and communication in the relationship. This counseling proceeded for 12 sessions and had a significant effect on reducing the stress in the relationship.

Nine months after the start of treatment, the husband had eliminated 95% of the repetitive behavior he engaged in at the urging of his wife. She had eliminated 90% of her avoidance behavior and was now going out of the house to shop, walk, visit family, and eat in restaurants. Her repetitive behavior, however, was only 50% improved. At this juncture, the patient's medication regimen was changed to clomipramine, gradually increasing the dose to 250 mg/day. Over the next 3 months, she had a significant response to behavior therapy and found it easier to resist the urges to repeat. Six months after the start of clomipramine therapy, her repetitive behavior was 75% improved; the patient has maintained this improvement, but has not been able to exceed this percentage.

Although clomipramine had a significant effect and made it easier for the patient to engage in ERP, it had no effect on the SPD, and she continued to meet all DSM-III criteria for this personality disorder. She also continued to have periodic incidents of "temporary insanity," which were sudden in onset, triggered by seemingly insignificant incidents, and ended as suddenly as they had begun.

The overall quality of her life and that of her husband had improved. She was able to engage in all behaviors inside and outside her home that were previously avoided, and her compulsions, although still troublesome at times, no longer interfered with her ability to function. A letter of gratitude written to the therapist by her daughter captures the extent of her improvement: "I would just like to let you know how pleasing it is for us to see how our mother has progressed . . . It really seems like a miracle by far. It has taken years, and finally there was light at the end of the tunnel. It is amazing to see her function at a somewhat "normal" capacity . . . She is able to enjoy life now, and we are able to enjoy it with her."

If this patient had been seen in 1997, after a trial of outpatient behavioral treatment and pharmacotherapy involving selective serotonin reuptake inhibitor medications, we would have referred her to the MGH-OCD Institute for intense residential treatment involving state-of-the-art behavioral, pharmacologic, and family therapy (see Chapter 25).

SUMMARY

These six cases are representative of the patients with OCD who are evaluated and treated at our unit and of our approach of using a combination of behavior therapy, pharmacotherapy, behavioral family and couples counseling, and other interventions that enhance ERP, which is a critical mode of therapy to overcoming the learned component of OCD.

We are not yet satisfied with our results with patients whose OCD symptoms are less phobic-like, for example, patients suffering from obsessional slowness, repetitive behaviors, symmetry concerns, or behaviors that must be performed until it feels "just right" or "complete." These OCD symptoms may be more tic-like, and it is unclear at this time whether or not ERP is the "most effective behavioral strategy." We are continuing to explore other strategies for treating these patients.

REFERENCES

1. Alexander JF, Barton C, Shaivo RS, et al: Systems behavioral intervention with families of delinquents: Therapist's characteristics, family behavior, and outcome, *J Consult Clin Psychol* 44:656–664, 1976.
2. Carkhuff RR, Truax CB: *Toward effective counseling and psychotherapy: Training and practice*, Chicago, 1967, Aldine Publishing.
3. Sweet AA: The therapist relationship in behavior therapy, *Clin Psychol Rev* 4:253–272, 1984.
4. Rabavilas AD, Boulougouris JC, Peressaki C: Therapist qualities related to outcome with exposure in-vivo in neurotic patient, *J Behav Ther Exp Psychol* 10:293–299, 1979.
5. Matthews AM, Johnston DW, Lancashire M, et al: Imaginal flooding and exposure to real phobic situations: Treatment outcome with agoraphobic patients, *Br J Psychiatry* 129:362–371, 1976.
6. Minichiello WE, In Gorol AH, May LA, Mulley AG, editors: *Primary care medicine*, Philadelphia, 1987a, JB Lippincott.
7. Rachman SJ, Hodgson RL, Marks IM: The treatment of chronic obsessional neurosis, *Behav Res Ther* 9:237–247, 1971.
8. Rachman SJ, Hodgson RJ: *Obsessions and compulsions*, Englewood Cliffs, 1980, Prentice-Hall.
9. Galassi JP, Galassi MD: *Assert yourself! How to be your own person*, New York, 1977, Human Science Press.
10. Minichiello WE, Baer L, Jenike MA: Schizotypal personality disorder: A poor prognostic indicator for behavior therapy in the treatment of obsessive-compulsive disorder, *J Anx Dis* 1:273–276, 1987b.
11. American Psychiatric Association: *Diagnostic and statistical manual of mental disorders*, ed 3, Washington, 1980, American Psychiatric Association.

21

Group and Family Treatment for Obsessive-Compulsive Disorder

Gail S. Steketee, Ph.D., Barbara L. Van Noppen, M.S.W., L.I.S.W.

As several chapters of this book confirm, the current psychosocial treatment of choice for obsessive-compulsive disorder (OCD) is behavioral therapy employing exposure to feared situations and prevention of ritualistic and avoidance behaviors.[1,2] Until recently, this exposure and response prevention (ERP) treatment had been conducted in an individual format; the rationale for this treatment and empirical findings regarding its effects are presented in Chapter 17 and will not be discussed here. Despite the relative benefits of this treatment, 20% to 25% of OCD patients who initially present for individual behavioral therapy refuse it, and of those who begin treatment, another 20% to 30% do not complete the program or are nonresponders.[3] More intensive programs may reduce the nonresponse rate, but not the refusal rate.[3] Thus, many patients continue to experience chronic symptoms that interfere with their personal, social, and family functions.

Although recent emphasis on the neurobiologic aspects of OCD has overshadowed the role of psychosocial factors, several recent studies have examined such factors in the development and treatment of OCD. Our clinical experience suggests that the response of the family support system (i.e., relatives and significant others) to OCD symptoms may be important in the prognosis and outcome of treatment. Family context may be especially relevant for behavior therapy nonresponders whose significant others' emotional responses toward the patient and the OCD symptoms are overly negative. Likewise, patients who live alone often need extra assistance to complete ERP homework assignments. Treatment in a group context, with or without family members, may be necessary for such patients.

In addition, in this time of growing concern with health care expenditures, time-limited group treatments hold considerable potential for reducing costs without sacrificing benefits. Group behavioral treatment (GBT) involves patients only, whereas multifamily behavioral treatment (MFBT) includes both patients and significant others. This chapter reviews the literature on these two modalities for treating OCD and presents brief descriptions of such groups in our Butler Hospital OCD clinic. More detailed case examples are available elsewhere.[4]

GROUP BEHAVIORAL TREATMENT

Many OCD patients never marry and have few social contacts. For example, Steketee, Grayson and Foa[5] reported that 37% of 75 adult OCD patients had never married and 25% were living with their parents. Men with OCD appear to be especially prone to remaining single, given reports that approximately 65% of men with OCD are unmarried[6-8] versus 27% of the U.S. male population.[9] The early onset age of OCD in many men contributes to the higher rate of nonmarriage, perhaps because of social isolation during critical teen years, when social skills are learned.[10]

Thus, GBT, with its readily available social networks, may be especially appropriate for OCD sufferers. A supportive group may provide a motivational boost for those sufferers who feel they cannot complete homework assignments without the accountability of the group and the compassion of other OCD patients. In his landmark writings on interpersonal group therapy, Yalom[11] identified "curative factors" common in groups: 1) instillation of hope; 2) imitative behavior; 3) imparting of information; 4) universality; 5) development of socializing techniques; 6) group cohesiveness; 7) catharsis; and 8) altruism. Some of these factors are powerful forces in behavioral treatment groups for OCD patients. In addition, Budman[12] recognized the pragmatic, economic, and motivation-enhancing reasons for developing time-limited models in group therapy.

The value of GBT has been reported for other anxiety disorders (e.g., panic disorder and agoraphobia)[13] and social phobia.[14] Several clinical researchers have investigated group treatments for OCD, although most studies are uncontrolled. These studies are summarized in Table 21-1 and are described in the following paragraphs. In an early uncontrolled study on GBT in OCD, Hand and Tichatzky[15] treated 17 OCD patients in three groups, targeting obsessive-compulsive symptoms, social interactions, and problem solving. The groups met for a minimum of 25 twice-weekly sessions and included *in vivo* exposure exercises, homework assignments, and attention to communication skills. Spouses and family members met in separate support group meetings. Therapist involvement was gradually withdrawn over 18 weeks, eventually resulting in an entirely self-help model. Despite the group format, Hand and Tichatzky's treatment was labor intensive for clinicians, and improvement in OCD symptoms and anxiety was variable among groups.

Epsie[16] employed group treatment for five OCD patients who had previously relapsed following individual behavioral treatment. Taylor and Sholomskas[17]

Table 21-1   Group Treatment for Obsessive-Compulsive Disorder

Study	Patients (n)	Sessions	Outcome
Hand and Tichatzky (1979)	17	25	Variable decrease in obsessive-compulsive disorder symptoms
Epsie (1986)	5	10	Successful outcome after individual behavior therapy failed
Taylor and Sholomskas (1993)	6	14	Benefits comparable to individual behavior therapy
Enright (1991)	24	9	Significant benefits for obsessive-compulsive disorder symptoms; 17% clinically improved[*]
Krone, Himle, and Nesse (1991)	36	7	Yale-Brown Obsessive-Compulsive Scale: 21 pretest, 16 posttest, 12 3-month follow-up
Van Noppen, et al (1993)	73	8–10	Yale-Brown Obsessive-Compulsive Scale: 22 pretest, 17 posttest, 16 6-month follow-up
Van Noppen, et al (1997)	17	10–12	Yale-Brown Obsessive-Compulsive Scale: 24 pretest, 17 posttest, 14.5 1-year follow-up; 43% clinically improved[*]
Fals-Stewart, Marks, and Schafer (1993)	30	24 group behavior therapy	Group behavior therapy = individual behavior therapy > relaxation
	31	24 individual behavior therapy	Yale-Brown Obsessive-Compulsive Scale: 22 pretest, 12 posttest, 14 6-month
	32	24 relaxation	follow-up

[*] Clinically significantly improved according to Jacobson & Truax's (1991) method.

co-led a group for six OCD patients. Treatment in both studies included 10 to 14 sessions of education, goal setting, behavioral skills training, ERP, and homework logs. Taylor and Sholomskas' group treatment included cognitive restructuring, whereas Epsie added two group follow-up sessions. In both case reports, benefits at the end of treatment and at follow-up were comparable with results reported in the individual behavioral treatment of OCD.

Enright[18] treated 24 patients in four groups for nine weekly 90-minute sessions, using a program similar to that previously described, except for the addition of assertiveness training. The patient dropout rate was modest at 11%, and attendance at GBT sessions was high (93%). Significant decreases were found in OCD symptoms, depressed and anxious mood, and functional impairment at posttest and at 6-month follow-up. However, only 17% of participants experienced clinically significant improvement (using a criterion of one standard deviation drop in obsessive-compulsive symptom scores). Thus, patients showed consistent benefit, but the amount of gain was generally not substantial. This study focused less on ERP during sessions than the other group clinical trials, perhaps accounting for the limited benefit.

Krone, Himle and Nesse[19] treated 36 OCD patients with a short 7-week group program that included education, instruction in cognitive and behavioral self-treatment, and therapist-directed ERP that occurred during group treatment sessions. An optional family psychoeducational session was provided. As in the Enright[18] study, significant reductions were found in obsessive-compulsive symptom scores; the Yale-Brown Obsessive Compulsive Scale (Y-BOCS)[20] scores dropped from a mean of 21 at baseline to a mean of 16 (the clinical cutoff line) at posttreatment, and to below clinical levels (mean = 12) at 3-month follow-up. Patient depression also decreased, particularly in those who were medicated, and improvement in OCD symptoms was independent of medication use. Thus, these investigators demonstrated very good gains for their large OCD sample in a short period of time.

Van Noppen, Pato, Marsland, and Rasmussen[21] provided group GBT to 73 outpatients with OCD who participated in 8 to 10 sessions of in-session group ERP cognitive exercises, and self-monitoring homework assignments. Mean Y-BOCS scores dropped from 22 at baseline to 17 at posttreatment, and 16 at 6-month follow-up. This group treatment package was further developed and tested on an additional 17 patients with OCD over 10 to 12 weekly group sessions, followed by six monthly group sessions (to assist in maintenance of gains).[22] After this longer treatment, mean Y-BOCS scores dropped from 24 baseline to 17 at posttreatment, and to 14.5 at 1-year follow-up. Approximately 75% of patients improved at least five points at posttest and follow-up, and clinically significant improvement was found in 43% of patients using Jacobson and Truax's[23] criterion. Patients also improved significantly in work, social, and family functioning posttreatment and 1 year later. This group therapy was well tolerated—few patients dropped out, and most reported being highly satisfied with the therapy.

Fals-Stewart, Marks, and Schafer[24] conducted the only controlled trial to date of GBT for OCD. They compared group ERP (n = 30) with comparable individual behavioral treatment (n = 31) and with an individual relaxation control treatment (n = 32). These investigators employed more sessions (24 over a 12-week period), making theirs the most intensive study of the group treatments reviewed here. Subjects in both group and individual exposure treatment conditions showed significant improvement in OCD symptoms, depression, and anxiety at both posttreatment and 6-month follow-up, whereas the control group improved only in anxiety. Mean Y-BOCS scores for GBT patients dropped from 22 at baseline to 12 at posttreatment, and 14 at follow-up; these results were comparable with those reported by Krone, et al[19] and Van Noppen, et al.[22] Mean Y-BOCS scores of individually treated patients were 20 at baseline, 12 at posttreatment, and 13 at 1-year follow-up. There were no significant differences in outcome between the group and individual treatment conditions, although individual therapy led to a somewhat more rapid change. It seems likely that the development of group cohesion may require a slightly longer period, possibly slowing initial gains until patients become comfortable with each other and motivated to engage in ERP homework. The investigators limited the generalization of their findings by excluding OCD patients with concurrent major depression and axis II diagnoses. It is therefore unknown how individuals with comorbidity, who comprise a large proportion of OCD clinic patients, would fare in this group treatment.

Comparisons of pre-effect and posteffect sizes using Cohen's d (another method for measuring the magnitude of the therapeutic impact) from studies using Y-BOCS data indicate that GBT produced very large effects that ranged from 0.79[19] to 2.69.[24] Effect sizes for individual behavior therapy have been very similar, ranging from 1.47[25] to 2.10.[24] Follow-up effect sizes using Y-BOCS scores also are similar for group (1.49 to 1.97) and individual (1.73 to 1.83) treatments.

In summary, behavioral treatment can be applied effectively using a group modality with results that are similar to individual treatment. This conclusion appears to be particularly true when the number of group sessions is comparable with that usually provided to individual patients (12 to 20 sessions). GBT for OCD appears to be a clinically successful and cost-effective alternative to standard individual treatment.

As Kobak, Rock, and Greist[26] noted and our own experience confirms, in addition to the lower cost, several aspects of GBT might enhance outcome beyond individual behavior therapy[27]: (1) the opportunity for clients to help other group members, thereby improving self-esteem and reducing demoralization and isolation; (2) vicarious learning from other members; (3) consensual reality testing regarding obsessive fears and compulsive behaviors; (4) role flexibility, allowing members to draw on personal experience to assist others and learn as patients; and (5) group cohesiveness that increases motivation to complete homework and achieve related goals.

Further controlled study of the benefits of clearly specified behavioral group intervention using ERP, cognitive strategies, and perhaps other adjunctive treatments is clearly needed. For the present, however, this mode of therapy may be valuable in clinical settings in which there are few behaviorally trained therapists and a sufficient patient flow to permit the establishment of groups for patients with OCD. We do not recommend combining OCD patients and those patients with other disorders in the same group, because the treatment of OCD is quite specialized, and patients with other diagnoses may have difficulty empathizing with the OCD patients' experience.

DESCRIPTION OF A GROUP BEHAVIORAL TREATMENT PROGRAM

Following is a description of the GBT program developed and tested at Butler Hospital, in Providence, Rhode Island. Table 21-2 summarizes this treatment program.

In our clinic, treatment begins when 6 to 10 patients have been referred for GBT. Patients are initially screened by an experienced clinician for diagnosis and interest in GBT. Patients are then evaluated by the group therapist to ensure appropriateness for group treatment and to collect symptom and general information. This process requires approximately two individual 1- to 1.5-hour, information-gathering sessions with the group therapist. In these meetings, historic and current information about the patient's OCD and other symptoms are collected along with information about previous mental health treatment and a general history of family and social relationships. Detailed information about the OCD symptoms is used to generate a hierarchy, which each patient later brings to the first group session. OCD and behavior therapy are defined, and the goals of GBT are outlined. Family members are invited to accompany the patient to part of the second information-gathering session to permit further psychoeducation and assessment of the family situation (although family members are not directly involved in GBT).

The GBT meets 2 hours for 12 consecutive weeks. At the first session, the therapist welcomes patients and asks members to introduce themselves. The agenda for all 12 sessions is then reviewed. The therapist discusses rules for confidentiality, requesting that any information revealed about a group member not be discussed with anyone outside the group. The therapist also arranges coverage between group sessions in case of a crisis and emphasizes the importance of consistent attendance. Questions such as "What do you hope to get out of this group?" are intended to encourage group members to examine their goals. Psychoeducational written material is provided, usually in the form of a handout about OCD, and patients are asked to read aloud from this handout. Alternatively, patients may be asked to purchase and read chapters from a self-help book selected by the therapist.[28] The material covered addresses the definition of OCD, phenomenology, course, comorbidity, personality traits, and overview of treatments, introducing the concepts of exposure and response prevention. Group members receive the self-rated version of the Y-BOCS Symptom Checklist and, to promote disclosure, patients are asked to read aloud sections of the checklist, enabling them to draw from their experience to provide examples for each symptom type.

Table 21-2   Group Behavioral Treatment for Obsessive-Compulsive Disorder

Group size: 8 to 10 patients with obsessive-compulsive disorder
Duration: 2 hours weekly for 12 weeks, 2 hours monthly for 6 months

Session 1

Introduction, goals, agenda, confidentiality
Yale-Brown Obsessive-Compulsive Scale symptom checklist
Obsessive-compulsive disorder handouts: etiology, course, demographics,
  treatments
Exposure homework form
Go-round selection of homework

Session 2

Check-in and go-round to report on homework and progress
Explanation of behavioral therapy techniques
Practice doing *in vivo* and imaginal exposure and response prevention
Go-round selection of homework

Session 3

Check-in and go-round
Neurobiology of obsessive-compulsive disorder
Practicing *in vivo* and imaginal exposure and response prevention
Go-round selection of homework

Sessions 4 through 12

Check-in and go-round
Practicing *in vivo* and imaginal exposure and response prevention
Go-round selection of homework

Sessions 15 through 19: monthly

Go-round to report on progress
Troubleshooting problem areas with group input
Formulate goals and methods for next month
Wrap-up

Session 20

Check-in and go-round
Review of progress
Discussion of termination of the group
Plans for future management of obsessive-compulsive disorder symptoms

---

This experience often permits members who have blamed themselves to observe others who suffer similar frustrations in their lives. The "curative" factors in this group process described by Yalom[11] are often effective in decreasing feelings of isolation, stigma, and shame, while universalizing problems, instilling hope, and using imitative behavior to promote change. Such sharing among patients produces a growing atmosphere of group cohesion and trust, paving the way for the use of ERP and modeling in the group. In addition, the heterogeneity of symptoms often promotes insight into OCD by facilitating greater participation in the *in vivo* exercises that leads to group consensus on normative behavior and beliefs. For example, it would be difficult to get a group of patients, all of whom had home-checking rituals, to leave their homes with only a single turn of a key in the lock. In the group setting, in which several other OCD patients do not share this symptom, patients must learn new normative rules. They also learn to appreciate the various forms of symptoms, enabling them to depersonalize the obsessive content.

After disclosing their own situations, patients select an item in the low-to-moderate discomfort range (35 to 45 out of 100 subjective units of discomfort [SUDS]) from their personal hierarchy to use during ERP homework. The therapist instructs group members to record their distress levels throughout the week when practicing this homework task. To keep group members on task, the clinician reminds patients of the time-limited nature of the therapy and the need to cover much ground in a relatively short time period.

The first item on the agenda of the subsequent sessions is a report from each member about the outcome of his or her homework assignment. Patients receive praise for their accomplishments and problem-solving feedback when they have experienced difficulties accomplishing the task or habituating to the feared context. Group input is intended to expand patients' awareness of alternatives and offer consensual validation of normative beliefs and behaviors. Humor often helps attenuate the intensity of fears. During this psychoeducational phase, the therapist also introduces the notion that although patients "feel" or "think" they have to perform their rituals, most group members have spoken in absolutes: "I have to check," "I have to straighten the magazines." This discrepancy is noted in later sessions to shift assumptions.

The therapist then provides a detailed overview of *in vivo* and imagined exposure, with examples of these techniques that are practiced in the group. An example is group members removing their wallets, shuffling around money and credit cards while reporting on their distress, putting the wallet away, continuing to monitor the distress, and then repeating the task. The therapist asks how other patients could tailor the challenge to make this an appropriate exposure task for their particular symptoms. For example, one member might pass around his wallet, allowing other group members to "contaminate" it, whereas another might open and close the wallet, allowing himself to think about "something bad happening" to a family member. A third might remove an item from an overstuffed wallet to discard it, whereas a fourth patient may look at pictures of his children and repeat a feared word aloud. All patients rehearse their exposure tasks and rate their discomfort levels until anxiety is reduced.

Such exposure practice sessions are often very lively and instructive in multiple ways for all concerned. Some very anxious patients appear to benefit greatly from the support, feedback, and encouragement of other patients to stay in the difficult situation. Most patients report that it is very helpful to observe others expose themselves and become increasingly anxious, and to see the discomfort recede after repeated and prolonged exposure. Thus, although therapist modeling has not been shown empirically to improve outcome, patients have reported that participant modeling was beneficial to them.[29] For homework, patients are asked to continue their in-group challenges and to add items from their hierarchies. The exposure homework practice and discomfort ratings are recorded on the homework forms and discussed the following week.

At the third and later sessions, patients begin by reporting on homework tasks. For psychoeducational purposes, we present a 15-minute videotape to provide information on the neurobiology of OCD, and appropriate medications and their effects. This videotape is followed by a brief discussion. The remainder of this session is devoted to exposure, with patients selecting items in the 50 to 60 range of discomfort from their hierarchies. As before, exposure exercises are modified to maximize the benefits for each group member. As group members become more comfortable in each other's presence, jokes become more common, and patients are able to laugh about the absurdity of their symptoms. All patients select homework assignments and receive feedback from the group to ensure that the tasks chosen are reasonable but challenging. This process is intended to increase individual patients' problem-solving options and to promote the use of various behavioral techniques. Imparting information and learning from other patients appears to be beneficial, as patients come to respect advice given by others "in the same boat" who have had success.

Subsequent sessions proceed in a similar fashion, with a report from each patient on homework successes and obstacles. The therapist quickly addresses any problems patients have encountered in completing homework assignments. Dropouts may occur during this early or middle phase if patients have not experienced any progress. Such dropout has been relatively infrequent in our experience, perhaps because the sense of competition among patients ("If Susan can do that, so can I!") is a powerful motivator. At times, group cohesion may become so well developed that patients take more risks to avoid disappointing other group members. Nonetheless, patients who select inappropriate challenges or engage in only brief exposures that do not allow habituation can become frustrated as others progress. To prevent dropout, which can discourage other group members, the therapist should look for warning signs that a patient has been repeatedly unsuccessful in employing ERP and then use *in vivo* group exercises to correct this experience.

As each session progresses, patients select items from their hierarchies that evoke increasing levels of distress. If possible, the most distressing stimulus should be introduced by session 8 to allow time for habituation. The group experience often becomes more interactive and patients press one another to tolerate anxiety. The therapist can encourage patients to change their manner of speaking about OCD symptoms to help alter the way they think and feel. For example, when group members describe a scenario as "I have to . . . ," the therapist corrects them, asking them to insert "I feel I have to" or "I think I have to." Over time, group members begin to catch each other doing this and take on the role of therapist, asking each other to correct the way they speak about obsessive-compulsive symptoms. Such interventions promote self-help strategies that encourage independent skills after formal treatment has ended. Often, a positive group experience convinces otherwise shy patients to become interested in joining self-help groups for people with OCD. Many patients have reported a sense of pride and self-worth in being able to help fellow OCD patients. This may be another active ingredient of GBT.

The final session is conducted in the same manner as those previously described, except that the therapist leaves sufficient time to address concerns and questions regarding the end of active treatment. Patients typically express fears that they will be unable to succeed without the group support. Responses to termination are varied, and the therapist must allow individual expressions of parting that do not lead the group too far from important tasks. Putting closure on weekly treatment sessions requires attention to manage the high level of intimacy in the group. The main focus is on fostering self-instruction and self-efficacy. Group members are asked to comment on the enormous changes they have observed in others and to identify the most helpful elements of the group treatment. Six monthly meeting dates are then scheduled and patients are encouraged to call for help between sessions as needed.

FAMILY TREATMENT INTERVENTIONS
The Effect of Obsessive-Compulsive Disorder on Families

Obsessive-compulsive disorder can have an adverse effect on family members' quality of life and interactions. Many families become dysfunctional as a result of a member's OCD and the family's involvement in his symptoms. Calvocoressi and colleagues[30] surveyed 34 family members of patients with OCD. Nearly one third of these family members reassured the patient three or more times per week, and a similar number participated in compulsion-related behaviors or took over activities that were the patient's responsibility. Many modified family and leisuretime routines and activities to accommodate the patient, usually to manage the patient's distress and potential anger. These accommodations also led family members to experience distress: 35% reported moderate distress and 23% reported severe or extreme distress. Shafran, Ralph, and Tallis[31] recorded the reactions of 98 family members (67% spouses or partners, 17% parents, 16% child, sibling, or other) of volunteers who scored high on obsessive-compulsive symptoms. Sixty percent of these relatives participated in rituals (e.g., checking, giving reassurance) or avoidance behavior to accommodate their afflicted family members. Only 10% of respondents experienced no interference in their lives from OCD, and 20% reported severe interference. More than half wanted assistance in the form of information, counseling, or discussion with other relatives of individuals with OCD. Thus, living with an OCD sufferer often leads families to try to reduce obsessive-compulsive fear and anxiety and also can result in frustration, anger, and guilt.

Family Responses to Obsessive-Compulsive Disorder Symptoms

Family responses to obsessive-compulsive symptoms range from families who give in to and assist in compulsions and avoidance, to those who completely oppose OCD behaviors.[32] Families who are entangled in the patient's OCD tend to fall on the accommodating end of the range, with few boundaries, poor limit setting, and avoidance of conflict in an effort to "keep the peace." Antagonistic families are rigid, demanding, intolerant of symptoms, and highly critical, generating feelings of loss of control and increased anxiety. Between these extremes are split families who are inconsistent in their response to symptomatology (i.e., one family member antagonistic, another understanding and indulgent, or erratic reactions within family members). Not surprisingly, both patients and family members often feel confused and anxious when faced with OCD. OCD puts stress on the patient and family members, along with accompanying guilt, blame, and social stigma. Guilty reactions from family members, especially parents, are common.[31,33] Some of the unfortunate consequences of guilt and frustration include preoccupation with the patient's needs and feeling burdened and increasingly isolated, as families remove themselves from usual social contacts.

Families with an OCD sufferer have difficulty functioning effectively. When members were assessed on family problem solving, communication, roles, affective responsiveness, affective involvement, behavior control, and global functioning, 52% scored in the unhealthy range of functioning on at least one of these dimensions.[32] Problems were common in the areas of affective responsiveness, role functioning, problem solving, and behavior control. Compared with control families, families of OCD patients had a higher percentage of unhealthy scores on all dimensions of family function except communication. Hibbs and colleagues[34] reported that nearly half of fathers and three quarters of mothers of children with OCD exhibited high levels of criticism or overinvolvement (called Expressed Emotion [EE]) with their children. These rates were two to three times higher than those found in parents of nonpsychiatric controls. Parents with high EE had more psychiatric diagnoses, more family conflict, and more marital discord.[34,35]

Most studies have indicated that married OCD sufferers are often dissatisfied with their marriages, although there is some disagreement within the literature.[36] Riggs, et al[37] found that level of marital distress was not associated with the severity of obsessive-compulsive symptoms nor with depression, but rather was modestly related to greater avoidance. It is not clear whether OCD symptoms adversely affect family functioning or whether poor family interactions exacerbate OCD symptoms.

Marital and Family Factors Predicting Treatment Outcome

Few studies have examined whether marital or family variables predict treatment outcome. Hafner[38] described five women with OCD who had relapsed after returning home to conflictual marriages. In a later report, he noted that spouse-aided behavioral therapy produced gains for another five women.[39] Similarly, Hoover and Insel[40] reported that 10 OCD sufferers relapsed somewhat on returning home to live with parents after behavioral therapy; separation from their parents contributed to further improvement.

Both Riggs, et al[37] and Emmelkamp, et al[41] found that patients in distressed marriages benefitted from behavioral treatment and that their outcome did not differ from patients who reported having good marriages. Thus, marital satisfaction did not predict whether patients improved during treatment. In addition, improvement in OCD patients did not provoke adjustment problems in their partners.[41] Interestingly, both studies also reported that successful behavior therapy led to improved marriages, although this did not persist in the Emmelkamp, et al study. Riggs and colleagues reported that 42% of 25 dissatisfied couples experienced improvement in marital satisfaction and reductions in demands and dependency. These two studies support earlier findings on small samples that exposure-based treatment for OCD and phobias improves both the anxiety targets and any marital problems.[42]

Steketee[43] found that poor social and family functioning and household interactions (characterized by anger and criticism) predicted fewer gains on OCD symptoms at 9-month follow-up. Conversely, patient-perceived positive interactions in the household were associated with more improvement. Perhaps relatives' criticism and expressed anger increased the patients' anxiety and guilt, thereby reducing ability to resist ritualizing. Relatives' beliefs that OCD patients were malingering and could "just stop" their rituals were strongly associated with poor outcome ($r = 0.55$, $p < 0.01$).

Emmelkamp, Kloek, and Blaauw[44] hypothesized that patients who lack coping skills or social support, or who experience criticism in the face of stressors, are likely to relapse. They suggested that OCD problems are further compounded when patients view their symptoms as a disease over which they have little control. Consistent with this model, Emmelkamp and colleagues found that the combination of EE ratings, avoidant coping style, and life events and daily hassles predicted relapse, although social support did not—a finding also reported by Steketee.[43] Criticism and hostility were evident at follow-up in three of their four relapse patients, although in neither of the two partial relapse patients.

Recently, Steketee and Chambless (unpublished) have obtained preliminary findings from an ongoing trial of family variables as predictors of behavioral treatment outcome in a sample of patients with OCD and agoraphobia. Patient-rated criticism and family hostility were associated with fewer benefits. These and earlier findings suggest that negative familial reactions and interactions with patients may have adverse effects on OCD patients' responsiveness to treatment. Of particular interest are findings of family members included in the therapy; these findings are discussed in the following paragraphs.

Family Involvement in Treatment

Emmelkamp and colleagues[44] recommended involving spouses or family members in treatment for OCD sufferers who have problems with social interaction. They suggested emphasizing empathic listening skills and communication training in individual and family group contexts. Such proposals have been pursued recently by other researchers as noted in the following paragraphs.

Support Groups

Support groups provide one avenue for involving family members in OCD treatment. Marks and colleagues[45] viewed family involvement in behavioral treatment of OCD as particularly important and instituted a mixed patient and relative group that met every few weeks while the patient participated in individual behavioral therapy. The benefits of combined patient/family or family-only support groups have also been reported by Black and Blum,[46] Cooper,[47] and Tynes, Salins, Skiba, and Winstead.[48] These groups usually included psychoeducation and social support for group members, both designed to increase hope, alleviate fear, and reassure patients and family members. Family groups typically discussed strategies for managing difficult problems such as reassurance seeking and requests to help in obsessive-compulsive behaviors.[45] Support groups that included both patients and significant others covered educational topics such as OCD symptoms, theories behind the development of OCD, treatment options, medications, complications, and relapse prevention.[48] Although no outcome data have been reported regarding the effects of family support groups on patient symptoms, participants reported satisfaction with these groups.

Family-Assisted Treatment

Several reports have included parents, spouses, or other family members assisting in behavior therapy for patients with OCD. Hafner[49] reported successful outcomes for five wives with OCD in distressed marriages by including spouses in the behavioral treatment. Similar benefits also have been reported for parental involvement in behavioral treatment of children,[50–52] adolescents, and adults.[39,40] For example, Hafner, et al[39] reported on a 16-year-old boy who did not improve after several attempts at behavioral treatment. When the boy's parents became involved in treatment, the family was able to express uncommunicated feelings and, after nine sessions, the boy's symptoms subsided. Thus, altering family communication style and learning alternative responses to the patient's OCD symptoms may facilitate gains.

In an uncontrolled trial, Thornicroft and colleagues[53] reported benefits for inpatients with OCD from efforts to reduce relatives' involvement in OCD symptoms and to teach relatives to monitor patient behavior and encourage self-exposure in a noncritical manner.[53] Family members were supervised by the therapist on the ward. The 45 patients participating in this treatment program (most of whom had OCD) experienced a 45% decrease in symptoms at discharge. A 60% reduction in symptoms and concomitant improvement in functioning was evident for 22 patients who were available at 6-month follow-up. These gains are impressive for an inpatient population that scored in the extreme range of disability from OCD symptoms.

Emmelkamp and colleagues[54] conducted two controlled studies of spouse-assisted ERP compared with individual behavior therapy. In the first study of 12 patients, spouse participation in therapy and homework assistance led to greater benefits than individual treatment, although this advantage did not persist at follow-up. In a later trial of a larger sample, spouse-aided exposure produced positive results, but the results were not better than individual behavior therapy either after treatment or at follow-up, despite improvement in marital satisfaction in the spouse-aided group.[41] In a later report, Emmelkamp, et al[44] particularly emphasized the need for empathic communication; thus it is possible that the failure to include formal training in family communication skills about patients' OCD symptoms might have reduced possible benefits from family treatment.

A controlled study of family-assisted behavioral treatment in 30 OCD patients in India produced conclusions different from those of Emmelkamp and colleagues.[55] Patients who were aided by a family member during treatment benefitted significantly more than those who received no family participation. Members of the family-treated group were also more likely to maintain their gains than individually treated patients, who relapsed more frequently. Nonanxious, firm family members proved especially effective in treatment. The greater intensity of treatment in the Indian trial (24 sessions twice weekly vs. eight sessions in 5 weeks in the Dutch study) may have contributed to the differences in outcome between these trials, as might the response styles of relatives from different cultures (i.e., Indian family members may have been less critical than their Dutch counterparts). Further, Mehta's[55] study included relatives other than spouses, possibly leading to different patient reactions.

Recently, Van Noppen and colleagues[56] tested the value of delivering behavioral treatment in a multifamily group format. This intervention is specifically aimed at reducing obsessive-compulsive symptoms, as well as changing dysfunctional communication patterns between family members that fuel obsessive-compulsive symptoms. The family group treatment incorporates psychoeducation, communication and problem-solving skills training, clarifying boundaries, social learning, and *in vivo* rehearsal of new behaviors, in the context of ERP with therapist and participant modeling. Such a multifamily group format is another potential strategy for reducing treatment costs and enhancing maintenance of gains in OCD treatment. In a recent uncontrolled trial[22] of 19 patients treated in this multifamilial group format, nine patients (47%) were clinically significantly improved in OCD severity scoring in the nonclinical range on the Y-BOCS at posttreatment, and 58% achieved this status at 1-year follow-up. Results were comparable with those achieved in individual behavior therapy. Poorer family role functioning and communication predicted less benefit on obsessive-compulsive symptoms, and poorer family functioning was associated with greater disability.

DESCRIPTION OF MULTIFAMILY BEHAVIORAL TREATMENT

Following is a description of the Multifamily Group Behavioral Treatment (MFBT) Program, developed and tested at the Butler Hospital OCD Clinic in Providence, Rhode Island. Table 21-3 outlines this therapy. A history and detailed description of patients' obsessive-compulsive symptoms are obtained during the two 60- to 90-minute individual information-gathering sessions with the therapist who will conduct the family group treatment. At least one of these sessions should be conducted with the patient alone to ensure that he or she has an opportunity to comment on the family situation and any concerns about these relationships. All or part of the second session should include relative(s) who will participate in the group. In this session, the therapist continues to collect information about symptoms, develop a hierarchy, and obtain any further information not already discussed about the patient's symptoms, history, and family history, especially since the onset of the OCD. Family groups usually include six or seven families to permit a family to drop out without disrupting the structure of the group. Groups usually range in size from 12 to 16 people. Because of the number of people in the room, cotherapy is often desirable, if this option is feasible in light of clinic costs.

At the outset of the MFBT group, initially high anticipatory anxiety is alleviated by providing structure, especially at the first session. However, the therapist also should allow room for individual expression, which will collectively determine the climate of the group with regard to blame, responsibility, overprotection, overinvolvement, distance, impotence, and denial. Once people begin talking, they are usually relieved to be with others who understand their plight, and it can be difficult to redirect informal conversation to begin the session. The therapist can carefully observe the level of interaction and content, as well as seating choices that could reveal alliances, conflicts, and level of trust within the group. As family members arrive, the therapist distributes name tags and begins the session with everyone seated in a circle. Each person introduces himself or herself and indicates what he or she hopes

Table 21-3 Multifamily Behavioral Treatment for Obsessive-Compulsive Disorder

Group size: 5 to 7 patients and their family members
Duration: 2 hours weekly for 12 weeks, 2 hours monthly for 6 months

Session 1

Introduction, goals, agenda, confidentiality
Yale-Brown Obsessive-Compulsive Scale symptom checklist
Obsessive-compulsive disorder handout: etiology, course, demographics, treatment
Exposure homework form
Go-round selection of homework

Session 2

Check-in and go-round to report on homework and progress
Explanation of behavioral therapy techniques
Practicing *in vivo* and imaginal exposure and response prevention
Go-round and selection of homework

Session 3

Check-in and go-round
Neurobiology of obsessive-compulsive disorder
Practicing *in vivo* and imaginal exposure and response prevention
Read "Family Guidelines" in *Learning to Live with OCD*
Go-round and selection of homework

Session 4 through 12

Check-in and go-round
Practice family behavioral contracting, *in vivo*
Practicing *in vivo* and imaginal exposure and response prevention
Go-round and selection of homework

Sessions 15 through 19: monthly

Review of obsessive-compulsive disorder symptoms in past month and family
relationships
Troubleshooting problem areas with group input
Formulate goals and strategies
Wrap-up

Session 20:

Check-in and go-round
Review of progress in family communication and obsessive-compulsive disorder
symptoms
Discussion of termination of the group
Plans for future management of obsessive-compulsive disorder symptoms and
family matters

to gain from the group. This facilitates participation and assists in establishing trust and group cohesiveness. The themes of the early MFBT groups usually entail such concerns as how to respond to excessive rituals, what constitutes OCD symptoms versus willfulness, and how other families cope with OCD.

A quick review of the "ground rules" clarifies group expectations about the duration of therapy, confidentiality (group members are asked not to discuss any personal information about members outside of the sessions), and notification of absence from the group. Group members are encouraged to contact the leader to discuss any feelings or issues that arise as a result of their group experience. The proposed agenda for the 12 weekly sessions and six monthly maintenance sessions is outlined. Thereafter, a handout (or assigned chapters from an OCD self-help book) is provided that includes the definitions of obsessions and compulsions, theories of etiology, course of illness, common coexisting disorders, and treatment. The Y-BOCS Symptom Checklist also is distributed and serves as a springboard for patients and family members to disclose their obsessive-compulsive symptoms and the behaviors that are typically hidden in shame. There is usually much relief as participants discover that other patients have had similar thoughts and experiences. Families enthusiastically compare experiences and are relieved to hear other relatives express their helplessness and decision to "just give in to keep the peace." Families discuss seemingly bizarre obsessive-compulsive symptoms in an atmosphere with little social stigma. Fears that loved ones are "going crazy" are quieted by meeting others with OCD who are "normal people."

As family members hear other people describe similar symptoms and feelings they have struggled with over many years, many begin to consider OCD a "real" disorder beyond the patient's control and begin to attend to the patient's comments with more objectivity. The notions of displaced aggression ("She's just doing it to spite me") and faulty parenting ("Was I overprotective?") can now be challenged in the multifamily context. The group often provides the first opportunity for some family members to discover the content of the patient's obsessions and the extent of compulsions or presence of mental rituals. Against this backdrop, a stress diathesis model of the pathogenesis of OCD is presented, incorporating genetic factors and familial and cultural factors pertaining to child development and parent-child interaction, family functioning, and overall levels of stress. Patients and their families often attempt to understand the patient's symptoms in psychodynamic terms because of prior therapy. Attempts to explain causation by analyzing the content of the obsessions should be pointed out as speculative and unhelpful in learning to manage the symptoms effectively. Some moments of silence are likely to occur as excitement dies down and family members try to come to terms with the illness.

Because medication often becomes the focus of conversation as patients compare notes on type, dosage, and side effects, the group must be reminded to save their questions for a later group session when a psychiatrist will be available. Some groups may express reluctance to concentrate on matters that provoke unpleasant emotional reactions by questioning the leader and others about other possible treatments for OCD. At this point, the leader can redirect group members with the comment that most people with OCD do get better by learning skills from ERP treatment, but that a complete cure is unrealistic. The leader can turn everyone's attention to selecting ERP homework challenges in a "go-round" fashion, with each patient selecting items that are relatively low on their hierarchies. Homework forms are distributed and instructions given, and the session formally ends with the therapist encouraging patients and relatives to view the first week as a practice time to begin ERP. Patients are instructed that if they do not experience any reduction in distress, they should modify the exposure challenge and work on one item until discomfort diminishes. Family members are reminded that one goal of treatment is to be involved in the OCD as little as possible, except in dangerous situations. Family members are requested to minimize their involvement without making any drastic changes in usual routines, until they learn to use behavioral contracting. The leader assigns patients to bring one or more hierarchy items to the next session for exposure practice. Further reading in a selected self-help text[28] can be assigned.

The second session begins with a review of what was accomplished in the previous session. Asking members about their thoughts, reactions, and questions provides continuity between sessions, enables members to "warm up," and conveys respect and appreciation for personal concerns. To prevent side-tracking, however, this discussion is kept brief and focused. Each patient then reports on homework completed during the week and the therapist collects homework forms, verifying that they were completed and reinforcing patients for the work. This also serves as a positive-feedback model for relatives. Patients report their level of anxiety during the exposure homework, which enables the clinician to discuss the benefits of prolonged exposure. If anxiety remains high, the therapist can comment on the patients' courage and perseverance without avoiding. When the homework is inadequately completed or reported, the therapist inquires about reasons for problems and encourages empathic confrontation to promote a corrective experience.

The majority of this second session is dedicated to a description of behavioral therapy and ERP techniques. The group leader asks members to explain what is meant by behavioral therapy, thereby assisting in the construction of a working definition. The therapist clarifies as follows: "Behavioral therapy provides tools for changing unwanted behaviors without analyzing the childhood history and meaning of the behaviors in detail." He or she then reviews the sequence of obsessions and compulsions, explaining how internal or external cues evoke obsessions, which then lead to feelings of anxiety and urges to ritualize. The techniques of direct and imagined ERP are described with examples. Patients practice by choosing an exposure homework task. Feedback and support from other group members serve to develop an optimal homework assignment. The group leader then translates the task into a form that can be rehearsed in the group, and everyone participates in this exposure challenge as described earlier for GBT. During this process, some patients benefit from observing others who are undisturbed by what for them is a very difficult task. Some discussion about the difference between observing outsiders compared with family members usually ensues, with expressions of frustration from relatives who have tried to help but have been rebuffed. This discussion often clears the air, in that patients have an opportunity to explain their difficulties and relatives receive understanding from other family members and often patients.

During in-session exposure, group members are asked to report anxiety every few minutes to illustrate the reporting requested for homework assignments. The unreasonableness of the fears, resultant anxiety, and compulsive behavior are identified by the therapist as hallmarks of OCD. Patients and relatives are encouraged to avoid "reasoning away" the obsessive concerns, because these obsessions are irrational in any case. The universal problem of reassurance seeking is identified as a ritual that is better handled with a kind refusal and redirection. Most families accept this easily, because they have experienced reassurance giving as "futile," "exhausting," and "frustrating." As patients and families experience this symptom during the session, the therapist encourages symptom identification and rehearsal of dismissal, distraction, and redirection. Patients often begin to develop better insight into both their OCD and misdirected reliance on family members to answer "the unanswerable."

At the end of the second session, the therapist instructs patients to continue the exposure from that day's session and add other homework items next on their hierarchies for practice at least 1 concentrated hour per day. When family members raise concerns about how to respond to the patient at times of intense obsessive-compulsive fears and rituals, the therapist acknowledges that all families are eager to have these dilemmas solved and that they will address these questions specifically at the next session. Families are encouraged to use what they have learned thus far to modify their responses and limit involvement in rituals, while communicating an appreciation of the patient's struggle.

For the third session, the group begins as usual with each patient reporting on homework task results. The members engage in troubleshooting for problems experienced in completing the ERP and homework forms. Frustrated patients can be encouraged with comments about progress to date and the need to be patient. As previously described for GBT, a brief videotaped lecture on the neurobiology of OCD is presented. Following the discussion of this tape, the therapist again asks patients to select exposure items with a discomfort level of approximately 50 to 60 SUDS. For example, for those patients with contamination fears, patients and family members take out an object to hold and touch the object or their "contaminated" hands directly to their face, hair, and clothing. Contact with the contaminant is continuous, and "spreading" of contamination is repeated every few minutes throughout the session, immediately prior to inquiring about the patient's discomfort level. During this time, family members also participate to provide a normative consensus. After approximately 1 hour of *in vivo* or imaginal exposure, the group's attention is shifted to "Guidelines for Living with OCD" in Van Noppen, et al's[56] *Learning to Live with OCD*. These guidelines are:

1. Recognize the signals that indicate a person is having problems.
2. Modify expectations during stressful times.
3. Measure progress according to the person's level of functioning.
4. Don't make day-to-day comparisons.
5. Give recognition for "small" improvements.
6. Create a strong, supportive home environment.
7. Keep communication clear and simple.
8. Stick to a behavioral contract.
9. Set limits, yet be sensitive to the person's mood.
10. Keep your family routine "normal."
11. Use humor.
12. Support the person's medication regimen.
13. Make separate time for other family members.
14. Be flexible!

As group members read aloud from sections of this booklet, the therapist asks families which reaction patterns best describe them. This promotes insight into family response patterns and the impact of these responses on the patient. For some, the accommodating pattern fits most closely, whereas others identify themselves as more frustrated and rejecting. Others oscillate between these, especially at times of frustration, sometimes leading to screaming fights over obsessive-compulsive symptoms. Other family members may respond to these family stories by noting how difficult it is to be consistent and to follow through on "threats." Patients are asked to reassess their behavioral homework task with the Family Guidelines in mind and to add other challenges if feasible. As patients and relatives become aware of the senselessness of their previous behaviors, they begin to make commitments to correct these patterns. Often, other family members remind relatives not to blame themselves for past mistakes, because they did not know what else to do at that time. Now with education and some tools, there is hope.

The first three sessions have provided patients and families with a clearer understanding of OCD. Next, they must learn how to cope more productively with obsessive-compulsive symptoms as a family using cognitive and behavioral techniques. This fourth session trains families in behavioral family contracting, which promotes family collaboration in subsequent sessions toward the joint goal of reducing OCD symptoms. As usual, each patient reports on homework during the week, with family members commenting on their role or observations. The therapists introduce behavioral contracting by asking the group what they believe this means. This leads gradually to a working definition that includes several components.

Each family identifies problem areas that result from demands of obsessive-compulsive symptoms. Examples are the imposition caused by OCD on others, family participation in rituals, excessive criticism of the patient, and assumption by family members of the patient's roles and responsibilities. The family's problems are defined in clear, behavioral terms. The group leader helps the family focus on and define one problem area for work. Using feedback from the group, family members explore behavioral response options and the possible consequences of each. Family members select the best response options. The leader facilitates a negotiation process between family members. This process consists of direct discussion of behavioral expectations among family members, using group suggestions and feedback. At this point, the family agrees on a contract that establishes the behavior therapy goal for the patient and the behavioral responses for family members. With the assistance of the group, the family assesses whether the solution is reasonable. If possible, the family rehearses the behavioral contract during the treatment session. The group evaluates the contract, adding suggestions based on observations of the family's ability to carry out the plan. If necessary, the family negotiates any modifications in the planned contract before moving on to the next family. All assignments are written on homework forms and contracts are recorded in writing.

The therapist suggests to family members that it is often useful to remind the patient that this agreement was made together, and it was everyone's responsibility to carry it out. However, although the contracts were meant to provide expectable guidelines for behavior in any given situation, they should be amenable to renegotiation and modification as needed. All families leave the session with a behavioral contract to practice and homework forms to record their progress. In a similar fashion as in the proceeding sessions, each patient commits to individual exposure homework and the family contract.

Several concepts are critical to effective behavioral contracting. Realistic expectations on the part of patient and family must be clearly defined. The family learns how to be supportive in ways that are therapeutic to the patient. The patient is given responsibility for therapy, which enhances his or her sense of control, motivation, and confidence. The limits of family members' responsibilities are clarified and family members are directed to refocus their attention on their own lives. Family group members are particularly useful in moderating the negotiations to decrease emotional tension between family members, encourage objective feedback during the behavioral task negotiation, and encourage clear and direct communication.

Later sessions of the MFBT group are devoted to reporting on homework and contracting outcomes, *in vivo* and imaginal ERP, practice in family contracting, self-monitoring distress levels, and homework planning. Family responses to OCD are discussed in greater detail, and greater disclosure about symptoms emerges. Group interaction becomes more intimate as families describe interpersonal conflicts that impede their attempts to manage obsessive-compulsive symptoms.

Families require support from the therapist and group members in their efforts "to help." Because many are unskilled at negotiating a family plan with the patient's consent, some well-intended family responses are likely to backfire, leaving patients feeling powerless. We have observed that some patients who complain about not having enough guidance or who try to push the group too quickly to contracting are often the ones who avoid committing themselves to a task when given the opportunity. These patients can consume considerable session time and must be politely confronted about their behavior and given permission to pass or to work on an exposure challenge of their own without family involvement. Thus, the decision to change is placed on the patient. The group coaches families to accept that they cannot force the patient to participate in treatment unless they are able to impose consequences that the family is prepared to carry out. The exposure homework must be the patient's choice. However, when a chosen task does not appear to be sufficiently challenging, the therapist can use group feedback to encourage a more meaningful one. In cases of parents and adolescent children with OCD, group members can prove instrumental in helping the adolescent accept family limits as reasonable and helping parents limit their interference, thereby allowing the teenager to engage in independent responsible behavior.

In each session, the therapist allows families to choose who would like to initiate the contracting. Cross-family modeling of behavioral contracts appears to be an important therapeutic factor in MFBT. Most family members are concerned about how much they should push the patient. Because applying force or ultimatums in the midst of rituals usually leads to more conflict and possible physical violence, families are advised to encourage resistance and discourage avoidance as previously agreed with the patient, but to "back off" if the patient's tension continues to mount. Rarely have we encountered the need for crisis intervention in or outside of sessions, although this remains a possibility for some patients and families.

As each family proceeds through behavioral contracting, each successive family incorporates what they have observed from the previous family. Through constant reevaluation of the behavioral contract outcome, families and patients become skillful at problem solving and decision making to cope with the "demands" of OCD. Another by-product of behavioral contracting is the clarification of roles. Throughout the later sessions, independently initiated ERP challenges and behavioral contracts occur with less therapist involvement. As such events occur, the therapist points out such successes to the group, stressing the importance of self-instruction and patients' and families' ability to use the techniques on their own. By session 11, the therapist ensures that each family has had an opportunity to review gains made and symptoms that require further work. As in GBT, patients' fears that they will be unable to maintain their improvement once the group ends are addressed by highlighting symptomatic improvement in OCD symptoms and increases in understanding gained through the MFBT. At this time, the therapist also reminds group members that monthly follow-up sessions will be scheduled to consolidate treatment gains. The therapist emphasizes that if patients anticipate stressors that might increase OCD symptoms (e.g., childbirth, job change, etc.), troubleshooting and preventative planning will be needed.

The twelfth and last weekly session begins as usual with review of homework, practice of ERP, and family behavioral contracting. As for GBT, the therapist addresses feelings of sadness and loss as part of ending the group and seeks to end on an optimistic note, with goals to be reported at the first monthly MFBT session. Six monthly sessions follow, using a format similar to weekly sessions: reviewing current symptom status, troubleshooting problem areas, and formulating monthly goals and strategies.

SUMMARY

Clinical research clearly has demonstrated that behavioral treatment by ERP is effective in reducing OCD symptoms. Yet, a large number of patients refuse or drop out of treatment, remain symptomatic following treatment, or experience loss of benefits once therapy has ended. In addition, the cost of providing individual behavioral treatment can be high. Individual and family treatments offered in group modalities offer promising alternatives to labor-intensive individual behavioral treatment. We have described in detail our 12-session groups, which meet weekly and include psychoeducation, exposure with modeling and response prevention, and homework assignments. Six monthly sessions follow the active phase of behavioral treatment to help consolidate gains and encourage independent problem solving regarding obsessive-compulsive symptoms.

Our clinical experience and recent research findings suggest that MFBT offers hope for patients who have not benefitted from standard individual behavior treatment for OCD and who are living with family members. Family members commonly participate in the symptoms of the OCD sufferer in some fashion, often in countertherapeutic ways. Multifamily GBT incorporates family members into behavioral treatment by examining family accommodation and teaching them and the OCD sufferer to negotiate contracts. The goal of this treatment is to encourage exposure and elimination of rituals to reduce anxiety, to provide education about family interaction and train families to contract with each other to reduce OCD symptoms, and to reduce family members' involvement in the patient's OCD. Such efforts can enable patients to consolidate their gains by establishing an environment that is supportive and firm, without being punitive or overly indulgent. Further study of both GBT and MFBT is warranted, because only one controlled trial of group treatment has been conducted for

OCD to date, and MFBT has not yet been studied in a controlled manner.

REFERENCES

1. Christensen H, Hadzi-Pavlovic D, Andrews G, Mattick R: Behavior therapy and tricyclic medication in the treatment of obsessive-compulsive disorder: A quantitative review, *J Consult Clin Psychol* 55:701–711, 1987.
2. Steketee G, Lam J: Obsessive compulsive disorder. In Giles TR, editor: *Handbook of effective psychotherapy: A comparative outcome approach*, New York, 1993, Plenum.
3. Foa EB, Steketee G, Grayson J, et al: Deliberate exposure and blocking of obsessive-compulsive rituals: Immediate and long term effects, *Behav Ther* 15:450–472, 1984.
4. Van Noppen B, Steketee G, Pato M: Group and multifamily behavioral treatments for OCD. In Hollander E, Stein OJ, editors: *Obsessive compulsive disorders: Diagnosis, etiology, treatment*, New York, 1997, Marcel Dekker.
5. Steketee G, Grayson JB, Foa EB: A comparison of characteristics of obsessive-compulsive disorder and other anxiety disorders, *J Anx Dis* 1:325–335, 1987.
6. Ingram IM: Obsessional illness in mental hospital patients, *J Ment Sci* 107:382–402.
7. Khanna S, Rajendra PN, Channabasavanna SM: Sociodemographic variables in obsessive compulsive disorder in India, *Int J Soc Psychiatry* 32:47–54, 1986.
8. Lo WH: A follow-up study of obsessional neurotics in Hong Kong Chinese, *Br J Psychiatry* 113:823–832, 1967.
9. US Bureau of Census, 1996.
10. Eisen J, Steketee G: Course of illness of OCD. In Dickstein LJ, Riba MB, Oldhan JM, editors: *Annual review of psychiatry*, vol 16, Washington, 1997, American Psychiatric Press.
11. Yalom ID: *The theory and practice of group psychotherapy,* New York, 1985, Basic Books.
12. Budman S, editor: *Forms of brief therapy,* New York, 1981, Guilford.
13. Telch MJ, Lucas JA, Schmidt NB, et al: Group cognitive behavioral treatment of panic disorder, *Behav Res Ther* 31:279–288, 1993.
14. Heimberg RG, Becker RE, Goldfinger K, Vermilyea JA: Treatment of social phobia by exposure, cognitive restructuring and homework assignments, *J Nerv Ment Dis* 173:236–245, 1985.
15. Hand I, Tichatzky M: Behavioral group therapy for obsessions and compulsions: First results of a pilot study. In Sjoden PO, Bates D, Dockens WS, editors: *Trends in behavior therapy*, New York, 1979, Academic Press, pp 269–297.
16. Epsie CA: The group treatment of obsessive-compulsive ritualizers: Behavioral management of identified patterns of relapse, *Behav Psychother* 14:21–33, 1986.
17. Taylor CJ, Sholomskas DE: *Group exposure and response prevention for OCD.* The annual meeting of the Anxiety Disorders Association of America, March 1993, Santa Monica, California.
18. Enright SJ: Group treatment for obsessive-compulsive disorder: An evaluation, *Behav Psychother* 19:183–192, 1991.
19. Krone KP, Himle JA, Nesse RM: A standardized behavioral group treatment pro-

gram for obsessive-compulsive disorder: Preliminary outcomes, *Behav Res Ther* 29:627–632, 1991.

20. Goodman WK, Price LH, Rasmussen SA: The Yale-Brown Obsessive Compulsive Scale. I. Development, use, and reliability, *Arch Gen Psychiatry* 46:1006–1011, 1989.

21. Van Noppen B, Pato MT, Marsland R, Rasmussen S: *Family function and family group treatment.* Paper presented at the American Psychiatric Association, May 1993, San Francisco, California.

22. Van Noppen B, Steketee G, McCorkle BH, Pato M: Group and multifamily behavioral treatment for obsessive compulsive disorder: A pilot study, *J Anx Dis* 11: 431–446, 1997.

23. Jacobson NS, Truax P: Clinical significance: A statistical approach to defining meaningful change in psychotherapy research, *J Consult Clin Psychol* 59:12–19, 1991.

24. Fals-Stewart W, Marks AP, Schafer J: A comparison of behavioral group therapy and individual behavior therapy in treating obsessive-compulsive disorder, *J Nerv Ment Dis* 181:189–193, 1993.

25. Steketee G, Chambless DL: Progress report for NIMH grant #44190, "Expressed Emotion in Anxiety Disorders," unpublished manuscript, 1994.

26. Kobak KA, Rock AL, Greist JH: Group behavior therapy for obsessive-compulsive disorder, *J Special Group Work* 20:26–32, 1995.

27. Van Noppen B, Steketee G: Individual group and multifamily cognitive behavioral treatment for OCD. In Pato M, Zohar J, editors: *Current treatments in OCD,* ed 2, Washington DC, in press, Psychiatric Press.

28. Steketee G, White K: *When once is not enough,* Oakland, 1990, New Harbinger.

29. Rachman S, Marks IM, Hodgson R: The treatment of obsessive-compulsive neurotics by modeling and flooding in vivo, *Behav Res Ther* 11:463–471, 1973.

30. Calvocoressi L, Lewis B, Harris M, et al: Family accommodation in obsessive-compulsive disorder, *Am J Psychiatry* 152:441–443, 1995.

31. Shafran R, Ralph J, Tallis F: Obsessive-compulsive symptoms and the family, *Bull Menninger Clin* 59:472–479, 1995.

32. Livingston-Van Noppen B, Rasmussen SA, Eisen J, McCartney L: Family function and treatment in obsessive-compulsive disorder. In Jenike M, Baer L, Minichiello WE, editor: *Obsessive-compulsive disorder: Theory and management,* St. Louis, 1990, Mosby–YearBook, pp 325–340.

33. Tynes LL, Salins C, Winstead DK: Obsessive compulsive patients: Familial frustration and criticism, *J Louisiana State Med Soc* 24–29, October 1990.

34. Hibbs ED, Hamburger SD, Lenane M, et al: Determinants of expressed emotion in families of disturbed and normal children, *J Psychol Psychiatry* 32:757–770, 1991.

35. Hibbs ED, Hamburger SD, Kruesi MJP, Lenane M: Factors affecting expressed emotion in parents of ill and normal children, *Am J Orthopsychiatry* 63:103–112, 1993.

36. Steketee G, Pruyn N: Family functioning in OCD. In Swinson RP, Antony MM, Rachman S, Richter MA, editors: *Obsessive compulsive disorder: Theory, research and treatment,* New York, in print, Guilford.

37. Riggs DS, Hiss H, Foa EB: Marital distress and the treatment of obsessive compulsive disorder. *Behav Ther* 23:585–597, 1992.

38. Hafner RJ: Marital interaction in persisting obsessive-compulsive disorders, *Austr New Z J Psychiatry* 16:171–178, 1982.

39. Hafner RJ, Gilchrist P, Bowling J, Kalucy R: The treatment of obsessional neurosis in a family setting, *Austr New Z J Psychiatry* 15:145–151, 1981.

40. Hoover CF, Insel T: Families of origin in obsessive-compulsive disorder, *J Nerv Ment Dis* 172:223–228, 1984.

41. Emmelkamp PMG, de Haan E, Hoogduin CAL: Marital adjustment and obsessive-compulsive disorder, *Br J Psychiatry* 156:55–60, 1990.

42. Cobb J, McDonald R, Marks I, Stern R: Marital versus exposure therapy: Psychological treatment of co-existing marital and phobic-obsessive problems, *Behav Anal Mod* 4:3–16, 1980.

43. Steketee G: Social support and treatment outcome of obsessive compulsive disorder at 9-month follow-up, *Behav Psychother* 21:81–95, 1993a.

44. Emmelkamp PMG, Kloek J, Blaauw E: Obsessive-compulsive disorders in principles and practice of relapse prevention. In Wilson PH, editor: *Principles and practice of relapse prevention*, New York, 1992, Guilford, pp 213–234.

45. Marks IM, Hodgson R, Rachman S: Treatment of chronic obsessive-compulsive neurosis by in-vivo exposure: A two-year follow-up and issues in treatment, *Br J Psychiatry* 127:349–364, 1975.

46. Black DW, Blum NS: Obsessive-compulsive disorder support groups: The Iowa model, *Comp Psychiatry* 33:65–71, 1992.

47. Cooper M: A group for families of obsessive-compulsive persons, *Fam Soc J Contemp Hum Serv* 301–307, May 1993.

48. Tynes LL, Salins C, Skiba W, Winstead DK: A psycho-educational and support group for obsessive-compulsive disorder patients and their significant others, *Comp Psychiatry* 33:197–201, 1992.

49. Hafner RJ: Anxiety disorders and family therapy, *Austr New Z J Fam Ther* 13:99–104, 1992.

50. Dalton P: Family treatment of an obsessive-compulsive child: A case report, *Fam Proc* 22:99–108, 1983.

51. Fine S: Family therapy: A behavioral approach to childhood obsessive compulsive neurosis, *Arch Gen Psychiatry* 28:695–697, 1973.

52. March JS, Mulle K, Herbel B: Behavioral psychotherapy for children and adolescents with obsessive-compulsive disorder: An open trial of a new protocol-driven treatment package, *J Am Acad Child Adolesc Psychiatry* 33:333–341, 1994.

53. Thornicroft G, Colson L, Marks IM: An inpatient behavioural psychotherapy unit description and audit, *Br J Psychiatry* 158:362–367, 1991.

54. Emmelkamp PMG, DeLange I: Spouse involvement in the treatment of obsessive-compulsive patients, *Behav Res Ther* 21:341–346, 1983.

55. Mehta M: A comparative study of family-based and patient-based behavioral management in obsessive-compulsive disorder, *Br J Psychiatry* 157:133–135, 1990.

56. Van Noppen B, Pato M, Rasmussen S: *Learning to live with OCD*, Milford, 1993, Obsessive Compulsive Foundation.

22

Drug Treatment of Obsessive-Compulsive Disorders

Michael A. Jenike, M.D.

We now have medications that have been well studied in adequately designed, controlled trials that predictably help more than half of obsessive-compulsive disorder (OCD) patients (Table 22-1). When sequential trials of these medications are given to individual patients, as many as 90% eventually have a clinically meaningful response. An important consideration, however, is the extent of change to be expected with effective pharmacotherapy for OCD: unlike affective disorders, OCD tends to respond to medication only partially, typically with a 30% to 60% symptom reduction, with patients tending to remain chronically symptomatic to some degree despite the best of pharmacologic interventions.[1] Nonetheless, patients usually experience this degree of improvement as quite significant. It is important to give a trial of behavior therapy to OCD patients who have improved with drug treatments, to maximize their potential for recovery and return to a normal lifestyle (see Chapters 17 and 19). For most patients, the combination of pharmacotherapy and behavior therapy represents optimal treatment.

The gold standard for the evaluation of a drug treatment is the double-blind, placebo-controlled trial. In such trials, patients are given either the active drug or an identically-appearing placebo so that neither the patient nor the investigator (hence "double-blind") knows whether the patient is taking active drug or placebo until the end of the experiment. Expectations and desires of both the clinician and patient are unable to influence the outcome of such a study, because it is expected that the placebo and active drug groups are affected equally, thus cancelling out such effects.

This type of randomized, prospective, placebo-controlled trial, which proved so useful in depression research, had been almost impossible to conduct until the last decade because of the small numbers of OCD patients available to any

Table 22-1 Typical Dosages of Medications Commonly Used to Treat
Obsessive-Compulsive Disorder*

Drug	Lowest Effective Dose (mg)	Typical High Dose (mg)
Fluoxetine (Prozac)	40	80
Clomipramine (Anafranil)	Unclear	250
Sertraline (Zoloft)	Unclear	200
Paroxetine (Paxil)	40	60
Fluvoxamine (Luvox)	Unclear	300

* These are recommended dosages based on results of multicenter controlled trials. In occasional individuals, very low dosages (i.e., 5 mg Prozac per day) are effective even if high dosages do not help.

one researcher. Now with a number of specialized clinics, large-scale trials are feasible. As the pharmaceutical industry realized the potential market for effective antiobsessional agents, companies invested millions of dollars in multicenter, placebo-controlled, double-blind trials of agents that are now on the United States market, including fluvoxamine (Luvox), sertraline (Zoloft), paroxetine (Paxil), fluoxetine (Prozac), and clomipramine (Anafranil).

A recent literature search[2] identified 28 controlled trials of medication for the treatment of OCD in adults (Tables 22-2, 22-3) and six such trials involving children and adolescents with OCD (Table 22-4). Of these trials, nine compared clomipramine to placebo and involved approximately 600 adults and 75 children or adolescents, making clomipramine the most extensively studied medication for the treatment of OCD. There also were four controlled trials comparing fluvoxamine with placebo involving approximately 260 patients. Two controlled trials, involving more than 400 subjects, compared sertraline with placebo, and two others compared various dosages of fluoxetine with placebo in 572 subjects. All of these trials demonstrated statistically and clinically significant improvements with the active drug compared with placebo. Improvements among individual patients ranged from an occasional complete cure to no effect whatsoever. For example, the Ciba-Geigy–sponsored multicenter trials of clomipramine reported that approximately 85% of patients taking clomipramine demonstrated some improvement, whereas fewer than 5% of patients taking placebo improved. Approximately 58% of the subjects who received clomipramine improved at least moderately. The mean decrease in symptoms of the patients receiving clomipramine was approximately 40% compared with 5% or less in those patients receiving placebo.

In addition to the previous studies that compared an active drug with placebo, there are a number of studies that compared two or more drugs head to head without a placebo (Table 22-3). Clomipramine and other serotonin reuptake inhibitors (SRIs) often have been compared in a controlled manner with

Table 22-2   Placebo-Controlled Trials of Drug Therapy for Obsessive-Compulsive Disorder—Adults

Study	Patients (n)	Drug Comparison	Comments
Clomipramine Collaborative Study Group	239	Clomipramine vs placebo	38% average decrease in symptoms with Clomipramine 3% average decrease in symptoms with placebo
Clomipramine Collaborative Study Group	281	Clomipramine vs placebo	44% average decrease in symptoms with Clomipramine 5% average decrease in symptoms with placebo
Greist et al, 1990*	32	Clomipramine vs placebo	73% of patients improved with clomipramine 6% of patients improved with placebo
Montgomery, 1980	14	Clomipramine vs placebo crossover	Clomipramine significantly better than placebo
Thoren et al, 1980	24	Clomipramine vs nortriptyline vs placebo	Clomipramine but not nortriptyline significantly superior to placebo
Jenike et al, 1989*	27	Clomipramine vs placebo	Clomipramine significantly better than placebo
Mavissakalian et al, 1985	12	Clomipramine (n = 7) vs placebo (n = 5)	Clomipramine significantly better than placebo
Karabanow, 1977	20	Clomipramine vs placebo	Clomipramine significantly superior to placebo
Greist et al, 1992	325	Sertraline vs placebo	Sertraline significantly superior to placebo
Chouinard et al, 1990	87	Sertraline vs placebo	Sertraline significantly superior to placebo
Jenike et al, 1990a**	19	Sertraline (n = 10) vs placebo (n = 9)	Sertraline was not significantly better than placebo (low power to detect a difference)
Goodman et al, 1989	42	Fluvoxamine vs placebo	Fluvoxamine significantly better than placebo
Jenike et al, 1990	38	Fluvoxamine vs placebo	Fluvoxamine significantly better than placebo
Perse et al, 1987	16	Fluvoxamine vs placebo	Fluvoxamine significantly better than placebo
Tollefson et al, 1994	355	Fluoxetine vs placebo	Fluoxetine (20, 40, 60 mg) significantly better than placebo
Montgomery et al, 1993	217	Fluoxetine vs placebo	Fluoxetine (40, 60 mg) significantly better than placebo Fluoxetine (20 mg) effects equal to placebo
Goodman et al, 1996	160	Fluvoxamine vs placebo	Fluvoxamine significantly better than placebo
Wheadon et al, 1993	348	Paroxetine vs placebo	Paroxetine (40, 60 mg) significantly better than placebo Paroxetine (20 mg) effects equal to placebo

* Included under "The Clomipramine Collaborative Study Group, 1992" report above.
** Included under "Chouinard et al, 1990" report above.

Table 22-3 Nonplacebo Controlled Trials of Drug Therapy for Obsessive-Compulsive Disorder—Adults

Study	Patients (n)	Drug Comparison	Results
Zhao, 1991	39	Clomipramine (n = 21) vs amitriptyline (n = 18)	95% of patients improved with clomipramine 56% of patients improved with amitriptyline (p < 0.01)
Pigott et al, 1990	11	Clomipramine vs fluoxetine	Comparable efficacy
Den Boer et al, 1987	6	Clomipramine vs fluvoxamine	Comparable efficacy
Cui, 1986	32	Clomipramine (n = 18) vs doxepin (n = 14)	78% of patients markedly improved with clomipramine 36% of patients markedly improved with doxepin
Lei, 1986	12	Crossover study of clomipramine vs imipramine	Clomipramine superior to imipramine (no data given in English abstract)
Volavka et al, 1985	16	Clomipramine (n = 8) vs imipramine (n = 8)	Clomipramine superior to imipramine
Zahn et al, 1984	12	Clomipramine vs clorgyline	Clomipramine superior to clorgyline
Insel et al, 1983	13	Clomipramine vs clorgyline	Clomipramine effective; clorgyline ineffective
Ananth et al, 1981	20	Clomipramine vs amitriptyline	Clomipramine significantly superior to amitriptyline
Goodman et al, 1990	40	Fluvoxamine (n = 21) vs desipramine (n = 19)	Fluvoxamine significantly better than desipramine
Freeman et al, 1994	66	Fluvoxamine vs clomipramine	Comparable efficacy
Bisserbe et al, 1995	168	Sertraline vs clomipramine	Comparable efficacy (fewer dropouts with sertraline)

Table 22-4 Controlled Trials of Drug Therapy for Obsessive-Compulsive Disorder—Children and Adolescents

Study	Patients (n)	Comparison	Results
DeVeaugh-Geiss et al, 1992	61 children and adolescents	Clomipramine vs placebo	37% average decrease in symptoms with Clomipramine 8% average decrease in symptoms with placebo
Flament et al, 1985 and 1985a	14 children	Clomipramine vs placebo crossover	Clomipramine significantly better than placebo
Rapoport et al, 1980	8 adolescents	Clomipramine vs desipramine vs placebo crossover	No significant difference between groups (but very low statistical power to detect a difference)
Leonard et al, 1991	26	Clomipramine substituted with desipramine in half of subjects	89% of patients receiving desipramine relapsed 18% of patients remaining on clomipramine relapsed
Leonard et al, 1988	48	Clomipramine vs desipramine	Clomipramine superior to desipramine 64% of patients relapsed when desipramine substituted for clomipramine
Riddle et al, 1992	14 children	Fluoxetine (n = 7) vs placebo (n = 7)	Fluoxetine significantly better than placebo

other antidepressant agents such as desipramine (three studies with 82 patients); imipramine (one study with 16 subjects); nortriptyline (one study with 24 subjects); amitriptyline (two studies with 59 subjects); clorgyline (two studies with 25 subjects); and doxepin (one study with 32 subjects). In each case, the drug that fell into the category of an SRI (e.g., clomipramine, fluvoxamine, fluoxetine, sertraline) was significantly better than the agent that was not in this category (e.g., desipramine, imipramine, clorgyline). Other controlled trials have compared two SRIs, for example, clomipramine with fluoxetine (one study with 11 subjects) and clomipramine with fluvoxamine (one study with six subjects). None of these studies found significant differences between SRIs in terms of efficacy. This finding may be the result of small numbers of subjects in these studies.

The Appendix to this chapter includes a drug pamphlet that was commissioned by the Obsessive-Compulsive Foundation that can be given to patients to answer common questions about OCD and specifically about medication treatments. Some topics include: What kinds of medications may help OCD? Do all antidepressants help OCD symptoms? How do we know these drugs are effective? Why do these drugs help? At what dosages are these drugs used? Are there side effects? Do antiobsessional medications cause long-term, irreversible side effects? What if I am afraid to take medications because of my obsessional fears about drugs? Can I get the drugs if I am poor? How long does it take antiobsessional medications to work? How helpful can I expect these medications to be? What about augmenting one drug with another? Will I have to take antiobsessional medications forever?

ANTIDEPRESSANT AND ANTIOBESSIONAL DRUGS

The main pharmacologic treatments for OCD involve the antidepressant drugs, especially those drugs with prominent serotonergic properties.[3,4] Terminology used for these drugs can be confusing. Anafranil is generally referred to as an serotonin reuptake inhibitor (SRI), whereas the other commonly used antiobsessional drugs such as Prozac, Sertraline, Luvox, and Paxil, are called *selective* serotonergic reuptake inhibitors (SSRIs), because they primarily have effects on serotonin, whereas Anafranil affects other neurotransmitter systems as well.

In addition to offering effective treatment for depressed OCD patients, these agents are useful for OCD patients who are not clinically depressed. Because a link between depression and OCD is frequently noted,[5–10] it is not surprising that antidepressants have been used extensively in this disorder. Case reports have suggested the occasional usefulness of almost all antidepressants in the treatment of patients with OCD (imipramine;[11–14] amitriptyline;[13,15] doxepin;[16,17] desipramine;[18] zimelidine;[19] fluoxetine;[20] trazodone;[21–23] fluvoxamine;[24] and citalopram).[25] All of these reports, however, involved a small number of cases without any controls. Responses were unpredictable and not clearly related to depression; there was, however, dramatic improvement in some cases.

As previously noted, there are now many carefully controlled trials demonstrating that some antidepressants are very effective agents, whereas others are ineffective in the treatment of patients with OCD. For example, in a placebo-controlled trial involving 37 patients Foa and colleagues[26,27] showed that imipramine reduced *depressive* symptoms in OCD patients, but that the drug did not specifically affect *OCD* symptoms in either depressed or nondepressed OCD patients.

Each of the main drugs reported to be helpful for OCD will be reviewed. First, agents that have been studied with more than one double-blind, placebo-controlled trial will be discussed, followed by agents that have been studied in a less rigorous manner. Toward the end of this chapter (see Table 22-6), an approach to the individual patient will be outlined that evaluates recommendations suggested by the wealth of data about drug treatment of OCD, which has accumulated over the past few decades.

WELL-STUDIED DRUGS

Clomipramine

There is much literature that details clomipramine (Anafranil)—a tricyclic antidepressant—as an effective treatment for OCD. Early anecdotal studies indicated that this drug might have specific antiobsessional properties apart from its antidepressant qualities.[28-42] A number of carefully controlled studies have confirmed that clomipramine is indeed superior to placebo in the treatment of OCD.[43-51]

Lopez-Ibor[28] gave clomipramine intravenously to 16 OCD patients and reported improvement over 2 to 5 days in 13 of the patients. Other experts reported similar findings.[29-35] Following these successes, other researchers attempted uncontrolled trials with oral clomipramine and reported mixed results. Some experts reported little improvement,[52] whereas others reported a good response.[36-38] Wyndowe and colleagues[39] noted that improvement in obsessions greatly exceeded improvement in anxiety, depression, and phobias, and Capstick[40] found that good results correlated with intravenous (IV) use of the drug, young age of the patient, presence of associated phobias, and presence of obsessions before the development of depression.

In a 4-week, randomized, double-blind trial, Ananth, et al[41] compared the efficacy of clomipramine with that of amitriptyline in 20 patients with severe OCD. Clomipramine, but not amitriptyline, produced statistically significant improvement in obsessive symptoms, depression, and anxiety. These researchers theorized that the lack of significant effect of amitriptyline on anxiety and depression may have been caused by the drug's inability to improve the primary obsessive symptoms, and that clomipramine has specific antiobsessional properties superior to those of amitriptyline.

Stroebel, et al[42] studied the effects of oral clomipramine (maximum dose, 300 mg/day) on obsessive symptoms in an open trial of 50 patients with various diagnoses and found that the overall success rate (reduction in obsessive symptoms) was 60% (30 patients). Of 15 patients with a primary diagnosis of OCD, 12 (80%) improved, whereas only 7 (41%) of 17 schizophrenic patients showed improvement. Patients who improved when taking clomipramine had a significantly higher depression scale score on the Minnesota Multiphasic Personality Inventory (MMPI) as compared with nonresponders. Patients generally began to show improvement 2 to 4 weeks after initiation of treatment and often continued to improve for up to 3 or 4 months. In only five patients, however, was there a complete remission of obsessive-compulsive symptoms. More often, the symptoms were greatly reduced; patients reported that ritualistic behavior could be resisted and obsessions mitigated. Twenty-five (83%) of the 30 successfully treated patients had previously been treated with adequate doses of other antidepressants for an average of 10 months without improvement in obsessive-compulsive symptoms, despite improvement in depression. These findings indicated that clomipramine may have a beneficial effect in the treatment of obsessive-compulsive symptomatology, regardless of the presence of other psychopathology. Unfortunately, the diagnostic criteria were not outlined in this report, and it has been documented that severe obsessive-compulsive patients are frequently mislabelled as schizophrenic.[53]

Thoren, et al[43,44] compared treatment with 150 mg of clomipramine (a fairly low dose) with 150 mg of nortriptyline and with placebo. Twenty-four patients were distributed among the three groups. Even with this relatively small sample size, a significant change was noted on an obsessive-compulsive subscale derived from the Comprehensive Psychiatric Rating Scale[55] (see Chapter 6). On this scale, 42% (10 of 24) of the clomipramine group showed improvement, 21% (5 of 24) of the nortriptyline group showed improvement, and the placebo group showed no change. The clomipramine-placebo difference was statistically significant. After a 5-week, double-blind trial, 22 of the patients were given an open trial of clomipramine and behavior therapy during which 11 (50%) of the patients improved, including three patients who failed to respond to nortriptyline. Interestingly, two of the patients who improved decided to stop taking the drug, preferring their symptoms to the demands of an asymptomatic state. This study suggested a substantial clomipramine effect; however, clomipramine did not produce improvement as measured on either the Leyton Obsessional Inventory[56] (see Chapter 6)—a standard scale for evaluating the severity of obsessional symptoms—or on social functioning scales.

Thoren, et al,[44] in an attempt to obtain a neurochemical correlate to clinical improvement of symptoms, measured spinal fluid concentration of monoamine metabolites before and during treatment with clomipramine, nortriptyline, and placebo in their OCD patients. It is well documented that when a monoamine reuptake inhibitor is given, the turnover of the respective amine is changed and this is reflected in a *decreased* concentration of its metabolite in the spinal fluid.[52] Nortriptyline, for example, is a preferential inhibitor of synaptic norepinephrine reuptake and produces a reduction of the norepinephrine metabolite 4-hydroxy-3-methoxyphenylglycol (MHPG) in the spinal fluid.[58] Zimelidine, a relatively selective serotonin reuptake blocker, causes a lowering of the spinal fluid level of the serotonin metabolite 5-hydroxyindoleacetic acid (5-HIAA).[59] Clomipramine was initially believed to be a pure SRI and because of its success in many patients, the so-called serotonin theory of OCD was developed (see Chapters 11 and 12). We now know that clomipramine is not a pure SRI and that its main metabolite, desmethylclomipramine, is a potent inhibitor of norepinephrine reuptake.[60] The plasma concentrations of the metabolite are almost always higher than those of the parent compound after oral administration.[57] In the study by Thoren, et al,[44] nortriptyline produced the predicted reduction in MHPG, clomipramine reduced both MHPG and 5-HIAA, and placebo treatment did not change the concentration of either metabolite. The change in 5-HIAA, but not that in MHPG, appeared to be important for the treatment outcome; there was a significant correlation between reduction in spinal 5-HIAA and effect on the two central OCD symptoms—rituals—and obsessive thoughts. Greater symptom reduction with clomipramine in the OCD patients was associated with a more pronounced lowering of 5-HIAA. This was in contrast to the pattern described in endogenous depression, where amelioration during clomipramine treatment has been found to be correlated with MHPG reduction, but not with 5-HIAA reduction.[60]

Marks, et al[45] later compared clomipramine with placebo in 47 outpatients and found modest yet significant improvement in self-rating scales, but no change in observer ratings in the clomipramine group after a 4-week study period. In this controlled study, all patients were admitted to the hospital for behavior therapy after the initial 4-week evaluations, with active drug or placebo continued. After intensive behavior therapy, all ratings of compulsions and mood showed significantly greater improvement for patients taking clomipramine than patients taking placebo. In those patients who were not depressed prior to the study, however, the investigators were unable to show any benefit of clomipramine over placebo; they concluded that clomipramine was useful only in OCD patients with concomitant depressed mood. Because there was no objective improvement in either placebo or active drug group before both groups entered behavior therapy, these results cannot be generalized to the drug-treatment-only situation. Marks and others had earlier shown that behavior therapy alone is a powerful and effective treatment of OCD (see Chapters 17, 19 and 20); however, this study neither proved nor disproved that longer treatment with clomipramine alone would yield improvement.[45]

Other carefully controlled, double-blind studies using clomipramine have been published,[46–51] which concur that clomipramine is more effective than placebo in reducing obsessional symptoms. In one of these studies, clomipramine was more effective than the monoamine oxidase inhibitor (MAOI) clorgyline;[48] and in another, clomipramine was possibly more effective than the tricyclic antidepressant amitriptyline.[41] In the above studies, clomipramine helped patients who had only obsessive thoughts and those with rituals.

One group studied the relationship between plasma levels of clomipramine and desmethylclomipramine and clinical response in obsessive-compulsive patients.[61] In general, the patient response was best in the middle range of plasma concentrations, demonstrating a therapeutic window or inverted U-curve, as has been well demonstrated with nortriptyline. However, the results of this study suggested that the response of compulsive ritualizers correlated with levels of plasma clomipramine, whereas depression response appeared to correlate better with plasma levels of desmethylclomipramine. As noted earlier by Thoren, et al[44] in OCD patients, during clomipramine treatment, both 5-HIAA (serotonergic metabolite) and MHPG (noradrenergic metabolite) concentrations are reduced in the spinal fluid. The extent of MHPG reduction correlated with the plasma concentration of the desmethyl metabolite, and the 5-HIAA reduction was a function of the plasma concentration of the parent compound. The latter association is not linear but U-shaped as previously mentioned; that is, both very low and very high concentrations of clomipramine are associated with a smaller reduction in 5-HIAA than are intermediate concentrations.[43,60]

Clomipramine is the only SRI that is currently available in an IV form. This preparation is commonly used to treat OCD and major depression in both outpatients and inpatients. There are some data suggesting that in OCD, IV-administered clomipramine reduces symptoms more quickly and is better tolerated than oral clomipramine. Warneke[62–64] reported moderate to marked improvement in nine patients toward the end of a trial of 14 daily infusions. Fallon, et al[65] reported a 39% average decrease in symptom scores in three of five patients with OCD after 14 consecutive weekday infusions. Of interest, patients unable to tolerate adequate doses of oral clomipramine easily tolerated IV clomipramine. Koran, et al[66] reported that five patients with OCD who were treated with gradually increasing doses of IV clomipramine improved to a marked degree within 4 weeks (i.e., almost twice as fast as patients in trials of oral clomipramine). Sallee, et al[67] reported a decrease of approximately 30% in OCD symptom scores in three adolescents within 36 hours of receiving two infusions of clomipramine (75 mg and 200 mg) over 2 days. In addition, patients unresponsive to oral clomipramine have subsequently benefited from IV clomipramine.[62,65] Recently, Koran, et al[68] conducted a randomized, double-blind, placebo-controlled trial of IV versus oral pulse loading of clomipramine in 15 patients with OCD. Seven subjects were randomly assigned to IV pulse-loaded clomipramine, and eight patients were assigned to orally pulse-loaded clomipramine. Patients received clomipramine 150 mg one day and another 200 mg 24 hours later. Within 5 days after the second pulse-loaded dose of clomipramine, six of the seven patients who were given IV drug experienced a marked decrease of 25% or greater in Yale-Brown Obsessive Compulsive

Scale (Y-BOCS) score, with a mean decrease of 41% for the six responders. Only one of the eight patients receiving oral drug responded. For patients who have not responded to oral drug, the majority of data indicate that some will respond to IV drug.

Occasionally, low doses of clomipramine given over short periods of time may result in significant improvement in symptoms, but usually to demonstrate a full effect, treatment should extend to at least 10 to 12 weeks and employ doses as high as 250 mg/day.

The strongest evidence of the efficacy of clomipramine in OCD comes from a large multicenter trial of clomipramine, which included 520 OCD patients in 21 centers funded by Ciba-Geigy Pharmaceutical Company in the United States.[50] Clomipramine was significantly more effective than placebo on the Y-BOCS and other scales. After 10 weeks of treatment, 58% of patients rated themselves much or very much improved when receiving clomipramine versus 3% of placebo-treated patients.

Clomipramine's side effects are primarily of an anticholinergic nature. Sexual difficulties (i.e., total or partial anorgasmia) are common,[69] and there is a small incidence of seizures at higher doses.[50] It is now well documented that seizures are very unlikely if the total daily dosage of clomipramine is kept at 250 mg/day or less. Most patients tolerate clomipramine well.

Fluoxetine

Fluoxetine (Prozac) became available in the U.S. market in 1987 and a number of open trials suggested that the drug had antiobsessional effects. Turner and colleagues[70] gave fluoxetine to 10 OCD patients and found that it reduced depressive symptoms but also had an effect (not statistically significant) on self-report measures of obsessions and ritualistic behavior. Fontaine, et al[71] performed a 9-week open trial of fluoxetine in nine OCD patients and reported a statistically significant improvement in obsessional symptoms. This group later reported a larger open trial in which 43 of 50 (86%) patients responded to fluoxetine doses, sometimes increased as high as 100 mg/day.

Jenike, et al[72] performed a 12-week open trial of fluoxetine in 61 OCD patients. Measuring improvement with the Y-BOCS, Maudsley Obsessive-Compulsive Inventory, and Beck Depression Inventory, they demonstrated significant improvement in OCD symptoms and depression; fluoxetine had similar effects on OCD in both the depressed and nondepressed subjects. Pigott, et al[73] evaluated fluoxetine using two separate experimental designs. In the first, using 11 OCD subjects, they compared fluoxetine with clomipramine in a randomized, double-blind, crossover paradigm. Over a 10-week treatment period, therapeutic effects were comparable for the two agents based on Y-BOCS scores. During a 4-week crossover phase with placebo, there were significant rates of relapse. In the second phase of the study, 21 patients stabilized on clomipramine with benefit and were crossed over to fluoxetine. Findings in the form of Y-BOCS scores were consistent with the conclusion that fluoxetine provides comparable efficacy with clomipramine in the treatment of OCD.

In the Lilly European fixed-dose OCD study, 217 OCD patients were treated with fluoxetine (20, 40, or 60 mg) or placebo in a double-blind manner for 8 weeks, 161 patients continuing the drug until the sixteenth week. Fluoxetine at a dose of 40 and 60 mg (but not 20 mg) was significantly superior to placebo.[74]

Another large multicenter, double-blind, placebo-controlled, 13-week study of fluoxetine in 355 OCD outpatients reported that 20 mg, 40 mg, and 60 mg of fluoxetine were statistically equally efficacious in the treatment of these patients, but that the 20-mg dose took longer to have an effect.[75] All dosages of fluoxetine were significantly superior to placebo on the Y-BOCS; however, a trend was noted suggesting greatest efficacy at 60 mg/day. Unfortunately, an 80-mg dosage was not included in this study, and, anecdotally, many investigators feel that larger dosages of this drug are more effective in most OCD patients.

Fluvoxamine

Fluvoxamine has been shown to be an effective antidepressant when compared in double-blind trials with clomipramine[76] and imipramine.[77–79] A unicyclic agent, fluvoxamine also possesses selective and potent effects on SRI and appears to be helpful in the treatment of severe OCD.[80–83] In one open trial,[82] 6 of 10 inpatients experienced clinically significant improvement, and in a controlled trial,[80] 9 of 21 OCD patients were much improved with fluvoxamine compared with no responders with placebo. However, because approximately 50% of the patients in this report had concurrent major depression, this controlled trial of fluvoxamine in OCD did not allow an adequate assessment of its antiobsessional properties separate from its antidepressant effects.[80] Other design problems confound the results of this study: treatment duration in this study was shorter than the 10 weeks usually required in trials of patients with OCD; the first 18 analyzable patients participated in only 6 weeks of double-blind treatment and the next 24 analyzable patients received 8 weeks of double-blind treatment. During this study, in addition to treatment with placebo or fluoxetine, patients attended individual psychotherapy sessions once weekly during which they were encouraged to resist their obsessions and compulsions.

In a more recent study of the efficacy of fluvoxamine in patients with OCD, no other treatments were allowed, depressed patients were excluded, and the double-blind portion of the study was continued for a full 10 weeks in all patients.[83] All subjects were outpatients who met *Diagnostic and Statistical Manual of Mental Disorders* (DSM-III-R) criteria for OCD, had suffered from OCD symptoms for at least 1 year, and were not depressed by clinical interview. To ensure that patients had significant OCD symptomatology, a minimum score of 7 on the National Institute of Mental Health (NIMH) Global Obsessive-Compulsive Scale (see Chapter 6) was required for entry into the study. Each patient had a baseline 17-item Hamilton Depression Rating Scale (HDRS)[84] score of 19 or less, and the score for item 1 ("depressed mood") was 2 or less. Thirty-eight of the 40 patients completed the study. The mean maximum dose during the study was 294 mg/day with 17 of the 18 patients who received fluvoxamine reaching the maximum dose of 300 mg; one could tolerate only 200 mg/day. Side effects were mild and consisted mainly of insomnia, nausea, fatigue, and headache. Overall, fluvoxamine had no serious side effects, and there were no clinically significant alterations in physical examination, laboratory findings, electrocardiogram (ECG), blood pressure, or pulse in any of the patients during the course of the study. Data analyses were conducted on 18 patients in the drug group and 20 patients in the placebo group. On the NIMH scale, the groups significantly differed only at week 10. On the CGI, the groups significantly differed both at week 6 and week 10. All comparisons favored the fluvoxamine group over placebo group.

In a large multicenter, double-blind, placebo-controlled trial Goodman, et al[85] studied 160 OCD patients. After a placebo washout phase, patients were randomized to treatment with placebo or fluvoxamine (100 to 300 mg/day) for 10 weeks. Seventy-eight patients in each group were evaluable for efficacy. Fluvoxamine was found to be significantly more effective than placebo as assessed by the Y-BOCS and other scales, with 33% of fluvoxamine-treated patients responding compared with 9% of those patients given placebo.

Sertraline

In the first study with OCD patients, Chouinard, et al[86] randomized 87 patients to either placebo or sertraline (50 to 200 mg/day) for 8 weeks. Sertraline was more effective than placebo and was well tolerated. In another study, sertraline was compared with placebo in a fixed-dose study with 325 nondepressed OCD patients who were randomized to 12 weeks of double-blind treatment with either placebo or 50, 100, or 200 mg of sertraline.[87] Sertraline had significantly greater effectiveness than placebo at all doses.

Paroxetine

Wheadon, et al[88] and Steiner, et al[89] reported the results of a 12-week, fixed-dose, multicenter study in 348 OCD patients. The subjects were randomized in a double-blind fashion to receive either 20, 40, or 60 mg paroxetine or placebo. The 40- and 60-mg doses were significantly better than placebo, whereas the 20-mg dose was not.

Which is the Best Drug for OCD?

A recent report,[87] which suggested that clomipramine was the best antiobsessional drug, used the statistical technique of metaanalysis, which is a crude way to compare different studies. These drugs were not compared in the same study, but the authors compared the results from four large multicenter, placebo-controlled trials of clomipramine (n = 520), fluoxetine (n = 355), fluvoxamine (n = 320), and sertraline (n = 325). For example, researchers looked at a study of clomipramine versus placebo, a study of sertraline versus placebo, and a study of fluoxetine versus placebo and statistically computed which drug was most effective compared with placebo. Another metaanalytic study from Europe[90] came to similar conclusions with an improvement rate over placebo on the Y-BOCS of 61% for clomipramine, 29% for fluoxetine, 28% for fluvoxamine, and 22% for sertraline. These authors commented that despite these statistical findings, when clomipramine was directly compared against fluoxetine and later against fluvoxamine, similar efficacy was demonstrated among all three drugs.

Metaanalysis is a very rough way to study drug effects. On careful examination of the data, it is clear that most of the studies were performed by the same centers, and that the first drug studied gave the best results and each subsequent drug gave poorer results. For example, sertraline was the last drug studied and gave the worst results. One possible explanation for this finding is that each subsequent study had sicker patients. For example, if a patient responded to clomipramine at any study site, he or she continued to receive the drug and did not go into the next drug study. If the patient failed to improve, he was placed into the next study, and on and on.

There are some data on head-to-head comparisons between drugs. Fluoxetine was compared with clomipramine by Pigott, et al[73] in 11 OCD patients in a 10-week crossover study. No significant differences were noted regarding the clinical efficacy. Researchers noted that some patients seemed to do better clinically with clomipramine, but that fluoxetine-treated patients reported fewer side effects.

Freeman, et al[91] compared the efficacy of fluvoxamine and clomipramine in a multicenter, randomized, double-blind, parallel-group comparison of 66 patients and found that both drugs were equally effective in the treatment of OCD. Both agents were well tolerated, and fluvoxamine produced fewer anticholinergic side effects and caused less sexual dysfunction than clomipramine, although fluvoxamine produced more reports of headache and insomnia.

On the other hand, in a 16-week, double-blind comparison of clomipramine and sertraline in 168 patients with OCD, side-effect dropouts on the former were substantially higher (26% vs. 11%).[92] Because of this, sertraline was more effective using the last observation analysis, whereas the drugs were similarly effective when the analysis was restricted to those patients who completed at least 4 weeks of treatment. Jefferson and Greist[93] speculated that perhaps 50 mg/day was too high a starting dose for clomipramine. This study found a robust 15-point improvement in Y-BOCS score for sertraline compared with less than 6 points in the U.S. multicenter study.[94]

It is likely that each of the five drugs (Table 22-1) that have been studied are roughly equally effective against OCD symptoms, although closure on comparative efficacy has not been reached. Clinical experience reports that any individual patient may have a good response to one or two of these drugs and no response to others. Thus, patients and doctors are left to try each drug at high dosage for approximately 3 months to determine which drug is best for any individual patient. Because nonresponse or partial response is common with OCD drug monotherapy, clinicians must frequently decide whether to switch to a different drug or to use an augmentation strategy. Thus far, no studies have directly compared the merits of a switch with those of augmentation. Fortunately, failure to respond to one OCD drug does not guarantee failure to respond to another, although it may decrease the likelihood of response. For example, in the fluvoxamine multicenter study,[95] 19% of patients who failed a previous trial with clomipramine or fluoxetine later responded to fluvoxamine. Because the results with a wide variety of augmentation strategies have not been overwhelmingly successful (see later in this chapter), some clinicians tend to switch to a different OCD drug when an adequate clinical trial has failed (no response or not tolerated) and to augment when there has been partial but less than satisfactory improvement.[93]

Dose and Duration of Drug Treatment

The treatment of OCD appears to be different from the treatment of depression, for which these same drugs are used. Although it is not uncommon when treating OCD to see statistically significant drug and placebo differences appearing as early as 2 to 3 weeks (2 weeks in the clomipramine and sertraline multicenter trials), clinical response may be delayed considerably longer (4 weeks in the fluoxetine and 6 weeks in the fluvoxamine multicenter trials); hence, a trial of 10 to 12 weeks is recommended before lack of efficacy is concluded.[93,96]

Regarding an adequate dose for OCD, the data are somewhat confusing. In the multicenter studies that employed fixed-dose comparisons, lower doses were often effective; therefore, some researchers recommend against rapid dosage escalation because side-effect dropouts are more common at higher doses. With regard to fluoxetine, in one study,[62] 20, 40, and 60 mg/day were equally effective with a trend favoring higher dosages, whereas dropouts resulting from adverse events were approximately four to five times greater in patients receiving 40 and 60 mg. In another large study,[74] 20 mg was no better than placebo. With paroxetine, however, 40 mg/day and 60 mg/day were more effective than placebo but 20 mg was not.[88] The results from the sertraline multicenter study were somewhat confusing because both 50 and 200 mg/day separated from placebo on all four efficacy measures, whereas 100 mg/day bested placebo on only one.[94]

Neither the clomipramine nor the fluvoxamine studies addressed the issue of minimum effective dose because each used a flexible dosage schedule. Jefferson and Greist[93] suspected that higher than necessary doses of OCD drugs are sometimes prescribed because clinicians become impatient if response is not immediately forthcoming. For example, Pato, et al,[97] successfully retreated patients who were maintained previously on 270 mg/day with a mean daily dose of only 165 mg/day.

There is general agreement that an OCD drug trial should not be considered complete until a patient has been treated with a minimally effective daily dose of the medication for 10 to 12 weeks (Table 22-1). There have been anecdotal reports of even higher doses being useful, so exceeding these recommendations remains a possibility, albeit a poorly documented one. In view of the increased risk of seizures with high blood levels of clomipramine, blood level monitoring is advised whenever higher doses are used.[93]

LESS-STUDIED DRUGS

Venlafaxine

In a recent study, 10 outpatients meeting DSM-IV criteria for OCD were treated openly with venlafaxine (Effexor); nine patients completed a 12-week course. Y-BOCS scores indicated that three patients (30%) experienced 35% or greater reduction in OCD symptom severity over the 12 weeks. As a group, the nine completers showed a statistically significant, but clinically modest, decrease in OCD symptom severity. The medication was well tolerated, although venlafaxine discontinuation caused withdrawal symptoms in four patients. Additional data, including a placebo-controlled trial, are needed to confirm the efficacy of venlafaxine for the treatment of OCD.

Trazodone

Hermesh, et al[98] reported improvement with trazodone in nine refractory OCD patients, whereas Pigott, et al[99] did not find it efficacious in a controlled study of 21 patients.

Monoamine Oxidase Inhibitors

As early as 1959, iproniazid was reported to produce marked improvement in patients who had obsessive-compulsive symptoms;[108] diagnostic criteria and symptoms, however, were not described in this study. Annesley[101] described a 49-year-old man with anxiety, phobias, disabling obsessions, and compulsive rituals, whose symptoms gradually remitted over a 6-week period after receiving phenelzine (Nardil). At 6-month follow-up, the study reported that the patient's improvement was maintained on a dose of 30 mg twice daily. Prior treatment failures included behavior therapy, electroconvulsive therapy, insulin therapy, phenothiazines, tricyclic antidepressants, benzodiazepines, and a neurosurgical procedure (bilateral rostral leucotomy).

Jain, et al[102] reported a 26-year-old man with anxiety, phobias, and disabling obsessive ruminations who responded to a monoamine oxidase inhibitor (MAOI) with a complete loss of symptoms over a 2-week period and was still symptom-free at 4-month follow-up. In another case report, a 48-year-old man with severe obsessive ruminative thoughts responded well to a combination of thought stopping (see Chapter 17) and tranylcypromine.[103] Rihmer, et al[104] reported a 50-year-old man with agoraphobia and severe anxiety associated with obsessive ruminations who responded to the MAOI nialamide. Jenike and colleagues[9,105] reported six more cases in which MAOI produced dramatic improvement and four cases in which there was no effect. In contrast to the patients in whom there was no improvement with MAOI, all of the cases reported in which MAOIs were effective had associated panic attacks or severe anxiety. Affective disease in patients or their families was not a good predictor of responsiveness to MAOI.

As noted earlier, Insel, et al[106] compared the efficacy of clomipramine and clorgyline, an MAOI, in a controlled crossover study of 13 OCD patients. Although clomipramine was effective, patients receiving clorgyline did not improve at all.

Vallejo, et al[107] conducted a controlled clinical trial on the efficacy of clomipramine and phenelzine in 30 OCD patients and reported improvement in both groups; however, the lack of placebo controls and the small size of the study groups limit the applicability of these findings.

In a recent 10-week, placebo-controlled trial of phenelzine versus fluoxetine in OCD patients meeting DSM-III-R criteria,[108] subjects were randomly assigned to receive either placebo, phenelzine (60 mg daily), or fluoxetine (80 mg daily). These dosages were achieved by the end of week 3 of the active phase of the study. Outcomes were assessed using standardized instruments to measure OCD, mood, and anxiety. There was a significant difference among the three treatments on one OCD scale, with fluoxetine-treated patients improving significantly more than those patients receiving placebo or phenelzine. A subgroup of OCD patients with symmetry obsessions did respond to phenelzine. This study provided no evidence to support the use of phenelzine in OCD except possibly in those patients with symmetry or other atypical obsessions. The authors found no support for the hypothesis that patients with high anxiety respond preferentially to phenelzine; however, patients with panic disorder were not included.

Based on these data, an MAOI trial is indicated in OCD patients who have not responded to adequate trials of the five major drugs (Table 22-1), especially when symmetry concerns or panic attacks are part of the clinical presentation. A full 5 weeks must intervene between stopping fluoxetine and 2 weeks with clomipramine, sertraline, paroxetine, fluvoxamine, or buspirone prior to starting an MAOI, because deaths have been reported when these drugs have been used in closer proximity.

Lithium Carbonate

A link between manic-depressive illness and OCD has been suggested,[8,109] and cycling obsessive-compulsive symptoms have been described, but there are very few reports on the successful use of lithium carbonate in OCD. One double-blind crossover trial of six OCD patients carried out in Denmark reported lithium was no more effective than placebo in symptom resolution.[110] On the other hand, there are a few case reports of OCD patients who improved with lithium carbonate.[109,111,112]

Obsessive-compulsive behaviors are sometimes found in patients suffering from bipolar affective disorder.[8,113] Although behavior therapy techniques of *in vivo* exposure and response prevention (ERP) are highly effective in treating these behaviors (see Chapters 17, 19, and 20), until recently there were no reports of their use in patients with bipolar disorder and concomitant OCD. A report of two patients who met criteria for both OCD and bipolar disorder and who were treated with a combination of therapist-aided and self-administered ERP demonstrated that behavior therapy was effective only after the major affective disorder was effectively controlled with the administration of lithium and neuroleptics.[113]

Anticonvulsants

Anticonvulsants have been little studied as treatments for OCD, but a few case reports suggest occasional efficacy.[114–116] Similarities between OCD patients and patients with temporal lobe epilepsy (TLE) have been noted[117] and "involuntary forced thinking" is well documented in TLE.[118,119]

In two studies, patients with electroencephalogram (EEG) abnormalities suggestive of epileptic foci were described.[114,120] Four "obsessional psychopaths" did respond to diphenylhydantoin, according to one report[121] in which diagnostic criteria were very unclear. In another study, only one of four subjects with temporal lobe EEG findings reported any improvement with carbamazepine.[114] A more recent study found that OCD symptoms did not respond to carbamazepine;[115] however, these patients were not selected on the basis of abnormal EEGs.

Attempting to identify a subgroup of OCD patients who would respond to carbamazepine, Khanna[116] studied subjects who showed some indication of temporal lobe dysfunction on EEG. In this study, seven patients were selected from approximately 50 OCD patients on the basis of EEG abnormalities that were considered to be indicative of a frontotemporal ictal discharge; abnormalities included spikes and sharp waves, periodic discharges, polymorphic delta, or hypsarrhythmia in the frontotemporal leads. Carbamazepine therapy of 200 mg/day was started and gradually increased to between 600 mg/day and 1,000 mg/day to maintain a therapeutic blood level for approximately a 12-week study period. Of the seven patients, two reported a reduction of greater than 50% in their clinical symptoms; there were, however, no significant differences on any of the outcome measures at the end of the 12-week trial. Both patients who were partial responders to carbamazepine had a history of coexistent clinical epilepsy. Khanna[116] hypothesized that the OCD symptoms were probably part of a complex partial seizure disorder in these carbamazepine-responsive patients.

Reference has been made to the ineffectiveness of another anticonvulsant, sodium valproate, in two cases of OCD.[122,123] In addition, a single case report demonstrating good antiobsessional effects from the benzodiazepine anticonvulsant clonazepam has surfaced.[124] We have just begun a small open trial of phenytoin for OCD, and very preliminary results are encouraging.[125]

The bulk of the evidence supports the idea that there may be a small subpopulation of OCD patients in whom anticonvulsant medication may be useful. In patients who suffer concomitant or past seizure disorders, the likelihood of a positive response may be higher.

Antipsychotic Agents

Under stress, the severe obsessional patient may appear psychotic—an observation that has prompted clinicians to attempt amelioration with neuroleptic drugs.[53] Patients commonly receive neuroleptics for many years, although there is no evidence that they have been of any help.

There are only a few case reports of success with these agents.[13,126–129] Most of these patients were atypical and some resembled the clinical picture of schizophrenia rather than classical OCD. It may be that the schizophrenic features were partly, or even substantially, responsible for the favorable outcomes.

In the absence of data on the efficacy of these older agents and the frequency of toxic side effects, their use can only be recommended for the more acutely disturbed obsessional patient. When these agents are tried, target symptoms should be identified and patients should be evaluated at regular intervals of not longer than 1 month; the neuroleptic should be discontinued if there is no definite improvement. The use of these older agents and the new generation of neuroleptics as potential augmentation agents for cyclic antidepressants is discussed in a later section of this chapter.

Anxiolytic Agents

Because OCD is considered one of the anxiety disorders in DSM-IV, it is not surprising that anxiolytics have been suggested in the treatment of OCD patients. The literature contains a few anecdotal reports of success with anxiolytic agents[13,120,124,130–134] and a few controlled trials[135,136] in which both diagnostic and outcome criteria were unclear. Once again, with one possible exception, there are no well-conducted studies addressing the use of anxiolytics in patients with OCD. Hewlett, et al[137] did perform a double-blind, randomized, multiple-crossover study of 28 OCD patients, which found that clonazepam was as effective as clomipramine and was superior to diphenhydramine that had been used as an active control drug. Most clinicians, however, believe that benzodiazepines are of little use in the treatment of obsessions or compulsions, but that these drugs do help with the anxiety that many OCD patients suffer. If antidepressants improve OCD, anxiety usually decreases without the use of anxiolytics.

Buspirone, an atypical anxiolytic with partial (5-HT$_{1A}$) serotonergic agonist properties, was ineffective in a small (n = 10) open trial.[138] However, in a random-assignment, double-blind crossover study, Pato and colleagues[139,140] studied 18 outpatients with OCD, comparing the efficacy of clomipramine and buspirone. The patients received up to 250 mg/day of clomipramine and up to 60 mg/day of buspirone. Clinical improvement was defined as a minimum of 20% improvement from baseline. Researchers found significant improvement in ratings of OCD and depression with both drugs over the 6-week course of phase 1 of the study, and there were no significant differences between clomipramine and buspirone. Phase 2 of the crossover design was not analyzed, as significant carryover effects were found. This trial has been interpreted to mean that buspirone was as effective as clomipramine, but the short-time course of the study and a wealth of anecdotal evidence suggest that this is not the case.

In view of the occasional spontaneous remission and often fluctuating course of OCD, it is difficult to make a strong case for the use of anxiolytic drugs on the basis of available data. There may, however, be a role for the novel anxiolytic, buspirone, as a primary treatment or more likely as an augmenting agent (see later section in this chapter). Further, because OCD is a chronic disorder, the use of anxiolytics for long periods raises questions of dependency brought about by long-term use of compounds from the benzodiazepine class.[4]

Tryptophan

Because a deficit in the serotonergic system is hypothesized in patients with OCD, the use of the serotonin precursor, tryptophan, is of interest. Most of the work on tryptophan has been performed by one group and results have not been replicated. Yaryura-Tobias and colleagues[141–143] reported a number of patients who improved with tryptophan.

The administration of tryptophan stimulates the enzyme that causes the breakdown of tryptophan; therefore, to be maximally effective, nicotinamide, and probably vitamins B$_6$ and C also should be administered. It is also likely that the administration of other large neutral amino acids should be controlled in the patient's diet and not administered in close proximity to doses of tryptophan.[144,145] The use of tryptophan as an augmenting agent is discussed later in this chapter.

Yohimbine

In an effort to investigate possibly abnormal adrenergic function in the pathogenesis of OCD, Rasmussen and associates[146] administered the alpha$_2$-adrenergic receptor antagonist yohimbine to 12 drug-free OCD patients and 12 healthy subjects and found no significant effect on OCD symptoms.

Oxytocin

Oxytocin is a neurosecretory nonapeptide, which is made by cells in part of the brain called the hypothalamus and is distributed to the central nervous system. It causes milk ejection and uterine contraction after babies are born. It also may help the mother forget the pain of childbirth. However, over the past decade, oxytocin has been found to have other purposes in the body, and the drug seems to be involved in grooming, thinking, and sexual behavior.

Lately, there has been some evidence that oxytocin is involved in some forms of OCD. For example, administration of oxytocin can increase self-grooming in rats; some experts have suggested that these behaviors may be similar to the repetitive handwashing and cleaning present in OCD. Oxytocin is elevated during the third trimester of pregnancy and after birth, and this is a time when many women report onset and worsening of OCD symptoms (see Chapter 5). It has further been suggested that obsessions regarding the safety of others and dirt and germs, as well as compulsions such as checking and cleaning, might be seen as pathologic correlates of normal maternal behavior. There is even a report that oxytocin is elevated in the cerebrospinal fluid of patients with OCD compared with age- and gender-matched normal control subjects and patients with Tourette's disorder.

In animals, oxytocin appears to be an amnestic neuropeptide that prevents the acquisition of conditioned behavior or facilitates its extinction in a way opposite to vasopressin.[147] Because compulsions are considered to be conditioned responses to anxiety-provoking events by behavior therapists, the possible beneficial activity of intranasal oxytocin was investigated. Ansseau, et al[147] administered intranasal oxytocin to a 55-year-old OCD patient over a 4-week period with resultant clear improvement in symptoms. Unfortunately, this improvement was concurrent with the development of severe memory disturbances, psychotic symptoms, and a marked decrease in plasma sodium and osmolality, which the authors theorized may have masked the OCD symptomatology. This initial trial was encouraging in terms of efficacy, but side effects will require close monitoring in future investigations.

Other experts have reported disappointing results when oxytocin was used to treat OCD.[148] This same group also found it ineffective for trichotillomania.[149] These authors have suggested that perhaps oxytocin given intranasally may not cross the blood-brain barrier and would therefore not be expected to affect repetitive behavior; also, 1 week of treatment may not be sufficient to effect a discernible change in symptoms.

Naltrexone and Naloxone

There are a number of self-harmful behaviors that are sometimes called compulsive even though they do not strictly fit into the category of OCD. These behaviors include repetitive self-injurious behavior and trichotillomania. Naltrexone and naloxone have been reported to be helpful for these behaviors.

There are conflicting reports, however, on the use of opiate antagonists in classical OCD.

Insel and Pickar[106] performed a double-blind, placebo-controlled trial of naloxone hydrochloride in two patients with OCD. They hypothesized that if obsessional patients with ruminative doubt had a deficit in an opiate-mediated capacity to register reward, this deficit would be manifested cognitively as a difficulty in reaching certainty. The opiate system has been suggested as a mediator of reward systems. The two subjects in this study specifically described the obsessional symptoms as spontaneous doubts that required repeated checks until a point of certainty was reached. Researchers administered IV naloxone at 0.3 mg/kg, a dose that is generally free from behavioral effects in normal subjects.[150] On a separate day, saline was similarly administered and both patients and raters were blind to the experimental condition. The first patient noticed no change after placebo administration, but when taking naloxone, he became acutely absorbed in checking rituals and was unable to reach certainty about the physical relationships of objects in the protocol room. He had considerable difficulty completing the ratings and this acute exacerbation continued for 24 hours. Similarly, the second patient noted no change with placebo, but became abruptly worse after naloxone with feelings that he could not reach a point of mastery of his intruding thoughts. In both cases, blind self- and observer-ratings corroborated spontaneous self-reports. Sandyk[151] reported improvement of severe OCD symptoms with a much lower dose of naloxone (0.01 mg/kg) in two patients who also had Tourette's disorder.

To further define the effects of modulating opiate function in OCD patients using a larger sample of subjects and a randomized, double-blind, placebo-controlled design, Keuler, et al[152] studied 13 medication-free outpatients with OCD. They used a 0.175-mg/kg dose of naloxone or placebo that was infused as a bolus in a randomized, double-blinded fashion. Ratings of OCD symptoms were made prior to infusion and at 1 and 2 hours postinfusion. Although 3 of the 13 subjects did experience an exacerbation of anxiety and OCD symptoms similar to that described by Insel and Pickar,[106] subjects as a group demonstrated no significant improvement or exacerbation relative to placebo on any rating scale. The authors speculated that these findings may reflect an underlying heterogeneity in OCD associated with differential responses to opiate blockade. These conflicting reports implicate endogenous opiates in the pathophysiology of obsessive doubt and resultant checking and may have further implications in terms of future research on opiate agonists as therapeutic agents in OCD. These results provide no clear evidence that OCD symptoms are modulated by opioid systems, but the effect of dosing (with lower dosages helpful for OCD symptoms) may be crucial. More work using a dose-response study is needed in this area to determine the role of opioid agents as treatments for OCD.

Naltrexone has been reported to decrease the frequency of self-injurious behavior in a dose-dependent fashion in some patients with mental retardation.[153]

Bystritsky and Strausser[154] reported a 46-year-old man with a complicated history that included partial complex seizures and grand mal seizures. He was said to have no evidence of a personality disorder and had had OCD since 16 years of age that consisted of avoiding "dirty" places and fears of contamination. He developed uncontrollable urges to drink his own and then his wife's urine, despite his wife's protests. After several months, his urges stopped, and he began to cut himself on his buttocks with a knife almost daily. Cutting produced a pleasurable feeling mixed with a feeling of guilt. On days when he had a seizure, he did not have any desire to cut himself. Fluoxetine, paroxetine, fluvoxamine, haloperidol, risperidone, and lithium had no effect on the cutting behaviors, and, in fact, increased the cutting. The patient began a treatment of naltrexone 25 mg twice daily, and the cutting and urges immediately stopped. After 2 days during which the patient did not cut himself, naltrexone was stopped for 1 day, resulting in an immediate resumption of cutting. Cutting stopped when naltrexone was restarted. Later, when the patient's OCD symptoms increased, he was restarted on fluoxetine, which improved OCD, but he resumed cutting, requiring an increase of naltrexone to 50 mg/day.

Even more convincing of the beneficial effect of opiate antagonists is a larger series of seven patients[155] with repetitive harmful behaviors accompanied by analgesia and dysphoria who were administered oral naltrexone 50 mg/day. All patients demonstrated persistent self-injurious behaviors prior to receiving the drug and mean follow-up after receiving naltrexone was 10.7 weeks. Six of the seven patients ceased the harmful behaviors entirely during naltrexone treatment. Two patients who discontinued naltrexone briefly experienced the rapid resumption of harmful behaviors, which again ceased after resumption of naltrexone. One patient exhibited superficial cutting on two occasions when receiving naltrexone, a rate that reflected a significant reduction from earlier behaviors.

There is a case report in which naltrexone significantly augmented an initial partial response to fluoxetine in a 45-year-old woman with a 33-year history of compulsive hair pulling.[156] Fluoxetine was administered open label, in a daily dose of 60 mg for 12 weeks; then naltrexone was added at a daily dose of 50 mg and continued for an additional 8 weeks. With the addition of naltrexone, the patient reported that she might initiate a hair-pulling episode, but reported experiencing little pleasure from it, and found it easy to stop; as a result, her hair began to grow in the affected areas for the first time in 15 years.

As previously mentioned, clomipramine has been clearly demonstrated to improve obsessional symptoms in at least some OCD patients; it also has been reported to potentiate the antinociceptive actions of opiates.[157]

These preliminary observations are consistent with the hypothesis that the endogenous opioid system is involved in cases of repetitive self-injurious behaviors that are accompanied by analgesia and dysphoria reduction. Placebo-controlled studies are needed to clearly answer the questions raised by these case reports.

Psychostimulants

D-amphetamine has been reported to provide brief but significant relief to patients with severe obsessions[10,158] and the mechanism may involve the opiate system because naloxone blocks D-amphetamine increases in activation and self-stimulation.[159]

Clonidine

Clonidine, an alpha$_2$-adrenergic agonist, has been reported as an effective treatment for OCD symptoms in the context of Tourette's disorder.[160] Despite reports of improvement in typical OCD patients with IV clonidine[161] and case reports of success with this drug when used alone[162] and as an augmenter with clomipramine,[161] our results with oral clonidine are not impressive. We found that only 3 of 17 patients had a minimal and not clinically significant improvement when clonidine was added to fluoxetine. Side effects with clonidine, consisting mainly of excessive sedation and unsteadiness, necessitated stopping the drug before a 1-month trial in more than 50% of the patients. Hollander, et al[161] also reported unimpressive results when clonidine was added to clomipramine in two patients.

Inositol

As previously noted, there is now considerable evidence that pharmacologic manipulation of the serotonergic system may help with OCD symptoms. Myoinositol is a ubiquitous carbohydrate that is present in large amounts in brain tissue and is involved in neuronal signaling and osmoregulation,[163] and the phosphatidylinositol cycle is the second messenger system for several neurotransmitters, including several subtypes of serotonin receptors.[164] In addition, desensitization of serotonin receptors is reversed by the addition of exogenous inositol.[165] There are reports that exogenous inositol was effective in controlled trials for patients with depression and panic, and recently a research group performed a double-blind, controlled crossover trial of 18 g/day of inositol versus placebo for 6 weeks each.[166] The subjects had significantly lower scores on the Y-BOCS when taking inositol than when taking placebo.

DRUG PLASMA LEVELS AND OUTCOME

In major depression, plasma levels of some antidepressants, such as nortriptyline, are meaningfully related to response to antidepressants, whereas the levels of SSRIs are not.[167] There are few data on the relationship of plasma levels of antiobsessional drugs and clinical improvement in OCD patients, and the relationships remain unclear. For example, with clomipramine, the relationship has been reported differently in various studies ranging from insignificant[168] to positive[48,61,169] to negative.[43,170] A large multicenter trial found no relationship between sertraline plasma levels and treatment outcome in OCD.[171]

In a multicenter trial, Koran and associates[176] examined the relationship between steady-state plasma levels of fluoxetine, its main metabolite norfluoxetine (measured after 7 weeks of treatment), and their sum, and clinical outcome as assessed with the Y-BOCS. The clinical assessments were obtained at baseline and after 13 weeks for 200 adult outpatients with moderately severe OCD treated with fluoxetine at 20 mg/day (n = 68), 40 mg/day (n = 64), and 60 mg/day (n = 68). As expected, they found that mean plasma levels of fluoxetine and norfluoxetine were statistically significantly higher with higher dose. However, there was no significant relationship for plasma level and change in OCD scores. Plasma levels of patients with a marked response were not significantly different from those patients who did not respond.

In summary, although it is generally felt that higher dosages of medications are more likely to benefit OCD patients, empirical support is lacking for this hypothesis based on plasma levels. There is probably little benefit in measuring plasma levels for most patients who can be better assessed by careful clinical monitoring of OCD symptoms and side effects.

TREATMENT-RESISTANT PATIENTS: AUGMENTATION STRATEGIES

The first task of the clinician faced with an OCD patient who has not responded to treatment is to obtain a careful, detailed history and determine if the patient has, in fact, received adequate treatment trials (Table 22-5). For each medication, dosage and length of trial must be elicited.[83] There is growing evidence that a full 10- to 12-week trial of potentially effective medications is required before assuming a drug to be ineffective. Also, specific behavioral techniques (ERP) that have been attempted should be noted. Other

Table 22-5   Some Common Reasons for Treatment Failure

Incorrect diagnosis (e.g., schizophrenia, obsessive-compulsive personality disorder)
Inadequate treatment
    Inappropriate or ineffective medication trials
    Medication trial too short
    Medication dosage too low
    No behavior therapy trial
Poor compliance
    Patient prefers sickness to health, cannot tolerate demands when well
    Unrecognized cognitive impairment
    Other concomitant psychiatric illness (e.g., schizophrenia, major depression, bipolar illness, etc.)
    Poor understanding of treatment plan by patient (e.g., only takes medication when feeling "stressed")

approaches such as simple relaxation, hypnosis, or biofeedback are not effective treatments for OCD (see Chapter 17).

We now know that if patients receive appropriate treatment, usually consisting of behavior therapy plus psychotropic medication, the majority will improve substantially (but rarely completely) within a few months.[145] In our clinical experience, the most common reason for lack of improvement was the use of ineffective modalities. Many patients primarily received psychodynamic psychotherapy, electroconvulsive therapy,[253] or neuroleptics without result. Despite the well-documented efficacy of behavioral therapies, it is still unusual for patients to arrive at our clinic having undergone even a cursory trial of ERP.

Even with good treatment, however, certain patients continue to be refractory. Predictors of treatment failure in behavior therapy for OCD include noncompliance with treatment, concomitant severe depression,[173] absence of rituals, fixed beliefs in necessity of rituals, presence of concomitant personality disorder,[174] and type of compulsive ritual. Patients with schizotypal and possibly other severe personality disorders (axis II in DSM-IV) also do poorly with pharmacotherapy.[175,176] Outcome studies and anecdotal evidence indicate that poor compliance with the behavioral treatment program is the most common reason for treatment failure with behavioral therapy for OCD.[177] Behavior therapy is more demanding of the patient than many other forms of psychotherapy, and the patient must comply with behavioral instructions both during treatment sessions and "homework" assignments. If the patient is inconsistent in doing this, treatment is unlikely to be successful. Severe depression also has been found as a negative predictor for improvement with behavior therapy of OCD,[173] possibly resulting from impaired learning abilities. In patients with major depression, the behavioral processes of physiologic habituation to the feared stimuli do not occur, regardless of the length of exposure.[178] Because most of the antiobsessional drugs also are powerful antidepressants, depression is not a negative predictive factor for drug outcome.

If a patient has severe obsessive thoughts without rituals, behavior therapy is unlikely to succeed. In these cases, pharmacotherapy is the treatment of choice. Patients who strongly hold the belief that their compulsive rituals are necessary to forestall future catastrophes (i.e., "overvalued ideas") have a poorer outcome with behavioral treatments.[173] For example, the patient who really believes that someone in his family will die if he does not wash his entire house every day is unlikely to give up the rituals with behavior therapy alone.

As previously noted, patients meeting DSM-IV criteria for both OCD and schizotypal personality disorder do not respond well to either behavior therapy or pharmacotherapy. The idea of concomitant schizotypal personality disorder as a negative prognostic indicator in OCD appears to have validity in light of the literature on treatment failure. This personality disorder encompasses several of the negative predictive factors reviewed earlier. Most noticeably, these patients may have strongly held beliefs that their rituals are necessary to prevent some terrible event. They also have difficulty complying with prescribed treatment and assigned record keeping. Rachman and Hodgson[179] have similarly found that the presence of an "abnormal personality" is a negative predictor of outcome in behavior therapy for OCD; more recently, Solyom, et al[180] reported a subcategory of patients with "obsessional psychosis," similar (perhaps identical) to the schizotypal subgroup, who also respond poorly to both behavior therapy and pharmacotherapy.

For a patient who meets criteria for schizotypal personality disorder, placement in a structured environment such as a day treatment center or halfway house during and after behavioral and pharmacologic treatments produces small decreases in patients' obsessive-compulsive symptoms, along with moderate improvements in overall function.

Patients with contamination fears and cleaning rituals appear to respond best to behavioral treatment.[179] Even when responsive to behavioral techniques, patients with checking rituals appear to improve more slowly than those with cleaning rituals.[181] A possible explanation for this difference is that many patients with checking rituals are unable to engage in the prescribed response prevention, especially those who check excessively at home.[179] In addition, patients with primary obsessional slowness often respond more slowly to behavior therapy than do patients with either cleaning or checking rituals.

Importance of Correct Diagnosis

Another reason for poor treatment outcome in OCD is inaccurate diagnosis. If a patient meets criteria for schizophrenia or suffers exclusively from obsessive-compulsive *personality* disorder (OCPD), the standard treatments for OCD may not be helpful. The currently accepted definition of OCD is given in the *Diagnostic and Statistical Manual of Mental Disorders* (DSM-IV) and is described in Chapter 1. Although patients diagnosed with OCPD may have some obsessions and minor compulsions associated with their perfectionism, indecisiveness, or procrastination, these rituals do not interfere with the patient's life to the extent that OCD does. However, some patients with OCD also have compulsive personality traits[182] and roughly 6%[183] meet DSM-III criteria for obsessive-compulsive personality disorder (see Chapters 4 and 27). With the change in diagnostic criteria in DSM-III-R, preliminary data have indicated that as many as 20% of OCD patients met criteria for OCPD (see Chapter 4).[184]

The differential diagnosis of OCD versus OCPD has important treatment implications. For example, although traditional psychotherapy produces little change in obsessions and compulsions in the context of OCD, it may be of value in the treatment of patients with OCPD (see Chapter 27).[145,185] Conversely, although behavior therapy and psychopharmacologic treatments have been found in controlled trials to be very effective for OCD, there is no evidence that these approaches are helpful for patients with OCPD.

Managing the Obsessive-Compulsive Disorder Patient Who is Unresponsive To Treatment

A flow sheet of possible treatment options is listed in Table 22-6. To outline a treatment plan for an OCD patient, it is necessary to have a clear idea of the problem, what exacerbates and what improves it, how it has evolved over the patient's life, and what other symptoms and difficulties exist concomitantly (see Chapter 30 for suggested evaluation). The clinical history and interview must reflect behavioral, psychodynamic, and family systems principles.

Table 22-6   Flow Sheet of Treatment Options for Obsessive-Compulsive Disorder[*]

1. Selective serotonin reuptake inhibitor trials for 12 weeks at full dosage or highest tolerated
   Fluoxetine trial—40 to 80 mg daily
   Clomipramine trial—to 250 mg daily
   Sertraline—to 200 mg
   Paroxetine—40 to 60 mg
   Fluvoxamine—to 300 mg
2. Try augmenting fluoxetine or clomipramine or sertraline or paroxetine or fluvoxamine
3. Try the other selective serotonin reuptake inhibitors (each drug for at least 12 weeks) with augmentation of each agent
4. Try venlafaxine to 375 mg for 3 months
5. Stop fluoxetine for 5 weeks or sertraline, fluvoxamine, clomipramine, venlafaxine, or paroxetine for 2 weeks
6. Monoamine oxidase inhibitor trial
7. Try augmenting monoamine oxidase inhibitors for 1 month (not buspirone)
8. Trials of experimental agents when available
9. Other medication trials (e.g., trazodone, imipramine, etc.)
10. If severe personality disorder present, consider halfway house or day treatment program
11. If patient is severely disabled, despite adequate treatment, consider psychosurgery
12. If poor compliance is a persistent problem, or patient prefers symptoms to being rid of them, or if patient also has obsessive-compulsive personality disorder or had early-onset OCD, consider concomitant psychodynamic psychotherapy

[*] *As soon as patient has at least a partial response to medication; if patient has rituals, begin behavior therapy of exposure and response prevention.*
Remain Flexible—change treatment approach if one is not successful. It is not unusual to have to try a few medications before a patient responds. **Drug trials should be continued for at least 12 weeks** before they are considered failures. Most of the time obsessive-compulsive disorder patients are slow to respond to medication, although occasionally one sees a very rapid response, especially with monoamine oxidase inhibitors.

To determine the appropriate treatment approach and understand the individual's potential for compliance, a thorough mental status examination is required. A depressed, manic, cognitively impaired, or psychotic patient requires a special treatment strategy. Behavioral treatments are unlikely to be effective until associated functional illnesses are well controlled. Also, alcoholic patients require treatment for alcoholism before they can comply with treatment aimed specifically at their obsessive-compulsive symptoms.

The importance of treating other concomitant psychiatric disorders, such as psychosis or depression, cannot be overemphasized. For example, as mentioned earlier, obsessive-compulsive behaviors are sometimes found in patients suffering from bipolar affective disorder[8,113] and one recent report[186] that used data from the ECA study found that approximately 21% of bipolar subjects had a lifetime diagnosis of OCD. Although behavior therapy techniques of *in vivo* ERP are highly effective in treating these behaviors, until recently there were no reports of their use in patients with bipolar disorder and concomitant OCD. A report of two patients from our clinic who met criteria for both disorders and who were treated with a combination of therapist-aided and self-administered ERP demonstrated that behavior therapy was effective only after their major affective disorder was effectively controlled with lithium and neuroleptics.[113]

Augmenting Antidepressants with Other Drugs

The majority of patients with OCD can now be helped with current pharmacologic and behavioral treatments. For example, with clomipramine alone, almost 60% of patients benefit at least moderately and approximately 85% benefit some from a 12-week trial.[187] Clinically, although considerable OCD symptoms may persist, many patients treated with clomipramine obtain a meaningful response with resultant improvement in social relationships, work performance, and overall function. The success of a number of serotonergic agents in treating patients with OCD lends partial support to a role for serotonin in this illness; however, because a number of patients fail to respond to these drugs, the role of other neurotransmitter systems must be considered in this disorder. This evidence suggests that partially effective drugs that primarily affect the serotonergic system might have their clinical effectiveness enhanced by the addition of other agents that have either different effects on the serotonergic system or affect other neurotransmitter systems (e.g., norepinephrine and dopamine). In addition, the brain's serotonergic system does not comprise a single type of receptor; there are many different receptor subtypes, each with its own agonists and antagonists. Thus, at least theoretically, it is likely that some patients fail to improve because only part of their proposed serotonergic abnormality is corrected by a particular drug.

Because of the previous findings and theoretic considerations, clinicians have been attempting to improve OCD symptoms in patients who are only partially responsive to serotonergic agents by adding other drugs as augmenters.

This strategy has been used with depressed patients for some years with agents such as lithium carbonate and triiodothyronine.

Lithium

Improvement in depressed patients has been demonstrated in tricyclic nonresponders after addition of lithium to the antidepressant.[188] This strategy has been attempted with refractory or partially responsive OCD patients. Rasmussen[189] reported a 22-year-old woman with classical OCD who did not respond to clomipramine alone, but who improved greatly a few days after lithium carbonate was added, with a stabilized blood level of 0.9 mEq/L. Feder[190] and Stern and Jenike[109] reported similar cases in which lithium potentiated ongoing treatment with clomipramine and imipramine, respectively. Eisenberg and Asnis[191] reported one patient who improved when lithium was added to ongoing desipramine. Golden and associates[192] reported two cases in which lithium augmentation improved response to clomipramine in one patient and doxepin in another. Another single case report by Howland[193] attested to the efficacy of lithium augmentation of fluoxetine.

On the other hand, Hermesh, et al[98] found that adding lithium to ongoing clomipramine was relatively ineffective in improving OCD symptoms, with only 1 of 10 patients having any response. Whether or not lithium augmentation of other cyclic antidepressants or monoamine oxidase inhibitors for obsessive-compulsive symptoms is helpful remains to be tested; however, Jenike[194] reported that only one of seven OCD patients receiving fluoxetine seemed to derive any additional benefit when lithium was added.

McDougle, et al[195] completed 2- and 4-week, double-blind, placebo-controlled trials of lithium augmentation of ongoing fluvoxamine in 20 and 10 OCD patients, respectively, who failed to respond to fluvoxamine alone. Although 2 weeks of double-blind lithium augmentation produced a small but statistically significant reduction in OCD symptoms, most patients did not have a clinically meaningful response. Further, there was no statistical or clinical improvement in OCD symptoms during the subsequent 4-week, double-blind, placebo-controlled trial of lithium augmentation. On the basis of treatment response criteria, only 18% and 0% of the patients responded to lithium augmentation of fluvoxamine during the 2- and 4-week treatment trials, respectively. McDougle, et al[195] noted that in light of the previously reported 44% response rate to lithium augmentation in treatment-resistant depressed patients taking fluvoxamine, the results of this study suggest that pathophysiologic differences may exist between OCD and depression and that the routine use of lithium augmentation in the management of patients with OCD who are refractory or only partially responsive to SRIs is not supported by their findings.

Pigott, et al[196] came to similar conclusions about the relative ineffectiveness of lithium in another small (n = 8) controlled crossover trial in which either lithium or L-triiodothyronine (T3) was blindly added to an ongoing trial of clomipramine in patients who had all been partial responders to clomipramine alone. Neither lithium carbonate nor T3 added anything to the clinical effect.

Suggesting a possible reason for the ineffectiveness of lithium augmentation in patients with OCD refractory to the selective serotonin 5-HT reuptake blockers, Blier and deMontigny[197] noted that with both *in vitro* techniques and *in vivo* electrophysiologic and microdialysis methods, lithium administration can enhance 5-HT release in the spinal cord, hypothalamus, and the hippocampus. However, negative results have consistently been shown on the capacity of lithium to enhance 5-HT release in the cerebral cortex. Moreover, the release of 5-HT evoked by electrical stimulations was decreased *ex vivo* in slices of the striatum after lithium treatment. Because OCD has recently been linked with abnormalities in the orbitofrontal cortex and striatum, it is thus likely that an increase in 5-HT neurotransmission did not occur in the patients in these critical regions, as a result of lithium addition.

Buspirone

Buspirone, an atypical anxiolytic with partial ($5\text{-}HT_{1A}$) serotonergic agonist properties, was approved in 1987 by the Food and Drug Administration for the treatment of anxiety. In addition to serotonergic effects, it has effects on dopamine-2 receptors in the central nervous system. Buspirone's major advantages versus the benzodiazepines are the lack of sedation or cognitive impairment and the low abuse or addiction potential.[198]

Several studies of buspirone augmentation in treating OCD have been published, with mixed results. Adding buspirone to an ongoing trial of fluoxetine has been reported to diminish OCD symptoms.[199-202] Alessi and Bos[202] reported a single case of an 11-year-old girl whose OCD symptoms improved when 30 mg/day of buspirone was added to ongoing fluoxetine treatment. Markovitz, et al[200,201] gave 11 OCD patients a prospective open-label trial of fluoxetine monotherapy followed by buspirone augmentation (up to 30 mg/day) and reported that the combination therapy was statistically superior to fluoxetine monotherapy. Jenike, et al[199] studied 20 patients treated with fluoxetine for OCD. Ten patients received fluoxetine for 12 weeks, with buspirone augmentation (up to 60 mg/day) for an additional 8 weeks. Ten additional consecutively treated patients received only fluoxetine. The authors used the Y-BOCS[203] and Beck Depression Inventory (BDI).[204] Patients taking buspirone and fluoxetine showed a significantly greater improvement on the Y-BOCS at the end of 2 months but not 1 month of buspirone augmentation. The results of this pilot study must be considered preliminary because of the small sample size, the lack of a double-blind design, and the retrospective nature of the control group. Blier and Bergeron[205] added buspirone to SRI plus pindolol in five OCD patients and found no further improvement in OCD symptoms.

In contrast to the previous open-label studies, several double-blinded studies have failed to show a statistically significant improvement in OCD symptoms with the addition of buspirone to other agents. Pigott, et al[206] studied 14 OCD patients who had received at least 3 months of treatment with clomipramine. Each patient was initially given placebo for 2 weeks and then treated with buspirone in a 10-week, double-blind study. Prior to the addition of buspirone, these patients had shown a partial but incomplete reduction (average, 28%) in OCD symptoms during clomipramine treatment alone. Although adjuvant buspirone treatment was well tolerated in most subjects, mean OCD and depressive symptoms, as evaluated by standardized rating scales (i.e., Y-BOCS, NIMH-OC), did not significantly change from baseline scores achieved on clomipramine treatment alone. The mean dose of buspirone was 57 +/– 7 mg/day. When the response of individual patients was examined, 4 (29%) of the 14 patients did have an additional 25% reduction of OCD symptoms after adjuvant buspirone treatment. Interestingly, 3 (21%) of 14 patients worsened more than 25% when buspirone was added. Pigott, et al[206] concluded that adjunctive buspirone therapy is not generally associated with significant further clinical improvement in OCD or depressive symptoms compared with clomipramine monotherapy, but that there may be a subgroup of patients who do benefit from adjuvant buspirone therapy; they did not speculate on or identify any factors in the drug-responsive patients that differentiated them from the nonresponders.

This study suffers from an obvious weakness in that buspirone and placebo were not compared head to head, and there was no even variation in the time that placebo was given (i.e., always the first 2 weeks) over the course of the study.

McDougle and colleagues[207] reported on 50 patients who were treated with fluvoxamine at doses up to 300 mg/day for OCD for 8 weeks. Thirty-three patients were determined to be refractory to treatment, with either a less than 35% reduction in Y-BOCS score or a Y-BOCS score of 16 or greater, no better than minimal improvement on a Clinical Global Improvement scale, or consensus of the investigators that the patient was unimproved. These 33 patients continued to receive the same dose of fluvoxamine, plus either placebo or buspirone at doses up to 60 mg/day for an additional 6 weeks. No significant improvement occurred with the addition of buspirone to fluvoxamine.

Grady, et al[208] studied 14 OCD patients who had been maintained on 80 mg/day of fluoxetine for at least 10 weeks. In a double-blind, crossover design, patients were given either buspirone (up to 60 mg/day) or placebo in addition to the fluoxetine for 8 weeks. There was no significant improvement (> 25%) from baseline on OCD ratings. Only one patient achieved a 25% reduction in symptoms when taking the buspirone augmentation.

Fenfluramine

Fenfluramine, an anorectic agent with serotonin reuptake blocking and releasing properties, has been reported in three cases to potentiate the effects of fluvoxamine when given on a daily basis at 30 to 45 mg/day.[161,209] Hollander, et al[210] gave an open trial of fenfluramine in doses of 20 to 60 mg/day to OCD patients who had only a partial response to fluoxetine, fluvoxamine, or clomipramine or were unable to tolerate therapeutic doses of these agents. Fenfluramine augmentation was well tolerated and resulted in a further decrease in obsessions and compulsions in six of the seven patients.

Antidepressants

Trazodone has been used as an augmenting agent[211,212]; it improved Y-BOCS scores by greater than 20% in 4 of 13 patients when it was added to ongoing fluoxetine. Almost one third of the patients who were augmented with trazodone, however, had to discontinue the medication because of excessive daily sedation, although the drug was given at bedtime.

Simeon, et al[213] reported adding fluoxetine (20 to 40 mg) to ongoing trials of clomipramine (25 to 50 mg) in six adolescents with OCD. Each of the six patients had either not improved or had developed intolerable side effects when taking clomipramine alone. Before fluoxetine was given, the mean daily dosage of clomipramine was only 92 mg (range, 50 to 175 mg) and the duration of treatment ranged from 3 to 32 weeks (mean, 17.5 weeks). In four patients, clomipramine dosage was reduced when fluoxetine was added because patients complained of adverse effects. Two anxious patients also received alprazolam. One patient improved moderately, and five improved markedly with combination treatment. The authors concluded that the combination of low doses of clomipramine plus fluoxetine resulted in greater clinical improvement with fewer adverse effects than did a trial of clomipramine alone.

It is important to keep in mind that all of the SSRIs can raise tricyclic (i.e., clomipramine) blood levels,[214] sometimes quite dramatically. Thus, it is important to begin augmentation with a low dose of clomipramine and very slowly increase the dose while closely monitoring efficacy and side effects.

Benzodiazepines

Benzodiazepines are often used as adjuncts to other medications and may be helpful in facilitating behavior therapy in patients who are unable to tolerate the anxiety produced by ERP techniques. We added clonazepam (0.5 mg two to three times daily) to ongoing fluoxetine in seven patients and only one improved more than 20% after the addition.

Beta Blockers

Recently, the addition of the 5-HT$_{1A}$/beta-adrenergic antagonist pindolol exerted a rapid therapeutic effect in depressed patients not responding to certain SRI or monoamine oxidase inhibitors.[215,216] Blier and Bergeron[205] explain the rationale for this approach: acute administration of SRI or MAOI suppresses the firing activity of midbrain 5-HT neurons because they enhance the availability of 5-HT in the vicinity of cell body 5-HT_{1A} autoreceptors, which exert a negative-feedback role on the firing rate of 5-HT neurons. However, firing activity gradually returns to normal as treatment is prolonged because of a desensitization of these 5-HT_{1A} autoreceptors. Because pindolol blocks these 5-HT_{1A} autoreceptors but not postsynaptic 5-HT_{1A} receptors in the limbic forebrain, it was postulated that pindolol addition may allow a normalization of the firing activity of 5-HT neurons in patients not responding to the SRI or MAOI, presumably because their 5-HT_{1A} autoreceptors had failed to desensitize.

Blier and Bergeron[205] treated 13 OCD patients, who had not responded to an SRI for at least 12 weeks, with pindolol 2.5 mg three times daily. These subjects were assessed weekly for 4 weeks using the Y-BOCS and other scales. None of the 13 patients reported untoward side effects. Of the 13 patients, although there was no significant group effect of pindolol addition with respect to OCD symptoms, four individuals had a marked improvement of OCD symptoms over the 4 weeks of pindolol addition (Y-BOCS score changes of 7, 8, 10, and 12). Of the four responders, three also met criteria for major depression.

These preliminary data indicate that there may be a role for pindolol augmentation, especially in those OCD patients who suffer from concomitant depression.

Tryptophan

Rasmussen[189] reported an OCD patient who had a partial response to clomipramine, which was dramatically boosted when 6 g/day of L-tryptophan was added. This patient relapsed when tryptophan was stopped and improved again when it was restarted. Whether tryptophan would boost the antiobsessional effects of other tricyclic antidepressants or MAOIs remains to be determined. Walinder and associates,[217] however, have demonstrated that L-tryptophan potentiates other tricyclic antidepressants in endogenously depressed patients.

Blier and Bergeron[205] added tryptophan at a dose of 2 g/day to SRI plus pindolol in nine OCD patients and found no further improvement in OCD symptoms. However, when the dose was increased to as high as 8 g/day, researchers noted that seven of the nine patients presented a clinically significant improvement with a decrease in Y-BOCS score of 5 or more. In fact, the mean decrement in Y-BOCS score for the treated patients was 36% over a 6-week period.

Steiner and Fontaine[218] reported five patients who developed a toxic reaction when fluoxetine and tryptophan were combined. All of the patients became agitated, and some developed nausea, worsening of OCD symptoms, abdominal cramps, headache, severe insomnia, aggressive behaviors, chills, and diarrhea. In all of these cases, fluoxetine alone was well tolerated, and the toxic reactions occurred after tryptophan was added in dosages ranging from 1 to 4 g/day. Similar reactions have occurred when clomipramine has been used in close proximity (i.e., within 1 month) to MAOI; these reactions have been compared with the serotonin syndrome seen in animals that have received 5-HT (serotonin) precursors pretreated with a drug that increases the availability of 5-HT in the brain.[219] These cases suggest the need for close monitoring when combinations of potent serotonin-enhancing agents are used.

Tryptophan is currently unavailable in the U.S. market because of its association with a potentially fatal illness called *eosinophilia myalgia syndrome* that appeared to have been caused by a contaminant. Despite identifying the source of the contaminated tryptophan to a single Japanese firm, tryptophan has not yet been reintroduced in most countries, even for use by prescription.

Neuroleptics

Although neuroleptic agents generally are not useful for patients with OCD, of interest is a report by Goodman, et al[24] of an open case series of 13 OCD patients in which eight patients were much improved after pimozide was added to ongoing fluvoxamine. McDougle, et al[220] presented data on the addition of neuroleptic (haloperidol or pimozide) to ongoing fluvoxamine treatment in 17 OCD patients (this study probably includes the same 13 patients as Goodman, et al). Nine of the patients improved to a clinically significant degree. Some of the patients were also taking lithium in combination with fluoxetine during this augmentation trial and its contribution to overall improvement is not clear, but none of the patients had significant improvement prior to neuroleptic augmentation. If neuroleptic augmentation is used, specific target symptoms should be identified, and if there is no improvement within a few months, the neuroleptic should be stopped because of the dangers of irreversible neurologic sequelae with these agents. There is some evidence that patients with tic-spectrum disorders (e.g., OCD and tics) are most likely to respond to neuroleptic augmentation.[221]

When the newer neuroleptics, such as clozapine and risperidone, are used alone without an SSRI, they may actually precipitate or worsen OCD symptoms.[222–228] Most, if not all, of these reports involve patients who had a primary diagnosis of schizophrenia.[220]

In 10 nonschizophrenic patients with classical OCD, clozapine monotherapy was not helpful in any patient,[229] but there was no worsening of OCD symptoms.

However, when risperidone (Risperdol) (1 mg/day), a novel combined D2 and 5-HT$_2$ receptor antagonist, was added to fluvoxamine being taken by three OCD patients who had failed to respond to at least 12 weeks of 250 to 300 mg/day, all three showed a significant improvement in their obsessive-compulsive symptoms as measured by the Y-BOCS with scores decreased by 43% to 65%.[230] The responses were maintained for up to 1-year follow-up. Other than mild or moderate sedation, no side effects were observed. Berigan and Harazin[231] reported a patient with compulsive tattooing who responded when risperidone was added to an SSRI, and Jacobsen[232] reported a small open trial in which risperidone augmentation was helpful.

In a larger open trial in which higher dosages (mean, 2.75 mg/day) were given, Saxena, et al[233] studied 21 OCD patients who had all failed to respond to at least one adequate trial of an SRI. In their study, five patients (24%) experienced side effects (most common, akathisia) that forced discontinuation of risperidone. Of the 16 patients who tolerated combined treatment, 14 (87%) had substantial reductions in obsessive-compulsive symptoms within 3 weeks. Patients with horrific mental imagery had the strongest and fastest response, often within a few days. Patients with comorbid psychotic disorders improved gradually over 2 to 3 weeks, whereas those with comorbid tic disorders had the poorest rate of response and highest rate of akathisia.

There are similar unpublished reports with the newer agent olanzapine (Zyprexia) used at a dose of 5 to 30 mg/day to augment SSRI therapy.

Because these novel antipsychotics cause less severe extrapyramidal side effects than older agents, they may now be preferred as neuroleptic augmenters.

Clinical Use of Augmenting Agents

Table 22-5 outlines some of the factors to consider when a patient fails to respond to antiobsessional medication and Table 22-6 presents a flow sheet of some treatment options that outline which augmenter drugs (Table 22-7) may be used.

Table 22-7 Potential Augmenting Agents for Treatment-Resistant Patients*

Alprazolam
Buspirone
Clonazepam
Clonidine
Clozapine
Cytomel
Haloperidol
Lithium
Methylphenidate
Nifedipine
Olanzapine
Pimozide
Pindolol
Risperidone
Trazodone
Tryptophan

* Add these to an ongoing trial of antiobsessional or antidepressant medication.

Prior to changing any antidepressant medication, it is worth trying to augment the response by adding each augmenting agent for a 2- to 8-week period. Based on published case reports and our anecdotal experience, this strategy will occasionally yield positive results. It would be nice if this chapter could be concluded with a list of preferred augmenting agents with hard data about which drug to use, what dose, and length of trial. Unfortunately, research in this area, although recently flourishing, is still in its infancy and definite recommendations must await further research.

It is important to keep in mind that even if large controlled trials indicate a lack of statistically significant improvement between augmented and nonaugmented groups, patients occasionally improve dramatically in such trials.

LENGTH OF TREATMENT

Patients who respond to pharmacotherapy are often reluctant to discontinue medication for fear that their symptoms will return. Our enthusiasm to withdraw patients from medication is tempered by the realization that there are no adequate guidelines indicating when to stop and which patients are likely to maintain their improvement without medication.

In one study[234] of 35 OCD patients who discontinued fluoxetine after a good response, only eight (23%) relapsed in the first year of follow-up without medication. However, in a double-blind, placebo-controlled study, Pato and colleagues[97] reported that 16 of 18 (89%) patients had substantial recurrence of obsessive-compulsive symptoms by the end of a 7-week placebo period. In addition, 11 patients had a significant increase in depressive symptoms. Treatment duration before discontinuation of clomipramine was not related to the frequency or severity of obsessive-compulsive or depressive symptom reappearance.

It is unclear why these two groups had such drastically different relapse rates. In the Pato, et al[97] study, none of the patients had concomitant behavior therapy, and clomipramine was tapered very rapidly (over 1 week); there was no mention of concomitant treatments by the other group. Behavior therapy that accompanies pharmacotherapy may not only increase the extent of symptom reduction but also may enhance the persistence of improvement after treatment discontinues. It seems unlikely that patients taking clomipramine would be more likely to relapse than those taking fluoxetine, but this is one possible explanation for the differences.

Based on clinical wisdom, many clinicians will attempt to keep significantly symptomatic patients on medication for 1 full year despite symptom reduction, often at a much-reduced dosage than was required for acute treatment. Medications should be very gradually tapered, perhaps by as little as 10 mg of fluoxetine or 50 mg of clomipramine every 2 months. When patients are doing well, it is important for them to undergo intensive behavior therapy. These recommendations are based on anecdotal evidence; definitive answers concerning the role of behavior therapy and rate of medication tapering in preventing relapse await further controlled studies.

MANAGING SEXUAL SIDE EFFECTS

Although the positive effects of SSRIs, clomipramine, and MAOIs are now well documented, there is a cost in terms of side effects. It is clear that more than 35% of patients on these drugs experience difficulties with sexual functioning. These problems usually involve diminished libido (although the opposite occasionally occurs) or orgasm problems in both genders. In men, inability to maintain an erection or even complete impotence may occur.

If the clinician does not specifically ask about sexual difficulties, it may appear that these side effects are quite rare, because patients are often embarrassed or more commonly, they do not think to blame medication for these problems and may attribute them to difficulties in their relationships. Sexual difficulties may be an unspoken cause of treatment noncompliance, and knowledge of the patient's sexual life may be a critical variable in drug compliance. To illustrate the magnitude of these problems, Monteiro[69] studied clomipramine and found that 96% of patients who took the drug developed anorgasmia. However, when a sexual dysfunction questionnaire was administered, only 36% of the 96% reported any type of sexual problem. When fluoxetine, sertraline, and paroxetine were first introduced, the reported incidence of sexual dysfunction was 2% to 9%; after careful questioning and improved case reporting, the incidence is now 30% to 40%.

It is not completely clear what the mechanism of these sexual difficulties is, but most of the evidence for anorgasmia supports the hypothesis that increased serotonergic activity is inhibitory to ejaculation and orgasm. The various serotonin-receptor subtypes may have different effects on sexual functioning; in particular, 5-HT_2 receptors are probably inhibitory, whereas other subtypes may be excitatory. This could account for the paradoxical effect of spontaneous orgasm in a small number of patients who have taken fluoxetine and clomipramine, although both of these drugs cause extreme difficulty with ejaculation in the typical patient. These inconsistent effects may be explained by activation of certain receptors in some, but not all, patients.[235]

The previous effects can sometimes be reversed by medication like cyproheptadine, a drug with antiserotonergic action, as shown in a number of case reports[236–240] and one double-blind study.[241] However, cyproheptadine can reverse the antidepressant effects of SSRIs,[239] and probably antiobsessional effects as well. In addition, it has significant sedative properties.

Recent reports[242,243] suggest that adding buspirone, a partial agonist of the 5-HT_{1A} autoreceptor, may have a beneficial effect of decreasing or reversing sexual dysfunctions induced by SSRIs.

Yohimbine, an alpha_2-adrenergic antagonist, also has been helpful for anorgasmia precipitated by SSRIs. It is probably best not to use in patients with comorbid panic disorder, excessive agitation, or hypertension.[235,243]

Bupropion is believed to have a predominantly adrenergic mechanism of action, and it has been reported to be successful in reversing fluoxetine-induced anorgasmia. Of interest, bupropion increases the sexual fantasy life in a cohort of women with hypoactive sexual desire; using the drug also may have a central effect that enhances libido as well as a peripheral effect that reverses SSRI–induced sexual dysfunction.[235]

In various case reports, dextroamphetamine, methylphenidate,[244] amantadine,[245–247] and even ginseng have all been useful for reversing anorgasmia.[235]

Reynolds[248] reported that nefazodone (Serzone), a drug with less than a 1% incidence of anorgasmia, partially reversed sertraline-induced anorgasmia in a 31-year-old man at a dose of 100 mg/day; lower doses were not helpful. At 150 mg taken 60 minutes before intercourse, the patient had a return of normal sexual functioning. At 6-month follow-up, the patient had no ill effects from the occasional addition of nefazodone to his continuing sertraline therapy. Reynolds noted that nefazodone has a relatively short half-life of only 2 to 4 hours and reaches peak serum levels 1 hour after oral dosing.

Sexual difficulties are sometimes managed through "drug holidays," in which patients are allowed to omit medications on the weekends to allow sexual activity. This practice may work when drugs are used that have a short half-life, such as sertraline, paroxetine, clomipramine, and fluvoxamine, but it will not work with drugs that have a very long half-life, such as fluoxetine.

A number of patients with drug-induced sexual dysfunction can be helped by a little-known technique of injection of the prostaglandin alprostadil into the corpus cavernosum of the penis (Caverject, Upjohn). This can produce an erection in some men with erectile dysfunction. Most men claim that this injection with a small-bore needle is almost painless. However, a recent report of using a pellet or microsuppository formulation that is used intraurethrally (MUSE [Medicated Urethral System for Erection] - Vivus) suggests that this technique may work as well without the need for injection. This is marketed as a sterile foil pouch containing a pellet 1.4 mm in diameter and 3 or 6 mm long within the stem of a hollow applicator, which is inserted 3 cm deep into the urethra. Pressing a button pushes the pellet into the urethra. In a double-blind, controlled trial of 461 alprostadil-treated patients, 299 (65%) reported that they had achieved successful intercourse at least once, compared with 95 (19%) of 500 patients who inserted placebo pellets. Results were similar, regardless of age or cause of impotence.[249] MUSE comes in four strengths that range in cost from $114 to $138 for 6 units.[250] The physician must determine the minimal effective dosage and check for hypotension before prescribing the drug for home use, because there is approximately a 3% incidence of hypotension when the agent is first used.

In terms of patient management, some guidelines can be gleaned from the available literature. First, it is crucial to elicit a reasonable patient sexual history and ask directly about difficulties with libido (sexual drive), orgasm, erection, and satisfaction with sexual activity. Be clear with patients up front that anti-obsessional and antidepressant medications are often associated with sexual difficulties. When identified, sexual problems sometimes can be lessened with simple dose reduction. Occasionally, these side effects diminish over time, but by no means in the majority of patients. Because there are now a number of effective antiobsessional drugs, it may be worth trying a switch to another drug; however, if patients have had a good response, they may be reluctant to do this. Patients may have sexual difficulties when taking one or two antiob-sessional agents and yet perform normally on others.

If for some reason you or the patient do not want to change the medication, several possible alternatives exist. Yohimbine is useful for anorgasmia except in patients with panic disorder, excessive agitation, or hypertension; it can be given at a dose of 10.8 mg (2 tablets) approximately 1 hour before intended intercourse. Other experts have recommended chronic use of yohimbine at 5.4 mg given three times a day.[235] Cyproheptadine also can be used on an as-needed basis, but it often causes drowsiness in patients. There also is the concern that it may reverse antiobsessional and antidepressant drug effects. Amantadine has been used on an as-needed basis and may be worth a try. Bupropion, given at a dose of 75 to 100 mg daily may correct SSRI–induced sexual dysfunction. If for some reason the patient cannot tolerate bupropion, 50 to 100 mg of trazodone can be given daily, especially for patients who have difficulties in developing and maintaining an erection.[235]

Sometimes combinations of these agents are used. For example, one report[235] advocated using bupropion starting at 37.5 mg on a regular basis (not as needed) and increasing the dose to 75 mg daily, sometimes in combination with 5.4 mg of yohimbine daily. Also, 10 mg of methylphenidate can be given daily on occasion, with beneficial results. Others recommend pemoline instead of methylphenidate as an adjunct, because this drug often reduces orgasm problems and has a half-life of 10 to 12 hours.

Caverject and MUSE systems may be helpful for some patients. More and more drug holidays are being advocated for the shorter-acting agents.

Above all, it is important to note the empirical nature of treating sexual difficulties and the need for flexibility (Table 22-8). Multiple approaches, including biologic and psychosocial, in an alliance with the physician, patient, and sexual partner, are required. There is no way to determine in advance which patients will have sexual difficulties and which approach will help them function. Several drugs and combinations may have to be tried. It also is important to monitor any concomitant medical problems or other medications that may have an effect on sexual functioning.

SUMMARY

There are algorithmic approaches[251] and consensus opinions[252] on methods of treating patients with OCD. It is important to keep in mind that the most likely effective augmenting tactic for any drug is to add concomitant behavior

Table 22-8 Management of Sexual Side Effects of Antiobsessional Drugs

Nonpharmacologic approaches
  Drug holidays (stop drug Friday and Saturday) for Zoloft, Paxil, Anafranil, and Luvox
  Not helpful for Prozac
Pharmacologic treatments
  Yohimbine (Yocan)
  Bupropion (Wellbutrin)
  Buspirone (Buspar)
  Cyproheptadine (Periactin)
  Dextroamphetamine (Dexedrine)
  Methylphenidate (Ritalin)
  Amantadine (Symmetrel)
  Nefazodone (Serzone)
Injection into penis of alprostadil (Caverject)
Insertion of suppository into penile urethra (MUSE)

therapy consisting of ERP. As in patients with treatment-resistant depressions, augmentation strategies are worth trying; that is, adding another drug to the treatment regimen when the patient has had no response or only a partial response to an initial drug. Prior to changing any antidepressant medication, it may be useful to add augmenting agents for a 2- to 8-week period each. Based on case reports and our anecdotal experience, this strategy will occasionally yield positive results. Although the overall percentage of responsive patients is small, occasionally patients have shown quite dramatic improvement, which justifies such trials before switching to another drug. Table 22-6 outlines one way of ordering the treatment options. Unfortunately, the optimum augmentation strategies remain undetermined, but much research is ongoing.

REFERENCES

1. White K, Cole J: Pharmacotherapy. In Bellack AS, Hersen M, editors: *Handbook of comparative treatments*, New York, 1990, John Wiley and Sons.
2. Jenike MA: Health care reform for Americans with severe mental illnesses: Report of the National Advisory Mental Health Council: Obsessive-compulsive disorder: Efficacy of specific treatments as assessed by controlled trials, *Psychopharmacol Bull* 29:487–499, 1993.
3. Goodman WK, Rasmussen SA, Foa EB, Price LH: Obsessive-compulsive disorder. In Prien RF, Robinson DS, editors: *Clinical evaluation of psychotropic drugs: Principles and guidelines*, New York, 1994, Raven Press.
4. Dolberg OT, Iancu I, Sasson Y, Zohar J: The pathogenesis and treatment of obsessive compulsive disorder, *Clin Neuropharmacol* 19:129–147, 1996.
5. Goodwin DW, Guze SB, Robins E: Follow-up studies in obsessional neurosis, *Arch Gen Psychiatry* 20:182–187, 1969.

6. Kendell RE, Discipio WJ: Obsessional symptoms and obsessional personality traits in patients with depressive illness, *Psychol Med* 1:65–72, 1970.
7. Vangaard T: Atypical endogenous depression, *Acta Psychiatr Scand Suppl* 267: 5–56, 1976.
8. Black A: The natural history of obsessional neurosis. In Beech HR, editor: *Obsessional states*, London, 1974, Methuen and Co.
9. Jenike MA, Surman OS, Cassem NH, et al: Monoamine oxidase inhibitors in obsessive-compulsive disorder, *J Clin Psychiatry* 44:131–132, 1983.
10. Insel TR, editor: *New findings in obsessive-compulsive disorder,* Washington, 1984, APA Press.
11. Geissman P, Kammerer T: L'imipramine dans la neurose obsessionelle: Etude de 39 cas, *Encephale* 53:369–382, 1964.
12. Angst J, Theobald W: *Tofranil,* Berne, 1980, Verlag Stampfl, pp 11–32.
13. Hussain MZ, Ahad A: Treatment of obsessive compulsive neurosis, *Can Med Assoc J* 103:648–650, 1970.
14. Turner SM, Hersen M, Bellack AS, et al: Behavioral and pharmacological treatment of obsessive-compulsive disorders, *J Nerv Ment Dis* 168:651–657, 1980.
15. Snyder S: Amitriptyline therapy of obsessive-compulsive neurosis, *J Clin Psychiatry* 41:286–289, 1980.
16. Ananth J, Solyom L, Solyom C, et al: Doxepin in the treatment of obsessive compulsive neurosis, *Psychosomatics* 16:185–187, 1975.
17. Bauer G, Nowak H: Doxepine: ein neues Antidepressivum Wirkungs-Verleich mit Amitriptyline, *Arzneimittelforsch* 19:1642–1646, 1969.
18. Gross M, Slater E, Roth M, editors: *Clinical psychiatry*, 1969, Bailliere Tindall and Casel.
19. Kahn RS, Westenberg HGM, Jolles J: Zimeledine treatment of obsessive-compulsive disorder, *Acta Psychiatr Scand* 69:259–261, 1984.
20. Fontaine R, Chouinard G, Iny L: An open clinical trial of zimelidine in the treatment of obsessive compulsive disorder, *Curr Ther Res* 37:326–332, 1985.
21. Prasad A: A double blind study of imipramine versus zimelidine in treatment of obsessive compulsive neurosis, *Pharmacopsychiatry* 17:61–62, 1984.
22. Lydiard RB: Obsessive-compulsive disorder successfully treated with trazodone, *Psychosomatics* 27:858–859, 1986.
23. Kim SW: Trazodone in the treatment of obsessive-compulsive disorder: A case report, *J Clin Psychopharmacol* 7:278–279, 1987.
24. Goodman WK, Price LH, Rasmussen SA, et al: Efficacy of fluvoxamine in obsessive-compulsive disorder: A double-blind comparison with placebo, *Arch Gen Psychiatry* 46:36–44, 1989.
25. White K, Keck PE, Lipinski J: Serotonin-uptake inhibitors in obsessive-compulsive disorder: A case report, *Comp Psychiatry* 27:211–214, 1986.
26. Foa EB, Steketee G, Kozak MJ, et al: Effects of imipramine on depression and obsessive-compulsive symptoms, *Psychiatr Res* 21:123–136, 1987.
27. Foa EB, Steketee G, Kozak MJ, et al: Imipramine and placebo in the treatment of obsessive-compulsives: Their effect on depression and on obsessional symptoms, *Psychopharmacol Bull* 23:8–11, 1987.
28. Lopez-Ibor JJ: Intravenous infusions of monochlorimipramine. Technique and results. In Proceedings of the Sixth International Congress of the CINP, Taragona,

April 1968. Exerpta Medica Foundation Int Congress Series No. 180, Amsterdam, 1969, pp 519–521.

29. DeVorvrie GV: Anafranil (G34586) in obsessive neurosis, *Acta Neurol Belg* 68:787–792, 1968.
30. Jiminez F: A clinical study of Anafranil in depressive, obsessional and schizophrenic patients, *Folia Neuropsiquat Sur Este Esp* 3:189, 1968.
31. Grabowski JR: Treatment of severe depression and obsessive depression with G3486, *Folia Med* 57:265–270, 1968.
32. Fernandez CE, Lopez-Ibor JJ: Monochlorimipramine in the treatment of psychiatric patients resistant to other therapies, *Actas Luso Esp Neurol Psiquiatr* 26: 119–147, 1967.
33. Rack PH: Clinical experience in the treatment of obsessed states, *J Int Med Res* 5(suppl 5):81–96, 1977.
34. Marshall WK, Micev V: Clomipramine in the treatment of obsessional illness and phobic anxiety states, *J Int Med Res* 1:403–412, 1973.
35. Yaryura-Tobias JA, Neziroglu MS, Bergman L: Clomipramine for obsessive compulsive neurosis: An organic approach, *Curr Ther Res* 20:541–548, 1976.
36. Yaryura-Tobias JA, Neziroglu MS: The action of clorimipramine in obsessive compulsive neurosis: A pilot study, *Curr Ther Res* 17:1, 1975.
37. Waxman D: A clinical trial of clomipramine and diazepam in the treatment of phobic and obsessional illness, *J Int Med Res* 5(suppl 5):99–110, 1977.
38. Coombe PD: Clomipramine and severe obsessive-compulsive neurosis, *Aust NZ J Psychiatry* 16:293–297, 1982.
39. Wyndowc J, Solyom L, Ananth J: Anafranil in obsessive compulsive neurosis, *Curr Ther Res* 18:611–617, 1975.
40. Capstick N: Clinical experience in the treatment of obsessional states, *J Int Med Res* 5(suppl 5):71, 1977.
41. Ananth J, Pecknold JC, van den Steen N, et al: Double-blind study of clomipramine and amitriptyline in obsessive neurosis, *Prog Neuropsychopharmacol* 5:257–262, 1981.
42. Stroebel CF, Szarek BL, Glueck BC: Use of clomipramine in treatment of obsessive-compulsive symptomatology, *J Clin Psychopharmacol* 4:98–100, 1984.
43. Thoren P, Åsberg M, Cronholm B, et al: Clomipramine treatment of obsessive compulsive disorder. I. A controlled clinical trial, *Arch Gen Psychiatry* 37:1281–1285, 1980.
44. Thoren P, Åsberg M, Cronholm B, et al: Clomipramine treatment of obsessive compulsive disorder. II, *Arch Gen Psychiatry* 37:1286–1294, 1980a.
45. Marks IM, Stern RS, Mawson D, et al: Clomipramine and exposure for obsessive compulsive rituals, *Br J Psychiatry* 136:1–25, 1980.
46. Montgomery SA: Clomipramine in obsessional neurosis: A placebo controlled trial, *Pharmacol Med* 1:189–192, 1980.
47. Ananth J, Solyom L, Bryntwick S, et al: Clomipramine therapy for obsessive compulsive neurosis, *Am J Psychiatry* 136:700–720, 1979.
48. Insel TR, Murphy DL, Cohen RM, et al: Obsessive-compulsive disorder. A double-blind trial of clomipramine and clorgyline, *Arch Gen Psychiatry* 40:605–612, 1983.
49. Jenike MA, Baer L, Summergrad P, et al: Obsessive-compulsive disorder: A double-blind, placebo-controlled trial of clomipramine in 30 patients, *Am J Psychiatry* 146:1328–1330, 1989.

50. DeVeaugh-Geiss J, Landau P, Katz R: Treatment of obsessive compulsive disorder with clomipramine, *Psych Ann* 19:97–101, 1989.
51. Greist JH, Jefferson JW, Rosenfeld R, et al: Clomipramine and obsessive-compulsive disorder: A placebo-controlled double-blind study in 32 patients, *J Clin Psychiatry,* in press, 1990.
52. Rapoport J, Elkins R, Mikkelsen A, et al: Clinical controlled trial of clorimipramine in adolescents with obsessive-compulsive disorder, *Psychopharmacol Bull* 3:61–63, 1980.
53. Carey RJ, Baer L, Jenike MA, et al: MMPI correlates of obsessive-compulsive disorder, *J Clin Psychiatry* 47:371–372, 1986.
54. Reference deleted in proofs.
55. Asberg M, Montgomery SA, Perris C, et al: A comprehensive psychopathological rating scale, *Acta Psychiatr Scand Suppl* 271:5–27, 1978.
56. Cooper J: The Leyton Obsessional Inventory, *Psychol Med* 1:48–64, 1970.
57. Asberg M, Thoren P, Bertilsson L: Psychopharmacologic treatment of obsessive-compulsive disorder. Clomipramine treatment of obsessive disorder—biochemical and clinical aspects, *Psychopharmacol Bull* 18:13–21, 1982.
58. Bertilsson L, Asberg M, Thoren P: Differential effect of clorimipramine and nor-triptyline on cerebrospinal fluid amines and metabolites of serotonin and noradrenaline in depression, *Eur J Clin Pharmacol* 7:365–368, 1974.
59. Bertilsson L, Tuck JR, Siwers B: Biochemical effects of zimelidine in man, *Eur J Clin Pharmacol* 18:483–487, 1980.
60. Traskman L, Asberg M, Bertilsson L, et al: Plasma levels of clorimipramine and its demethyl-metabolite during treatment of depression. Differential biochemical and clinical effects of the two compounds. *Clin Pharmacol Ther* 26:600–610, 1979.
61. Stern RS, Marks IM, Mawson D, et al: Clomipramine and exposure for compulsive rituals: II. Plasma levels, side effects and outcome, *Br J Psychiatry* 136: 161–166, 1980.
62. Warneke LB: The use of intravenous chlorimipramine in the treatment of obsessive compulsive disorder, *Can J Psychiatry* 29:135–141, 1984.
63. Warneke LB: Intravenous chlorimipramine in the treatment of obsessional disorder in adolescence: Case report, *J Clin Psychiatry* 46:100–103, 1985.
64. Warneke LB: Intravenous chlorimipramine in obsessive-compulsive disorder, *Can J Psychiatry* 34:853–859, 1989.
65. Fallon BA, Campeas R, Schneier FR, et al: Open trial of intravenous clomipramine in five treatment-refractory patients with obsessive-compulsive disorder, *J Neuropsychiatr Clin Neurosci* 4:70–75, 1992.
66. Koran LM, Faravelli C, Pallanti S: Intravenous clomipramine for obsessive-compulsive disorder, *J Clin Psychopharmacol* 14:216–218, 1994.
67. Sallee FR, Pollock BG, Perel JM, et al: Intravenous pulse loading of clomipramine in adolescents with depression, *Psychopharmacol Bull* 25:114–118, 1989.
68. Koran LM, Salee FR, Pallanti S: Rapid benefit of intravenous pulse loading of clomipramine in obsessive-compulsive disorder, *Am J Psychiatry* 154:396–401, 1997.
69. Monteiro WO, Noshirvani HF, Marks IM, et al: Anorgasmia from clomipramine in obsessive-compulsive disorder: A controlled trial, *Br J Psychiatry* 151:107–112, 1987.

70. Turner SM, Jacob RG, Beidel DC, et al: Fluoxetine treatment of obsessive-compulsive disorder, *J Clin Psychopharmacol* 5:207–212, 1985.
71. Fontaine R, Chouinard G: An open clinical trial of fluoxetine in the treatment of obsessive-compulsive disorder, *J Clin Psychopharmacol* 6:98–101, 1986.
72. Jenike MA, Buttolph L, Baer L, et al: Fluoxetine in obsessive-compulsive disorder: A positive open trial, *Am J Psychiatry* 146:909–911, 1989a.
73. Pigott TA, Pato MT, Bernstein SE: Controlled comparisons of clomipramine and fluoxetine in the treatment of obsessive compulsive disorder. Behavioral and biological results, *Arch Gen Psychiatry* 47:926–932, 1990.
74. Montgomery SA, McIntyre A, Osterheider M, et al: A double-blind, placebo-controlled study of fluoxetine in patients with DSM-III-R obsessive-compulsive disorder. The Lilly European OCD Study Group, *Eur Neuropsychopharmacol* 3:143–152, 1993.
75. Tollefson GD, Rampey AH, Potvin JH, et al: A multicenter investigation of fixed-dose fluoxetine in the treatment of obsessive-compulsive disorder, *Arch Gen Psychiatry* 51:559–567, 1994.
76. Coleman BS, Block BA: Fluvoxamine maleate, a serotonergic antidepressant: A comparison with chlorimipramine, *Prog Neuropsychopharmacol Biol Psychiatry* 6:475–478, 1982.
77. Itil TM, Shrivastava RK, Mukherjee S, et al: A double-blind placebo-controlled study of fluvoxamine and imipramine in out-patients with primary depression, *Br J Clin Pharmacol* 15:433S–438S, 1983.
78. Guy W, Wilson WH, Ban TA, et al: A double-blind clinical trial of fluvoxamine and imipramine in patients with primary depression, *Drug Dev Res* 4:143–153, 1984.
79. Guelfi JD, Dreyfus JF, Pichot P: A double-blind controlled clinical trial comparing fluvoxamine with imipramine, *Br J Clin Pharmacol* 15:411S–417S, 1983.
80. Reference deleted in proofs.
81. Perse TL, Greist JH, Jefferson JW, et al: Fluvoxamine treatment of obsessive-compulsive disorder, *Am J Psychiatry* 144:1543–1548, 1987.
82. Goodman WK, Price LH, Rasmussen SA, et al: The Yale-Brown Obsessive Compulsive Scale (Y-BOCS): Part I. Development, use, and reliability, *Arch Gen Psychiatry* 46:1006–1011, 1989.
83. Jenike MA, Baer L, Greist JH: Clomipramine vs. fluoxetine in obsessive-compulsive disorder: A retrospective comparison of side effects and efficacy, *J Clin Psychopharmacol* 10:122–124, 1990.
84. Hamilton M: A rating scale for depression, *J Neurol Neurosurg Psychiatry* 23:56–62, 1960.
85. Goodman WK, Kozak MJ, Liebowitz M, White KL: Treatment of obsessive-compulsive disorder with fluvoxamine: A multicentre, double-blind, placebo-controlled trial, *Int Clin Psychopharmacol* 11:21–29, 1996.
86. Chouinard G, Goodman W, Greist J, et al: Results of a double-blind placebo controlled trial using a new serotonin uptake inhibitor, sertraline, in obsessive-compulsive disorder, *Psychopharmacol Bull* 26:279–284, 1991.
87. Greist J, Chouinard G, DuBoff E, et al: Double-blind comparison of three doses of sertraline and placebo in the treatment of outpatients with obsessive compulsive disorder, 9th World Congress of Psychiatry, June 1993, Rio de Janeiro.
88. Wheadon DE, Bushnell WD, Steiner M: A fixed dose comparison of 20, 40, or

60 mg of paroxetine to placebo in the treatment of OCD. Presented at the 1993 Annual Meeting of the American College of Neuropsychopharmacology, December 1993, Honolulu.

89. Steiner M, Oakes R, Gergel IP, Wheadon DE: Predictors of response to paroxetine therapy in OCD. Presented at the 1994 Annual Meeting, American Psychiatric Association, May 1994, Philadelphia.

90. Piccinelli M, Pini S, Bellantuono C, Wilkinson G: Efficacy of drug treatment in obsessive compulsive disorder: A meta-analytic review, *Br J Psychiatry* 166: 424–443, 1995.

91. Freeman CPL, Trimble MR, Deatin JFK, et al: Fluvoxamine versus clomipramine in the treatment of OCD: A multicenter, randomized, double-blind, parallel-group comparison, *J Clin Psychiatry* 55:301–305, 1994.

92. Bisserbe JC, Wiseman RL, Goldberg MS, et al: A double-blind comparison of sertraline and clomipramine in outpatients with OCD. American Psychiatric Association Annual Meeting, 1995, New Research Abstracts 173.

93. Jefferson JW, Greist JH: The pharmacotherapy of obsessive-compulsive disorder, *Psychiatr Ann* 26:202–209, 1996.

94. Greist JH, Jefferson JW, Kobak KA, et al: Efficacy and tolerability of serotonin transport inhibitors in obsessive-compulsive disorder, *Arch Gen Psychiatry* 52:53–60, 1995.

95. Rasmussen SA, Goodman WK, Greist JH, et al: Fluvoxamine in the treatment of obsessive-compulsive disorder: A multicenter double-blind placebo-controlled study in outpatients, *Am J Psychiatry,* in press.

96. Rasmussen SA, Eisen JL, Pato MT: Current issues in the pharmacologic management of obsessive compulsive disorder, *J Clin Psychiatry* 54(suppl 6):4–9, 1993.

97. Pato MT, Zohar-Kadouch R, Zohar J, et al: Return of symptoms after discontinuation of clomipramine in patients with obsessive-compulsive disorder, *Am J Psychiatry* 145:1521–1525, 1988.

98. Hermesh H, Aizenberg D, Munitz H: Trazodone treatment of clomipramine-resistant obsessive-compulsive disorder, *Clin Neuropharmacol* 13:322–328, 1990.

99. Pigott TA, L'Heureux F, Rubenstein CS, et al: Double-blind, placebo-controlled study of trazodone in patients with obsessive-compulsive disorder, *J Clin Psychopharmacol* 12:156–162, 1992.

100. Joel SW: Twenty month study of iproniazid therapy, *Dis Nerv Syst* 20:1–4, 1959.

101. Annesley PT: Nardil response in a chronic obsessive compulsive, *Br J Psychiatry* 115:748, 1969.

102. Jain VK, Swinson RP, Thomas JE: Phenelzine in obsessional neurosis, *Br J Psychiatry* 117:237–238, 1970.

103. Swinson RP: Response to tranylcypromine and thought stopping in obsessional disorder, *Br J Psychiatry* 144:425–427, 1984.

104. Rihmer Z, Szantok, Arato M, et al: Response of phobic disorders with obsessive symptoms to MAO inhibitors, *Am J Psychiatry* 139:1374, 1982.

105. Jenike MA: Rapid response of severe obsessive-compulsive disorder to tranylcypromine, *Am J Psychiatry* 138:1249–1250, 1981.

106. Insel TR, Pickar D: Naloxone administration in obsessive-compulsive disorder: Report of two cases, *Am J Psychiatry* 140:1219–1220, 1983.

107. Vallejo J, Olivaes J, Marcos T, et al: Clomipramine versus phenelzine in obsessive compulsive disorder: A controlled clinical trial, *Br J Psychiatry* 161:665–670, 1992.

108. Jenike MA, Baer L, Minichiello WE, et al: A placebo controlled trial of fluoxetine and phenelzine for obsessive compulsive disorder, *Am J Psychiatry* 154:1261–1264, 1997.

109. Stern TA, Jenike MA: Treatment of obsessive-compulsive disorder with lithium carbonate, *Psychosomatics* 24:671–673, 1983.

110. Geisler A, Schou M: Lithium ved tvangsneuroser, *Nord Psychiatr Tidsskr* 23:493–495, 1970.

111. Forssman H, Walinder J: Lithium treatment of atypical indication, *Acta Psychiatr Scand Suppl* 207:34–40, 1969.

112. Van Putten T, Sander DG: Lithium in treatment failures, *J Nerv Ment Dis* 161:255–264, 1975.

113. Baer L, Minichiello WE, Jenike MA: Behavioral treatment of obsessive-compulsive disorder with concomitant bipolar affective disorder, *Am J Psychiatry* 142:358–360, 1985.

114. Jenike MA, Brotman AW: The EEG in obsessive compulsive disorder, *J Clin Psychiatry* 45:122–124, 1984.

115. Joffe RT, Swinson RP: Carbamazepine in obsessive-compulsive disorder, *Biol Psychiatry* 22:1169–1171, 1987.

116. Khanna S: Carbamazepine in obsessive-compulsive disorder, *Clin Neuropharmacol* 11:478–481, 1988.

117. Jenike MA: Obsessive-compulsive disorder: A question of a neurologic lesion, *Comp Psychiatry* 25:298–304, 1984.

118. Brickner RM, Rosen AA, Munro R: Physiological aspects of the obsessive state, *Psychosom Med* 2:369–383, 1940.

119. Hill A, Mitchell W: Epileptic amnesia, *Folia Psychiatr Neurol Jpn* 56:718, 1953.

120. Epstein AW, Bailine SH: Sleep and dream studies in obsessional neurosis with particular reference to epileptic states, *Biol Psychiatry* 3:149–158, 1971.

121. Pacella BL, Polantin P, Nagler SH: Clinical and EEG studies in obsessive compulsive states, *Am J Psychiatry* 100:830–838, 1944.

122. McElroy SL, Keck PE, Pope HG: Sodium valproate: Its use in primary psychiatric disorders, *J Clin Psychopharmacol* 7:16–24, 1987.

123. McElroy SL, Pope HG, editors: *Use of anticonvulsants in psychiatry: Recent advances,* Clifton, 1988, Oxford Health Care.

124. Bodkin A, White K: Clonazepam in the treatment of obsessive compulsive disorder, *J Clin Psychiatry* 50:265–256, 1989.

125. O'Sullivan R, Jenike MA, Dreyfus: personal communication, 1997.

126. Altschuler M: Massive doses of trifluoperazine in the treatment of compulsive rituals, *Am J Psychiatry* 119:367, 1962.

127. O'Regan B: Treatment of obsessive compulsive disorder (letter), *Can Med Assoc J* 103:648–650, 1970.

128. O'Regan B: Treatment of obsessive compulsive neurosis with haloperidol, *Can Med Assoc J* 103:167–168, 1970a.

129. Rivers-Buckeley N, Hollender MH: Successful treatment of obsessive-compulsive disorder with loxapine, *Am J Psychiatry* 139:1345–1346, 1982.

130. Breitner C: Drug therapy in obsessional states and other psychiatric problems, *Dis Nerv Syst* 21(suppl):31–35, 1960.

131. Bethume HC: A new compound in the treatment of severe anxiety states: Report on the use of diazepam, *N Engl J Med* 63:153–156, 1964.

132. Tesar GE, Jenike MA: Alprazolam as treatment for a case of obsessive-compulsive disorder, *Am J Psychiatry* 141:689–690, 1984.

133. Tollefson G: Alprazolam in the treatment of obsessive symptoms, *J Clin Psychopharmacol* 5:39–42, 1985.

134. Hewlett WA, Vinogradov S, Argas WS: Clonazepam treatment of obsessions and compulsions, *J Clin Psychiatry* 51:158–161, 1990.

135. Venkoba Rao A: A controlled trial with Valium in obsessive compulsive states, *J Indian Med Assoc* 42:564–567, 1964.

136. Orvin GH: Treatment of the phobic obsessive compulsive patient with oxazepam, an improved benzodiazepine compound, *Psychosomatics* 8:278–280, 1967.

137. Hewlett WA, Vinogradov S, Agras WS: Clomipramine, clonazepam, and clonidine treatment of obsessive-compulsive disorder, *J Clin Psychopharmacol* 12(6): 420–430, 1992.

138. Jenike MA, Baer L: Buspirone in obsessive-compulsive disorder: An open trial, *Am J Psychiatry* 145:1285–1286, 1988.

139. Pato MT, Pigott TA, Hill JL, et al: Clomipramine versus buspirone in OCD: A controlled trial. New Research Symposium, American Psychiatric Association Meeting, May 1989, San Francisco.

140. Pato MT, Pigott TA, Hill JL, et al: Controlled comparison of buspirone and clomipramine in obsessive compulsive disorder, *Am J Psychiatry* 148:127–129, 1991.

141. Yaryura-Tobias JA, Bhagavan HN: L-tryptophan in obsessive-compulsive disorders, *Am J Psychiatry* 134:1298–1299, 1977.

142. Yaryura-Tobias JA, Neziroglu MS, Bhagavan H: Obsessive-compulsive disorders: A serotonergic hypothesis. In Saletu B, Berner P, Hollister L, editors: *Neuropsychopharmacology: Proceedings of the 11th Congress of the CINP,* Oxford, 1979, Pergamon Press, pp 117–125.

143. Yaryura-Tobias JA: Tryptophan may be adjuvant to obsessive-compulsive therapy, *Clin Psychiatr News* p 16, September 1981.

144. Cole JO, Hartmann E, Brigham P: L-tryptophan: Clinical studies, *McLean Hosp J* 5:37–71, 1980.

145. Jenike MA, Baer L, Minichiello WE, et al: Concomitant obsessive-compulsive disorder and schizotypal personality disorder, *Am J Psychiatry* 143:530–533, 1986.

146. Rasmussen SA, Goodman WK, Woods SW, et al: Effects of yohimbine in obsessive compulsive disorder, *Psychopharmacology* 93:308–313, 1987.

147. Ansseau M, Legros JJ, Mormont C, et al: Intranasal oxytocin in obsessive-compulsive disorder, *Psychoneuroendocrinology* 12:231–236, 1987.

148. Epperson CN, McDougle CJ, Price LH: Intranasal oxytocin in obsessive compulsive disorder, *Biol Psychiatry* 40:547–549, 1996.

149. Epperson CN, McDougle CJ, Price LH: Intranasal oxytocin in trichotillomania, *Biol Psychiatry* 40:559–561, 1996a.

150. Pickar D, Cohen MR, Nabbed D, et al: Clinical studies of the endogenous opioid system, *Biol Psychiatry* 17:1243–1276, 1982.

151. Sandyk R: Naloxone abolishes obsessive-compulsive behavior in Tourette's syndrome, *Intern J Neurosci* 35:93–94, 1987.
152. Keuler DJ, Altemus M, Michelson D, et al: Behavioral effects of naloxone infusion in obsessive compulsive disorder, *Biol Psychiatry* 40:154–156, 1996.
153. Herman BH, Arthur-Smith A, Hammock MK, et al: Naltrexone decreases self-injurious behavior, *Ann Neurol* 22:550–552, 1987.
154. Bystritsky A, Strausser BP: Treatment of obsessive compulsive cutting behavior with naltrexone, *J Clin Psychiatry* 57:423–424, 1996.
155. Roth AS, Ostroff RB, Hoffman RE: Naltrexone as a treatment for repetitive self-injurious behavior: An open-label trial, *J Clin Psychiatry* 57:233–237, 1996.
156. Carrion VG: Naltrexone for the treatment of trichotillomania: A case report, *J Clin Psychopharmacol* 15:444–445, 1995.
157. Sewell RDE, Lee RL: Opiate receptors, endorphins, and drug therapy, *Postgrad Med J* 56(suppl 1):2530, 1980.
158. Insel TR, Hamilton J, Guttmacher L, et al: D-Amphetamine in obsessive compulsive disorder, *Psychopharmacology* 80:231–235, 1983.
159. Segal DS, Brown RG, Arnsten A, et al: Characteristics of beta endorphin-induced behavioral activation and immobilization. In Usdin E, Bunney WE Jr, Kline NS, editors: *Endorphins in mental health research*, New York, 1979, Oxford University Press.
160. Cohen DJ, Detlor J, Young JG, Shaywitz BA: Clonidine ameliorates Gilles de la Tourette syndrome, *Arch Gen Psychiatry* 37:1350–1357, 1980.
161. Hollander E, Fay M, Liebowitz MR: Clonidine and clomipramine in obsessive-compulsive disorder, *Am J Psychiatry* 145:388–389, 1988.
162. Knesevich JW: Successful treatment of obsessive-compulsive disorder with clonidine, *J Clin Psychopharmacol* 7:278–279, 1982.
163. Vadnal R, Parthasarathy L, Parthasarathy R: Role of inositol in the treatment of psychiatric disorders: basic and clinical aspects, *CNS Drugs* 7(1):6–16, 1997.
164. Hoyter D, Clarke DE, Fozard PR, et al: VII International Union of Pharmacology classification of receptors for 5-hydroxytryptamine (serotonin), *Pharmacol Rev* 46:157–203, 1994.
165. Rahman S, Neumrn RS: Myo-inositol reduces serotonin (5-HT2) receptor induced homologous and heterologous desensitization, *Brain Res* 631:349–351, 1993.
166. Fux M, Levine J, Aviv A, Belmaker RH: Inositol treatment of obsessive compulsive disorder, *Am J Psychiatry* 153:1219–1221, 1996.
167. Depression Guideline Panel: *Depression in Primary Care, Volume 2: Treatment of Major Depression,* Rockville 1993, US Department of Health and Human Services Agency for Health Care Policy and Research, AHCPR Publication 93-0551.
168. Kasvikis Y, Marks IM: Clomipramine in obsessive compulsive ritualizers treated with exposure therapy: Relations between dose, plasma levels, outcome and side effects, *Psychopharmacol* (Berl) 95:113–118, 1988.
169. Mavissakalian MR, Jones B, Olson S, Perel JM: Clomipramine in obsessive compulsive disorder: clinical response and plasma levels, *J Clin Psychopharmacol* 10:261–268, 1990.
170. Flament MF, Rapoport JL, Berg CJ, et al: Clomipramine treatment of childhood obsessive compulsive disorder: A double-blind controlled study, *Arch Gen Psy-*

chiatry 42:977–983, 1985.

171. Greist J, Chouinard G, DuBoff E, et al: Double-blind comparison of three doses of sertraline and placebo in the treatment of outpatients with obsessive compulsive disorder, *Arch Gen Psychiatry* 52:53–60, 1995a.

172. Koran LM, Cain JW, Dominguez RA, et al: Are fluoxetine plasma levels related to outcome in obsessive-compulsive disorder? *Am J Psychiatry* 153;1450–1454, 1996.

173. Foa EB: Failure in treating obsessive-compulsives, *Behav Res Ther* 17:169–176, 1979.

174. Minichiello WE, Baer L, Jenike MA: Schizotypal personality disorder: A poor prognostic indicator for behavior therapy in the treatment of obsessive-compulsive disorder, *J Anx Dis* 1:273–276, 1987.

175. Jenike MA, Baer L, Minichiello WE, et al: Concomitant obsessive-compulsive disorder and schizotypal personality disorder: A poor prognostic indicator, *Arch Gen Psychiatry* 43:296, 1986a.

176. Jenike MA, Baer L, Minichiello WE: *Obsessive-compulsive disorders: Theory and management*, Littleton, 1986b, PSG Publishing.

177. Marks IM: Review of behavioral psychotherapy, I: Obsessive-compulsive disorders, *Am J Psychiatry* 138:584–592, 1981.

178. Lader M, Wing L: Physiological measures in agitated and retarded depressed patients, *J Psychiatr Res* 7:89–100, 1969.

179. Rachman SJ, Hodgson RJ: *Obsessions and compulsions,* Englewood Cliffs, 1980, Prentice-Hall.

180. Solyom L, DiNicola VF, Phil M, et al: Is there an obsessive psychosis? Aetiological and prognostic factors of an atypical form of obsessive-compulsive neurosis, *Can J Psychiatry* 30:372–380, 1985.

181. Foa EB, Goldstein A: Continuous exposure and strict response prevention in the treatment of obsessive-compulsive neurosis, *Behav Ther* 17:169–176, 1978.

182. Rasmussen SA, Tsuang MT: Epidemiology and clinical features of obsessive-compulsive disorder. In Jenike MA, Baer L, Minichiello WE, editors: *Obsessive compulsive disorders: Theory and management*, Littleton, 1986, PSG Publishing, pp 23–44.

183. Baer L, Jenike MA, Ricciardi JN, et al: Standardized assessment of personality disorders in obsessive-compulsive disorder, *Arch Gen Psychiatry,* 47:826–837, 1990.

184. Baer L, Jenike MA, Personality disorders obsessive-compulsive disorders and effect of treatment. In Jenike MA, editor: *Psychiatric Clinics of North America, Obsessional disorders,* Philadelphia, 1992, WB Saunders.

185. Salzman L: *Obsessional personality,* New York, 1969, Science House.

186. Chen YW, Dilsaver SC: Comorbidity for obsessive-compulsive disorder in bipolar and unipolar disorders, *Psychiatr Res* 59:57–64, 1995.

187. Clomipramine Collaborative Study Group: Efficacy of clomipramine in OCD: Results of a multicenter double-blind trial, *Arch Gen Psychiatry* 48:730–738, 1991.

188. DeMontigny C, Grunberg F, Mayer A, et al: Lithium induces rapid relief of depression in tricyclic antidepressant drug non-responders, *Br J Psychiatry* 138: 252–256, 1981.

189. Rasmussen SA: Lithium and tryptophan augmentation in clomipramine-resistant

obsessive-compulsive disorder, *Am J Psychiatry* 141:1283–1285, 1984.

190. Feder R: Lithium augmentation of clomipramine, *J Clin Psychiatry* 49:458, 1988.

191. Eisenberg J, Asnis G: Lithium as an adjunct treatment in obsessive-compulsive disorder, *Am J Psychiatry* 142:662, 1985.

192. Golden RN, Morris JE, Sack DA: Combined lithium-tricyclic treatment of obsessive-compulsive disorder, *Biol Psychiatry* 23:181–185, 1988.

193. Howland RH: Lithium augmentation of fluoxetine in the treatment of OCD and major depression: A case report, *Can J Psychiatry* 36:154–155, 1991.

194. Jenike MA: Augmentation strategies for treatment-resistant obsessive-compulsive disorder, *Harv Rev Psychiatry* 1:17–26, 1993a.

195. McDougle CJ, Price LH, Goodman WK, et al: A controlled trial of lithium augmentation in fluvoxamine-refractory obsessive compulsive disorder: Lack of efficacy, *J Clin Psychopharmacol* 11:175–184, 1991.

196. Pigott TA, Pato MT, L'Heureux F, et al: A controlled comparison of adjuvant lithium carbonate or thyroid hormone in clomipramine-treated patients with obsessive compulsive disorder, *J Clin Psychopharmacol* 11:242–248, 1991.

197. Blier P, deMontigny C: Short-term lithium administration enhances serotonergic neurotransmission electrophysiological evidence in the rat CNS, *Eur J Pharmacol* 113:69–79, 1985.

198. Harvey KV, Balon R: Augmentation with buspirone: A review, *Ann Clin Psychiatry* 7:3:143–147, 1995.

199. Jenike MA, Baer L, Buttolph L: Buspirone augmentation of fluoxetine in patients with obsessive-compulsive disorder, *J Clin Psychiatry* 1:13–14, 1991.

200. Markovitz PJ, Stagno SJ, Calabrese JR: Buspirone augmentation of fluoxetine in obsessive-compulsive disorder, Biological Psychiatry Annual Meeting, May 1989, San Francisco, Abstract #379.

201. Markovitz PJ, Stagno SJ, Calabrese JR: Buspirone augmentation of fluoxetine on obsessive-compulsive disorder, *Am J Psychiatry* 147:798–800, 1990.

202. Alessi N, Bos T: Buspirone augmentation of fluoxetine in a depressed child with obsessive-compulsive disorder, *Am J Psychiatry* 148:1605–1606, 1991.

203. Goodman WK, Price LH, Rasmussen SA, et al: The Yale-Brown Obsessive Compulsive Scale (Y-BOCS): Part II. Validity. *Arch Gen Psychiatry* 46:1012–1018, 1989.

204. Beck AT, Ward CH, Mendelson M: An inventory for measuring depression, *Arch Gen Psychiatry* 41:561–571, 1961.

205. Blier P, Bergeron P: Sequential administration of augmentation strategies in treatment-resistant obsessive-compulsive disorder: Preliminary findings, *Int Clin Psychopharmacol* 11:37–44, 1996.

206. Pigott TA, L'Heureux F, Hill JL, et al: A double-blind study of adjuvant buspirone hydrochloride in clomipramine-treated patients with obsessive-compulsive disorder, *J Clin Psychopharmacol* 12:11–18, 1992.

207. McDougle CJ, Goodman WK, Leckman JF, et al: Limited therapeutic effect of addition of buspirone in fluvoxamine-refractory obsessive compulsive disorder, *Am J Psychiatry* 150:647–649, 1993.

208. Grady TA, Pigott TA, L'Heureux F, et al: Double-blind study of adjuvant buspirone for fluoxetine-treated patients with obsessive compulsive disorder, *Am J Psychiatry* 150:819–821, 1993.

209. Judd FK, Chua P, Lynch C, Norman T: Fenfluramine augmentation of clomipramine treatment of obsessive compulsive disorder, *Aust N Z J Psychiatry* 25: 412–414, 1991.

210. Hollander E, DeCaria CM, Schneier FR, et al: Fenfluramine augmentation of serotonin reuptake blockade antiobsessional treatment, *J Clin Psychiatry* 51:119–123, 1990.

211. Jenike MA: Approaches to the patient with treatment-refractory obsessive-compulsive disorder, *J Clin Psychiatry* 51(2, suppl):15–21, 1990c.

212. Jenike MA: Management of patients with treatment-resistant obsessive-compulsive disorder. In Pato MT, Zohar J, editors: *Obsessive-compulsive disorders*, Washington, 1991, APA Press, pp 135–156.

213. Simeon JG, Thatte S, Wiggins D: Treatment of adolescent obsessive-compulsive disorder with a clomipramine-fluoxetine combination, *Psychopharmacol Bull* 26:285–290, 1990.

214. Szegedi A, Wetzel H, Leal M, et al: Combination treatment with clomipramine and fluvoxamine: Drug monitoring, safety, and tolerability data, *J Clin Psychiatry* 57:257–264, 1996.

215. Artigas F, Perez V, Alvarez E: Pindolol induces a rapid improvement of depressed patients treated with serotonin uptake inhibitors, *Arch Gen Psychiatry* 51:248–251, 1994.

216. Blier P, Bergeron R: Effectiveness of pindolol with selected antidepressant drugs in the treatment of major depression, *J Clin Psychopharmacol* 15:217–222, 1995.

217. Walinder J, Skott A, Carlsson A, et al: Potentiation of the antidepressant action of clomipramine by tryptophan, *Arch Gen Psychiatry* 33:1384–1389, 1976.

218. Steiner W, Fontaine R: Toxic reaction following the combined administration of fluoxetine and L-tryptophan: Five case reports, *Biol Psychiatry* 21:1067–1071, 1986.

219. Insel TR, Roy BF, Cohen RM, et al: Possible development of the serotonin syndrome in man, *Am J Psychiatry* 139:954–955, 1982.

220. McDougle CJ, Epperson CN, Price LH: Obsessive-compulsive symptoms with neuroleptics, *J Am Acad Child Adolesc Psychiatry* 35:837, 1996.

221. McDougle CJ, Goodman WK, Price LH, et al: Neuroleptic addition in fluvoxamine-refractory obsessive compulsive disorder: An open case series, *Am J Psychiatry* 147:552–554, 1991a.

222. Nassir-Ghaemi S, et al: Is there a relationship between clozapine and obsessive-compulsive disorder? A retrospective chart review, *Comp Psychiatry* 36:267–270, 1995.

223. Eales MJ, Layeni AO: Exacerbation of obsessive compulsive symptoms associated with clozapine, *Br J Psychiatry* 164:687–688, 1994.

224. Patil VJ: Development of transient obsessive compulsive symptoms during treatment with clozapine, *Am J Psychiatry* 149:272, 1992.

225. Patel VJ, Tandon R: Development of obsessive compulsive symptoms during clozapine treatment, *Am J Psychiatry* 159:836, 1993.

226. Baker RW, et al: Emergence of obsessive compulsive symptoms during treatment with clozapine, *J Clin Psychiatry* 53:12, 1992.

227. Kopala L, Honer WG: Risperidone, serotonergic mechanisms and obsessive compulsive symptoms in schizophrenia, *Am J Psychiatry* 151:11, 1994.

228. Toren P, Samuel E, Weizman R, et al: Case study: Emergence of transient com-

pulsive symptoms during treatment with clothiapine, *J Am Acad Child Adolesc Psychiatry* 34:1469–1472, 1995.

229. McDougle CJ, Barr LC, Goodman WK, et al: Lack of efficacy of clozapine monotherapy in refractory obsessive-compulsive disorder, *Am J Psychiatry* 152:1812–1814, 1995.

230. McDougle CJ, Fleischmann RL, Epperson CN, et al: Risperidone addition in fluvoxamine-refractory obsessive-compulsive disorder: Three cases, *J Clin Psychiatry* 56:526–528, 1995a.

231. Berigan TR, Harazin JS: Response to risperidone addition in fluvoxamine-refractory obsessive-compulsive disorder: Three cases, *J Clin Psychiatry* 57:594–595, 1996.

232. Jacobsen FM: Risperidone in the treatment of affective illness and obsessive-compulsive disorder, *J Clin Psychiatry* 56:423–429, 1995.

233. Saxena S, Wang D, Bystritsky A, Baxter LR: Risperidone augmentation of SRI treatment for refractory obsessive-compulsive disorder, *J Clin Psychiatry* 57: 303–306, 1996.

234. Fontaine R, Chouinard G: Fluoxetine in the long-term maintenance treatment of obsessive-compulsive disorder, *Psychiatr Ann* 19:88–91, 1989.

235. Seagraves RT, Thompson TL, Wise T: Sexual dysfunction and antidepressants, *J Clin Psychiatry* Intercom: The Experts Converse. August, 1996.

236. McCormick S, Olin J, Brotman AW: Reversal of fluoxetine-induced anorgasmia by cyproheptadine in two patients, *J Clin Psychiatry* 51:383–384, 1990.

237. Arnott S, Nutt D: Successful treatment of fluvoxamine-induced anorgasmia by cyproheptadine, *Br J Psychiatry* 164:838–839, 1994.

238. Seagraves RT: Reversing anorgasmia associated with serotonin uptake inhibitors (questions and answers), *JAMA* 266:2279, 1991.

239. Feder R: Reversal of antidepressant activity of fluoxetine by cyproheptadine in three patients, *J Clin Psychiatry* 52:163–164, 1991.

240. Goldbloom DS, Kennedy SH: Adverse interaction of fluoxetine and cyproheptadine in two patients with bulimia nervosa, *J Clin Psychiatry* 52:261–262, 1991.

241. Steele TE, Howell EF: Cyproheptadine for imipramine-induced anorgasmia, *J Clin Psychopharmacol* 6:326–327, 1986.

242. Norden MJ: Buspirone treatment of sexual dysfunction associated with selective serotonin reuptake inhibitors, *Depression* 2:109–112, 1994.

243. Seagraves RT: Treatment of drug-induced anorgasmia, *Br J Psychiatry* 165:554, 1994.

244. Bartlik BD, Kaplan PM, Koscis JH: Primary psychiatry, 2(10):13, 1995.

245. Balogh S, Hendricks SE, Kang J: Treatment of fluoxetine-induced anorgasmia with amantadine, *J Clin Psychiatry* 53:212–213, 1992.

246. Balon R: Intermittent amantadine for fluoxetine-induced anorgasmia, *J Sex Mar Ther* 22(4):290–292, 1996.

247. Masand S, Reddy N, Gregory R: SSRI-induced sexual dysfunction successfully treated with amantadine, *Depression* 2:319–321, 1994–95.

248. Reynolds RD: Sertraline-induced anorgasmia treated with intermittent nefazodone, *J Clin Psychiatry* 58:89, 1997.

249. Padma-Nathan H, Hellstrom WT, Kaiser FE, et al: Treatment of men with erectile dysfunction with transurethral alprostodil, *N Engl J Med* 336:1–7, 1997.

250. Intraurethral alprostadil for impotence, *Med Lett* 39:32, 1997.
251. Jefferson JW, Altemus M, Jenike MA, et al: Algorithm for the treatment of obsessive-compulsive disorder, *Psychopharmacol Bull* 31(3):487–490, 1995.
252. The Expert Consensus Guideline: Treatment of obsessive-compulsive disorder, *J Clin Psychiatry* 58:(suppl 4), 1997.
253. APA Task Force Report No. 14 on Electroconvulsive Therapy. Washington, American Psychiatric Association, 1978.

APPENDIX: DRUG TREATMENT OF OBSESSIVE-COMPULSIVE DISORDER IN ADULTS
Introduction and Acknowledgments

This pamphlet was commissioned by the Obsessive-Compulsive Foundation as a service for OCD patients and their family members. The purpose is to provide concise information about drug treatments of OCD and to answer frequently asked questions. You can obtain a copy of this pamphlet directly from the Obsessive-Compulsive Foundation or give the patient a copy of this section of this book.

It is important to acknowledge that the answers in this book are the opinions of the author, but that they are for the most part backed up by solid clinical studies. In the case in which recommendations are based solely on the author's clinical experience, it will be so stated.

Overview

Obsessive-compulsive disorder is a potentially devastating illness that can result in considerable social and economic disability for both afflicted patients and their family members. OCD is usually treated with a combination of specific behavioral therapies, called exposure and response prevention (ERP), and medications. It is important to note that many psychoactive medications are not likely to help OCD symptoms, but that a number of partially effective drugs have now been carefully evaluated. The treatment, however, for most OCD patients should involve the combination of behavior therapy with medications. This pamphlet will focus on medications but is not meant to diminish the importance of behavior therapy.

What Kinds of Medications May Help Obsessive-Compulsive Disorder?

The majority of the drugs that help OCD are classified as antidepressants. It is important to note that depression commonly results from the disability produced by OCD and that doctors can treat both the OCD and depression with the same medication.

There also are a number of disorders that are possibly related to OCD, such as compulsive gambling and sexual behaviors, trichotillomania, body dysmorphic disorder, compulsive eating, nail biting, and compulsive spending. There is some evidence that the medications and behavior therapies discussed in this pamphlet will help some of these patients, but more research is needed in this area to give firm recommendations.

Do All Antidepressants Help Obsessive-Compulsive Disorder Symptoms?

No! Some commonly used antidepressants have no effect whatsoever on OCD symptoms. Drugs, such as imipramine (Tofranil) or amitriptyline (Elavil), which are good antidepressants, only rarely improve OCD symptoms.

Which Drugs Help Obsessive-Compulsive Disorder and How Do We Know These Drugs are Effective?

There are five drugs found useful in very good, double-blind (i.e., both physician and patient are unaware of whether patient is receiving drug or placebo [inert sugar pill]), placebo-controlled (i.e., approximately half of the patients receive drug and the other half placebo or inactive pill) studies. This method is a very good way to evaluate drugs, because improvements can be evaluated in an unbiased manner and drug effectiveness can be accurately determined.

The five drugs that are effective in such studies include: fluvoxamine (Luvox), fluoxetine (Prozac), sertraline (Zoloft), paroxetine (Paxil), and clomipramine (Anafranil). Anafranil has been around the longest and is the best studied throughout the world, but there is growing evidence that the other drugs are as effective.

In addition to these carefully studied drugs, there are hundreds of case reports of other drugs occasionally being helpful. There are small series of patients reported that suggest that venlafaxine (Effexor) may also be somewhat effective, but large-scale controlled trials are lacking.

Why Do These Drugs Help?

It remains unclear as to why these particular drugs help OCD, whereas similar drugs do not. Each has potent effects on a particular neurotransmitter, or chemical messenger, in the brain called *serotonin*. It appears that potent effects on brain serotonin are necessary (but not sufficient) to produce improvement in OCD. Serotonin is one of several neurotransmitter chemicals that nerve cells in the brain use in communicating with one another. Unlike some other neurotransmitters, the receptors are not localized in a few specific areas of the brain; hence, its uptake and release affects much of our mental life, including OCD and depression.

Neurotransmitters such as serotonin are active when they are present in the "gap" (referring to the synaptic cleft) between nerve cells. Transmission is ended by a process in which the chemicals are taken back up into the transmitting cell. The antiobsessional drugs are called *serotonin reuptake inhibitors* or SRIs; these drugs work by slowing the reuptake of serotonin, thus making it more available to the receiving cell and prolonging its effect on the brain. We think that this increased serotonin produces changes, over a period of a few weeks, in receptors (areas in which serotonin attaches) in some of the membranes of the nerves. We also believe that these receptors may be abnormal in patients with OCD and that the changes that occur in them because of these medications at least partly reverse the OCD symptoms. This is only part of how drugs work; it is very likely that other brain chemicals, in addition to serotonin, are involved. In fact, when activity in the brain's serotonergic system is altered, this changes the activity of other brain systems.

Experiments have been performed with drugs that directly stimulate components of the serotonin system in the brain, and it was found that such so-called serotonergic agonists actually make OCD symptoms worse. However, after patients are successfully treated for OCD, these agonists do not worsen OCD symptoms, thus suggesting that there may be some changes in the brain's serotonergic system with effective drug treatment that somehow result in improvement in symptoms.

Don't worry if this does not make sense to you. Researchers do not know how the drugs work and that is why this is so confusing. The good news is that we do know, after decades of research, how to treat patients, although we do not know exactly why our treatments work.

At What Dosages Are These Drugs Used?

As a general rule, it appears that for most people, high dosages of these drugs are required to obtain antiobsessional effects. The studies performed to date suggest that the following dosages may be necessary: Luvox (up to 300 mg/day), Prozac (40–80 mg/day), Zoloft (up to 200 mg/day), Paxil (40–60 mg/day), Anafranil (up to 250 mg/day). Where a lower dosage is listed, at least some of the studies have suggested that a dose lower than the minimum was not significantly better than placebo.

I also have seen a very small number of patients who have not responded to large dosages of each of these medications, but who improved on extremely low doses, such as 5 to 10 mg/day of Prozac or 25 mg/day of Anafranil. These patients have not been carefully studied and, to my knowledge, these low-dosage responders are not reported in the psychiatric literature. If patients fail to improve with high dosages of these medications, it is probably worth a trial of a very low dose.

Are There Side Effects?

Each of these drugs has side effects, and it is quite unusual for an individual patient not to have one or more side effects. As with all drugs, the patient and physician must weigh the benefits of the drug against the side effects. It is important for the patient to be open and forceful about problems that may be caused by the medication. Sometimes just an adjustment in dosage or switch in the time of day that one takes the medication is all that is required.

Luvox, Prozac, Paxil, and Zoloft are called SSRIs, or selective serotonin reuptake inhibitors; Anafranil is an older tricyclic antidepressant or SRI (serotonin reuptake inhibitor) that has effects on other chemical messengers besides serotonin and is thus not selective for serotonin. All of these drugs commonly produce sexual side effects in both genders that may range from lowered sexual drive to delayed ability to have an orgasm to complete inability to have an erection or orgasm. Interestingly, there is an uncommon side effect that has been reported in which patients have spontaneous orgasms while yawning. This effect must be quite uncommon, because no patient has ever told me of such a symptom, and when patients yawn in my office, they always look bored, not excited. Occasionally, patients report increased interest in sexual activity. Although it may seem embarrassing, the patient should tell the physician about sexual difficulties so that he or she can help figure out how best to deal with them. These side effects are so common that the psychiatrist will not be surprised. There recently have been a few reports of patients who were having sexual difficulties while taking these drugs and who stopped taking them on Fridays and Saturdays and were able to at least enjoy successful sexual activity on the weekends. Thus far, it appears that this approach has not produced a relapse in symptoms, but this may be reported as people try this more often. Also, this approach has not been as effective with Prozac, because it is such a long-acting compound.

SSRIs also commonly cause nausea, inability to sit still, sleepiness (in some individuals), insomnia in others, and a heightened sense of energy. The tricyclic Anafranil may cause pronounced effects such as drowsiness, dry mouth, racing heart, memory problems, concentration difficulties, and urination difficulties (mostly in men). Sometimes weight gain is a problem, and a strict diet may be needed if appetite is increased. There are many other less common side effects from these drugs that the physician may discuss with the patient. As a general rule, these drugs are very safe, even with long-term use, and all of the side effects completely reverse when the drugs are stopped; thus, there is no evidence that they do permanent damage to the body.

What If I Cannot Tolerate Even the Smallest Pill Size of the Medication?

Occasionally, patients are very sensitive to medications and cannot tolerate even the lowest dosage that comes in pills. Many of the pills can be broken in half to allow for lower dosages. There is also a liquid form of Prozac that has allowed many patients to gradually increase the dosage to therapeutic levels. Often if patients can start at very low dosages (e.g., 1 to 2 mg/day) and very slowly increase the dose, they will eventually be able to tolerate the medication. This technique has proven so successful for many people that there is now a "fan club" of those helped by this approach.

Many patients have been able to use liquid Prozac. For example, one woman who was started on Prozac 20 mg/day complained of very bothersome side effects such as increased anxiety, shakiness, and terrible insomnia. She also believed it had made her OCD worse. In addition, she had horrible side effects from even 12.5 mg of Anafranil, and later with low dosages of Paxil and Zoloft. She then started 1 to 2 mg/day of liquid Prozac, which she learned about from other patients over a computer bulletin board. She felt no side effects, and over a period of a few weeks, she raised her dosage to 20 mg/day, again without the previous side effects that she had felt when taking this dose previously. She continued to increase the Prozac to 60 mg/day over a few months, and her OCD improved quite dramatically.

Thus, careful and gradual increases in dosage with liquid medication may allow some medication-sensitive patients to reach therapeutic levels.

Do Antiobsessional Medications Cause Long-Term, Irreversible Side Effects?

As far as we know, there are no irreversible side effects caused by the standard antiobsessional drugs. Many patients have used these drugs for years without difficulties. Some of the drugs that are occasionally used—such as the antipsychotic (or sometimes called neuroleptic) drugs like haloperidol (Haldol), chlorpromazine (Thorazine), thioridazine (Mellaril), and trifluoperazine (Stelazine)—can produce irreversible neurologic problems, such as persistent tremor or tongue thrusting. These drugs are best avoided in patients with the usual forms of OCD; if these drugs are used, it should generally be for only a few weeks. Occasionally, patients need to remain on these potentially troublesome drugs for longer periods of time. For example, in OCD patients that also have tics (brief muscle jerks, such as repetitive eye blinks, nervous cough, or shoulder shrugs), there is evidence that very low doses of these neuroleptic drugs added to ongoing SRI medication help OCD symptoms. In OCD patients without tics, there is no evidence that neuroleptics are helpful and are best avoided. There are newer neuroleptic agents, such as olanzapine (Zyprexa) and risperidone (Risperdol), that may have fewer of these types of neurologic problems and may be helpful when added to SRI treatment. These new drugs should not be used alone, because they have been associated with worsening of OCD symptoms when not taken in combination with an SRI.

Who Should Not Take Antiobsessional Medications?

In general, we try not to give antiobsessional medications to pregnant or breastfeeding women. Because we do not clearly understand the long-term effects of these drugs on a fetus or infant, this is the most prudent course of action. If severe OCD cannot be controlled any other way, however, these medications seem to be safe and many pregnant women have taken them without difficulty. If there were risk to the fetus, it is likely that most of the risk would be during the first 3 months of pregnancy when the baby's brain is developing. Some OCD patients are able to use the behavioral techniques of ERP to avoid medications at least during the initial 3 months of pregnancy. If the OCD is very severe, the patient may need to take a medication throughout the course of pregnancy.

In very elderly patients, it is best to avoid Anafranil as the initial drug, because it has side effects that can interfere with thinking and can cause or worsen confusion in the elderly. Some of the other antiobsessional drugs, such as Prozac, Zoloft, Luvox, and Paxil, can be used in the elderly, but greatly reduced dosages are usually needed.

Although these drugs can be taken by patients with heart disorders, special caution is required, and close monitoring with frequent cardiograms may be necessary.

Should a Patient Take Antiobsessional Medications Only When He or She is Feeling Stressed?

No. This is a common mistake. These medications are meant to be taken on a regular daily basis to maintain a constant level in the bloodstream. They are not taken like the typical antianxiety agents—when the patient feels upset or anxious. It is best not to miss dosages if possible. Having said this, it is unlikely that any adverse effect on OCD will occur if a daily dose is missed occasionally; sometimes missed dosages are prescribed by the doctor to help manage troublesome side effects, such as sexual dysfunction.

What Kind of Doctor Should a Patient Look for to Prescribe These Antiobsessional Medications?

Although any licensed physician can legally prescribe these drugs, it is probably best to deal directly with a board-certified psychiatrist who understands OCD. A list of psychiatrists with special interest in OCD can be obtained from the Obsessive-Compulsive Foundation. Keep in mind, however, that these are physicians who have expressed an interest in OCD and that the Foundation has not evaluated them in any way. Legally, they are obligated to list any psychiatrist who expresses an interest in the disorder. It also is important to find a psychiatrist who is a psychopharmacologist, that is, one who has special knowledge about the use of drugs to treat psychiatric disorders.

What if the Patient Feels Failure Because He or She Needs Help of a Drug?

A useful way of thinking about the use of medication for OCD is to compare the illness with a common medical disorder such as diabetes. There is growing evidence that OCD is, in fact, a neurologic or medical illness and not simply a result of some problem in the environment or of improper upbringing. As with the diabetic patient who needs insulin to live a normal life, some

OCD patients need anticompulsive medication to function normally; diabetics also often feel angry and upset about taking insulin. There is no evidence that OCD is a result of anything that the patient has done, and it is best to consider the disorder a chemical or neurologic disorder affecting a part of the brain.

What If the Patient is Afraid to Take Medications Because of Obsessional Fears About Drugs?

Usually with reassurance from a doctor that the patient can trust, fears can be overcome. If the patient still refuses to take medication, behavior therapy can be started, and part of the therapy can focus on the reluctance to take medication. Our experience indicates that the combination of medication and behavior therapy maximizes chances for improvement.

How Much Does it Cost to Take These Drugs?

Unfortunately, these drugs are very expensive and can cost the patient up to $6 or $7 per day for larger doses. When the patent expires on each of these drugs, other companies can make generic forms of each drug, and then the prices fall.

Why are These Drugs so Expensive?

One can think of many sinister reasons why pharmaceutical companies charge so much for these medications, but we must keep in mind that it costs millions of dollars to bring a single drug to market in the United States. Most drugs do not make it to the market and represent a lost investment; however, if the pharmaceutical companies do not try out new agents, no progress in this area is likely. These companies spend millions in research trying to identify new compounds that may have therapeutic value. Without pharmaceutical companies, there would likely be few, if any, advances in clinical pharmacology in the United States, and we would not have new drugs available to us. Pharmaceutical companies also are heavily involved in promoting awareness of the various diseases, including OCD, for which they have a medication. These promotions (television, radio, print) are of benefit to patients, because this is often the manner in which they discover that they have OCD, that the affliction has a name, and that it can be treated. Pharmaceutical companies have even been active in promoting nondrug treatments, such as behavior therapy, when they have nothing to gain financially. They also sponsor educational programs for physicians and have been instrumental in spreading the knowledge base about OCD to both physicians and patients. These companies have been financial backers of organizations such as the National Obsessive-Compulsive Foundation.

Can a patient get drugs if he or she is poor?

Often pharmaceutical company representatives visit physicians and leave free samples of medications. Physicians may give these samples to patients who cannot afford the expense of the medications.

In addition, each of the pharmaceutical companies involved in the production of the five primary antiobsessional drugs offers free drugs to patients who are truly poor. The Pharmaceutical Manufacturers Association publishes a directory of programs for those patients who cannot afford medications. Physicians can request a copy of the guide by calling (800) PMA-INFO. To get more information on each company's programs, the patient or physician can contact the indigent patient program at the following companies directly:

- **Luvox:** Solvay Patient Assistance Program, 800-788-9277
- **Prozac:** Lilly Cares Program, 800-545-6962
- **Paxil:** SmithKline Paxil Access To Care Program, 800-546-0420 (patient requests); 215-751-5722 (physician requests)
- **Zoloft:** Pfizer Indigent Patient Program, 800-646-4455
- **Anafranil:** Ciba-Geigy Patient Support Program, 800-257-3273; 908-277-5849

How Long Does it Take Antiobsessional Medications to Work?

It is important not to give up on a medication until the patient has been taking it at a therapeutic dose for 10 to 12 weeks. Many patients feel no positive effects for the first few weeks of treatment, but then they may improve greatly. Unfortunately, during the early part of treatment, patients may have only side effects and no positive results, and sometimes physicians forget to tell patients about this lag in response. We do not know why medications take so long to work for OCD. The patient should keep in mind that even many psychiatrists give up on the medications after 4 to 6 weeks, because this is the time it takes for depressed patients to improve. Thus, the patient may have to remind the psychiatrist to keep him on the medication longer.

How Helpful Can the Patient Expect These Medications to Be?

In the large studies that have been performed, approximately 75% to 85% of the patients experience some improvement. Approximately 50% to 60% of patients in each trial had at least a moderate response to medication. Some patients have no response at all. If a patient does not respond to the first medication, it is important to try the next. I have seen patients who have had no response to three medications, who had a wonderful response to the next one. There also are techniques of combining medications that may increase the response magnitude and rate. One patient wrote to me: "Seeking an effective medication for OCD is a lot like dating to find a mate; don't be afraid to shop around and try different meds till you find one that works for you!"

What About Augmenting One Drug with Another?

The best augmenting technique is to add behavior therapy to ongoing drug treatment. However, to boost a drug's effect, we sometimes combine two or more medications together. For example, some people respond to combining Luvox or Prozac with Anafranil. It is important for the physician to keep in mind that the blood level in a patient taking Anafranil can be dramatically increased by adding one of the other drugs, so it is important to keep the dose of Anafranil low, at least during the initial stages of treatment. Sometimes blood levels are helpful, but most of the time a good clinician can follow side effects and symptom reduction to find the correct dosage.

Other drugs are sometimes combined with ongoing SRI medications. Some that have commonly been used include: buspirone (Buspar), lithium carbonate (Eskalith), clonazepam (Klonopin), methylphenidate (Ritalin), fenfluramine (Pondamin), and other antidepressants (e.g., trazodone, bupropion, desipramine, etc). The controlled trials that have been performed with these augmenting agents have been largely disappointing, but because occasional patients respond to the addition of a second drug, clinicians frequently try this technique.

Are There Other Medications That Can Be Used to Treat OCD?

Yes, there are drugs that are occasionally helpful in individual patients besides those already mentioned. For example, some patients may be helped by drugs called *monoamine oxidase inhibitors* (MAOI) (e.g., Nardil [phenelzine], Parnate [tranylcypromine]) that work in a different way than the previously mentioned drugs. These drugs inhibit one of the enzymes that degrades the chemical messengers in the nerve gaps, thereby lengthening the time that the messenger can be active. There is some anecdotal evidence that OCD patients who also have panic attacks or prominent concerns with symmetry may be more likely to improve with MAOIs. With these drugs, certain foods and medications cannot be taken with them or potentially fatal reactions can occur. These drugs are particularly dangerous in combination with SRI medications and must be stopped for at least 2 weeks (5 weeks for Prozac, which is longer lasting) prior to starting MAOIs.

The other antidepressants occasionally help, but chances of this are quite small.

Will the Patient Have to Take Antiobsessional Medications Forever?

No one knows yet how long patients should take these medications once they have been effective. Some patients are able to discontinue medications after a 6- to 12-month treatment period. However, it does appear that more than half of OCD patients (and maybe many more) will need to take at least a low dosage of medication for years, perhaps even for life. It seems likely that the risk of relapse will be lower if patients learn to use behavior therapy techniques when they are doing well on medications, and if medication is tapered very slowly (even over several months). The behavioral techniques may enable patients to control any symptoms that return when they stop taking medication. Typically, after medications are stopped, symptoms do not return immediately, but may return within weeks to months.

When one of these drugs is working and then discontinued and symptoms return, the vast majority of patients have a good response on reinstitution of the medication. However, I have now seen some patients who did not respond when the discontinued drug was restarted.

Can Patients Drink Alcohol When Taking Medication?

Many patients drink alcohol when taking these medications and tolerate it well. It is important to keep in mind that alcohol may have a greater effect on individuals who are taking medication—that is, one drink could affect an individual as if it were two drinks, and so on. Also, it is not known if alcohol can counteract some of the therapeutic effects of the medication, so it may be worth not drinking alcohol during the first few months after starting medication.

Do Patients Need Other Treatments in Addition to Medications?

As noted earlier, most psychiatrists and behavior therapists today believe that combining behavior therapy, consisting of ERP, and medication is the most effective approach.

What is Behavior Therapy?

Traditional psychotherapy, which is aimed at helping the patient develop insight into his or her problem, is generally not helpful specifically for OCD symptoms themselves. However, traditional psychotherapy may be beneficial as part of a treatment package for patients who have been ill and isolated for many years or for those patients whose illness started at an early age. On the other hand, behavior therapy consisting of techniques called ERP is effective for many people with OCD. In this approach, the patient is deliberately and voluntarily exposed to feared objects or ideas, either directly or by imagination (the *exposure* component), and then is discouraged or prevented (with the patient's permission) from carrying out the usual compulsive response (the *response prevention* component). For example, a compulsive hand washer may be urged to touch an object believed to be contaminated and then may be denied the opportunity to wash for several hours. When the treatment works well, the patient gradually experiences less anxiety from the obsessive thoughts and is able to do without the compulsive actions for extended periods of time.

Studies of behavior therapy for OCD have found it to produce lasting benefits. To achieve the best results, a combination of factors is necessary: (1) the therapist should be well trained in the specific method developed; (2) the patient must be highly motivated; and (3) the patient's family must be cooperative. In addition to therapist visits, the patient must be faithful in fulfilling homework assignments. For those patients who complete the course of treatment, the improvements can be significant.

With a combination of drug and behavioral therapy, the majority of OCD patients will be able to function well in both their work and social lives. The ongoing search for causes, together with research on treatment, promises to yield even more hope for people with OCD and their families.

How are Obsessive-Compulsive Disorder and Depression Related?

Approximately two thirds of OCD patients also have suffered at least one major depression in their lives. Approximately one third of patients are depressed when they present for treatment. Some experts believe the OCD causes the depression, whereas others believe the OCD and depression simply tend to coexist. Most patients tell me that their OCD symptoms came first, and depression began when they were unable to handle the OCD.

What are Some Signs of Depression?

Signs of depression include loss of appetite; weight loss; early morning awakenings; lack of energy; too much or too little sleep; sadness; crying, especially without knowing why; suicidal thoughts; feelings of hopelessness; feelings of helplessness; lack of interest in things that formerly interested the person; and lack of enjoyment of life.

The presence of one or more of these symptoms does not necessarily indicate the presence of depression, but if several symptoms are present, the patient may be depressed.

What if the Patient's Obsessive-Compulsive Disorder Gets Better But He or She Remains Depressed?

It sometimes happens that OCD improves and depression persists. Occasionally, a second drug is added to combat the depression; sometimes the doctor can assist the patient in finding other reasons why depression persists.

23

Hoarding: Clinical Aspects and Treatment Strategies

Randy O. Frost, Ph.D., Gail S. Steketee, Ph.D.

HOARDING SYMPTOMS AND FEATURES

Hoarding behavior is most commonly associated with the collection and storage of food items among rodents, small animals, and birds.[1] Among these creatures, food hoarding is a normal part of the life cycle and can be stimulated in predictable ways.[2-4] Although nonfood hoarding occurs in some nonhuman species, the phenomenon is unusual and not well studied.[5,6] The relationship between nonhuman and human hoarding is uncertain, although Smith[7] has suggested some similarities. Virtually no research exists on the hoarding of food in humans and, until recently, only clinical descriptions of nonfood hoarding among humans could be found. Hoarding behavior has been observed in a variety of disorders, including anorexia nervosa,[8] organic mental disorders,[9] psychotic disorders,[10] obsessive-compulsive personality disorder (OCPD),[11] and mental retardation.[12] However, the majority of research links hoarding to obsessive-compulsive disorder (OCD).

Definition of Hoarding

Although it is widely recognized as a symptom of OCD, hoarding is not described in the *Diagnostic and Statistical Manual of Mental Disorders* (DSM-IV)[11] in this context. DSM-IV presents hoarding in the context of OCPD in which it is defined as the inability to discard worthless or worn-out things, even though they have no sentimental value. Hoarding is defined in the same way on the Yale-Brown Obsessive-Compulsive Scale Checklist (Y-BOCS).[13] Until recently, little attention has been given to this type of compulsion in the research literature, despite the fact that it appears difficult to treat.[14]

Because both the DSM-IV and Y-BOCS definitions of hoarding appear inadequate, Frost and Gross[15] proposed a refined definition of hoarding as, "the acquisition of, and failure to discard possessions which appear to be useless or of limited value" (p. 367). Several features of this definition are noteworthy.

The definition of hoarding includes acquisition[15-17] because most hoarders actively acquire possessions. We have found that hoarders often buy extra possessions "just in case" they might need them in the future.[15] For example, one of our study participants bought and kept more than 30 bottles of shampoo; if her hoard fell below that number, she felt compelled to buy more. Another participant had rooms full of "gifts" that she had purchased over several decades. She did not know to whom she would give them, but they were "good buys" that she couldn't pass up. A third had accumulated an entire room full of unworn clothing with the sales tags still attached.

The absence of sentimentality as an exclusion criterion is a second feature of this definition. Although both DSM-IV and the Y-BOCS suggest that hoarding involves only nonsentimental saving, several studies dispute this assumption. For example, Furby found that ordinary people save possessions for either instrumental reasons (i.e., because they have a need for them) or for sentimental reasons (because they are emotionally attached to them).[18] These are the most frequent reasons for saving among hoarders as well.[15] Clinical observations have consistently described hoarding as, in part, an overemotional attachment to possessions.[8,15,19,20] Further, hoarders develop a greater emotional attachment to their possessions than nonhoarders,[16] and these emotional reasons are part of why they hoard.[15] Indeed, this feature appeared so prominently among our study participants, that we made it a major component of our cognitive-behavioral model of hoarding (see following paragraphs, and Frost and Hartl[21]).

One difficulty with our proposed definition is that it does not distinguish between hoarding as a behavior and hoarding as a clinical symptom. That is, *how much* does one have to hoard to constitute a symptom of OCD? In one of our first hoarding studies, we placed an ad in the local newspaper asking for "packrats" or "chronic savers" to participate in our research, and we received more than 100 calls. Although all these people considered themselves hoarders, our home visits found that many did not have a clinical problem associated with their hoarding. In our subsequent research, we found that the reasons for saving possessions and the types of things saved by hoarders were no different than those of nonhoarders.[15] Hoarders endorsed the same reasons for saving described by Furby[18] as reasons for saving in the general population. We also asked self-identified hoarders and control subjects to rate 80 possessions on the extent to which they saved each one.[15] (The 80-possession list was generated in an earlier investigation of frequently saved things, such as clothes, magazines, and bags, as well as less frequently saved items, such as old appliances, flower pots, and shoe laces.) From this list, we ranked items in each group and calculated a Spearman Rank Order correlation. The correlation between the groups was high (rho = 0.79, p < 0.001), suggesting that hoarders save the same kinds of things as nonhoarders, but in larger quantities.

To clarify the distinction between clinical and nonclinical levels of hoarding, Frost and Hartl[21] proposed a three-part definition of clinical hoarding: (1) the acquisition of, and failure to discard, a large number of possessions that appear to be useless or of limited value; (2) living spaces sufficiently cluttered so as to preclude activities for which those spaces were designed; and (3) significant distress or impairment in functioning caused by the hoarding. This definition ties the notion of hoarding to clutter, which is the most common associated functional deficit.

Hoarding, Obsessive-Compulsive Disorder, and Obsessive-Compulsive Personality Disorder

Is hoarding a characteristic of OCD, OCPD, or both? Because hoarding is one of the diagnostic criteria for OCPD, it is reasonable to assume that it would be correlated with other OCPD diagnostic criteria and with global measures of OCPD. To test this hypothesis, Frost and Gross[15] administered a self-report measure of hoarding; measures of other OCPD characteristics such as perfectionism, excessive job involvement, restricted affect, rigidity, generosity, and authoritarianism; and a global measure of OCPD to a sample of college students. We found that hoarding was not correlated with a general measure of OCPD, nor was it correlated in the predicted direction with most of the specific OCPD characteristics (the only predicted significant relationship being between hoarding and perfectionism). In a follow-up study, Frost, et al[17] examined hoarding, perfectionism, and general OCPD traits in a group of self-identified hoarders compared with community volunteers matched for age and gender. Although hoarders scored significantly higher on hoarding scale scores and perfectionism, they did not significantly differ from community members on the global measure of OCPD.

A number of studies have attempted to measure the covariation of OCPD symptoms,[22] but only one of these has attempted to objectively measure hoarding behavior. Heatherington and Brackbill[23] told a group of children that they could keep any rocks put into their box from a pile in the experimental room. Rocks were selected based on the assumption that they were "transitional objects" representing money or feces. The number of rocks they kept was the operational definition of hoarding. The number of rocks taken and kept was correlated with other tests of parsimony. Unfortunately, no attempt was made to independently verify the reliability or validity of this measure of hoarding. The findings from our studies, plus the scant evidence on the covariation of hoarding and other OCPD characteristics, lead us to question whether hoarding is truly a symptom of OCPD.

Is hoarding a symptom of OCD? If so, it should be correlated with other measures of OCD. Frost and Gross[15] found that a hoarding scale was significantly correlated with nearly all subscales from three different measures of OCD symptoms among college students and a community sample. They also found that self-identified hoarders had significantly higher scores on nearly all OCD subscales compared with a group of matched controls. Subsequently, Frost, et al[17] found that the hoarding scale was significantly correlated with the Y-BOCS total score in a sample of college women. Further, when participants in this study were divided into subclinical compulsives and noncompulsives based on their scores on an obsessive-compulsive inventory, the subclinical compulsives more frequently identified hoarding as a target symptom on the Y-BOCS than noncompulsives.

In another study, we compared the Y-BOCS scores of a sample of self-identified and screened hoarders to a matched control group. The mean Y-BOCS total score for the hoarding group was significantly higher than that of the matched controls. (The mean Y-BOCS total for the hoarding group was 16.5, which indicated a clinical OCD severity in this undiagnosed population.) These findings strongly suggest that hoarding is closely associated with OCD symptomatology.

Associated Features of Hoarding

Prevalence estimates of hoarding symptoms in OCD patients range widely. Rasmussen and Eisen[24] reported that 18% of 200 adult OCD patients had hoarding compulsions. Rapoport[25] found that 11% of 70 children with OCD had hoarding symptoms, and in a later study, it was reported that 42% (10 of 24) of children with OCD had hoarding as a pronounced symptom.[26] However, because no definition of hoarding was provided in these studies, the findings are somewhat unclear. We used the Y-BOCS Checklist and found endorsement of hoarding obsessions in 31% and hoarding compulsions in 26% of 39 outpatients in treatment for OCD.[17] Thus, it appears that hoarding symptoms typically occur in one quarter to one third of OCD patients. No studies have documented the frequency with which hoarding is a primary symptom.

Greenberg[19] suggested that the onset of problematic hoarding occurs in the patient's early twenties. However, this estimate was based on only four patients, two of whom reported hoarding symptoms in childhood. Among 32 hoarders, Frost and Gross[15] noted that 66% recalled hoarding behavior in childhood and an additional 25% reported onset in the teens or early twenties. A significantly greater number of hoarders reported excessive saving among first-degree relatives (84%) than did nonhoarders (54%). Interestingly, the hoarding patients were more often unmarried compared with nonhoarders in this study—similar to findings from other OCD populations.[14] Nothing is known about the gender ratio of compulsive hoarding, although Frost and Gross[15] found no gender differences on hoarding scale scores.

Although little research exists on the symptom of hoarding, the nature of acquisition tendencies was once a popular topic in psychology. William James[28] believed acquisitiveness was an instinct commonly found in the general population. Other early theorists incorporated hoarding into theories of psychopathology. Fromm[27] described hoarding as one aspect of character, a way in which people related to the world around them. He described a "hoarding orientation," which represents one type of "nonproductive character" in which security depends on acquiring and saving things. For Freud,[29] the hoarding of money reflected the parsimony component of the anal triad. Jones[30] elaborated on Freud's notion of hoarding by including the hoarding of other possessions. Bender and Schilder[31] suggested that hoarding in children is a precursor to the development of obsessions. Likewise, Adams[32] described it as a background characteristic from which OCD develops. Other psychoanalytic writers (e.g., Salzman[33]) suggested that hoarding develops from perfectionistic strivings to gain control over the environment. To achieve perfect control, the hoarder must not throw out anything that might be needed in the future. Thus, because one cannot be certain of exactly what might be needed in the future, the safest course of action is to save everything. In a slightly different vein, Rapoport[25] suggested that hoarding is a "fixed-action pattern" (p. 280) resulting from evolutionary development. Similar to nesting in animals, this behavior is innate and released by certain hormonal changes.

Despite the longevity of some of these theories, they have failed to generate research that supports or refutes them and have failed to generate treatment programs directed at compulsive hoarding. Prior to 1993, most of the available information on hoarding came from case studies. Greenberg[19] described four cases of compulsive hoarding. In each case, despite debilitating symptoms, patients strongly resisted changing the hoarding behavior, and attempts by family members to discard possessions were met with intense anger and threats of violence. Frankenburg[8] described an anorexic patient who hoarded "bits of paper and styrofoam, toothpaste tube caps, screws, and nails (p. 57)." As with other hoarding patients, she had plans to use each of these possessions, and consistent with Fromm's[27] observation, she felt "safe" only when she was surrounded by her possessions.

A COGNITIVE-BEHAVIORAL MODEL OF COMPULSIVE HOARDING

Based on our recent research using nonclinical samples,[15–17] on interviews of people suffering from this condition,[15] and on attempts to change hoarding behavior,[34] we propose a cognitive-behavioral model of compulsive hoarding[21] as a guide for future research and treatment. It is a preliminary model, in that many of the features are hypotheses that are, as yet, untested. The model is phenomenologic in nature, in that it outlines a number of experiential and behavioral features associated with hoarding. We make no assumptions about how these features develop, but hypothesize how they are related to each other and to hoarding behavior.

In this model, we view hoarding as a multifaceted problem that stems from four types of deficits or difficulties: (1) information-processing deficits; (2) problems with emotional attachments to possessions; (3) behavioral avoidance; and (4) erroneous or distorted beliefs about the nature or importance of possessions. These deficits or difficulties overlap in significant ways. Each of these facets is discussed together with the pertinent research in the following paragraphs.

Information-Processing Deficits

Deficits in information processing in compulsive hoarding encompass three general and overlapping cognitive functions: (1) decision making; (2) categorization/organization; and (3) memory. These deficits appear to be general, because they are not limited to saving or hoarding. These functions are closely related to one another and can be difficult to separate.

Decision Making

The clinical literature suggests that indecisiveness is a hallmark of compulsive hoarding. Case descriptions typically note the difficulty these people have in making general decisions,[20,35] not merely decisions about what to save and what to throw away. In studies of college students, community volunteers, and self-identified hoarders, we have found substantial correlations between general indecisiveness (unrelated to hoarding) and measures of compulsive hoarding.[15,36] Deciding what to wear in the morning, what to order at a restaurant, and what task to perform next are all troublesome decisions for compulsive hoarders. Warren and Ostrom[20] suggested that the indecisiveness shown by compulsive hoarders may be a way of avoiding mistakes. Consistent with this hypothesis, we found hoarding to be correlated with the perfectionistic concern over making mistakes.[15] As with the findings regarding indecisiveness, this relationship existed in student, community, and self-identified hoarder samples. Perhaps hoarding is an avoidance behavior closely related to indecisiveness and perfectionism[15] (i.e., saving a possession allows the hoarder to avoid the decision required to throw it away, thereby avoiding the worry that a mistake has been made). The general indecisiveness displayed by compulsive hoarders forms the backdrop for specific difficulties in deciding whether or not to save a possession, and if saved, where to put it.

Categorization/Organization

Another information-processing deficit that may be related to compulsive hoarding is categorizing and organizing information. Reed[37] has suggested and other investigators[38-41] have found support for the hypothesis that obsessionals have more complex concepts. They define category boundaries so narrowly that few items fit within them, a feature labelled *underinclusion*, and thus many categories are required to classify personal possessions. This has several implications for compulsive hoarders. First, each possession may be seen as belonging to its own category (i.e., so unique that nothing else is like it and nothing can substitute for it). Such a view makes it difficult to discard anything. Second, because each possession is unique and complex, it is impossible to decide that a class of objects (e.g., old newspapers) is unimportant and can be discarded without closely examining each one. All important aspects of each possession must be examined before discarding. Third, because each possession is unique, it cannot be categorized with similar objects, and thus there is no way to organize possessions.

An example of this phenomenon can be seen in the arrangement of a hoarder's books. The hoarder begins to read a book but must stop to do something else. The book cannot be returned to the shelf because it is now in a different category—books being actively read. It is placed on the coffee table. Next, a cookbook is consulted for dinner, and it too cannot be returned to the shelf, because it is being used. It is deposited on the back of the couch. The dictionary used next cannot be reshelved, lest the person forget the word he looked up. This process is repeated until there are books everywhere, none of which can be returned to its shelf because they are all different in their own category. Their new position in the room has meaning because each position represents a different category, and an idiosyncratic sort of organization exists, but the ultimate result is clutter and chaos.

The finite amount of space available means that possessions must be piled on top of one another until there are large mounds of unrelated objects. From this chaos, a sort of temporal organization emerges. The hoarder may have a sense of where things are placed based on when they entered the pile. Hoarders trying to sort through a pile often pick up a possession and, not being sure what to do with it say, "I'll set it here for now," placing it somewhere nearby. This is repeated until the piles are so large and numerous that they begin merging (or collapsing) into one large pile. With each new attempt to organize and discard, everything in the pile is examined and moved to the new pile or repositioned in the old pile. The end result is that the pile has been "churned" but no real progress has been made.

Another organizational problem is the mixing of important and unimportant possessions. A typical pile contains everything from paychecks to gum wrappers. We have observed that hoarders have trouble determining the relative importance of possessions, because when a possession is picked up and examined, its value increases. Whatever is "in sight" becomes more important. Judgments about discarding or organizing that are based on the value of a possession are thus difficult to make. When being examined by the hoarder, everything seems "very important." In the treatment of hoarding, we recommend the creation of a small number of categories into which objects from a hoarding pile can be placed (e.g., save, discard, to go through later). One of our participants created a fourth category, an "immediate to-go-through" box. In it she placed possessions from a pile on her couch that she deemed essential to go through right away (i.e., before our next session). At the next session she had not gone through the box and could not remember what was in it, so she created *another* category she called "immediate-immediate to-go-through." This box contained the same sorts of things that went into the immediate to-go-through box, but these seemed even more important. The only difference between the objects in these two boxes was that she had handled one group of items more recently and they had therefore become more important to her.

The mixing of important and unimportant objects in a hoarding pile creates complications when trying to excavate the pile. The hoarder's wish to closely review everything before discarding it has some basis in reality. For example, some of our research participants found envelopes full of cash (up to $100) among decades-old newspapers. Such occurrences reinforce the hoarder's belief that he must carefully scrutinize everything before discarding it.

Memory

Some evidence suggests that OCD patients and nonclinical compulsive checkers suffer from subtle memory deficits.[42–44] In addition, OCD patients and nonclinical checkers show less confidence in their memories.[44,45] Similar memory problems have been observed with compulsive hoarders.[21] Frost and Hartl[21] suggested that two aspects of memory are salient: (1) confidence in memory and (2) beliefs about the importance of remembering or recording information. For example, one of our participants saved newspapers because she was convinced she would not remember the information they contained. Saving the newspapers allowed her to feel that she still retained the information, even though she could not remember it. Frost and Longo[46] recently examined several hypotheses regarding memory functioning in compulsive hoarders. Participants scoring high or low on the hoarding scale were given the Wechsler Memory Scale-Revised and a measure of the extent to which they would rely on (have confidence in) their memory. The findings failed to reveal any actual memory deficits, but did reveal significantly lower confidence in memory among hoarders.

Beliefs about memory have been hypothesized to influence memory processes themselves (e.g., Andersson[47]). In the case of hoarding, these beliefs may be important determinants of saving behavior. In addition to believing that things must be saved lest they be forgotten, hoarders also seem to believe that if an object is out of sight, it will be forgotten. The concern reported by one of our participants about using a filing system was, "If I put it with this stuff [into a filing system], I won't remember it!" This suggests that visual cueing is an important memory aid for compulsive hoarders, and this element may explain why hoarders create piles of objects in living areas and why things in sight take on greater value. Difficulties like these suggest that hoarding is a problem not only of saving, but also of organizing possessions.

Why hoarders believe it is important to remember everything is unclear. It may be that they believe the negative consequences of not remembering are more likely and more severe than do nonhoarders. The high levels of perfectionism seen among compulsive hoarders[15] may be partly responsible for these beliefs. Perhaps forgetting is interpreted as a mistake or failure that provokes distress. Lack of confidence in memory among compulsive hoarders may manifest itself in checking rituals. The extent to which the hoarding or checking is the primary symptom may be difficult to determine. Further research on the relationship between checking and hoarding is necessary to sort out these questions.

Emotional Attachment Problems

We have already noted that hoarded items are saved for both nonsentimental and sentimental reasons. Case studies and anecdotal reports of compulsive hoarding frequently note extreme emotional attachments to possessions.[8,19,20,34] From these accounts, it appears that many hoarders see their possessions as extensions of themselves. When other people touch or move them, the hoarder feels violated.[16]

Several empirical studies also have demonstrated the extent to which possessions are saved for sentimental reasons. Frost and Gross[15] found that hoarders reported more sentimental saving than nonhoarders, and greater emotional attachment to possessions. In a subsequent study, Frost, et al[16] found evidence for two types of excessive emotional attachment to possessions among compulsive hoarders: sentimental and security-based. In the former, possessions serve as meaningful reminders of important past events. They become extensions of the self, not to be discarded without careful consideration, because getting rid of such a possession feels like the loss of a close friend. Possessions also provide a source of comfort and security, signaling a safe environment (see Fromm[27]).[48,49] For example, after a particularly stressful day, one hoarder remarked, "I just want to go home and gather my treasures around me." The thought of throwing away these possessions violates this feeling of safety. In a test of these emotional attachment hypotheses, Frost, et al[16] found that among both college student and community samples, hoarding severity was correlated with a measure of sentimental attachment to possessions and the extent to which possessions provided emotional comfort.

Such attachment also appears to occur among hoarders when they are acquiring new possessions. Buying objects seems to provide hoarders with some degree of comfort, even if the items are frivolous. The relationship between compulsive hoarding and compulsive shopping is unclear, although such a relationship has been hypothesized.[21]

Behavioral Avoidance

A third prominent feature of compulsive hoarding is behavioral avoidance. Saving possessions allows the hoarder to avoid the loss of objects that may be needed someday, that may be of use to others, or that are aesthetically pleasing. Hoarding also prevents emotional upset associated with discarding (losing) possessions with sentimental or safety signal value. Although it is clear that these situations are avoided, it is still not entirely clear why. Perhaps the significant variable here is the fear of losing something that is not entirely tangible. Hoarders who save newspapers, for instance, fear losing not so much the paper itself or the stories that they have read, but information that *may* be there. O'Connor and Robillard[50] described people with OCD as creating a fiction ("I may be contaminated") and trying to bend the real world to match the fiction (trying to wash away germs that are not there). This idea is applicable here. Hoarders may manufacture an idea that something very important is embodied in this possession. With newspapers, it may be information. With junk mail, it may be opportunities. Used envelopes may represent a part of their life. Saving these things means avoiding such losses. Likewise, excessive buying of unneeded items may seem to prevent the loss of a good bargain. Relatedly, one of our research participants noted that imagining all the newspapers that are published in the world made her very uncomfortable because of all the information that is lost to her forever.

In addition, hoarders save to avoid decision making—a difficult and unpleasant chore—perhaps because of their excessive concern over mistakes.[15] The overly complex concepts of compulsive hoarders require consideration of many details and for some extensive checking and reading rituals. Simply saving the item avoids this time-consuming and onerous process. In some instances, decision making is more troublesome than actually discarding the possession. On several occasions, we have observed patients with very high anxiety in anticipation of making a decision to discard something, but once the decision is made, the anxiety subsides quickly and thoughts about the object itself play a very small role.

As mentioned earlier, hoarding involves not only the inability to discard objects of limited value, but also a problem in organizing possessions. Without a workable organizational scheme, decisions about where to put things are problematic, especially when coupled with fears of losing information, opportunities, or parts of oneself. Putting everything in a pile to be sorted later avoids this problem, and leaving things in sight avoids the worry that they will be forgotten if they are filed away. Unfortunately, however, the creation of an effective filing system may not resolve fears of loss, as in the case of one client who still reported feeling that filed papers were lost to her despite her newfound ability to locate them using her organizing scheme.

Beliefs About the Nature of Possessions

Underlying many hoarding behaviors is a set of beliefs about the nature and meaning of possessions. Many of these beliefs are experienced by patients with other OCD symptoms (see Chapter 18), but in patients with hoarding tendencies, they have a specific connection to possessions. Several of these beliefs have already been mentioned: (1) beliefs about the necessity of perfection and excessive concern over mistakes; (2) beliefs about responsibility; (3) beliefs about control over possessions; (4) beliefs about emotional attachments to possessions; and (5) beliefs about memory. Each of these beliefs is related to an overestimation of catastrophe or loss. Distorted beliefs about the probability and severity of negative consequences if possessions are discarded or placed out of sight may be a key feature connecting these distorted thoughts. For example, beliefs about memory and the usefulness of keeping important things in sight also appear to influence hoarding behavior. Other types of beliefs are discussed in the following paragraphs.

Perfectionism

As mentioned previously, compulsive hoarders score higher on measures of perfectionism, especially concern over mistakes.[15] It also has been suggested that hoarders have a fundamental belief that perfection is not only possible, but expected.[21] For example, Frost and Hartl[21] described a woman who reported two concerns when trying to discard newspapers. First, she was concerned that she had not read them thoroughly, and second, she couldn't remember what she had read. She believed that it was possible to read the paper and remember everything "perfectly." Failure to do so seemed a catastrophe. Saving the newspapers allowed her to continue the fiction (erroneous belief) that perfect paper reading was possible and to avoid the failure associated with not reading the paper perfectly.

Need for Control

Frost, et al[16] found hoarding to be associated with an exaggerated need for control over possessions. Hoarders were less willing to share possessions with others or to have others touch or use their possessions. Unauthorized touching or moving of possessions can prompt extreme anger among compulsive hoarders.[19] This need for control may be associated with other features. For instance, if someone else touches a possession, it may remove some of the safety signal value of the possession, similar to an object becoming contaminated. Because possessions are often believed to be extensions of the self, it may seem to the hoarder that he is personally being violated when someone touches his things. This feature has obvious implications for treatment, which will be discussed shortly.

Responsibility

Beliefs about the nature of responsibility toward possessions also may play a role in the development and maintenance of hoarding behavior. Frost, et al[16] reported that hoarders felt more responsible for preparing to meet future needs than did nonhoarders. This behavior also was reflected in the fact that hoarders carry more "just-in-case" items in their pockets, purses, and cars than do non-hoarders.[15] If they can imagine a situation in which an object they possess (or could possess) can be used, hoarders appear to feel responsible for attaining and saving that object in case that situation arises.

A second type of responsibility is for the proper care and use of possessions. Discarding a possession that still has a use—even a remote one—leads hoarders to feel guilty about waste. Frost, et al[16] found that hoarders reported these thoughts more frequently than did nonhoarders. Specifically, thoughts such as, "Ownership carries with it a responsibility to use a possession properly," "I must take precautions to protect my possessions from harm," and "I feel guilty if I don't use something for a long time," were reported more frequently by hoarders than by nonhoarders.

Emotional Comfort

In addition to these beliefs, a fourth set of beliefs has to do with beliefs about emotional comfort. Beliefs such as, "Without my possession, I will be vulnerable," "Throwing something away means losing a part of my life," and "My possessions provide me with emotional comfort," characterize compulsive hoarders[16] and undoubtedly make discarding possessions more difficult.

TREATMENT FOR COMPULSIVE HOARDING

At present, very little information is available about the treatment outcomes of patients with hoarding problems. Most single-case and anecdotal reports[9,19] have been descriptive rather than treatment-oriented, noting a tendency among hoarders to be disinterested in changing their behaviors. Occasionally, treatment outcome studies of patients with OCD have made passing reference to the difficulty in treatment of hoarding[14] or to refusal, dropout, or treatment failure of those patients with hoarding symptoms.[55] However, Baer[53] and Foa and Wilson[54] anecdotally described cases of women with hoarding symptoms who made substantial progress in reducing these symptoms by using a behavioral program of gradual exposure to discarding.

Based on an early version of our hoarding model, Frost and Hartl[34] developed a preliminary treatment strategy and applied it in a single case study, using a multiple-baseline design.

Case 1

A 53-year-old woman had suffered from compulsive hoarding since childhood. She had one drug trial—a serotonin reuptake inhibitor (SRI) with limited success—and side effects resulted in discontinuation. Her hoarding behavior was so severe that no room in her house could be used in any normal way.

Because her kitchen table was covered, her family ate with their plates on their laps. Several rooms had only small pathways, with possessions piled halfway to the ceiling everywhere else.

Our treatment strategy had three main components. The first of these was training in decision making and organizational skills for the management of possessions. For many hoarders, the idea of trying to discard possessions is too frightening, but being more organized and decisive is a goal they will agree to and strive to achieve. In this case, decision-making training involved category creation and moving designated possessions to storage with a goal of creating uncluttered living space. This training was performed in the context of weekly excavation sessions with homework between sessions. The second component was exposure to discarding and the associated experiences that saving things allowed her to avoid (i.e., decision making, emotional upset, etc.). Cognitive restructuring of hoarding-related beliefs was the third component of the treatment. Excavation sessions provided an *in vivo* context for cognitive restructuring of beliefs related to saving behaviors (i.e., perfectionism, responsibility, control over possessions, memory, and emotional attachment to possessions).

Treatment progressed with each room being completed before moving to the next. Within each excavation session, a four-step process was used, which included identifying a target area to work on, creating a small number of categories into which possessions were placed, excavation of the area, and physical moving of the items in each category to their proper destination. To assess the severity of hoarding, we calculated two clutter ratios (CRs) for each room in the house before treatment and again when each room was excavated. Floor CRs were calculated by dividing the square footage of floor space that was cluttered by the square footage of total floor space not occupied by furniture. Furniture CRs were calculated by dividing the square footage of cluttered furniture tops by the total square footage of furniture tops minus decorative items. To gain some perspective on normal CRs, a small pilot study was undertaken in which CRs of four nonhoarding individuals were calculated. The mean CRs from this sample for both floor and furniture tops were less than 0.05.

At pretest, this patient's floor CRs ranged from 0.23 to 0.78 with a mean of 0.54. Furniture CRs ranged from 0.53 to 1.0 with a mean of 0.85. Over 18 months and 35 sessions, seven rooms were excavated. When each room was excavated, the CRs declined substantially. Immediately after excavation, the mean CR for floors for all seven rooms was 0.02 and for furniture tops it was 0.05–ratios that were quite normal. The CRs of rooms completed early in the treatment were maintained throughout the 18 months.

The results of this case study indicate that it is possible to significantly alter severe hoarding behavior using a framework consistent with the cognitive-behavioral model outlined earlier. Based on this model of hoarding and the results of this case study, we have generated a treatment program for compulsive hoarding.[54] We are in the process of refining and testing the intervention, which can be administered either by an individual therapist treating a patient in the home or in a group format supplemented with a paraprofessional helper holding excavation sessions in the patient's home. The treatment assumes that the therapist is familiar with this cognitive-behavioral model of compulsive hoarding, and that the patient accepts the basic goals and procedures of treatment. Outlined below are the assessment procedures, treatment goals, treatment rules, a description of the excavation sessions, and a brief overview of cognitive restructuring.

Assessment

A great deal of information about the patient's hoarding behavior is essential for designing this treatment program. Much of this information can be gathered from initial interviews. The types of information needed include the following:

- What types of possessions are saved?
- What are the reasons for saving each type of possession?
- Where are saved items kept? Is there some form of organization?
- What is the actual amount of clutter? Spaces in the house should be evaluated in terms of their usability. Note parts of the house that are unusable because of clutter.
- Are family members involved? How does the problem affect relationships with family or friends?
- How are items acquired? Note how new items enter the house and where they go when they do.
- Does the patient have decision-making problems? A careful analysis of the nature and extent of decision-making problems and the creation of effective decision-making strategies are crucial.
- What avoidance behaviors are evident? A careful analysis of all of the things that are avoided by saving is necessary.
- How much anxiety or discomfort regarding hoarding is experienced during a typical day and during attempts to organize and discard possessions? This information is critical for setting up excavation sessions and hierarchies for discarding, and for determining the course of habituation to discarding.
- What is the patient's hoarding history and previous treatment? Circumstances surrounding the onset of hoarding and the results of previous attempts at treatment for the problem behavior may be helpful.

In addition to this information, standardized assessments also are useful. The Y-BOCS provides an overall index of severity of the problem. We recommend the use of a modified Y-BOCS in which the clinician inquires about the hoarding symptoms rather than all OCD symptoms. We also have developed a Hoarding Severity Scale and a Hoarding Cognitions Inventory to provide additional information on the severity and range of thoughts and beliefs associated with hoarding.* Psychomatic data supporting the reliability and validity of these measures are pending.

Finally, a behavioral assessment of hoarding severity is necessary. As noted earlier, we have used CRs to provide baseline information about the severity of the hoarding problem and to track the progress during treatment. As described earlier, two clutter ratios are useful, one for floor space and one for furniture tops. Photographs or videotapes of rooms also can help in the calculation of these ratios after the initial room measurements are made.

Treatment Goals

A careful discussion of concrete goals is essential prior to beginning treatment. Most severe hoarders are reluctant to enter a treatment program in which the only goal is to discard the possessions they have spent their lives collecting. Thus, in this treatment program, the discarding of possessions is a lesser goal at the outset of treatment and gains importance as it becomes apparent to the patient that the most important goals cannot be reached without discarding. The first and primary goal of this treatment program is the *creation of uncluttered living space*. The most troublesome aspect of compulsive hoarding is that clutter interferes with the ability to use interior living spaces. Most people who suffer from compulsive hoarding can readily agree to such a goal. Even if no change occurs in the acquisition and saving by a hoarding patient, if he is able to maintain uncluttered living spaces in his home, the treatment will have been useful.

A related goal is to *increase the appropriate use of space*. Severe hoarders may not have used most parts of their houses for years. Establishing a regular pattern of use will facilitate the maintenance of a clutter-free house. For instance, patients must learn to use the kitchen table for food preparation or sit-down meals. If it is not used in this way, the table may once again become a space to store hoarded objects.

To excavate and maintain an uncluttered home, it is necessary for a hoarder to *improve decision-making skills,* and to *develop an organizational plan* for the home. The strategy we have adopted is to create with the patient a small number of categories for each type of possession. Then all possessions are placed into one of these categories. Each category has a designated location once excavation is performed. For example, because most compulsive hoarders have difficulty with books, we often begin with books and require that every book in a room go into one of three categories: (1) sell or donate; (2) store; and (3) display. The sell-or-donate books are placed in a box and moved to a designated location out of the main living area. The books to be stored are also placed in a box, labelled, and placed in a designated storage location. Books to display are put on a bookshelf. If the display category is larger than the bookshelf, the extra books are treated like books to store, but are labelled

---

* These scales are available from the authors.

"display" so they may be readily identified when bookshelf space becomes available. Limiting the number of categories makes these first decisions easier and the organizational plan clear. Other types of possessions usually require more elaborate filing systems (e.g., letters, documents, etc.).

Discarding unneeded possessions is a more difficult goal. Most hoarders recognize that they must be more selective about what they keep, but fear they will lose control over what is saved and what is discarded. This is especially problematic in cases in which family members have discarded some possessions against the patient's wishes. In this treatment, we emphasize that the volume of possessions does not matter. What matters instead is that appropriate living space exists in the home. In their efforts to achieve the first several goals, hoarders begin to change their perspective about how much they "need" to keep. One strategy we have found helpful is asking hoarders to think about the clutter in their house as a loss of control. Then, we request that they think about "temporarily suspending" their normal saving behavior to gain control over the clutter. This allows them to view the discarding of possessions as serving a greater purpose (i.e., giving them a sense of control over the hoarding). As the patient gains some experience at discarding, the prospect of discarding unneeded possessions becomes a more palatable therapeutic goal.

Reducing the accumulation of new possessions is a necessary goal of this treatment. Because many hoarding patients engage in compulsive shopping or trash picking in an effort to accumulate new possessions, it is important to understand the value that these possessions have for the hoarder. Understanding the instrumental or sentimental value of each type of acquisition enables the therapist to design specific exposure and response prevention (ERP) strategies as well as cognitive interventions. If the patient accumulates possessions from certain places (e.g., tag sales, dumpsters), the therapist can accompany the patient to these sites, identify desired items, and stay until the patient habituates to the feeling of "needing" to acquire the possession. It is important to emphasize the distinction between objective need and the feeling of need. If a patient can learn this distinction, managing the "feeling" of need may be easier.

Familiarizing patients with the nature of OCD hoarding and the model on which this treatment is based helps them develop confidence in their ability to tolerate the discomfort associated with hoarding. Education regarding OCD hoarding also gives patients a sense of optimism and empowerment. Finally, *developing skill of self-instruction and cognitive correction* of faulty thinking about saving possessions is an essential part of this treatment. The exact nature of these skills and suggestions for developing them are presented in the following paragraphs.

Treatment Rules

The history of interpersonal relationships for someone with a hoarding problem is invariably intertwined with the relationships they have with their possessions. Most hoarders have had family or friends attempt to "help" them with their hoarding problem and actively resist this help because they usually involve offers to make decisions about what to save and to do the discarding for the hoarder. In considering treatment, the hoarder often has only these negative experiences of "helpers" on which to reflect. To make the treatment and the therapist's role clear, specifically defined rules of behavior for the therapist are necessary. Likewise, to make the importance of the procedures clear, a defined set of rules for the patient to follow is necessary. We propose the following six treatment rules.

1. *The therapist may not touch or throw away anything without explicit permission.* Knowing that the therapist will not touch a possession without permission helps to develop trust and confidence in a cooperative patient-therapist relationship. This is not an easy rule to follow. The impulse to pick things up and discard or organize them is strong when the goal is to remove clutter. However, if the rule is violated, the trust between the therapist and patient also will be violated. There may be some exceptions to this rule if the patient has contamination fears or obsessions about others disturbing their possessions. In this case, a change in the rule should be negotiated and the rationale for doing so should be clear to both patient and therapist.

2. *All decisions regarding saving, discarding, and organizing are made by the patient.* Because part of the problem of compulsive hoarding has to do with inability to make decisions of this sort, making decisions for these patients will not help. Indeed, one of the goals for the treatment is to teach the patient how to make decisions.

3. *Any possession touched by the patient during an excavation session should be placed in a final location.* The excavation sessions should enable the patient to learn the most efficient way of organizing and discarding to prevent behaviors that have led to the clutter problem. One of the most prominent of these is "churning." We use the Only Handle It Once (OHIO) rule: Whenever a possession is picked up, it cannot go back onto the pile. It must go into one of the categories generated prior to the excavation (or in some cases, a new category).

4. *Categories for possessions must be established before handling them.* Before each excavation session, a small number of categories must be established by the patient and therapist. This is essential for the development of efficient decision making and organization of possessions.

5. *Treatment should proceed systematically.* Like the excavation sessions themselves, it is important that the treatment sequences be systematic and well organized, so the patient will know what needs to be done and when. Many hoarders spend hours trying to organize and discard with little success, because their efforts are unfocused and produce little visible benefit. They may spend 30 minutes in one room and 30 minutes in another room and in the end see no progress. Thus, it is important that treatment should focus on one area

or room until it is complete before moving to the next. More easily categorized objects (e.g., books) should be first, and should progress to more difficult ones (documents). Focus first on spaces in which progress will be readily observable and have the most desired functional effect for the patient (e.g., able to eat comfortably or sit in favorite chair).

6. *Flexible and creative strategies are to be applied as needed to make steady progress.* There will invariably be unforeseen problems in trying to excavate a house full of possessions. It may be necessary, for instance, to temporarily redefine some areas of the home as storage rather than living space, until more actual storage space becomes available later in the treatment.

Excavation Sessions

Before beginning the first excavation session, the patient should understand the model of hoarding and the objectives of the treatment. The excavation sessions are designed to create *in vivo* opportunities for the patient and therapist to encounter each of the problems outlined in the model. These sessions have clear-cut steps to help the patient structure similar excavation homework between sessions. Such structure helps the patient avoid some of the difficulties encountered in previous attempts to clear the house. The specific steps for each excavation session are outlined in the following list.

- Step 1. Select a target area (e.g., kitchen table).
- Step 2. Assess types of possessions in the target area.
- Step 3. Determine hierarchy of items within target area.
- Step 4. Select type of possession with which to begin.
- Step 5. Create categories and a filing system for this possession type.
- Step 6. Begin excavating.
- Step 7. Continue until target area is clear.
- Step 8. Plan for appropriate use of cleared space.
- Step 9. Plan for preventing new clutter to this area.

Cognitive Restructuring

During excavation sessions, there is ample time to explore the belief systems underlying hoarding behavior. The therapist should encourage the patient to verbalize thoughts and feelings when excavating to understand specific decision-making problems and erroneous beliefs regarding saving and discarding. A "stream of consciousness" instruction facilitates this process. It is important to help the patient recognize his characteristic thought processes and develop ways of challenging these beliefs. The most common themes encountered are perfectionism, responsibility, control, emotional attachment, and beliefs about memory. A variety of techniques are useful here to challenge these thoughts and the excessive value placed on possessions. These cognitive techniques are described elsewhere[52] (see Chapter 18).

During these sessions, it is important that the therapist not express disappointment or negative feedback regarding decisions made by the patient. Such expressions are likely to increase shame and disappointment and decrease motivation. It also is important not to engage in extended arguments with the patient about a decision to save something. A Socratic approach that encourages the patient to question his or her reason for saving something is preferable. These instances also may provide opportunities to remind patients of the goals in treatment, especially the need to create usable living spaces and to establish decision-making rules and categories for saving.

Behavioral experiments to test the patient's beliefs and reactions also are helpful in the process of cognitive restructuring. Most hoarders show excessive attachment to possessions that have little instrumental value and are not reminders of special times. They believe they will not be able to tolerate discarding such a possession. A behavioral experiment to test this hypothesis by discarding such an item reveals not only the strength of this feeling, but also the amount of time it takes to habituate to a decision to discard such a possession. The outcome of such an experiment also will clearly show the patient that his or her "feeling" of being unable to stand it is inaccurate.

SUMMARY

Obsessive-compulsive hoarding is a little-studied phenomenon. This chapter reviews the existing literature on this topic, presents a cognitive-behavioral model of compulsive hoarding, and outlines a treatment program for this problem. The literature review suggests a change in the definition of compulsive hoarding most commonly used so as not to exclude possessions saved for sentimental reasons. Compulsive hoarding was defined here as having three parts: (1) the acquisition of, and failure to discard, a large number of possessions that appear to be useless or of limited value; (2) living spaces sufficiently cluttered so as to preclude activities for which those spaces were designed; and (3) significant distress or impairment in function caused by the hoarding. The cognitive-behavioral model of compulsive hoarding emphasizes four major factors: (1) information-processing deficits; (2) problems with emotional attachments to possessions; (3) behavioral avoidance; and (4) erroneous or distorted beliefs about the nature or importance of possessions. The individual and group treatment program outlined emphasizes the creation of uncluttered living space, the appropriate use of uncluttered space, improvement in decision-making skills, and the creation of an organizational plan for possessions. As treatment progresses, more emphasis is placed on discarding and reducing accumulation. The treatment is conducted in the context of highly structured excavation sessions during which exposure and cognitive restructuring can take place.

REFERENCES

1. Honig WK: Structure and function in the spatial memory of animals. In Abraham WC, Corballis M, White KG, editors: *Memory mechanisms: A tribute to GV Goddard*, Hillsdale, 1991, Lawrence Erlbaum.
2. Anderson C: Imagination and expectation: The effect of imagining scripts on personal intentions, *J Personal Soc Psychol* 45:293–305, 1983.
3. Kolb B: Prefrontal lesions alter eating and hoarding behavior in rats, *Physiol Behav* 12:507–511, 1974.
4. Lanier DL, Estep DQ, Dewsbury DA: Food hoarding in muroid rodents, *Behav Biol* 11:177–187, 1974.
5. Wallace RJ: Tail-hoarding in the albino rat, *Anim Behav* 24:176–180, 1976.
6. Wallace RJ: Hoarding of inedible objects by albino rats, *Behav Neurol Biol* 23: 409–414, 1978.
7. Smith JP: *Mammalian behavior: The theory and the science*, Tuckahoe, 1990, Bench Mark Books.
8. Frankenburg F: Hoarding in anorexia nervosa, *Br J Med Psychol* 57:57–60, 1984.
9. Greenberg D, Witztum E, Levy A: Hoarding as a psychiatric symptom, *J Clin Psychiatry* 51:417–421, 1990.
10. Luchins DJ, et al: Repetitive behaviors in chronically institutionalized schizophrenic patients, *Schizophr Res* 8:119–123, 1992.
11. American Psychiatric Association: *Diagnostic and statistical manual of mental disorders*, ed 4, Washington, 1994, American Psychiatric Association Press.
12. van Houten R, Rolider A: Recreating the scene: An effective way to provide delayed punishment for inappropriate motor behavior, *J Appl Behav Anal* 21:187–192, 1988.
13. Goodman WK, et al: The Yale-Brown Obsessive Compulsive Scale: I. Development, use, and reliability, *Arch Gen Psychiatry* 46:1006–1011, 1989.
14. Steketee G: *Treatment of obsessive compulsive disorder*, New York, 1993, Guilford Press.
15. Frost RO, Gross RC: The hoarding of possessions, *Behav Res Ther* 31:367–381, 1993.
16. Frost RO, et al: The value of possessions in compulsive hoarding, *Behav Res Ther* 33:897–902, 1995.
17. Frost RO, Krause M, Steketee G: Hoarding and obsessive compulsive symptoms, *Behav Mod* 20:116–132, 1996.
18. Furby L: Possessions: Toward a theory of their meaning and function throughout the life cycle. In Bates PB, editor: *Life span development and behavior*, vol 1, New York, 1978, Academic Press.
19. Greenberg D: Compulsive hoarding, *Am J Psychother* XLI:409–416, 1987.
20. Warren LW, Ostrom JC: Pack rats: World class savers, *Psychol Today* 22:58–62, 1988.
21. Frost RO, Hartl T: A cognitive-behavioral model of compulsive hoarding, *Behav Res Ther* 34:341–350, 1996.
22. Pollak J: Obsessive-compulsive personality: Theoretical and clinical perspectives and recent research findings, *J Personal Dis* 1:248–262, 1987.
23. Heatherington EM, Brackbill Y: Etiology and covariation of obstinacy, orderliness and parsimony in young children, *Child Dev* 34:919–943, 1963.

24. Rasmussen SA, Eisen JL: Clinical features and phenomenology of obsessive-compulsive disorder, *Psychiatr Ann* 19:67–73, 1989.
25. Rapoport JL: *The boy who couldn't stop washing: The experience and treatment of obsessive-compulsive disorder*, New York, 1989, EP Dutton.
26. Leonard HL, et al: Childhood rituals: Normal development or obsessive-compulsive symptoms? *J Am Acad Child Adolesc Psychiatry* 29:17–23, 1990.
27. Fromm E: *Man for himself: An inquiry into the psychology of ethics*, New York, 1947, Rinehart.
28. James W: *The principals of psychology*, vol 2, New York, 1918, Dover Publications.
29. Freud S: *Collected papers*, vol 2, London, 1908, Hogarth.
30. Jones E: Anal erotic character traits, 1912. In Jones E, editor: *Papers on psychoanalysis*, London, 1938, Tindall & Cox.
31. Bender L, Schilder P: Impulsions: A specific disorder of the behavior of children, *Arch Neurol Psychiatry* 44:990–1008, 1940.
32. Adams PL: *Obsessive children*, New York, 1973, Brunner/Mazel.
33. Salzman L: *The obsessive personality: Origins, dynamics, and therapy*, New York, 1973, Jason Aronson.
34. Frost RO, Hartl T: Treatment of compulsive hoarding: A multiple baseline single case design. Paper presented at the annual meeting of the Association for the Advancement of Behavior Therapy, Washington, 1995.
35. Shafran R, Tallis F: Obsessive-compulsive hoarding: Three cases suggesting the primacy of learning and cognition, Unpublished manuscript, 1995.
36. Frost RO, Shows DL: The nature and measurement of compulsive indecisiveness, *Behav Res Ther* 31:683–692, 1993.
37. Reed GF: *Obsessional experience and compulsive behavior: A cognitive-structural approach*, New York, 1985, Academic Press.
38. Frost RO, et al: Information processing among non-clinical compulsives, *Behav Res Ther* 26:275–277, 1988.
39. Persons J, Foa E: Processing of fearful and neutral information by obsessive-compulsives, *Behav Res Ther* 22:259–265, 1984.
40. Reed GF: Under-inclusion—A characteristic of obsessional personality disorder: I, *Br J Psychiatry* 115:781–785, 1969a.
41. Reed GF: Under-inclusion—A characteristic of obsessional personality disorder: II, *Br J Psychiatry* 115:787–790, 1969b.
42. Boone KB, et al: Neuropsychological characteristics of nondepressed adults with obsessive-compulsive disorder, *Neuropsychiatr Neuropsychol Behav Neurol* 4: 96–109, 1991.
43. Christensen KL, et al: Neuropsychological performance in obsessive-compulsive disorder, *Biol Psychiatry* 31:4–18, 1992.
44. Sher KJ, Frost RO, Otto R: Cognitive deficits in compulsive checkers: An exploratory study, *Behav Res Ther* 21:357–363, 1983.
45. McNally RJ, Kohlbeck PA: Reality monitoring in obsessive-compulsive disorder, *Res Ther* 31:249–253, 1993.
46. Frost RO, Longo C: Memory deficits in compulsive hoarding, Unpublished manuscript, 1996.
47. Andersson M, Krebs JR: On the evolution of hoarding behaviour, *Anim Behav* 26:707–711, 1978.

48. Rachman S: The modification of agoraphobic avoidance behaviour: Some fresh possibilities, *Behav Res Ther* 21:567–574, 1983.
49. Sartory G, Master D, Rachman S: Safety-signal therapy in agoraphobics: A preliminary test, *Behav Res Ther* 27:205–210, 1989.
50. O'Connor K, Robillard S: Inference processes in obsessive-compulsive disorder: Some clinical observations, *Behav Res Ther* 33:887–896, 1995.
51. Freeston MH, Rheaume J, Ladouceur R: Correcting faulty appraisals of obsessional thoughts, *Behav Res Ther* 34:433–446, 1996.
52. Frost RO, Steketee G: Individual treatment manual for compulsive hoarding, Unpublished treatment manual, 1996.
53. Baer L: *Getting control: Overcoming your obsessions and compulsions*, Boston, 1991, Little, Brown, & Co.
54. Foa EB, Wilson R: *Stop obsessing*, New York, 1991, Bantam.
55. Ball SG, Baer L, Otto MW: Symptom subtypes of obsessive-compulsive disorder in behavioral treatment studies: A quantitative review, *Behav Res Ther* 34:47–51, 1996. (revised May 21, 1997).

24

Religion, Scrupulosity, and Obsessive-Compulsive Disorder

Joseph W. Ciarrocchi, Ph.D.

I was lost in a momentary reverie while writing this chapter when the phone rang. The caller from 1,000 miles away told me he had a degree in theology and suffered from chronic obsessive-compulsive disorder (OCD). He was seeking referral to a therapist who was both knowledgeable about OCD and open to the religious dimension. He explained that his current therapist was sufficiently informed about OCD, yet seemed unable to handle the religious symptoms. This clinical vignette is common when OCD intersects with religious symptoms in persons of faith.

There are at least three reasons for clinicians to attend to the religious dimensions of OCD.

1. *Clinical assessment requires an individualized cultural formulation for each patient.* Just as failing to attend to a person's ethnic, gender, or socio-economic status would miss essential information, so too does failing to attend to religious orientation. Indeed the *Diagnostic and Statistical Manual of Mental Disorders* (DSM-IV) requires that we understand exactly how religious culture affects each of the following areas[1]: (1) the person's conceptualization of the problem; (2) the therapist's ability to understand the person's symptoms; (3) the therapist's ability to communicate clearly with the person; and (4) the development and implementation of the treatment plan. This chapter describes how the religious dimension of OCD affects each of these crucial areas and requires clinical understanding beyond expertise in such common nonreligious symptoms as checking and cleaning.

2. *Current ethical regulations direct clinicians to recognize and respect the person's individual beliefs.* For example, the code of ethics of the American Psychological Association requires nonjudgmental respect for, and noninterference with, individual religious beliefs.[2] When clinicians see religious symp-

toms in persons with OCD, ethical concerns oblige them to approach the symptoms with care and sensitivity. A person's faith is part of his or her core understanding of the universe and the self. Believers view attempts to "modify" these "responses" by even well-intentioned therapists as "explaining away" their religious beliefs. Naturally, this generates resistance to any treatment plan.

3. *Researchers and clinicians now agree that the more intractable symptoms in OCD often fall under the rubric of overvalued ideas.*[3] Overvalued ideas occupy a midway point between reality and delusion—ideas firmly held but with a tinge of uncertainty as to their truth. Religious obsessions and compulsions, because they involve the ethical dimension for people, frequently fall into this category of overvalued ideas. People with OCD may sense the irrationality of their anxiety-driven religious behavior, yet cannot give themselves permission to act against the religious compulsions. Accurate assessment of overvalued ideas is essential to developing motivational and treatment planning strategies. Because exposure-based treatment simultaneously induces fear and challenges faith in religious OCD symptoms, the therapist who proceeds without taking this into consideration may meet with powerful resistance.

BARRIERS TO UNDERSTANDING RELIGIOUS SYMPTOMS IN OCD

Despite the importance of attending to the religious dimensions of OCD, barriers exist between clinicians and patients who attempt this complex task. Although a lengthy discussion of the historical tension between mental health and religion is beyond the scope of this chapter, at least four such barriers are worth discussing.

The Diversity of Religious Practices

In the United States alone scholars identify 1,730 primary religious bodies, each with its own definable set of beliefs and practices.[4] New York City alone has scores of language groups, many with their own religious culture. In light of this diversity, not even the most dedicated student could possibly become familiar with the entire range of religious beliefs in most communities.

Hermeneutic or Language Barriers

The different languages of theology and psychology can create barriers to understanding and, in turn, to treatment. An example is the word "conscience." Psychology, influenced by Freud, views conscience as an *emotional* faculty; when one acts contrary to conscience, the resulting feeling is guilt for having broken the rules. (In psychoanalytic terms, these rules reflect the operating of the superego.)

In many moral theology systems (particularly those influenced by Aristotle or epistemologic realism), conscience is seen as a *judgment,* an act of reason to discern the moral nature of a particular behavior.

Clinicians often focus on the destructive nature of an overly rigid and punitive "conscience" with its attendant paralyzing guilt. But religious individuals see "conscience" as an essential cognitive act in making ethical decisions. Thus, therapists tend to help patients eliminate the damaging features of "conscience," while religious ministers tend to value "conscience" as an ethical guide.

Religious OCD sufferers can easily get caught in a trap between the equivocal uses of the word "conscience." Already beset with anxiety over life's uncertainties, their confusion may intensify if they believe the therapist is trying to mitigate the strength of their "conscience."

Religiosity Gap

Many studies have documented a large disparity between therapists and the general population regarding participation in organized religion. Bergin pointed out that many more therapists than members of the general population no longer participate in the religious tradition in which they were raised.[5] This high rate of "apostasy," to use Bergin's language, means that many therapists have left behind institutional religion. For example, half of American psychologists responded "none" when asked what religion they belong to, a rate considerably lower than average for Americans.[6] This disparity may raise countertransference issues that training programs seldom address.

Ethical Dilemmas

Ethical dilemmas often emerge for both patient and therapist in the treatment of OCD. For example, telling a woman who is bombarded with blasphemous intrusive thoughts in church to stop attending church services might be effective from a solution-focused viewpoint. However, if she then begins to obsess about going to Hell for missing church, the new symptoms are iatrogenic.

Advice about sexual behavior may also complicate OCD treatment. Obsessions about refraining from masturbation may cause the therapist to recommend engaging in the behavior. Two negative outcomes can result: (1) the patient may leave treatment because the advice violates conscience, or (2) guilt may intensify after complying with the advice.

Ethical dilemmas in OCD are a two-way street, because like their patients, therapists need to believe that treatment is consistent with their own values. For therapists who maintain that OCD symptoms are surface manifestations of intrapsychic conflicts, a frontal assault on the symptoms may seem unethical because it does not get at the "real" problem. Belief in symptom substitution poses other therapeutic riddles with potential ethical implications. For example, as a trainee at an outpatient VA Mental Health Clinic, I was instructed by a staff psychiatrist not to attempt to "take away all the phobias" of an OCD patient. By implication, the "real" problem may have manifested itself in an even more destructive way had I done so. Therapists with such belief systems may find behavioral approaches alone to be unethical.

SCRUPULOSITY IN THE HISTORY OF PASTORAL CARE

In traditional Christianity, pastoral theology and pastoral care are, respectively, the conceptual and applied domains of individual spiritual care. These fields provide guidelines for the community's religious leaders to minister to the individual needs of its members. Originally derived from moral theology, these disciplines have long addressed patterns of religious behavior that we recognize today as OCD under the term "scrupulosity."

Derived from the diminutive for the Latin word meaning a small, sharp stone, "scrupulosity" alluded to either making too much of a small matter, or the discomfort associated with walking with such a sharp stone in your shoe. Scrupulosity, then, came to mean both the cause (excessive conscientiousness) and effect (the psychic pain from such an outlook) of the condition. Gradually, tradition shortened it to simply "seeing sin where there is none."

Although scrupulosity takes a number of forms in religious life, it is important to see *doubt* as the key ingredient in all. Similarly, the French refer to OCD as "the doubting disease."

Specific content questions about beliefs or dogma are typical with scrupulosity. All ministers deal regularly with questions of faith in all congregations (e.g., "Could Jesus be God?" "Is there life after death?" "How could there be a God given the fact of the Holocaust?"). What distinguishes scrupulosity from normal questioning and intellectual curiosity is the inability to resolve doubt. OCD sufferers become caught in an endless loop of reasoning from first premises to conclusions and back again, never reaching a final conclusion.

Another area of religious practice in which scrupulosity is encountered is spiritual direction. Some religious groups encourage this practice in which a member who is well schooled in the spiritual life guides others, either individually or in groups. Historically, spiritual directors cautioned their directees about scrupulous practices. Monks, for example, might manifest scrupulous behavior through restriction of food or drink, endless repetitive prayers, wearing of hair shirts, or self-flagellation with chains, never believing they had done enough.

In the moral realm, two features are common:

1. Excessive guilt over moral transgressions manifests itself in the belief that one's sin is so great it cannot be forgiven. Sometimes the "sin" is trivial or, even worse, unknown. In the seventeenth century the renowned English spiritual writer, John Bunyan, believed he had committed the "unpardonable sin" against the Holy Spirit, even though he could not name his transgression.[7] I once met a twentieth century counterpart to Bunyan. He was a young man who had this same obsession after listening to tapes on the topic of unpardonable sins by Reverend Jimmy Swaggart. His father was contacting religious scholars who might have some idea what the sin referred to, even looking for those who could read Aramaic, the supposed conversational language of Jesus.

Those who repeatedly request forgiveness for sins without feeling assurance of forgiveness also fall into this category. In the Catholic practice of confession, bringing up "old" sins and believing that one did not confess properly also are examples of scrupulosity.

2. Following rules rigidly with no sense of proportion or an inability to adjust rules to fit changing circumstances. A Jewish man who suffered from OCD told the following story: One Saturday during the U.S. Great Depression, his grandfather was walking to synagogue and happened upon a $10 bill on the ground, which surpassed a week's income at the time. His interpretation of religious law forbade him to pick up money on the Sabbath. Instead, he put his foot on the money and stood there until the Sabbath ended at sundown, when he picked it up and went home, never having attended services.

Clergy developed pastoral strategies that rested on their moral theology tradition to care for persons with scrupulosity. To highlight the connection between these practices and modern behavior therapy, we need to review pastoral care's conceptual model.

Two general points are relevant for the relationship between scrupulosity and OCD. First, an ancient principle held that "one cannot act with a doubtful conscience." The reasoning is that, in true doubt, one could be doing evil as easily as doing good. This position pervades the debate over the morality of abortion, which continues to divide many today. As far back as the Middle Ages, Christian, Jewish, and Islamic theologians were divided about the point at which a person exists *in utero*. The principle of never acting in a doubtful situation means that direct abortion is illicit because it could constitute killing an innocent person.

But ambiguity in moral behavior is common, so how should one act in unclear situations? To help, scholastic theology developed the notion of a *probable* conscience (under "correct" in Table 24-1). When absolute values were not at issue and choice had a degree of reason behind it, the person could act with probable certitude. To modern thinkers "probable certitude" may seem an oxymoron, but theologians in the late Middle Ages appreciated that some degree of uncertainty attends many everyday human choices and they devised guidelines for discerning sensible reasoning at such moments.

Some historical attempts to apply this reasoning became far-fetched through the discipline of casuistry (i.e., moral reasoning based on the study of ethical cases). This reached its nadir when the great French mathematician and philosopher Blaise Pascal pilloried it, yet ironically, ethicists of late have returned to using aspects of casuistry in grappling with thorny problems in biomedical ethics.[8]

Pastoral theology called scrupulosity a form of erroneous conscience that could take two forms: lax or scrupulous. Lax conscience means "I see an act as acceptable when it is really wrong" (e.g., a World War II German soldier kills an innocent Jewish child because he was "following orders"). Scrupulous

Table 24-1   Moral Theology Tradition Types of Conscience

Correct	Erroneous	Doubtful
Certain	Lax	
Probable	Scrupulous	

conscience means judging behavior to be wrong when it is really permissible (e.g., a monk refuses to touch his genitals with his own hand when washing for fear of illicit sexual stimulation).

Armed with a conceptual model that views scrupulosity as erroneous, pastoral ministers evolved a number of prescient strategies in recognizing they had to circumvent three behavioral tendencies in scrupulous persons: (1) the tendency repeatedly to seek reassurance (e.g., "Are you sure I can do x?"); (2) the tendency to repeat religious practices, often in an attempt to "get them right"; and (3) the Catholic tradition of using confession repetitively to seek reassurance of forgiveness. Manuals written for confessors as far back as the sixteenth century provided strategies for ministering to the scrupulous:

1. The person has a duty to act contrary to the scruples. This follows from the position that a scrupulous conscience, in fact, is an erroneous conscience, and must be corrected. St. Ignatius Loyola developed the maxim for this, *agere contra*, meaning "do the opposite." If the impulse is to repeat something, don't; if the impulse is to avoid an activity, do it.

2. When the scrupulous person is uncertain as to what would be correct behavior in a situation, he or she should imitate a "prudent person."

3. Even though the person will doubt the advice given by a spiritual advisor or minister, he or she must blindly obey.

4. When the person desires to avoid situations or events that trigger scrupulous feelings or tendencies, he or she faces them directly. A traditional manual recommends:

> If impure thoughts arise by his looking at innocent objects or persons, he may look attentively at such things and becomingly at such persons, and pay no attention to the resulting emotions.[9]

5. The scrupulous person must stop using religious practices in a repetitive, ritualistic manner. For example, the personal confessors of both Martin Luther and Saint Ignatius Loyola forbade them to bring up past sins in their confessions.

Readers familiar with modern behavior therapy treatment for OCD will recognize the ecclesiastical applications of techniques such as exposure and response prevention (ERP) and modeling.

ASSESSMENT OF RELIGIOUS SYMPTOMS IN OCD

This section and the next presuppose some understanding of standard behavioral approaches such as ERP and theoretic rationale (see Chapter 17). Comprehensive treatment also assumes that the therapist is knowledgeable about issues of medication referral and the literature on the effectiveness of behavioral and pharmacologic treatments of OCD, alone or in combination (see Chapter 22).

Scrupulosity Types

Figure 24-1 illustrates three types of scrupulosity:

1. *Emotional scrupulosity* refers to what we recognize today as OCD.
2. *Developmental scrupulosity* emerges naturally during adolescence or young adulthood, or as part of a conversion experience. In adolescence, youngsters may develop a heightened religious sensitivity, which evolves into a moral or spiritual perfectionism and leads to a preoccupation with such issues as world hunger, peace, sexual impropriety, and intimacy with God. Religious obsessions and compulsions are common in this phase. Most people mature out of religious obsessive-compulsive symptoms with the help of patient mentors.

Another form of developmental scrupulosity occurs for some who undergo a religious conversion. Both Martin Luther and Ignatius Loyola experienced this behavior. St. Ignatius could not step on two pieces of straw if they formed a cross, lest he show disrespect to Christ crucified. Both, as previously noted, irritated their confessors with their ritualistic use of the sacrament of Confession. (How intriguing from a psychologic standpoint that the central historic figures in the Protestant Reformation and the Catholic Counter-Reformation both suffered from scrupulosity.) As with adolescent scrupulosity, appropriate religious consultation usually alleviates the condition.

3. *Environmental scrupulosity* has a strong situational component and has to be carefully taught, to borrow a lyric from Oscar Hammerstein. This form is usually transmitted by subgroups within religious traditions who teach the necessity of strict legalistic conformity to spiritual or moral values. These subgroups transmit ethical guidelines that exceed the received norms of the majority. For example, one community of Italian monks places stiff-bristled scrub brushes in the shower stalls so monks need not touch their genitals when washing. Another woman has accepted the view of her religious educators that sex is, in itself, inherently nasty and disgusting, even if permitted in marriage; when she has sex with her husband, she puts her Bible in a drawer so as to not mix religious and sexual images in her mind. Another Catholic man still cannot eat meat on Fridays because a priest told him that the church expected sacrifice from people, even though the law has changed.

Pastoral interventions for environmental scrupulosity require mentoring similar to that discussed for developmental scrupulosity. However, attending

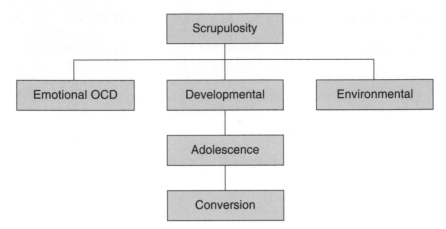

Fig. 24-1   Scrupulosity types.

to the environment is equally important, because those people unable to remove themselves from social influences that are supportive of scrupulous practices may have difficulty in their recovery.

Behavioral Assessment of Scrupulosity

Dealing with scrupulosity through behavior therapy requires understanding the functional distinction between obsessions and compulsions. DSM-IV now codifies obsessions and compulsions according to behavioral typology (i.e., an obsession is an unwanted thought, image, feeling, impulse, or behavior that *triggers* anxiety, whereas a compulsion is a thought, image, or act that *relieves* anxiety). Obsessions are anxiogenic; compulsions are anxiolytic. One challenge in treating scrupulosity is distinguishing obsessions from compulsions, particularly if the clinician is unfamiliar with the person's religious tradition. Because exposure therapy with response prevention requires an accurate assessment, if the clinician is unsure, consultation with a religious expert in the patient's tradition may be helpful.

As is the case for nonreligious symptoms, purely cognitive events present the most difficulty in assessment (e.g., mental prayer). Subjective experience in prayer for scrupulous persons may alternately focus on obsessions or compulsions so that only detailed assessment can provide a functional distinction. For example, a woman has thoughts about the devil when she prays in church. To combat these, she closes her eyes and prays harder, but then her thoughts become sexually blasphemous and she prays for forgiveness. Next, she tries to distract herself by thinking about going to a movie after church, but this triggers guilt for not praying properly and allowing worldly ideas to intrude. So she prays for forgiveness, which, in turn, leads to thoughts about the devil, because she believes she may go to Hell for her sins.

These cognitive obsessions and compulsions are frequently entangled. The clinician must help this woman categorize her mental events into either intrusive, unwanted thoughts (obsessions) or mental acts in response to these thoughts (compulsions). Whether one is treating someone who compulsively checks electric outlets or compulsively prays in response to intrusive images, therapy requires knowing which stimuli require exposure and which require prevention.

To further confuse matters, clinicians may be unclear as to whether particular religious practices are authentic expressions of faith or part of the illness. Psychiatrist Daniel Greenberg has outlined five helpful principles to help clinicians evaluate their own "index of suspicion" about a particular religious practice related to OCD.[10]

1. Practices that are beyond the requirements of the law (e.g., when members act "more Catholic than the Pope"). If a ritual requires abstaining from food or drink, the scrupulous person may begin to believe that swallowing saliva is sinful.

2. Beliefs or practices that have a narrow focus, or attention paid in prayer to "getting it right," rather than to a way of developing a relationship with God.

3. Scruples that interfere with standard religious practice, such as when members stop attending church or synagogue because of intrusive blasphemous thoughts.

4. Ignoring the essential, such as when performing a ritual perfectly consumes significant amounts of time and energy, but charity toward the less fortunate has no attraction.

5. Religious symptoms resemble typical OCD symptoms, such as an emphasis on checking or repeating prayers, religious rituals, or seeking spiritual guidance. Similarly, nonreligious symptoms of OCD are common in cases of scrupulosity.

TREATMENT OF RELIGIOUS SYMPTOMS IN OCD

As described in Chapter 17, the core of behavioral treatment of OCD is ERP. Step-by-step guidelines are also available.[11–14] Following are examples of exposure for religious symptoms and a discussion of dealing with resistance based on religious grounds.

Once patient and therapist have distinguished religious obsessions from compulsions, the stage is set.

Case 1

The following is an exposure scene used by a woman with OCD who became guilt-ridden and prayed compulsively whenever she had negative feelings or thoughts about annoying personal habits of her husband or children. Because the words, "I hate x when he or she . . . ," triggered intense anxiety, she recorded the following on audiotape in the therapist's office.

I hate Bill (*husband*) when he doesn't clean up his dishes at the dinner table. I hate him when he sits in front of the television all day. I hate him when he sulks for an entire afternoon. I hate him when he does not ask me how my day went. I hate Phoebe (*daughter*) when she answers back to me. I hate her when she throws all her dirty clothes in a heap on the floor instead of the hamper. I hate her when she teases her little brother. I hate Ryan (*son*) when he doesn't wipe his tennis shoes off after playing in the mud. I hate him when he won't fall asleep when I put him down and keeps asking for me to read him a story.

The audiotape included variations on these themes and lasted approximately 20 minutes. As she made the tape, she recognized that her complaints were exaggerated, and that the events were really only annoyances. But because her distress was high in response to the words "I hate," and to experiencing negative feelings toward family members, combining the words with annoying events provided a double exposure. After playing the tape at home several times a day, she reported that negative feelings no longer triggered compulsive praying, even when she experienced twinges of guilt.

Case 2

A 37-year-old homosexual Baptist man who lived a celibate life was plagued by constant worries around intrusive sexual thoughts. Although he was physically attracted only to adult men, he had severe obsessions of pedophilia. Whenever he saw a handsome young man, he began to worry that he might not be older than 18 years of age. He was so concerned about having sexual thoughts toward underage boys that he avoided looking at *any* man who was not obviously older than approximately 30 years of age. This obsession was most bothersome during church services, because the notion of having sexual thoughts about minors in church was horrific. As a result, he gazed with a fixed stare at the minister, lest his eyes wander and he be guilty of the sin of pedophilia.

Stage 1 of his exposure program involved obtaining a large department store catalogue. Therapist and patient then went through the fashions for adult men, selecting approximately 10 pictures of men modeling business wear, casual wear, and beach attire. The patient then rank-ordered the pictures according to the degree of distress each picture generated, from least to most anxiety-provoking, with no large gaps in anxiety between any two pictures. Exposure then began in the therapist's office with the patient staring at the least anxiety-provoking picture until anxiety was sufficiently reduced. This process continued until desensitization was achieved for all the pictures.

Stage 2 used the same catalogue, but this time the pictures were selected from the adolescent fashion section. Again, the patient chose a range of pictures from dress clothes to beachwear, and exposure then proceeded in the same manner as described earlier. During both stages, the patient continued exposure trials at home, although it took several weeks of *in vitro* sessions before he had sufficient self-confidence to try it on his own.

Stage 3 involved *in vivo* exposure in natural environments. Now instead of avoiding looking at young men, the patient was instructed to actively seek them out and to look at them in a natural way.

Stage 4 involved performing the same *in vivo* exposure with adolescent men, and stage 5 involved purposely looking at young men and teenage boys during church services. (Television programs often provide useful exposure trials, because scenes that scrupulous people avoid are readily available.)

Problems in Behavioral Treatment

The largest problem in treating religious OCD symptoms is gaining patient compliance to engage in exposure treatment. DiClemente and Prochaska,[15] in their transtheoretic model of behavior change, aptly comment on the importance of determining a patient's motivational stage in the success of treatment. Although ERP is the state-of-the-art procedure for changing OCD symptoms, if patients refuse to try it, no change will occur.

Religious-based resistance to exposure is usually caused by the patient's belief that the recommended procedure is morally objectionable. Some patients claim that therapists are not sufficiently familiar with their religious tradition and thus unwittingly suggest objectionable practices. Others may suspect that most therapists are antireligious and are intentionally trying to convert patients to their way of thinking.

Others conflate certain acts of thinking, imagining, and feeling with moral value. The prototype of this was the infamous *Playboy* magazine interview of President Jimmy Carter wherein he confessed to the sin of "having lust in his heart." Carter was giving a common interpretation to the gospel saying of Jesus,

"You have heard it said, 'You shall not commit adultery.' But I say to you, everyone who looks at a woman with lust has already committed adultery with her in his heart." (Matthew 5:27–28)[16]

Imagine the torment of an OCD sufferer continually *needing to decide* whether every look at an attractive person constitutes looking with lust. People with scrupulosity view some of their thoughts and feelings to be the equivalent of acting out the deed. This holds for emotions such as anger, jealousy, and sexual feelings. As a result, a patient may believe that an exposure exercise such as looking at pictures of attractive women in a catalogue constitutes "adultery of the heart," and be unwilling to comply with it.

Clinicians can easily fall into the trap of attempting to persuade the patient of the moral or psychologic harmlessness of the exercise, such as when clinicians with religious knowledge try to engage the patient in discussing ways of interpreting biblical sayings. However, this strategy is a waste of time, because it assumes that the patient's resistance is rational.

Clinicians should consider three approaches to patient resistance to exposure strategies.

1. Greenberg and colleagues[17] advise patients to bring a list of their exposure tasks to their religious advisor and ask, "Is it permissible for me to do . . .?" The adviser then comments on which tasks are permissible and which are objectionable. This highlights the importance of therapists' positive professional relationship with religious leaders and their desire to work in consultation with them.

2. Emphasize the internal logic of the exposure procedure itself. For example, when completing exposure tasks such as those related to blasphemy as described earlier, patients may worry that the goal is to desensitize them to committing sin, whatever the type of sin under discussion. They may then react with abhorrence to the notion that they are becoming desensitized to appalling acts such as blasphemy, pedophilia, adultery, or thievery. Some patients can comprehend my explanation to them that these acts are genuinely despicable, to me as well as to them! But their disorder is not about a willingness to commit these acts, but their inability to think about them, which paralyzes them with anxiety and guilt. I explain that although most of us can avoid these behaviors, none of us can avoid thinking about them at times. So the goal of exposure is simply to desensitize them to the fear of thinking about thinking.

3. The strongest resistance to exposure strategies may arise in patients who conflate internal imagery or feelings with sinful acts. Even after obtaining permission from religious advisors, some patients still refuse or are unable to comply. A patient might resist, for example, the catalogue-picture exposure described earlier, because of the belief that lustful feelings will emerge during the experience and this behavior would be sinful. I deal with such resistance by an emotion-regulation strategy used for the treatment of borderline personality disorder. Linehan[18] applied concepts from Buddhist spiritual practices (i.e., mindfulness) and Gestalt therapy (i.e., sensory awareness) to assist patients who feel overwhelmed by emotions. The strategy is to face the negative emotions "with a wise mind," while observing, describing, and remaining nonjudgmental about the experience. In adapting this strategy to OCD, I refer to it as the "reporter strategy," because newspaper reporters attempt to present the facts objectively, without influence of their emotional reactions, even though they remain aware of such reactions. A full description of this strategy can be found in my book, *The Doubting Disease*.[19] Patients who use this technique learn that there is no necessary connection between the presence of the threatening stimuli and the intentional willing of immoral behavior. For those

patients disturbed by the risk of sexual arousal, I note that such a strategy creates a "spectator" role, which actually decreases sexual arousal.[20]

Other clinicians have applied this "acceptance" modality to a wide range of emotional problems, including anxiety disorders, substance abuse, and paraphilia. LoPiccolo's[21] description of this technique in treating paraphilia comes close to my use of mindfulness with scrupulosity. I also have borrowed Marlatt's term[22] *urge surfing* as a visual metaphor suggesting to patients that feelings are transient if they will only give themselves permission to step back and observe them. A theoretic rationale for the use of exposure and acceptance in OCD is the "white-bear" phenomenon. (The Russian novelist, Leo Tolstoy, described how his older brother would avoid playing with him by telling Tolstoy to stand in a corner until he was no longer thinking about white bears.) Research demonstrates that suppressing thoughts actually increases their frequency.[23] Urge surfing, mindfulness, or responding as a reporter teaches that thoughts, feelings, and images have a natural history of creation, endurance, and decay. The goal of such acceptance is to conclude that ultimately there is nothing to fear.

SUMMARY

This chapter illustrates the application of empirically validated behavioral treatments for OCD patients whose religious symptoms are prominent. Two key points were emphasized. First, scrupulosity, similar to other overvalued ideas, is often treatment resistant. Second, dealing with this resistance is compounded by the cultural barriers often present between patient and clinician when issues touch on personal religious beliefs.

Several motivational strategies may help increase treatment compliance with empirically validated interventions. These strategies include enlisting religious advisors as consultants for patients and teaching mindfulness and acceptance to reduce moral fears surrounding exposure techniques. Research is needed to assess the clinical effectiveness of these interventions.

Although strong religious belief and emotional pain may be strong in some OCD patients, this does not warrant a general indictment of religious faith. In fact, contrary to the opinion of some experts,[24] there is a modest positive relationship between religious belief and mental health. How modest? Nearly as strong as the effect size of psychotherapy![25]

Schwartz' distinction between form and content in psychopathology may help clinicians maintain objectivity when dealing with scrupulosity.[26] The form of the disorder is often diagnostically relevant, whereas the content is multidetermined. Telling children to wash their hands before eating does not cause compulsive handwashing any more than reading the Bible causes scrupulosity. Religious belief does not cause a person with schizophrenia to have the delusion of being the Blessed Virgin any more than the study of European history causes the delusion of being Napoleon. Rather, these cultural experiences can influence the content of the disorder, the shape of the symptoms, and personal reactions to them. OCD draws its arsenal from the individual's life experiences—whatever they may be.

REFERENCES

1. American Psychiatric Association: *Diagnostic and statistical manual of mental disorders*, ed 4, Washington, 1994, American Psychiatric Press.
2. Ethical principles of psychologists and code of conduct, *Am Psych* 47:1597–1611, 1992.
3. Foa EB, et al: Success and failure in the behavioral treatment of obsessive-compulsives, *J Cons Clin Psych* 51:287–297, 1983.
4. Melton JG: *Encyclopedia of American religions*, ed 4, Detroit, 1993, Gale Research.
5. Bergin AE: Values and religious issues in psychotherapy and mental health, *Am Psych* 46:394–403, 1991.
6. Shafranske E: Religious beliefs, affiliations and practices of clinical psychologists. In Shafranske E, editor: *Religion and the clinical practice of psychology*, Washington, 1996, American Psychological Association, pp 149–164.
7. Bunyan J: *Grace abounding: To the chief of sinners*, Westfield, 1988, Christian Library.
8. Jonsen AR, Toulmin S: *The abuse of casuistry: A history of moral reasoning*, Berkeley, 1988, University of California Press.
9. Jone H, Adelman U: *Moral theology*, Westminister, 1959, The Newman Press.
10. Greenberg D: Are religious compulsions religious or compulsive? *Am J Psychiatry* 38:524–532, 1984.
11. Baer L: *Getting control: Overcoming your obsessions and compulsions*, New York, 1992, Penguin.
12. Foa EB, Wilson R: *Stop obsessing: How to overcome your obsessions and compulsions*, New York, 1991, Bantam Books.
13. Steketee G: *The treatment of obsessive compulsive disorder*, New York, 1996, Guilford Press.
14. Steketee G, White K: *When once is not enough: Help for obsessive compulsives*, Oakland, 1990, New Harbinger Publications.
15. Prochaska JO, Norcross JC, Diclemente CC: *Changing for good*, New York, 1994, Avon.
16. *The new American Bible*, Mission Hills, 1986, Benziger Publishing Company.
17. Greenberg D, Witzum E, Pisante J: Scrupulosity: Religious attitudes and clinical presentation, *Br J Med Psychiatry* 60:29–37, 1987.
18. Linehan MM: *Skills training manual for treating borderline personality disorders*, New York, 1993, Guilford Press.
19. Ciarrocchi JW: *The doubting disease*, New York, 1995, Paulist Press.
20. Masters WH, Johnson VE: *Human sexual inadequacy*, Boston, 1970, Little Brown.
21. LoPiccolo J: Acceptance and broad spectrum treatment of paraphilias. In Hayes S, et al, editors: *Acceptance and change: Content and context in psychotherapy*, Reno, 1994, Context Press, pp 149–170.

22. Marlatt GA: Addiction and acceptance. In Hayes S, et al, editors: *Acceptance and change: Content and context in psychotherapy*, Reno, 1994, Context Press, pp 175–197.

23. Wegner D: *White bears and other unwanted thoughts: Suppression, obsession, and the psychology of mental control*, New York, 1989, Viking.

24. Ellis A: *The case against religion*, New York, 1983, The Institute for Rational-Emotive Therapy.

25. Bergin AE: Religiosity and mental health: A critical reevaluation and meta-analysis, *Prof Psych Res Pract*, 14:170–184, 1983.

26. Schwartz JM: *Brain lock: Free yourself from obsessive-compulsive behavior*, New York, 1996, Regan Books.

25

Inpatient and Home-Based Treatment of Obsessive-Compulsive Disorder

B. Steven Willis, Ph.D., Johan Rosqvist, M.S.W., Denise Egan, M.S., Diane Baney, R.N., M.B.A., Peter Manzo, M.S.W.

As more effective psychopharmacologic, cognitive, and behavioral therapies for obsessive-compulsive disorder (OCD) become available, the problem of treating patients who are unresponsive to the standard outpatient application of these therapies remains. Although the efficacy of behavioral treatment for OCD was on psychiatric inpatient units,[1-4] the effectiveness of behavioral techniques is enhanced when applied in the environment in which the feared stimuli naturally occur.[5-9] As a result, two models of treatment—hospital-based and home-based—have been proposed to support patients with treatment-resistant OCD.

HOSPITAL-BASED TREATMENT

As noted earlier, Meyer[2] first demonstrated the effectiveness of exposure and response prevention (ERP) for OCD in an inpatient psychiatric hospital. Following a functional analysis of the obsessions and compulsions, nursing staff blocked the patients from performing their rituals (i.e., response prevention), and the patients were gradually exposed to more stressful stimuli (exposure). Exposure therapy was aided by the therapist's first modeling how to perform the exposure task and then cueing the patient to do as the therapist had done. Because subsequent research has demonstrated that ERP can be carried out in outpatient settings, and similar positive results have been found in inpatient settings,[10] the question is: "Is there any remaining need for hospital-based OCD treatment today?"

Steketee[8] suggested that inpatient OCD treatment be arranged if the patient is: (1) unable to carry out ERP without constant supervision; (2) severely depressed and potentially suicidal, thus requiring medication and supervision; (3) without supportive family members to assist in the home. Frank[11] provided similar reasons to consider inpatient behavioral treatment: (1) the patient is severely depressed and unable to function in daily life; (2) necessary treatment may be too intense to be carried out in outpatient settings; (3) outpatient therapy has failed; or (4) there is potential for symptom relief in a shorter period of time. Pollard[12] recently listed similar criteria for inpatient admission: (1) outpatient treatment is unsafe; (2) outpatient treatment is impractical; and (3) outpatient treatment has failed. Finally, Calvocoressi, et al[13] listed the following reasons for admission to a generic psychiatric unit at Yale University: (1) noncompliance with outpatient treatment; (2) disruption of the home environment by interfering symptoms; (3) inability to manage self-care; and (4) potentially self-injurious behavior.

Pollard, et al[4] described the difficulty of managing OCD on generic psychiatric hospital units: (1) poor execution of behavior therapy recommendations; (2) lack of regard for behavioral variables when making clinical and administrative decisions; (3) the mix of diagnoses commonly found on generic units; (4) frequent invasions of privacy; and (5) inconsistent staff-patient interactions. Steketee[8] urged the behavior therapist who intends to conduct ERP in an inpatient setting to be prepared to spend a considerable amount of time describing and monitoring the course of treatment with all staff members who will be in contact with the patient. Similarly, Frank[11] suggested that the efficacy of inpatient care for treatment-resistant OCD is enhanced when the program provides comprehensive evaluation and treatment recommendations; expert behavioral treatment; experienced staff; family education and intervention; and ERP provided in an intense fashion by well-trained staff. The milieu consists of patients with anxiety disorders, and close attention is paid to follow-up treatment. Pollard, et al[4] stressed the importance of autonomous hospital units to be staffed by trained personnel whose primary task is to provide high-quality behavior therapy.

Drummond[14] describes the management of treatment-resistant OCD on a behavioral inpatient unit. The 49 inpatients in this study were unresponsive to previous therapy (including clinic or generic hospital interventions) or experienced gains that had not generalized to home from previous treatments. The program included intensive inpatient ERP supplemented by behavioral trials in the community. At 19-month follow-up, 63% of the patients reported an average of 40% reduction of rituals. Drummond concluded that "inpatient treatment of OCD in a specialized unit can result in lasting improvements in patients who have previously failed to respond to behavioral therapy."

Thornicroft, et al[15] described an inpatient behavioral unit in London that specialized in the treatment of OCD. Patients were assisted by unit staff in blocking rituals and gradually exposing themselves to increasingly difficult obsessional material. As treatment progressed, the patients spent longer periods engaging in ERP outside of the hospital. Buchanan, et al[16] reported the results of 127 patients treated on this unit over a 3-year period. Discharged patients were offered continued outpatient behavioral therapy. The mean percentage of improvement for all patients was 44%. Of patients remaining in outpatient treatment at 3, 6, 9, and 12 months, mean improvements were between 60% and 62%. Patients who were employed or living with a family member when in treatment complied better with treatment. Multiple regression methods showed that improvement in symptoms was associated with the patient's: (1) never being previously treated; (2) being employed when in treatment; (3) having a fear of contamination; (4) practicing overt rituals; (5) showing absence of depression; and (6) living with a family member.

Levendusky, et al[17] described a behaviorally oriented inpatient unit in Belmont, Massachusetts, that treated OCD and other disorders. The unit provided individual ERP, normalization strategies, individualized behavioral contracts, a menu of therapeutic groups, and a view of the patient as a colleague in the treatment process. Pollard, et al[4] also described the workings of a behaviorally oriented inpatient unit in St. Louis and stressed the importance of involving patients as active participants in the treatment process, an active milieu, intense individual behavioral therapy, family therapy, and discharge planning. Outcome data reported by Pollard, et al[4] suggest that a majority of patients experienced moderate to complete symptom improvement on a variety of measures. Both behavioral programs served a variety of psychiatric populations. Each set of authors stressed active participation of patients in the creation of their treatment plans, an active group-based milieu, individual behavior therapy, family therapy, relapse prevention, and active discharge planning.

All of the behavioral inpatient programs described previously included *in vivo* ERP as part of the behavioral treatments.

Increased severity of patients admitted to generic psychiatric units perceived compromises in the types of services offered, and decreasing lengths of inpatient stay as a result of managed care, combined with the elimination of elective admissions, limits the choice of inpatient treatment for OCD patients and the type of treatment they will receive following admission.[17-20] The goal of most generic psychiatric inpatient units today is to stabilize patients who are in acute psychiatric crisis; these units are not intended as a site for intensive behavioral treatment.[17]

"When hospitalization on a specialized behavioral therapy unit is not possible, patients with primary obsessive-compulsive disorder may require treatment on a general psychiatric ward."[13] The authors describe effective treatment of 77 OCD patients on a generic psychiatric research unit in New Haven, which focused on pharmacologic treatment over a 7-year period. The authors suggest that, with modest modifications of standard inpatient practice, OCD can be treated in a generic inpatient unit without specialized staff if treatment goals remain modest (i.e., thorough OCD–specific assessment, management of OCD and comorbid symptoms, and the development of a comprehensive discharge plan). All patients received physical and neurologic examinations and specialized assessment based on presenting symptoms. A psychosocial assessment was completed to identify functional deficits and stress-inducing components of the patient's environment. The specifics of the patient's obsessions and compulsions and his or her ability to participate in behavioral treatment were assessed via clinical interview and standardized measures. Symptom management was accomplished with pharmacologic interventions and aid in normalizing the behavior through behavioral contracting or direct assistance by staff. Patients were encouraged (but not required) to participate in behavior therapy. There were no behavior therapists or formal behavior therapy groups in the unit. Family members were informed of the behavioral management program and asked to support the treatment plan.

In the generic unit described by Calvocoressi, et al,[13] patients reportedly caused disruptions in the milieu because of strong control and dependency needs. Conflicts occurred among staff members regarding the patients' control over their OCD symptoms and among other patients who became angry at the amount of staff time and attention devoted to these OCD patients. Education of staff about OCD patients' dependency needs and control issues and engaging the support of other patients were reported to improve both milieu conditions and treatment for OCD patients.

Although inpatient care has generally not been found superior to outpatient care OCD,[5,10] inpatient treatment may be a viable treatment option when a patient's symptoms fail to respond to standard interventions or when concomitant illness or safety cannot be managed in an outpatient setting.[12,21] On the other hand, the decision to admit an OCD patient to hospital requires careful consideration of the person's situation. Steketee[8] indicated the difficulty of generalizing treatment gains unless arrangements have been made for assistance with behavioral techniques in the natural setting. Also, for some patients (e.g., those who check and hoard), hospitalization may remove them from feared stimuli and make behavioral therapy difficult to carry out in the inpatient setting.[8] Premature discharge from specialized OCD units has occurred in the rare cases in which a patient engaged in threatening or self-injurious behavior or had consumed alcohol.[14] Severe depression or the presence of character pathology complicates the inpatient treatment of OCD symptoms.[4,14] In the absence of specialized behavioral units, generic psychiatric units can provide the necessary structure to assess, normalize behavior, develop a comprehensive outpatient treatment plan, and ensure the safety of the patient. The hallmark of all effective inpatient care is the development of a comprehensive discharge plan.

Today, most psychiatric hospitals provide various levels of care, including locked inpatient units, open-door inpatient units, day and evening programs, and residential programs. Inpatient care is typically heavily staffed with nurses, physicians, and nurse assistants. Other levels of care tend to employ counselors and have fewer nursing staff members. Psychologists, social workers, and rehabilitation therapists can be found at any level of care. Inpatient care is typically reserved for persons who are in an acute crisis. The other levels of care usually are provided for patients who are not in crisis, but have not yet returned to a level of functioning in which they can profit from outpatient care. These levels of care are recent innovations, and the effectiveness has not been adequately documented. Programs that specialize in the treatment of OCD are listed in the Appendix, and an updated list is available from the Obsessive-Compulsive Foundation. These programs provide (or are affiliated with programs that provide) intensive treatment models in inpatient, day program, or residential settings.[22]

Conclusions

When seeking psychiatric hospitalization for an OCD patient, it is essential to clarify the goals for the admission. If it is a matter of safety or one of managing the exacerbation of manic, depressive, or psychotic symptoms, most generic psychiatric units can stabilize symptoms and help patients through a crisis. On the other hand, if what is needed is intensive behavior therapy, few inpatient units currently provide the type and length of treatment that are necessary for that patient. It has been our experience that inpatient treatment, in any but a few specialty programs, results in disappointment for the patient seeking OCD symptom relief. In some cases, the hospitalization produces a negative iatrogenic effect, especially if the exacerbation of symptoms was a first-time occurrence. The following cases are illustrative of situations in which hospitalization yielded deleterious consequences.

Case 1

This patient sought admission for obsessions that he might stab or sexually abuse his newborn child. His rituals involved reassurance seeking. Prior to the birth of his child, his obsessions had involved acting on unwanted impulses to harm a friend or loved one. His ritual involved frequent reassurance from the clergy. These "new" obsessions distressed the patient to the point that he was seriously considering suicide. He was admitted to an inpatient unit within 50 yards of a behavioral unit that treated OCD. The physician in charge of his case believed that OCD was a psychotic disorder, that behavior therapy would lead to the release of the patient's psychotic core, and that the patient required individual, supportive, dynamic therapy to deal with his probable history of childhood sexual trauma. The patient was discharged and within hours readmitted; because the previous unit was full, he was placed on the behavioral treatment unit. A trial of antidepressant medication and ERP, which was started in the hospital and continued after discharge to an outpatient setting, produced an 80% improvement in symptoms calculated on the Yale-Brown Obsessive-Compulsive Scale (Y-BOCS) and allowed the patient to enjoy a normal relationship with his child.

Case 2

The patient obsessed that he might harm himself and suffered from panic attacks. His insurance company required that he be evaluated by an independent crisis team. When the patient was in the midst of a panic attack, a neighbor thought the patient was having a heart attack and called an ambulance. When waiting at the emergency room for his insurance to be verified and for the crisis team to arrive, the patient told an attendant he was afraid he might harm himself. The emergency room staff notified the crisis team, which instructed the emergency room staff to restrain the patient until they arrived. When the team arrived, they admitted the patient to an inpatient unit where he was placed in a quiet room. Several days later, he was discharged with an inappropriate diagnosis of borderline personality disorder. He eventually responded positively to cognitive behavioral and psychopharmacologic treatment.

One psychiatric hospital ward that had previously provided behavioral interventions altered its treatment philosophy when the new physician in charge regarded behavioral therapy as a "laughing stock." Subsequent OCD patient admissions to the unit were not provided with intensive behavior therapy, did not receive an OCD–specific evaluation, and the milieu was not arranged to normalize behavior. As a result, many subsequent OCD patients were inappropriately diagnosed with personality disorders because of the difficulty they had in complying with milieu requirements.

As an example, we were asked to consult on a woman with OCD who had spent many weeks on a generic "short-term" psychiatric unit and would not use the showers or sinks on the unit. Because she had not yet undergone a trial of behavior therapy or lengthy trials of antiobsessional agents, we suggested these approaches. The physician in charge refused to return our calls, and the patient was eventually diagnosed with a primary axis II diagnosis and discharged.

Conversely, we also have had many experiences in which inpatient hospitalization on a generic psychiatric unit produced positive results. These results were found when a treating physician or psychologist either was personally familiar with current treatments of OCD or sought out consultation with OCD specialists. The following cases demonstrate this point.

Case 3

This man, who had severe OCD and a psychotic disorder, had been in a Massachusetts state hospital for many years. His treatment team stabilized his psychotic symptoms and taught him independent living skills. They then arranged for him to receive short-term intensive treatment for his OCD in our residential program. The procedures that were developed on the generic psychiatric unit were of such a high quality that we made only minor adjustments in his program. After 3 weeks of OCD–specific treatment, he moved to a supervised apartment that had been arranged by his inpatient team.

Case 4

This man suffered from OCD and manic-depressive illness. He had responded well to treatment for his OCD but suffered an exacerbation of his depression. His medications were successfully adjusted in a generic inpatient setting. Although the unit was not equipped to conduct ERP, they assisted the patient in maintaining a normalized routine, and he has now been stable for many years.

Another case demonstrates the potential efficacy of short-term, generic psychiatric admission for assessment and arrangement of aftercare.

Case 5

A woman was suffering from serious diabetes, which required her to maintain a regular diet and stable body weight. She had suffered from mild contamination obsessions for many years and had never sought treatment, but recently, her condition had suddenly worsened. She was admitted to a generic psychiatric unit at a university hospital. The inpatient team decided that the patient required an intensive trial of behavior therapy to help her eat; because the generic unit did not have those resources, the patient was referred to an OCD specialty unit where she responded positively to treatment.

As previously noted, thoughtful discharge and aftercare planning is critical with these patients.[4,13,23] Hospitalization and other forms of intensive treatment rarely, if ever, produce a complete cure for severe OCD. Sophisticated OCD–specific programs routinely include relapse prevention and structured follow-up care to solidify treatment gains.[24] Failure to prepare or follow-through with an adequate aftercare plan often results in return of symptoms. Conversely, adherence to a well thought-out discharge plan prevents relapse and ensures the continuing reduction of symptoms and psychosocial problems associated with these symptoms. Competent behavior therapy, psychopharmacology, family therapy, and adjunctive therapies are critical following hospital-based treatment for severe OCD, as demonstrated by the following case example.

Case 6

A young man was hospitalized in a generic unit for major depression, obsessions that grave harm would come to his family, and rituals of tapping and counting. His inpatient treatment progressed smoothly, because the social worker on the unit had participated in several OCD workshops and enlisted unit staff to help the patient perform ERP. Because the patient's insurance company required that he be treated as an outpatient by a provider on their panel, the social worker contacted a psychologist who was listed as a behavior therapist by the insurance company and made an appointment for the patient. The psychologist attempted a trial of relaxation training and assertiveness training, and suggested to the patient that, when he was obsessing, he should practice deep-muscle relaxation techniques. The patient relapsed and was readmitted several months later. As a result, the inpatient social worker now questions all behavior therapists about their training and experience in working with people with OCD (especially their familiarity with ERP) before a referral is made.

Another example demonstrates how institutional policies and procedures can result in poor discharge planning. A short-term, generic psychiatric unit was praised by hospital administration and insurance companies for the efficiency and speed with which it triaged and stabilized psychiatric patients. But as a result, OCD patients were routinely referred back to their outpatient therapists (regardless of the therapists' skills in treating OCD), without any suggestion of behavioral consultation because senior staff on the unit did not regard consultation as part of their responsibility.

It has been our experience that most outpatient treators, regardless of their theoretic orientation, have the best interests of their patients in mind. They typically use consultation and supervision to hone their behavioral therapy skills or cooperate with a behavior therapist performing concurrent therapy. However, as we seek aftercare for our patients, we have become increasingly alarmed by therapists who identify themselves, on preferred-provider lists, as behavior therapists. Often, these therapists, only after cursory questioning, are found incompetent in these methods. Some therapists identify themselves as behaviorally oriented after simply taking a course in relaxation training, reading a book or article on behavior therapy, or attending a seminar on the cognitive therapy of depression. One psychologist, referred to us via an HMO preferred-provider list, informed us that he was a behavior therapist; when asked if he practiced ERP, he did not know what the treatment involved and was aghast when we explained it to him. He then told us he would read a book about OCD before the patient arrived. We did not make the referral.

In seeking competent behavioral therapy as part of a comprehensive discharge plan, several questions should be asked to determine if a potential therapist is familiar with the treatment of OCD: (1) Did the therapist train in a setting in which he received instruction and supervision in behavior therapy? (2) Has the therapist received supervision in the delivery of ERP and habit reversal? (3) How many OCD sufferers has the professional treated? and (4) If the therapist did not train in a behavioral program, has he or she received supervision in behavior therapy (ERP, habit reversal, cognitive behavioral therapy) following "conversion" to behaviorism? We have supervised several professionals who were not behaviorally oriented but who were seeking respecialization in OCD–specific behavior therapy. Although these professionals were dedicated to their patients and were interested in developing new skills, they also were feeling pressure to develop behavioral skills—otherwise, they would not be accepted as providers by insurance carriers.

We also have been faced with the difficulty of finding a behavior therapist competent to treat OCD located in the patient's home area. A listing of therapists who identify themselves as behavior therapists is maintained by the Obsessive-Compulsive Foundation and the Association for the Advancement of Behavior Therapy.

Discharge plans also should address ways of overcoming barriers to effective reintegration into the community. These barriers can include family discord; problems with housing, employment, or socialization; concomitant physical and psychiatric illness; and discrimination against persons with neurobehavioral disorders. Of critical importance, in any discharge plan, are specific relapse-prevention strategies and securing of competent psychopharmocologic follow-up.

It has been our experience that if effective generic inpatient units meet the criteria described by Calvocoressi, et al,[23] they can serve as starting points for competent OCD–specific treatment and as a safe haven when patients are in crisis. When an inpatient unit either either does not meet these criteria or suffers from the pitfalls described by Pollard,[4] inpatient treatment is likely to be problematic for an OCD sufferer. As a result, intensive treatment in OCD specialty programs holds the greatest promise for positive outcome in severe OCD.

HOME- AND COMMUNITY-BASED TREATMENT

Following a combination of *in vivo* ERP, 75% to 85% of patients have fewer symptoms of OCD and their gains are maintained over time.[8,25] Van den Hout, et al[10] reported that there is nothing that intensive inpatient treatment of OCD adds to the effect of a well thought-out, outpatient protocol. Similarly, some authors feel that self-directed in vivo ERP is just as effective clinically as therapist-controlled *in vivo* ERP, and it is more cost effective (Emmelcamp, et al, 1988).

However, a recent metaanalysis found that therapist-supervised ERP is more effective than self-controlled exposure, and that complete response prevention paired with exposure is more effective than partial or no response prevention.[26] Although Mehta[27] reported that adding a family member as a coach during ERP improved overall functioning, Emmelkamp, et al[28] found this practice did not add to the effectiveness of self-directed ERP. Clearly, for the majority of persons who suffer from OCD, self-guided exposure is the treatment of choice. But, for the minority of people who do not respond to competently designed and carried-out self-directed ERP, coaching can add to the effectiveness of these techniques.

Steketee[8] developed a comprehensive therapist manual for conducting therapist-aided *in vivo* behavior therapy; this manual is an invaluable resource for the design, implementation, and fading of therapist-guided behavioral therapy. Following her treatment approach, therapist guidance is phased out until the patient is able to engage in self-guided *in vivo* ERP. It has been our experience that the most effective outpatient behavioral treatment of OCD usually begins with the behavior therapist conducting an assessment in the environment in which symptoms occur, and then providing direct assistance and coaching in ERP in that environment (gradually fading out support as the patient gains skills and self-confidence). Problems occur when the patient is unable to follow through with self-directed exposure, the environment is not supportive, or clinical management is time consuming. Colleagues have reported that, because of increasing demands in outpatient clinics and decreasing funding for therapy, they are typically unable to conduct assessment or therapy in natural settings. The distance and time required to conduct home- and community-based treatment also can be prohibitive. When OCD symptoms persist and severely impact the patient's life, or concomitant psychiatric and psychosocial problems are severe, home care can aid in behavioral and tertiary care.

Behavioral Home- and Community-Based Services

When self-directed *in vivo* ERP has not provided adequate symptom relief, constructing of supports in the natural environment can add to the gains acquired through behavioral therapy. For example, one patient feared he would not have adequate information should he witness a terrible auto accident and obsessed that if an accident occurred, he would be called upon to bear witness in court. When driving, he ritualistically wrote the license plate numbers of all autos that were exceeding the speed limit, but after several near accidents, he resorted to recording these numbers on a portable tape recorder. Several nights a week, he arrived home late because of following a car until he could read the plate number. In behavioral therapy, this patient created a hierarchy of roads that triggered his obsessions. However, he was unable to drive on his most frightening routes without pulling off to the side of the road and writing plate numbers in the dirt. After several failed attempts to complete driving exposures on the more frightening roadways, his therapist accompanied him. Then, when the patient asked the therapist if she also had seen an example of reckless driving, the therapist replied that she was not paying attention. Further, the patient did not write or record any numbers during these coached exposures. Next, the patient's brother and girlfriend visited the therapist to learn how to coach him during driving exposures. Eventually, he was able to complete the exposures without coaching, and he is now doing quite well. This example demonstrates how fading-out supports in the natural environment can ultimately lead to self-directed ERP.

Another patient obsessed that he would act on unwanted impulses, such as jumping from high places, throwing objects from high places and striking others, and hitting the young or the elderly. His mental rituals involved logical undoing and prayers. He had had multiple psychiatric hospitalizations but had not profited from self-directed ERP. With the help of his therapist, he recorded several repeating-loop audiotapes containing his obsessions. He next accompanied his therapist to bridges, overpasses, and places where children and the elderly gathered, and he listened to the tape when looking down from a bridge or sitting in a park where children were playing. The patient was eventually able to complete these exposures without coaching and has been living and working in the community for several years without the need for hospitalization.

We have found that when (1) supportive friends or family are not available; (2) the amount of time required to effectively assist the patient is greater than the therapist can provide; or (3) the financial resources of the patient do not allow adequate therapist involvement, it is helpful to set up a home-based treatment program to assist the patient with inadequate response to self-directed ERP.[29]

In our home-based program, Willis[29] is summarized:

1. A referral is received. Problems are identified by the referring parties. The prospective patient is contacted. An initial office visit is scheduled (if possible). If an office visit is not possible, the initial contact is made in the patient's home.

2. A licensed professional completes an *in vivo* behavioral and systems evaluation. Problems are observed and interviews conducted in the patient's home environment.

3. Based on a perusal of records, contact with other treators, input from the patient and family, payor requirements, and the professional's evaluation, a behavioral treatment plan is developed. The treatment plan specifies the goals of the treatment, how those goals will be achieved, timelines for each of the goals, and the cost of the treatment. The treatment plan serves as a contract between the patient and the treators.

4. When cognitive and behavioral technologies are being applied, psychologic assistants provide a majority of in-home and other community-based services. The number and purpose of the in-home visits are negotiated as part of the treatment contract.

5. Psychologic assistants monitor specific components of the treatment contract and report to the professional staff.

6. Objective measures are negotiated as part of the treatment contract and used to monitor progress.

7. Relapse-prevention strategies are developed and implemented to help minimize the potential return of problem behaviors.

8. The patient continues to meet with the professional staff person on a routine basis to refine the treatment plan. Psychologic assistants have a minimum of a Bachelor's degree in a human services–related field and receive ongoing supervision and training. They conduct two sessions per week, with exposures lasting at least 90 minutes. Initial results are encouraging, with an average decrease in symptoms reported at 60% in Y-BOCS scores.

The following are examples of home- and community-based treatment.

A woman entered our home-based program after numerous failed trials of self-guided *in vivo* ERP and numerous psychopharmacologic trials. She obsessed that she would be contaminated by dust that had been contaminated with animal feces. She engaged in extensive handwashing and checking rituals and avoided leaving her home. At the end of 12 weeks of two sessions per week of ERP, she reported an 80% reduction in symptoms as measured by the Y-BOCS. Following home-based treatment, she continued in traditional outpatient self-guided ERP and was able to seek employment for the first time in many years.

A man entered our home-based program following several hospitalizations and several failed outpatient behavioral and psychopharmacologic treatments. He experienced severe obsessions about catching deadly viruses and practiced handwashing rituals. Following 24 sessions of coached ERP, his symptoms had been reduced by 75% on the Y-BOCS, and he was able to continue self-guided ERP with an outpatient therapist.

Home- and community-based treatment for treatment-resistant OCD becomes more complex as other problems facing the patient worsen, interfering with straightforward ERP (e.g., alcohol abuse, family violence, child neglect and abuse, and the loss of economic and social supports). In some cases, patients are able to make gains, but maintained only with continued home-based contacts.

Case 7

This patient obsessed that she might leave a valuable possession behind whenever she moved from one area to another. She engaged in checking rituals, often taking many hours to simply move from room to room or getting in and out of an automobile. She was unable to work, lived with a family member, had not left the house for many months, and was receiving disability insurance payments. She had unsuccessfully tried self-guided ERP, cognitive therapy, and psychopharmacology. After 1 year in home-based treatment, the patient was able to drive to a vocational rehabilitation program, and after 2 years, she was working full-time and living in her own apartment. However, fading out her home-based sessions to fewer than once per week repeatedly resulted in a symptom relapse severe enough to keep her housebound again. After 3 years, she still gets one home visit per week and is stable.

Case 8

This man obsessed that items in his home must be placed in order and that rugs and furniture must be lined up symmetrically. He had not improved with behavioral outpatient treatment. During a home visit, both he and his wife were found to be intoxicated. The psychologic assistant informed the supervising psychologist who then made the next home visit. During the course of the visit, it became apparent that when drinking, the patient used corporal punishment with his 5-year-old child. With the couple's knowledge, the psychologist informed the child protection agency and remained with the family until the investigator arrived and the child was found not to have been physically harmed. Both parents were then required to attend a parenting class, to use positive parenting techniques in the home, to begin couples therapy with the psychologist, and to be evaluated for substance-abuse treatment. Home-based treatment for OCD also continued.

As this patient's case demonstrates, when psychosocial issues become more complex, concomitant psychiatric and physical illness more severe, and OCD symptoms more debilitating, *in vivo* behavioral coaching may become part of a menu of more complex tertiary home-care treatment.

TERTIARY HOME CARE

Marks, et al[1] reported better treatment outcome for severely mentally ill patients with home-care treatment than with either inpatient or outpatient care. Home-based treatment was reported to be more cost effective and to produce greater patient and family satisfaction and adjustment. However, community-based care did not work "miracles" in these patients. Although there were improvements, there also were setbacks, such as patients who refused medications and home-based patients who still required substantial care, even after interventions as long as 20 months. Marks, et al[1] reported that this model of home-based treatment reduced crisis hospital admissions by 80%.

Visiting Nurses Associations and home health care agencies can assist patients with complex medical conditions and management sometimes necessary in the treatment of severe concomitant psychiatric illness. In our experience, these types of agencies are not expert in behavioral psychology, but they provide a variety of other valuable services.

One patient had severe OCD and a thought disorder but had done well with home-based behavioral treatment for his OCD symptoms. His psychotic disorder had been in remission for many years, and he lived with his parents, spent his days at a structured workshop, and had an array of supportive friends. However, after his mother's death and his father's serious illness, he lost the support he needed to live independently. A nurse, who specialized in independent living, assisted the patient in finding an apartment with a compatible roommate, and in developing shopping and budgeting skills, and other independent living skills via behavioral skills training in the community.

This woman suffered from severe OCD, which had improved after home-based intervention. Still, because of severe deficits in social skills, she was unable to find a job. Although she worked with a psychologic assistant to develop new patterns of communication, she continued to have difficulty finding a job. Finally, through a vocational rehabilitation program, a job coach was secured through a home healthcare agency, who helped the patient secure and maintain a job.

When acute family dysfunction, serious personality disorders, or drug or alcohol abuse is present, home-based behavioral interventions for OCD may be delayed until tertiary home care or other interventions have decreased the impact of these problems. Although there are yet no controlled studies that assess the impact of home-based care on OCD, a pilot study funded by the Obsessive-Compulsive Foundation is ongoing at our site.

Massachusetts General Hospital Obsessive-Compulsive Disorder Institute

We recently developed the Massachusetts General Hospital OCD (MGH OCD) Institute as a clinical arm of the MGH OCD Clinic to provide a comprehensive program that integrates somatic, behavioral, and milieu treatment for refractory OCD and its most common comorbid conditions. The Institute mission is to serve as a national and regional center to advance clinical care, the teaching and training of professionals, and the exporting of somatic, behavioral, and programmatic interventions for severe, treatment-resistant OCD. The program grew out of a need to provide treatment for persons with severe OCD who were not profiting from outpatient therapies.

The Institute consists of five levels of care: (1) residential; (2) day program; (3) evening treatment; (4) outpatient; and (5) home-based treatment. Seventeen patients are served in the residential program, and five patients are treated in the day and evening programs.

Milieu

The milieu is constructed to stress the proactive involvement of the patient in treatment. This involvement is achieved by viewing the patient as a colleague in the treatment process, rather than a passive recipient of treatment.

Decisions regarding treatment as well as policies and procedures are made through collaboration between staff and patients.

Therapeutic Contracts: Self-Directed Treatment Plans

Each patient completes a therapeutic contract detailing the treatment plan for the week. Patients are assisted in constructing contracts via feedback from staff and other patients. At the end of the week, the patient receives feedback from staff and patients about progress and effort. Patients complete weekly measures of their symptoms and improvement and report the results on their contracts. Patients define the problem they are addressing that week, the solution to the problem, short-term objectives that break the problem down into smaller components, and the action steps necessary to accomplish their objectives.

Behavior Therapy

Each patient is assigned a behavior therapist who meets with the patient individually several times per week. The behavior therapist is responsible for devising an individualized behavioral program as a guideline to ensure a consistent coaching approach by staff or other patients. The behavior program details the patient's obsessions and compulsions, provides a menu of ERP tactics, outlines instructions for cognitive and behavioral techniques, details instructions for group leaders, and provides other information necessary to assist the patient in overcoming symptoms. The behavior therapist assists the patient in completing ERP, creating relapse-prevention strategies, developing more effective social skills, applying cognitive-behavioral tactics, and practicing psychosocial problem solving. In addition to the individual meetings with the behavior therapist, the patient also engages in daily ERP exercises with the direct care staff, both individually and in groups.

Patients are assisted in adhering to a normalized schedule of therapeutic activities, self-care, social events, and community-based activities through a variety of methods. Using the behavior program as a guide, staff and other patients actively coach patients who are having difficulty blocking rituals or normalizing their behavior. Patients routinely engage in ERP in community settings, either through self-exposure or coaching by staff or other patients. Imaginal techniques are frequently paired with *in vivo* ERP strategies.

Patients receive cognitive-behavioral interventions in individual and group formats.[30] Motivational interviewing techniques also are applied in group and individual sessions.[31] Incorporated within each therapeutic contract and behavioral program, relapse-prevention strategies are stressed in both individual sessions and in a therapeutic group setting.[24] Each patient also attends a daily ERP group and a group designed to help the patient develop coping skills and response-prevention strategies. The development of social skills, including assertiveness, is stressed through ongoing interactions with direct care staff, behavioral therapists, and in group discussions.[32]

Somatic Treatment

Patients meet with a psychiatrist at least once per week. Psychiatrists also attend the contract review group and medication management group, and take an active role in interacting with patients in the milieu. Unit nurses meet with each patient on a weekly basis to review the medication regime, discuss side effects, and provide education. Both psychiatrists and nurses take an active role in the provision of behavioral and psychosocial interventions; their contacts are both formal and informal. Patients can access the medical staff on an as-needed basis. All medical staff are thoroughly trained in behavioral techniques. Pharmacologic treatments are tailored for patients with treatment-resistant OCD and play an integral role in the program.[33] Patients who have received psychosurgical interventions are admitted directly from surgical units. Patients scheduled for surgery are encouraged to engage in the program before and after surgery.

Social Work

The social worker provides a bridge to the family and assists in the development of discharge plans. Social workers take an active role in negotiating insurance coverage and assisting patients in finding outpatient treatment. Social workers also provide individual behavioral and dynamic therapy and conduct a variety of therapy groups. Social workers lead multifamily groups that allow patients and their families to identify more effective ways of managing OCD symptoms.[34] Additional social work–led groups include discharge planning, women's issues, and coping skills groups.

Group Therapies

Patients attend five to six therapy groups per day. The group therapy program provides a forum for therapies targeting motivation; compliance; decreasing behavioral symptoms of other axis I and axis II disorders; increasing normalized family, work, and social functioning; presenting education and support; and offering additional vehicles for cognitive and behavioral therapies. The following is a sampling of groups not previously listed.

Treatment Planning Group

At the beginning of each day, residents and day patients meet with staff for a treatment planning group. Individual appointments, exposures, groups, chores, and other events are placed on a daily activity schedule. Patients also outline specific goals for the day and rate their anxiety using objective measures. Work in this group is guided toward learning time management skills and daily planning.

Self-Assessment

The group meets at the end of each day. Participants assess whether or not they attained their daily goals and how they have worked toward meeting the objectives on their contracts, and rate their anxiety using objective measures. Patients receive feedback from their peers and program staff.

Contract Workshop

The group meets once a week. The goal of the group is to provide an opportunity for the resident to brainstorm weekly goals and action steps for the following week's therapeutic contract. Emphasis is placed on the translation of these ideas into objective, measurable goals.

Contract Setting

The group meets at the beginning of each week. Patients are prepared with a rough draft of their therapeutic contract, which was developed in contract workshop, and present the contract to the group. Incorporating feedback from the milieu, residents finalize their contract and post it publicly.

Contract Review

The group meets at the end of each week. Patients read their contract, report on whether they have made progress on their weekly objectives and report their scores on measures of OCD and overall improvement. The participants then receive feedback from residents, day patients, and staff.

Dialectic Behavior Therapy

This group focuses on acquisition of skills such as self-management, emotion regulation, and mindfulness for patients with borderline personality disorder. Goals include decreasing suicidal and self-injurious behaviors, decreasing behaviors that interfere with achieving goals, and increasing behavioral skills.[35]

Patient Government

Patients meet once a week, brainstorm ideas to improve the program, and develop lists of concerns. Minutes prepared by a patient are distributed through e-mail to all administrators and staff.

Community Meeting

Residents and staff meet on a weekly basis to discuss and develop solutions to issues that affect the community. Minutes of this meeting are included in the Patient Government Meeting minutes for distribution to all residents and staff. A variety of groups stress the development of social and recreational skills, housekeeping and cooking skills, and other independent living and interpersonal skills.

Counseling Staff

All members of the counseling staff must hold at least a Bachelor's degree in a human service–related field, and some positions require a Master's level degree. All counselors participate in a rigorous orientation and training, which includes not only the specifics of working with OCD, but also supportive counseling techniques, cognitive and behavioral therapy, crisis prevention and intervention, cardiopulmonary resuscitation, and group leadership skills. Counselors are available 24 hours a day and provide a significant presence on the milieu. They provide both individual and group interventions.

Technology

The MGH OCD Institute is constantly refining a computerized system that is used to focus on positive outcomes through well-defined and empirically monitored goals and objectives. Patients have access to a networked computer system through which they can use e-mail, access the Internet, and compose therapeutic contracts. All patients are given e-mail accounts so that they can be in touch with their treators, other residents, and people outside the program. The e-mail is used as an ongoing "Town Meeting" for patients and staff to share ideas and suggestions about improving the program. Computer, telephone, Internet, and video technologies are being tested as methods to improve relapse-prevention programs after discharge.

Continuum of Care

The program's clinical staff evaluate all patients for admission to the program. Although many patients require the most intensive residential level of care because of the severity of their symptoms, some patients are able to use the program only during the day or evening when residing elsewhere. Patients also have access to home-based coaching from behavior therapists and counselors. The goal is to move patients to less acute levels and toward more normalized functioning.

SUMMARY

The factors associated with positive response to the treatment of severe OCD have not widely been studied.[16] The MGH OCD Institute is committed to the refinement of existing treatments for OCD and concomitant conditions and the integration of new approaches as they evolve. Several approaches to longer-term behavioral and psychosocial treatment offer promise. At the Providence, Rhode Island, program, Rich Marshland, R.N. offers a program that enables patients to live and receive behavior therapy within a family setting. This approach has been borrowed by the MGH OCD Institute, which plans to develop a network of mentor homes to provide intensive behavior therapy in a normal family environment. Other directions for future programs include treatments geared toward children and adolescents who suffer from treatment-resistant OCD, further refinement of home-based services, integration of a menu of interventions for comorbid conditions, and long-term supportive housing.

REFERENCES

1. Marks IM, Connolly J, Muijen M, et al: Home-based versus hospital-based care for people with serious mental illness, *Br J Psychiatry* 165:179–194, 1994.
2. Meyer V: Modifications of expectations in cases with obsessional rituals, *Behav Res Ther* 4:273–280, 1966.
3. Meyer V, Levy R, Schrurer A: The behavioral treatment of obsessive-compulsive disorders. In Beech HR, editor: *Obsessional states*, London, 1974, Methuen.
4. Pollard CA, Merkel WT, Obermeir HJ: Inpatient behavior therapy: The St. Louis University model, *J Behav Ther Exp Psychiatry* 17(4):233–243, 1986.
5. Foa EB, Steketee G, Grayson JB, et al: Deliberate exposure and blocking of obsessive-compulsive rituals: Immediate and long-term effects, *Behav Ther* 15:450–472, 1984.
6. Hooguduin CAL, Hoogduin WA: The outpatient treatment of patients with an obsessional-compulsive disorder, *Behav Res Ther* 22(4):455–459, 1984.
7. Shappiro L, Steketee G: Obsessive compulsive disorder. In Bellack A, Hersen M, editors: *Handbook of behavior therapy in psychiatric settings*, New York, 1993, Plenum Press.
8. Steketee GS: *Treatment of obsessive compulsive disorder: Treatment manuals for practitioners,* New York, 1993, Guilford Press.
9. Dar R, Greist JH: Behavior therapy for obsessive compulsive disorder, *Psychiatr Clin North Am* 15(4):885–894, 1992.
10. van den Hout M, Emmelkamp P, Kraykamp H, et al: Behavioral treatment of obsessive-compulsives: Inpatient vs. outpatient, *Behav Res Ther* 26(4):331–332, 1988.
11. Frank M: Inpatient behavioral treatment, *OCD News* 4(2):1–2,4–5, 1990.
12. Pollard CA: Inpatient treatment of refractory obsessive-compulsive disorder. In Goodman W, Maser J, Rudorfer M, editors: *Treatment challenges in OCD*, in press, Lawerence Earlbaum Associates.
13. Calvocoressi L, McDougle CI, Wasylink S, et al: Inpatient treatment of patients with severe obsessive-compulsive disorder, *Hosp Comm Psychiatry* 44(12): 1150–1154, 1993.
14. Drummond LM: The treatment of severe, chronic, resistant obsessive-compulsive disorder: An evaluation of an in-patient programme using behavioral psychotherapy in combination with other treatments, *Br J Psychiatry* 163:223–229, 1993.
15. Thornicroft G, Colson L, Marks I: An in-patient behavioral psychotherapy unit. Description and audit, *Br J Psychiatry* 158:362–367, 1991.
16. Buchanan AW, Meng KS, Marks IM: What predicts improvement and compliance during the behavioral treatment of obsessive compulsive disorder, *Anxiety* 2:22–27, 1996.
17. Levendusky PG, Willis BS, Ghinassi FA: The therapeutic contracting program: A comprehensive continuum of care model, *Psychiatr Q* 65(3):189–208, 1994.
18. Canton C, Gralnick A: A review of issues surrounding length of psychiatric hospitalization, *Hosp Comm Psychiatry* 858–863, 1987.

19. Mezzick J, Coffman G: Factors influencing length of hospital stay, *Hosp Comm Psychiatry* 36:1262–1270, 1985.
20. Craig TJ: Economic and inpatient care, *Psychiatr Ann* 18:75–79, 1988.
21. Levendusky PG, Willis BS, Berglas S: The therapeutic contracting program: A comprehensive cognitive behavior therapy model. In Corrigan P, Liberman R, editors: *Behavior therapy in psychiatric hospitals*, New York, 1993, Springer.
22. Broatch J: Personal communication, 1997.
23. Calvocoressi, et al. 1986.
24. Hiss H, Foa EB, Kozak MJ: Relapse prevention program for treatment of obsessive-compulsive disorder, *J Consult Clin Psychol* 62(4):801–808, 1994.
25. van Oppen P: *Obsessive compulsive disorder: Issues in assessment and treatment*, Netherlands, 1994, Vrije University Press (?).
26. Abramowitz JS: Variants of exposure and response prevention in the treatment of obsessive-compulsive disorder: A meta-analysis, *Behav Ther* 27:583–600, 1996.
27. Mehta M: A comparative study of family-based care for people with serious mental illness, *Br J Psychiatry* 157:133–135, 1990.
28. Emmelkamp PMG, de Haan E, Hoogduin CAL: Marital adjustment and obsessive-compulsive disorder, *Br J Psychiatry* 156:55–60, 1990.
29. Willis BS: Home based behavioral treatment of obsessive compulsive disorder, *OCD News* 12:23, 1994.
30. van Oppen P, Haan ED, Balkom AJLM, et al: Cognitive therapy and exposure in vivo in treatment of obsessive compulsive disorder, *Behav Res Ther* 33(4):379–390, 1995.
31. Miller WR, Rollnick S: *Motivational interviewing*, New York, 1991, Guilford Press.
32. Emmelcamp PMG, Bouman TK, Scholing A: *Anxiety disorders: A practitioner's guide*, New York, 1992, Wiley.
33. Jenike MA, Rauch SL: Managing the patient with treatment-resistant obsessive compulsive disorder: Current strategies, *J Clin Psychiatry* 55(suppl 3):11–17, 1994.
34. Livingston-Van Noppen B, Rasumussen SA, Eisen J, et al: Family function and treatment in obsessive-compulsive disorder. In Jenike MA, Baer L, Minichiello WE, editors: *Obsessive compulsive disorders, theory and management*, Chicago, 1990, Year Book.
35. Linehan MM: *Cognitive-behavioral treatment of borderline personality disorder*, New York, 1993, Guilford Press.

APPENDIX

As intensive care for psychiatric illness and neurobehavioral disorders evolves, several sites have continued to provide specialized treatment for OCD. These settings attempt to provide the intensity of care that the general public assumes is part and parcel of inpatient psychiatric units, but in truth rarely is. As programs continue to evolve, consumers are advised to contact the Obsessive-Compulsive Foundation (203-878-5669) for updated lists and descriptions of programs that target OCD-specific treatment.

The Obsessive-Compulsive Foundation currently lists six intensive treatment programs for OCD:

1. Anxiety Disorders Center at St. Louis Behavioral Medicine Institute in St. Louis, Missouri. A continuum of care program for anxiety disorders that includes a behaviorally oriented inpatient unit. The program has been in existence for many years.
2. A day program for OCD at the University of California at Los Angeles. The program provides a variety of group and individual therapies. Patients are provided with cognitive, behavioral, rehabilitation, skills training, and a variety of other services.
3. OCD–specific day program at the Medical College of Philadelphia. The first OCD–specific program in the United States, the program offers high-quality individualized behavior therapy and follow-up.
4. A multifaceted program at Brown University that includes day treatment within both a generic and women's day programs. Brown has a long history of quality services for OCD. There is also a strong specialty in body dysmorphic disorder and family treatment.
5. Behavioral program for OCD that is affiliated with a generic psychiatric inpatient unit on Long Island, New York. This program has demonstrated a long-term commitment to the delivery of empirically based behavioral therapy.
6. Massachusetts General Hospital's OCD Institute, a multilevel program with residential, day, outpatient, and home-based programs specifically for people with OCD. The program provides intensive milieu, psychopharmacologic and individualized behavioral, cognitive, family, and dynamic treatments in a supportive community atmosphere.

Each of these programs has a commitment to the delivery of empirically validated treatments and the development of more effective interventions. Most have evolved as clinical service units from well-established research programs. Relapse prevention, family involvement, and discharge planning are included in all programs. Several include groups and milieus that are tailored specifically for persons with OCD.

When seeking inpatient, partial hospital, or day treatment for obsessions and compulsions, the following list of criteria should guide the consumer in his or her choice of treatment sites:

1. Is psychopharmocology provided by a clinician with experience working with OCD patients?
2. Is there a behavioral therapist on staff with experience in the use of ERP, habit reversal, and cognitive-behavioral therapy? Is the behavior therapist familiar with relapse-prevention strategies and the current OCD research, including the newer evolving cognitive techniques?
3. Is the behavior plan developed by the patient and behavior therapist transmitted to and carried out by direct care staff? How frequently will the patient meet with the behavior therapist?
4. Are family members included in the treatment process?
5. Is there a specific treatment plan tied to clinical goals? Is the length of stay tied to clinical gain?
6. Are arrangements made for aftercare and relapse prevention?
7. Are group therapies targeted toward the needs of persons with OCD?
8. Does the program provide services or referral for services that help patients return to work and address psychosocial and relationship issues?

If the above criteria are not met, the program does not provide OCD–specific treatment. The program may help in a crisis situation but does not include state-of-the-art treatments for OCD.

26

Neurosurgical Treatment of Obsessive-Compulsive Disorder

Michael A. Jenike, M.D., Scott L. Rauch, M.D.,
Lee Baer, Ph.D., Steven A. Rasmussen, M.D.

Despite major advances in our understanding of appropriate medication and behavioral therapies to treat patients with obsessive-compulsive disorder (OCD), there remain a very small number of patients who are not only refractory to all conventional treatments, but also are extremely ill and essentially nonfunctional. For such treatment-refractory and severely ill OCD patients, clinicians are obligated to consider any treatments, even neurosurgical options, that could possibly provide some relief. For more than a decade, the Massachusetts General Hospital OCD (MGH OCD) Clinic staff had not referred any OCD patients for neurosurgery, despite having one of the main centers performing these procedures in the same hospital. Conceptually, it did not seem logical that removing a small piece of brain tissue could improve the lives of such severely ill patients. We also were aware of the controversial nature of these procedures and did not wish to become involved unless there were likely to be tangible rewards for our patients. However, as our clinic followed an increasing number of patients, the population of refractory patients grew, and we eventually felt obliged to more fully investigate potential benefits of these operations. Our guiding principle has been: "Would I refer a close family member for such an operation or would I undergo it myself?" If, after careful consideration of the available data, we could not answer affirmatively, we would not recommend this option to our patients. Our retrospective[1] and prospective[2] reviews of the outcomes and complications of one of these operations (cingulotomy) gave us some reason for optimism.

Surprisingly, in reviewing the neurosurgical literature, we found that OCD is one of the most commonly reported psychiatric disorders treated by neurosurgery.[3] Modern stereotactic surgical interventions produce lesions only millimeters in diameter, which are placed with great precision in brain structures that may be important for symptom production. The clinician who is contemplating neurosurgical intervention for an otherwise intractable OCD patient will need to know general selection guidelines, indications and contraindications, the procedures available, their probable outcome, the hazards involved, what preoperative work-up is needed, and the rationale behind neurosurgery for OCD.

It is of utmost importance to remember that the data are far from conclusive; that there remains much controversy; that not all of the published reports seem equally credible; and that there have been no controlled trials for these operations, which may have a significant placebo effect.

Several methodologic issues must be borne in mind when interpreting studies from this field. Many earlier reports are problematic in that: (1) these studies are retrospective; (2) diagnostic criteria have changed in the many years during which the studies were carried out; and (3) outcome assessment instruments with documented validity and reliability were not typically used. Because these interventions are performed at only a few centers, very few physicians are experienced in the field. Accordingly, it is common that the same clinician who was responsible for selection and treatment of the patients also determined clinical outcome, sometimes after only a short period of observation.

Neurosurgical procedures are now routinely performed for intractable pain, Parkinson's disease, and uncontrollable epileptic seizures. However, only a few centers in the world have kept surgery as a therapeutic option for intractable mental illness.[4] Each center tends to favor one particular type of operation, often determined by local tradition rather than by comparison of the relative merits of different methods. There are a considerable number of challenges in comparing two treatments of modest and similar efficacy in a heterogeneous disorder such as OCD. For example, high variance and probable small differences in response lead to a very low predicted effect size, and consequently an adequately powered study would require huge numbers of subjects to detect small differences. This is all the more impractical given the relatively small number of subjects who are appropriate for these procedures. This is one of many reasons why no meaningful head-to-head comparisons have been performed to date. Neurosurgical intervention for mental illness is prohibited or not available in some countries, and citizens of these countries have to go abroad for treatment. The operations most often reported in the treatment of refractory OCD are subcaudate tractotomy, limbic leucotomy, cingulotomy, and capsulotomy.

PATIENT SELECTION

Most clinicians agree that evidence must be well documented that the illness is causing considerable suffering and that the patient's psychosocial functioning is significantly reduced. Some of the severely ill candidates for such operations appear to suffer from a malignant form of OCD referred to by various terms such as *obsessional psychosis*[5–7] or *schizoobsessive state*,[7a] and most have comorbid conditions such as severe depression, body dysmorphic disorder, panic disorder, or personality disorders.

Most surgical candidates have failed all available and appropriate psychotropic medication trials as well as behavioral treatments. Each patient should have had adequate trials (at least 10 weeks at maximally tolerated dose) of clomipramine, fluoxetine, fluvoxamine, sertraline, paroxetine (some require only a minimum of three of these drug trials), and a monoamine oxidase inhibitor (MAOI) and augmentation of at least one of the previous drugs for 1 month with at least two of the following: lithium, clonazepam, or buspirone. If a patient has tics, a trial of augmentation with a low-dose neuroleptic should be performed.[8] With recent preliminary data suggesting that venlafaxine may be helpful for OCD,[9] this should perhaps be added to the list of required medication trials. All patients also must have had an extended trial of behavior therapy consisting of a minimum of 20 hours of exposure and response prevention (ERP). The illness must have been subject to intensive psychiatric treatment for a sufficient period of time to confirm that it is, indeed, clearly refractory to standard treatment; in practice, most centers define this as a minimum of 5 years of intensive treatment. Patients that meet these criteria may be candidates for neurosurgical intervention (Table 26-1).

Contraindications (Table 26-2) also must be taken into consideration. For the most part, these are not absolute contraindications, and considerable clinical judgment and experience must be exercised in each case to determine which patients are reasonable candidates. The use of multidisciplinary committees to evaluate these complicated patients is crucial to ensure that patients meet inclusion and exclusion criteria, to eliminate potential bias on the part of the treating clinicians, and to make certain that patients fully comprehend potential risks and benefits. The committee reviews each applicant's past psychiatric and treatment history in detail to ensure that all inclusion and exclusion criteria are satisfied and adjudicates all cases in which questions arise (e.g., whether a patient who has been through all the medication trials but, because of the illness, is unable to comply with reasonable trials of behavior therapy, should be allowed to undergo the operation). If the initial review of case material suggests that the patient may be an appropriate candidate, the committee performs an on-site assessment of the patient and meets with the patient's family before a final determination is made.

TYPES OF OPERATIONS

As noted earlier, the four procedures commonly used to treat severely ill OCD patients include subcaudate tractotomy, limbic leucotomy, cingulotomy, and capsulotomy. The majority of these procedures are stereotactic interventions in which a device called a *stereotactic frame* is employed to permit high

Table 26-1   Indications for Neurosurgical Intervention

1. The patient fulfills the diagnostic criteria for obsessive-compulsive disorder.
2. The duration of illness exceeds 5 years.
3. The disorder is causing substantial suffering.
4. The disorder is causing substantial reduction in the patient's psychosocial functioning.
5. Current treatment options tried systematically have either been without appreciable effect on the symptoms or discontinued because of intolerable side effects.
6. The prognosis, without neurosurgical intervention, is considered poor.
7. The patient gives informed consent.
8. The patient agrees to participate in the preoperative evaluation program.
9. The patient agrees to participate in the postoperative rehabilitation program.
10. There is a referring physician in the patient's local area willing to accept responsibility for the postoperative, long-term management of the patient.

accuracy (± 1 mm in three dimensions) in placing bilateral lesions in intended targets, as determined by neuroradiologic imaging. The operation may be performed under local anesthesia with light sedation. When the targets are being lesioned, patients do not report subjective sensations. Neurosurgeons often prefer to err on the conservative side by creating initial lesions that are quite small and performing a second intervention if warranted clinically.

Subcaudate Tractotomy

The main indication for subcaudate tractotomy is not OCD, but rather unresponsive affective disorder.[10,11] As of 1991, 1,200 psychiatric patients were reported to have undergone this procedure.[12] Subcaudate tractotomy was developed in London. Unlike most other operations in which heated electrodes are used to make the lesions, this procedure created lesions by means of beta radioactive 90-Yttrium rods, 1 mm wide and 7 mm long, inserted stereotactically into the target area.[11,13,14] The half-life of the beta-emitter is approximately 60 hours, so eventually the rods became inert. They were arranged as an array in two or three rows covering a volume approximately 20 mm wide, 18 mm long, and 5 mm thick. This technique is no longer used, and the yttrium rods are no longer manufactured. Some surgeons have continued to make this lesion via other conventional means (e.g., by thermocoagulation), as in part of limbic leucotomy. Under general anesthesia, bilateral burr holes, 16 mm in diameter, are made just above the frontal sinuses and 15 mm from the midline. The targets, visualized by means of a ventriculogram, are located beneath the head of the caudate nucleus, in a brain region called the *substantia innominata*. In the first few postoperative weeks, the patient may suffer from episodes of confusion.

There are a few reports on the efficacy of this procedure in OCD patients. Strom-Olsen and Carlisle[15] published results of 20 OCD patients who under-

Table 26-2 Relative Contraindications for Neurosurgical Intervention

1. Patient age below 18 or above 65 years
2. The patient has another (current or lifetime) axis I diagnosis (e.g., organic brain syndrome, delusional disorder, or current or recent alcohol or drug abuse) that substantially complicates function, treatment, or the patient's ability to comply with treatment, or leads to serious adverse events such as overdosage, suicide attempts, etc. Some centers include somatoform disorders as a contraindication.
3. A complicating current axis II diagnosis from Cluster A (e.g., paranoid personality disorder) or B (e.g., borderline, antisocial, or histrionic personality disorder) may constitute a relative contraindication. A current Cluster C personality disorder (e.g., avoidant or obsessive-compulsive personality disorder) is generally not a contraindication because it may, in fact, disappear with successful treatment of the coexistent obsessive-compulsive disorder.
4. The patient has a current axis III diagnosis with brain pathology, such as moderate or marked cerebral atrophy, stroke, or tumor, or has undergone previous neurosurgical procedures that might produce complications.

went operation in the 1960s. Ten of these patients were either completely recovered or had slight residual symptoms without need for further postoperative treatment.[16] However, the authors noted that four of these patients later relapsed. Göktepe, et al[11] later reported on 18 OCD patients, 50% of whom reported total recovery or minimal symptoms. In these reports, there was a low rate of postoperative epilepsy and of adverse behaviors such as overeating, volubility, and extravagance.

In summary, clinical improvement was reported in approximately 50% of the 38 OCD patients who had undergone this operation. The minimum period of follow-up was 1 year. These reports did not include discussion of possible long-term effects from the radioactivity caused by the implanted Yttrium seeds.[16]

Cingulotomy

Cingulotomy and capsulotomy are the most commonly reported surgical procedures for anxiety disorders.[17] Cingulotomy has been the neurosurgical approach of choice over the past 20 years in the United States and Canada for intractable pain, major depression,[18–20] and OCD.[3,11] Cingulotomy is relatively benign, having a very low incidence of complications and transient or late side effects. It is not unusual, however, for a second operation (in which the initial lesion is enlarged) to be necessary. This procedure is usually performed 6 months to 1 year after the initial procedure, when it is clear that no further benefit may be expected. The operation is performed under local or general anesthesia and involves only minimal hair shaving just behind the anterior hairline, usually causing no significant postoperative cosmetic problem. Bilateral burr holes, approximately 12 mm in diameter, are made and magnetic resonance imaging (MRI) is used to visualize the targets. Electrodes are introduced stereotactically into two adjacent targets in the cingulate bundle on each side. Lesions are then created by the radiofrequency-induced heating of the tip of the electrodes to 80° to 85° centigrade for 100 seconds.[19,21,22]

One of the earliest reports of this operation was by Whitty, et al[22a] in which five obsessional patients underwent open cingulotomy and four reportedly improved. The pronounced side effects on personality and behavior common with frontal lobotomy were not found with cingulotomy. Kullberg[23] later reported that 4 of 13 patients improved after undergoing cingulotomy. Foltz and White[24] modified the operation by using the stereotactic method that was later used by Ballantine and colleagues,[19] who reported that of 32 OCD patients, 25% were found to be functionally well and another 31% were markedly improved at follow-up. Side effects of this procedure included a 1% incidence of epilepsy controllable with anticonvulsant medication. There was no evidence of behavioral, emotional, or intellectual side effects.

Jenike and coworkers[1] retrospectively evaluated 33 OCD patients who had undergone cingulotomy at Massachusetts General Hospital over a 25-year period. Using the Yale-Brown Obsessive Compulsive Scale (Y-BOCS) as the dependent measure and very conservative criteria, the authors estimated that at least 25% to 30% of the patients "benefited substantially from the intervention." Several patients attributed improvement primarily to postsurgical drug or behavioral treatments. Excluding those subjects, as many as 30% to 40% of these severely disabled patients believed they benefitted substantially from the cingulotomy alone, and another 10% maintained that the surgery had augmented subsequent treatments. These operations were often performed before the common usage of serotonin reuptake inhibitors (SRIs) and behavior therapy; however, with improved efficacy of nonsurgical treatment for OCD, future patients will likely be an even more refractory population than in previous studies.

In a later prospective study,[2] 18 severely ill OCD patients who had failed modern treatments and undergone bilateral anterior cingulotomy were assessed before and 6 months after surgery (using the Y-BOCS). Five patients (28%) met conservative criteria for treatment response, and three others (16%) were possible responders. The group improved significantly in mean functional status and no serious adverse effects were found. In a disorder that characteristically waxes and wanes, fluctuation in level of improvement is to be expected, but with such severely ill patients, it is unlikely that they would improve significantly unless the intervention was helpful.

Limbic Leucotomy

In this multitarget procedure developed by Kelly and coworkers in 1973 in the United Kingdom, the subcaudate tractotomy lesions described previously are produced, but targets in the cingulum also are lesioned; hence, this operation is basically a combination of the two previously described procedures.

The proponents of this operation feel that lesions in both sites produce better results in OCD than lesions in either area alone.[25–27] After hair shaving, and under local or generalized anesthesia, bilateral burr holes are made 9.5 cm posterior to the nasion and 15 mm from the midline. Again, a ventriculogram is used to visualize the targets. Intraoperative stimulation of autonomic responses may be used to verify the accuracy of target placement, at least in the substantia innominata site,[25,28] although its usefulness has been questioned.[29] The limbic leucotomy lesions are produced by means of radiofrequency-heated electrodes. Side effects include transient postoperative confusion and headache.

Mitchell-Heggs, et al[25] reported that 89% of 27 OCD patients of whom were improved 1 year postoperatively. This figure was disputed by Bartlett and Bridges,[13] who noted that the 89% improvement rate included patients with significant residual symptoms.[16] Transient side effects included headache, confusion, and perseverative behaviors, but no long-term personality changes or seizures. Including the previous patients, Kelley[27] later provided an additional review of patients treated by limbic leucotomy and reported that 84% of 49 patients were improved at a mean of 20 months postoperatively.

Capsulotomy

Developed at the Karolinska Institute in Sweden more than three decades ago, this procedure has been used for the treatment of refractory anxiety disorders including OCD and has recently been performed by U.S. neurosurgeons. Two surgical techniques for capsulotomy have been described—the radiofrequency (RF) thermolesion and the radiosurgical, or gamma, capsulotomy.

Unfortunately, it remains unknown where precisely in the internal capsule the lesions should be made for optimal results for OCD, and an open trial is now under way with the gamma knife in an effort to determine this location.[29]

The RF thermolesion procedure, developed by the Swedish neurosurgeon Lars Leksell,[30–33] is performed under local anesthesia and light sedation. The coordinates of the target in the anterior limb of the internal capsule are determined with MRI. Small bilateral burr holes are made just behind the coronary suture, and monopolar electrodes with a diameter of 1.5 mm are inserted into the target area. Thermolesions are produced by heating the uninsulated tip of the electrode to approximately 75° centigrade for 75 seconds, creating a lesion approximately 4 mm wide and 15 to 18 mm long. Patients report no subjective sensations when the lesions are being produced. Postoperative headache is uncommon. As with other procedures in current use (with the possible exception of cingulotomy), a mild decrease in initiative and motivation may be noted during the first 2 to 3 postoperative months after RF capsulotomy. This appears to correlate with circumlesional edema, as determined with MRI, and disappears with resolution of edema.[34] From 3 months onward, initiative and motivation have usually returned to preoperative levels, except in a few patients who had large lesions and who continued to be somewhat apathetic for lengthy periods of time.

The first report of the efficacy of this procedure for OCD was by Herner,[35] who found either "good" or "fair" outcomes in 78% of 18 patients. Bingley, et al[30] reported that at a mean follow-up of 35 months, 71% of 35 patients were either "free of symptoms" or "much improved." Of interest, of 24 patients unable to work preoperatively, 20 resumed work postoperatively. Kullberg, et al[23] reported that 10 of 13 patients improved with capsulotomy compared with only 4 of 13 cingulotomy patients. There was one serious side effect of capsulotomy in one patient who reportedly lost impulse control and became aggressive. In addition, several patients treated with capsulotomy demonstrated personality changes consisting of emotional shallowness, loss of initiative, diminution of inhibition, and mood elevation.[27] Fodstad, et al[35] reported another two OCD patients who improved after capsulotomy.

In the radiosurgical, or gamma capsulotomy, technique, also developed by Leksell and coworkers,[33,37,38] lesions are produced by cross-firing of approximately 200 narrow beams of 60-Cobalt gamma irradiation from a stereotactic gamma unit. Craniotomy and shaving are unnecessary. Although the biologic effect of any individual gamma beam is negligible, at the point of focus, the effects are combined to produce a radiosurgical lesion. This method has been successfully used for more than 20 years in the treatment of acoustic neuromas, arteriovenous malformations, cancer pain, craniopharyngiomas, pituitary adenomas, and other deep-seated pathologic processes. Gamma capsulotomy patients are not hospitalized for postoperative care. As yet, the experience with gamma capsulotomy is considerably less extensive than that with the RF technique.[32,33] The risk for radiation-induced malignancy is not elevated following this form of irradiation; no such case has been observed in the two decades during which the procedure has been used.

In an ongoing investigation of gamma capsulotomy, with a small number of OCD patients, it appears that there is progressive improvement in OCD symptoms over 18-month follow-up with a mean decrement in Y-BOCS scores of approximately one third and similar improvement in depression and anxiety scores. It is important to keep in mind, however, that other postoperative treatments were not controlled, and some of the patients had very intensive behavior therapy after the operation. For example, two patients who were the best responders actually lived in the home of an experienced behavior therapist involved in the study for several months after the operation. If these two patients are removed from the data analysis, the assessment of group outcome is not nearly as good.

With the advent of such new technology, it is now clinically and ethically feasible to perform a sham operation as a control condition. With the gamma knife, we are able to overcome logistic challenges that had previously prevented an ethical controlled trial. With this technique, a small lesion can be precisely localized in specific regions of the brain without opening the cranium. Our group has proposed to study 48 OCD patients randomly assigned to receive either anterior capsulotomy (n = 24) or a sham procedure (n = 24). During the sham condition, each of the radiation ports is blocked with lead inserts by a research technician so that even the surgeon is unaware if the ports are open or closed when the operation is performed. Investigators performing examinations and patients will remain blind to surgical condition. Clinical questionnaires, structured interviews, neuropsychologic testing, and neuroimaging techniques (i.e., morphometric MRI) will be used to evaluate patients both prior to operation and again 6 months later to follow treatment response, adverse effects, and structural changes that may correlate with postoperative clinical improvement. At the 6-month point, the treatment code (i.e., capsulotomy or sham procedure) will be broken and the patient then offered the capsulotomy operation if he or she received the sham procedure initially. This study has been approved by three Institutional Review Boards (Massachusetts General Hospital, Brown University, and Rhode Island Hospital) and will likely begin when the optimal lesion site in the anterior capsule has been determined in our currently ongoing dose-finding trial.

WHICH IS THE BEST OPERATION FOR OBSESSIVE-COMPULSIVE DISORDER?

Unfortunately, there have been few comparison studies of these operations. In addition, diagnostic criteria for OCD were not consistent across the studies, outcome standards varied among research groups, and complications were not always reported. Strikingly, there are essentially no negative reports of neurosurgical procedures in the medical literature, suggesting that only favorable or partly positive reports have been published. Keeping these variables and uncertainties in mind, it appears at first glance that limbic leucotomy has been more effective than the other procedures, but the group reporting these data may have been more liberal about their definitions of improvement than the other researchers. Certainly, no definitive conclusions about which procedure is best can be drawn without further research.

For reasons discussed in the following paragraphs, most studies have not had control groups. Many investigators have instead compiled data from different reports, an approach marred by the obvious shortcoming that the procedures, including assessments of outcome and observation time, all vary considerably among studies. Moreover, outcome cannot be independently ascertained from some reports, because the results are not given in sufficient detail. This makes direct comparison across studies difficult to interpret.

Some patients with only limited response to surgery report that treatment modalities that were ineffective before surgery seemed to give patients at least some symptom relief postoperatively.[1,39] This important information requires further study but offers some hope to the patient who has had a poor response to surgery alone.

RISKS OF SURGERY

Operative complications include infection, hemorrhage, epileptic seizure, and weight gain. Despite occasional complications, Ballantine, et al[19] reported no deaths in their series of 696 cingulotomies performed in patients with various psychiatric disorders over a 25-year period. Although infection and intracerebral hemorrhage cannot always be avoided, their sequelae can, provided that treatment is instituted immediately. The incidence of hemiplegia has been estimated at 0.03% following cingulotomy;[19] these only occurred during the pre-MRI-guidance era, and were the result of injecting air into the ventricles. No such events have happened in conjunction with contemporary methods of cingulotomy. No case of hemiplegia has been reported in subcaudate tractotomy, limbic leucotomy, or capsulotomy. The risk of postoperative epilepsy following these interventions has been estimated at less than 1%,[1,19,21,40] and these were usually easily controlled with antiseizure medications. Several authors have reported weight gain in capsulotomized patients,[30,39] but it is unknown whether this phenomenon is specific for capsulotomy or occurs after other procedures as well.

The risk of neurosurgery for severe OCD compares favorably with that of stereotactic operations for nonpsychiatric illnesses; in one study of 243 consecutive stereotactic interventions for various neurologic illnesses, 15 complications were noted, including one death.[41]

Cognitive Alterations

The risk of negative effects on cognitive functioning following modern procedures has been carefully investigated by several independent researchers who evaluated patients before and after cingulotomy,[21,42–44] subcaudate tractotomy,[11,13] limbic leucotomy,[25,27] and capsulotomy.[30,31,35,45–47] Using various psychometric tests preoperatively and postoperatively, the authors found no evidence of reduced intellectual function related to surgery. On the contrary, patients tended to achieve better test results after operation—a finding for which several explanations have been advanced, including improved concentration ability, freedom from drugs, and practice effects from retaking the tests.

One group[19] noted that an independent study of a cohort of their cingulotomy patients was performed for the U.S. government by the Department of Psychology at the Massachusetts Institute of Technology, with reports indicating no evidence of lasting neurologic, intellectual, personality, or behavioral deficits after cingulotomy.[42,44] In fact, a comparison of preoperative and postoperative scores revealed modest gains in the Wechsler IQ ratings. The only apparent irreversible decrement identified by these investigators was a decrease in performance on the Taylor Complex Figure Test in patients more than 40 years of age.

Although not demonstrable with conventional tests, neurosurgical intervention may give rise to frontal lobe dysfunction. Therefore, it is important to evaluate the surgical candidate's cognitive functions; a patient with preoperative abnormal or borderline test scores may run an elevated risk for postoperative changes.

Personality Alteration

It is interesting that side effects may, in fact, also occur in patients who do not undergo surgery. In their prospective, controlled study comparing the efficacy of intensive nonsurgical treatment with that of modified bimedial leucotomy in OCD, Tan and coworkers[47a] noted brusqueness and irritability (six patients), apathy, laziness, and general blunting (two patients) among the 13 controls. In other words, symptoms and signs often regarded as "postoperative" side effects also appeared in the nonsurgery group.

According to anecdotal evidence, negative personality changes following current surgical procedures are rare. Because the interventions may be expected to influence, directly or indirectly, frontal lobe function and, hence, personality, more research is needed in this area. With regard to subcaudate tractotomy, tests were administered, but only at follow-up.[11] Kelly[27] gave the Leyton Obsessional Inventory (LOI) to 26 OCD patients before and at 20 months after limbic leucotomy and found significant changes in obsessive features in the direction of normality. Unfortunately, the validity of the LOI is not well established.

A widely used personality instrument, the Eysenck Personality Inventory, was administered prospectively to 15 patients undergoing capsulotomy,[30,38] and in no cases were negative personality changes observed after capsulotomy.

It is well known that impulsiveness is one of the most conspicuous symptoms of frontal lobe dysfunction.[48] For this reason, a method likely to detect negative personality changes following surgery must detect impulsiveness and related features such as psychopathy, hostility, and aggressiveness. One such instrument is the Karolinska Scales of Personality (KSP), developed by Schalling and coworkers.[49] It contains scales measuring traits related to frontal lobe function and scales reflecting different dimensions of anxiety-proneness. A large number of studies have been performed by independent investigators who have shown the KSP to differentiate between diagnostic subgroups and to correlate significantly with biologic markers for vulnerability to certain psychopathologic conditions. Mindus and Nyman[46] gave the KSP to 24 consecutive patients before and at 1 year after RF capsulotomy. Before surgery, deviant scores were obtained on 5 of the 15 KSP scales, four of which are scales related to anxiety-proneness. At 1 year after capsulotomy, statistically significant decreases were noted on eight of the scales with normal scores on all but two scales (which remained borderline). In particular, the scores on scales related to impulsiveness, psychopathy, hostility, and aggressiveness were within the normal range. Negative personality changes are not likely to occur after modern surgical procedures.[50]

It must be remembered, however, that these conclusions are based on observations made on subject groups and do not preclude that negative changes could occur in individual patients.

Suicide

In the review by Waziri,[51] only 3% of the patients were reported to be worse or dead at follow-up. Among the dead was one suicide. It is important, however, to keep in mind that suicide may be a complication of surgical procedures, at least in very depressed OCD patients; Jenike, et al[1] found that 4 of 33 patients who had undergone cingulotomy for OCD had died by suicide at follow-up that averaged 13 years. According to these patient records, each patient who had committed suicide had been noted to suffer from severe depression with prominent suicidal ruminations when he or she was first evaluated for cingulotomy. Although they all met criteria for OCD, they had extensive comorbid disease. None of the OCD patients who were not suicidal at baseline assessment became suicidal after the operation. It remains possible that disappointment secondary to failure of this "last-resort" treatment could have contributed to suicide in these predisposed patients. Ballantine, et al discussed in more detail the issue of suicide in psychiatric patients who have undergone cingulotomy.[19]

Because patients with a poor response to surgery may be at increased risk for suicide,[1] these individuals should be informed of two things: (1) treatments that were ineffective before surgery might be helpful when tried postoperatively; and (2) neurosurgeons prefer to err on the conservative side, creating only small initial lesions, permitting a second intervention if warranted clinically.

RISK OF NONINTERVENTION

In most surgical studies, patients had a duration of illness averaging more than 15 years. This tells something of the prognosis. The risk for social, somatic, and mental complications (including suicide) in this group of patients cannot be overrated. A small number of patients have been described who were eligible for intervention but never operated on for different reasons.[19,39] Their conditions remained the same, and some eventually committed suicide. The physician with a patient with malignant OCD, in whom all therapeutic options have been exhausted, has the delicate task of weighing the risk of intervention against the risk of nonintervention. Deferring the decision to operate on a given patient may not spare him or her complications.

POSTOPERATIVE CARE

A postoperative treatment program should be instituted early, preferably under the guidance of the referring physician or someone else who knows the patient well. Behavioral treatment with ERP should be reinstituted shortly after the operation (see Chapter 17).

NEUROBIOLOGIC RATIONALE FOR OPERATIONS

Despite many hypotheses, it remains unknown why these operations might improve symptoms in some patients and not others. No reliable predictors have been identified of which OCD patients might improve overall or if a specific operation may help one type of patient. It appears that different surgical approaches all have the common objective of severing interconnections between the orbitomedial areas of the frontal lobes and limbic or thalamic structures. In humans, it has been shown that lesions in the substantia innominata following subcaudate tractotomy cause extensive degeneration in the ventral portion of the internal capsule.[52] The fiber tract degeneration can be traced back to the dorsomedial nucleus of the thalamus, which has extensive interconnections with various parts of the limbic system.[53,54] These observations indicate that lesions in one region may affect the function of other brain regions. Conversely, there is evidence to show that different approaches may affect similar clinical conditions. For example, lesions in the anterior cingulate cortex (as in cingulotomy), the substantia innominata (as in subcaudate tractotomy), the orbitofrontal-thalamic tract (as in capsulotomy), or the midline thalamic nuclei (as in certain forms of thalamotomy)[55] have all been associated with improvement in OCD symptoms. In other words, although different surgical interventions have different stereotactic targets, they might directly or indirectly affect the same brain system(s).

Despite the lack of a specific, identified brain abnormality in OCD, there is growing evidence that the syndrome has a biologic cause (see Rauch and Jenike[56,57] and Chapters 11 and 12). Only recently have morphometric MRI analyses revealed that OCD patients (only studied in women thus far) have diminished brain white matter compared with carefully matched control subjects.[58,59] It remains intuitively appealing to search for underlying localized brain pathology; however, current thinking has shifted away from ascribing complex functions such as speech or associative memory to individual areas of the brain. Instead, circuits in many different areas of the brain are called upon to interact simultaneously using parallel distributed processing.[60,61] This shift in thinking has been bolstered by neuroanatomic techniques that have demonstrated a highly complex interconnectivity between widespread areas of the brain. Abnormalities in frontal lobe and basal ganglia structure and function[56,57,62–69] in patients with OCD have led to hypotheses about the disorder's pathogenesis, which emphasize possible aberrations in the neural circuits that connect these regions.[70–72] For more extensive discussions of the neurobiology of OCD, see Chapters 11 and 12.

As noted previously, the surgical literature provides considerable anecdotal evidence for lessening OCD symptoms in some patients following cingulotomy, limbic leucotomy, subcaudate tractotomy, and anterior capsulotomy. All of these procedures interrupt connections among the frontal lobes, basal ganglia, and limbic system.

Preliminary evidence suggests that OCD patients do not improve immediately after surgery, but that several weeks to months are required for positive clinical effects to be fully manifested. This delay in efficacy may be caused by secondary nerve degeneration or metabolic alterations in brain areas outside the region that is actually lesioned. Morphometric MRI may be used to assess gross volumetric changes in areas distant from the lesion site; MR spectroscopic measurement of N-acetyl-aspartate (NAA; a putative index of neuronal integrity) may allow for serial assessment of downstream effects following surgical lesions.

The proposed pathogenetic imbalance of these brain region functions appears to be somehow counteracted by neurosurgical intervention, the net effect experienced by some patients as symptom relief.

SUMMARY

The data on neurosurgery for intractable and malignant OCD are far from conclusive. There remains much controversy, and not all of the published reports seem equally credible. There also have been no controlled trials for these operations, which may have a significant placebo effect. It is prudent to convey this uncertainty to patients so that they have an accurate perspective. If misconceptions about these operations are perpetuated, some patients will not perform the considerable work needed to improve with behavior therapy, because they feel there is an easier way; other patients (or their psychiatrists) may reject the option of neurosurgical treatment presumptively on false premises.

We cannot be sure that rater bias was eliminated in any of the studies that have been reviewed or that the open treatment of patients with surgical procedures might not have affected the postoperative assessment to some degree. The theoretic ideal of a randomized, double-blind trial would be required to solve these problems; however, the feasibility and ethics of such a study have been discussed. The gamma knife now allows a controlled trial to be undertaken; until now, we had to rely on a more traditional method of evaluation by objectively reviewing the responses of patients who had already received these treatments.

Progressive improvement over time has been reported after some of these surgical procedures, and there is anecdotal evidence that other treatments, including pharmacotherapy and behavior therapy, are more likely to be successful after operation than before. Because the vast majority of patients who have undergone surgery were severely and chronically disabled, it is quite possible that these procedures were helpful in alleviating some of their symptoms, and the results of the cumulative studies strongly support the need for continued research in this area. It is currently impossible to determine which surgical procedure is best for a particular patient. Head-to-head comparison studies are not yet available, and it may be years until we have comparative data. Until such data are available, clinicians should work with the surgical team that is closest to them.

When nonsurgical treatments have failed, there is evidence that at least partial, and often significant, relief can be obtained in some OCD patients by surgery. In the future, it will be important to maximize our understanding of these procedures. When the technology is available, patients should be prospectively studied, before and after surgery, with single photon emission computed tomography or positron-emission tomography and MRI. As previously noted, usually patients do not benefit immediately; a few weeks to months are required for optimal improvement. Sequential scans might allow researchers to follow the course of metabolic and structural lesions in an effort to understand what parts of the brain are affected in patients who respond and also in those patients who are not helped. With modern technology, it is possible that lesion site and size can be correlated with clinical outcome, and that the course of downstream neuronal degeneration remote from the lesion itself can be followed. The identification of clinical subgroups of patients with a particularly high (or low) likelihood of improvement after a neurosurgical procedure also merits further study.

REFERENCES

1. Jenike MA, Baer L, Ballantine HT, et al: Cingulotomy for refractory obsessive-compulsive disorder. A long term follow-up of 33 patients, *Arch Gen Psychiatry* 48:548–555, 1991.
2. Baer L, Rauch SL, Ballantine HT, et al: Cingulotomy for intractable obsessive-compulsive disorder: Prospective long-term follow-up of 18 patients, *Arch Gen Psychiatry* 52:384–392, 1995.
3. Mindus P, Jenike MA: Neurosurgical treatment of malignant obsessive-compulsive disorder. In Jenike MA, editor: *Psychiatric clinics of North America: Obsessional disorders*, vol 15, no 4, Philadelphia, 1992, WB Saunders, pp 921–938.
4. Snaith P: The case for psychosurgery (letter), *Br J Hosp Med* 8:147, 1987.
5. Insel TR, Akiskal HS: Obsessive-compulsive disorder with psychotic features: A phenomenologic analysis, *Am J Psychiatry* 143:1527, 1986.
6. Robinson S, Winnik HZ, Weiss AA: Obsessive psychosis: Justification for a separate clinical entity, *Isr Ann Psychiatry* 30:372, 1976.
7. Solyom L, DiNicola VF, Phil M, et al: Is there an obsessive psychosis? Aetiological and prognostic factors of an atypical form of obsessive-compulsive neurosis, *Can J Psychiatry* 30:372, 1985.
7a. Jenike MA, Baer L, Minichiello al: Coexistent obsessive-compulsive disorder and schicotype personality disorder: a poor prognostic indicator, *Arch Gen Psychiatry* 43:296, 1986.
8. McDougle CJ, Goodman WK, Price LH, et al: Neuroleptic addition in fluvoxamine-refractory obsessive-compulsive disorder: An open case series, *Am J Psychiatry* 147:552–554, 1990.
9. Rauch SL, O'Sullivan RL, Jenike MA: Open treatment of obsessive-compulsive disorder with venlafaxine: A series of ten cases, *J Clin Psychopharm* 16:81–84, 1996.
10. Lovett LM, Shaw DM: Outcome in bipolar affective disorder after stereotactic tractotomy, *Br J Psychiatry* 151:113, 1987.

11. Göktepe EO, Young LB, Bridges PK: A further review of the results of stereotactic subcaudate tractotomy, *Br J Psychiatry* 126:270, 1975.
12. Malizia A: Indications for psychosurgery [Abstract S-13-12-02], *Biol Psychiatry* (suppl 11S), 1991.
13. Bartlett JR, Bridges PK: The extended subcaudate tractotomy lesion. In Sweet WH, Obrador S, Martin-Rodriguez JG, editors: *Neurosurgical treatment in psychiatry, pain, and epilepsy*, Baltimore, 1977, University Park Press, p 387.
14. Knight GC: Bifrontal stereotaxic tractotomy in the substantia innominata: An experience of 450 cases. In Hitchcock E, Laitinen L, Vaernet K, editors: *Psychosurgery*, Springfield, 1972, Charles C. Thomas, p 269.
15. Strom-Olsen R, Carlisle S: Bi-frontal stereotactic tractotomy: A follow-up study of its effects on 210 patients, *Br J Psychiatry* 118:141–154, 1971.
16. Chiocca EA, Martuza RL: Neurosurgical therapy of obsessive-compulsive disorder. In Jenike MA, Baer L, Minichiello WE, editors: *Obsessive-compulsive disorders: Theory and management*, Chicago, 1990, Year Book Medical Publishers, p. 283.
17. See reference 51.
18. Ballantine HT Jr, Levy BS, Dagi TF, et al: Cingulotomy for psychiatric illness: report of 13 years' experience. In Sweet W, Obrador S, Martin-Rodriguez JG, editors: *Neurosurgical treatment in psychiatry, pain and epilepsy*, Baltimore, 1977, University Park Press, p 333.
19. Ballantine HT Jr, Bouckoms AJ, Thomas EK, et al: Treatment of psychiatric illness by stereotactic cingulotomy, *Biol Psychiatry* 22:807–819, 1987.
20. Bouckoms AJ: The role of stereotactic cingulotomy in the treatment of intractable depression. In Amsterdam JA, editor: *Advances in neuropsychiatry and psychopharmacology 2: Refractory depression*, New York, 1991, Raven Press, p 2.
21. Ballantine HT Jr: Neurosurgery for behavioral disorders. In Wilkins RH, Rengachary SS, editors: *Neurosurgery*, New York, 1985, Elsevier/North Holland Biomedical Press, p 2527.
22. Martuza RL, Chiocca EA, Jenike MA, et al: Stereotactic radiofrequency thermal cingulotomy for obsessive-compulsive disorder, *J Neuropsych Clin Neurosci* 2: 331–336, 1990.
22a. Whitty CWM, Duffield JE, Tow PM, et al: Anterior cingulectomy in the treatment of mental disease, *Lancet* 1:475–481, 1952.
23. Kullberg G: Differences in effects of capsulotomy and cingulotomy. In Sweet WH, Obrador WS, Martin-Rodriguez JG, editors: *Neurosurgical treatment in psychiatry, pain, and epilepsy*, Baltimore, 1977, University Park Press, pp 301–308.
24. Foltz EL, White LE: Pain relief by frontal cingulotomy, *J Neurosurg* 19:89, 1962.
25. Mitchell-Heggs N, Kelly D, Richardson A: Stereotactic limbic leucotomy–a follow-up at 16 months, *Br J Psychiatry* 128:226–240, 1976.
26. Richardson A: Stereotactic limbic leucotomy. Surgical technique, *Postgrad Med J* 49:860, 1973.
27. Kelly D: *Anxiety and emotions. Physiological basis and treatment*, Springfield, 1980, Charles C. Thomas.
28. Kelly D: Physiological changes during operations on the limbic system in man, *Cond Reflex* 7:127, 1972.

29. Poynton A, Bridges PK, Bartlett JR: Psychosurgery in Britain now, *Br J Neurosurg* 2:297, 1988.
30. Bingley T, Leksell L, Meyerson BA, et al: Long term results of stereotactic capsulotomy in chronic obsessive-compulsive neurosis. In Sweet WH, Obrador S, Martin-Rodriguez JG, editors: *Neurosurgical treatment in psychiatry*, Baltimore, 1977, University Park Press, p 287.
31. Burzaco J: Stereotactic surgery in the treatment of obsessive-compulsive neurosis. In Perris C, Struwe G, Jansson B, editors: *Biological psychiatry*, Amsterdam, 1981, Elsevier/North Holland Biomedical Press, p 1103.
32. Meyerson BA, Mindus P: Capsulotomy as treatment of anxiety disorders. In Lunsford LD, editor: *Modern stereotactic neurosurgery*, Boston, 1988, Martinus Nijhoff, p 353.
33. Mindus P, Bergström K, Levander SE, et al: Magnetic resonance images related to clinical outcome after psychosurgical intervention in severe anxiety disorder, *J Neurol Neurosurg Psychiatry* 50:1288, 1987.
34. Mindus P, Unpublished results.
35. Herner T: Treatment of mental disorders with frontal stereotactic thermo-lesions. A follow-up of 116 cases, *Acta Psychiatr Scand* (suppl)36, 1961.
36. Fodstad H, Strandman E, Karlsson B, et al: Treatment of chronic obsessive-compulsive states with stereotactic anterior capsulotomy or cingulotomy, *Acta Neurochir* 62:1–23, 1982.
37. Leksell L, Backlund EO: Stereotactic gamma capsulotomy. In Hitchcock ER, Ballantine HT Jr, Meyerson BA, editors: *Modern concepts in psychiatric surgery*, Amsterdam, 1979, Elsevier/North Holland Biomedical Press, p 213.
38. Rylander G: Stereotactic radiosurgery in anxiety and obsessive-compulsive states: Psychiatric aspects. In Hitchcock ER, Ballantine HT Jr, Meyerson BA, editors: *Modern concepts in psychiatric surgery*, Amsterdam, 1979, Elsevier/North Holland Biomedical Press, p 235.
39. Mindus P: *Capsulotomy in anxiety disorders. A multidisciplinary study*, Thesis, Stockholm, 1991, Karolinska Institute.
40. Bingley T, Person A: EEG studies on patients with chronic obsessive-compulsive neurosis before and after psychosurgery, *Electronenc Clin Neurophys* 44:691, 1978.
41. Blaauw G, Braakman R: Pitfalls in diagnostic stereotactic brain surgery, *Acta Neurosurg* (suppl)42:161, 1988.
42. Corkin S: A prospective study of cingulotomy. In Valenstein ES, editor: *The psychosurgery debate*, San Francisco, 1980, WH Freeman & Co, p 264.
43. Corkin S, Hebben N: Subjective estimates of chronic pain before and after psychosurgery or treatment in a pain unit. Paper presented at the Third World Congress on Pain of the International Association for the Study of Pain, Edinburgh, Scotland, 1981.
44. Corkin S, Twitchell TE, Sullivan EV: Safety and efficacy of cingulotomy for pain and psychiatric disorder. In Hitchcock ER, Ballantine HT, Myerson BA, editors: *Modern concepts in psychiatric surgery*, New York, 1979, Elsevier/North Holland, pp 253–272.
45. Vasko T, Kullberg G: Results of psychological testing of cognitive functions in patients undergoing stereotactic psychiatric surgery. In Hitchcock ER, Ballantine

HT Jr, Meyerson BA, editors: *Modern concepts in psychiatric surgery*, Amsterdam, 1979, Elsevier/North Holland Biomedical Press, p 303.

46. Mindus P, Nyman H: Normalization of personality characteristics in patients with incapacitating anxiety disorders after capsulotomy, *Acta Psychiatr Scand* 83: 283–291, 1991.

47. Sweet WH, Meyerson BA: Neurosurgical aspects of primary affective disorders. In Youmans JR, editor: *Neurological surgery*, Philadelphia, 1990, WB Saunders.

47a. Tan E, Marks IM, Marset P: Bi-medial leucotomy in obsessive-compulsive neurosis: a controlled serial inquiry, *Br J Psychiatry* 118:155, 1971.

48. Stuss DT, Benson DF: Personality and emotion. In Stuss DT, Benson DF, editors: *The frontal lobes*, New York, 1986, Raven Press, p 121.

49. Schalling D, Åsberg M, Edman G, et al: Markers of vulnerability to psychopathy: Temperament traits associated with platelet MAO activity, *Acta Psychiatr Scand* 16:172, 1987.

50. Mindus P, Nyman H, Rosenquist A, et al: Aspects of personality in patients with anxiety disorders undergoing capsulotomy, *Acta Neurochir Suppl* 44:138, 1988.

51. Waziri R: Psychosurgery for anxiety and obsessive-compulsive disorders. In Noyes R Jr, Roth M, Burrows GD, editors: *Handbook of anxiety. Treatment of anxiety*, Amsterdam, 1990, Elsevier Science Publishers.

52. Corsellis J, Jack AB: Neuropathological observations on yttrium implants and on undercutting in the orbito-frontal areas of the brain. In Laitinen LV, Livingston KE, editors: *Surgical approaches in psychiatry*, Baltimore, 1973, University Park Press, p 90.

53. Modell JG, Mountz JM, Curtis GC, et al: Neurophysiologic dysfunction in basal ganglia/limbic striatal and thalamocortical circuits as a pathogenetic mechanism of obsessive-compulsive disorder, *J Neuropsychiatry* 1:27–36, 1989.

54. Nauta WJH: Circuitous connections linking cerebral cortex, limbic system, and corpus striatum. In Doane BK, Livingston KE, editors: *The limbic system. Functional organization and clinical disorders*, 1986, p 43.

55. Hassler R, Dieckman G: Relief of obsessive-compulsive disorders, phobias and tics by stereotactic coagulation of the rostral intralaminar and medial-thalamic nuclei. In Laitinen LV, Livingston KE, editors: *Surgical approaches in psychiatry*, Baltimore, 1973, University Park Press, p 206.

56. Rauch SL, Jenike MA: Neurobiological models of obsessive-compulsive disorder, *Psychosomatics* 34:20–32, 1993.

57. Rauch SL, Jenike MA: Neural mechanisms of obsessive-compulsive disorder, *Curr Rev Mood Anx Dis* 1:84–94, 1997.

58. Breiter HCR, Filipek PA, Kennedy KN, et al: Retrocallosal white matter abnormalities in patients with obsessive-compulsive disorder, *Arch Gen Psychiatry* 51:663–664, 1994.

59. Jenike MA, Breiter HCR, Baer L, et al: Cerebral structural abnormalities in patients with obsessive-compulsive disorder: A quantitative morphometric magnetic resonance imaging study, *Arch Gen Psychiatry* 53:625–632, 1996.

60. Alexander GE, DeLong MR, Strick PL: Parallel organization of functionally segregated circuits linking basal ganglia and cortex, *Ann Rev Neurosci* 9:357–381, 1986.

61. Alexander GE, Crutcher MD, DeLong MR: Basal ganglia-thalamocortical circuits: Parallel substrates for motor, oculomotor, "prefrontal" and "limbic" functions,

Prog Brain Res 85:119–146, 1990.
62. Ward CD: Transient feelings of compulsion caused by hemispheric lesions: Three cases, *J Neurol Neurosurg Psychiatry* 51:266–268, 1988.
63. Luxenberg JS, Swedo SE, Flament MF, et al: Neuroanatomical abnormalities in obsessive-compulsive disorder detected with quantitative X-ray computed tomography, *Am J Psychiatry* 145:1089–1093, 1988.
64. LaPlane E, Levasseur M, Pillon B, et al: Obsessions-compulsions and behavioural changes with bilateral basal ganglia lesions: A neuropsychological, magnetic resonance imaging and positron tomography study, *Brain* 112:699–725, 1989.
65. Nordahl TE, Benkelfat C, Semple WE, et al: Cerebral glucose metabolic rates in obsessive-compulsive disorder, *Neuropsychopharmacology* 2:23–28, 1989.
66. Jenike MA, Baer L, Minichiello WE, editors: *Obsessive-compulsive disorders: Theory and management*, ed 2, Chicago, 1990, Year Book Medical Publishers.
67. Weilburg JB, Mesulam MM, Weintraub S, et al: Focal striatal abnormalities in a patient with obsessive-compulsive disorder, *Arch Neurol* 46:233–235, 1989.
68. Kellner CH, Jolley RR, Holgate RC, et al: Brain MRI in obsessive-compulsive disorder, *Psychiatr Res* 36:45–49, 1991.
69. Rauch SL, Jenike MA, Alpert NM, et al: Regional cerebral blood flow measured during symptom provocation in obsessive-compulsive disorder using 15-O labeled CO_2 and positron emission tomography, *Arch Gen Psychiatry* 1:62–70, 1994.
70. Baxter LJ, Schwartz JM, Mazziotta JC, et al: Cerebral glucose metabolic rates in nondepressed patients with obsessive-compulsive disorder, *Am J Psychiatry* 145:1560–1563, 1988.
71. Baxter LR, Phelps ME, Mazziotta JC, et al: Local cerebral glucose metabolic rates in obsessive-compulsive disorder, *Arch Gen Psychiatry* 44:211–218, 1987.
72. Baxter LR, Schwartz JM, Bergman KS, et al: Caudate glucose metabolic rate changes with both drug and behavior therapy for OCD, *Arch Gen Psychiatry* 49:681–689, 1992.

27

Psychotherapy of Obsessive-Compulsive Personality Disorder

Michael A. Jenike, M.D.

The treatment of patients suffering from obsessive-compulsive disorder (OCD) is a superb example of the need to integrate various approaches to maximize patient outcome. It is very unusual for OCD patients to respond fully to either psychotherapeutic or pharmacologic approaches; for optimal response, patients must generally receive medication in combination with particular behavior therapies. This approach can be expected to improve the condition of most patients substantially, and occasionally completely, within a few months. What then is the role of psychotherapy in the treatment of these patients?

Traditional psychodynamic psychotherapy is not an effective treatment for obsessions and/or rituals occurring in patients meeting criteria for OCD as defined in the *Diagnostic and Statistical Manual of Mental Disorders* (DSM-IV); there are no reports in the modern psychiatric literature of patients who stopped ritualizing when treated with this method alone. Traditional psychodynamic psychotherapy, however, may be helpful for patients with obsessive-compulsive *personality* disorder (OCPD). Conversely, there is no evidence that behavioral therapy and medications are helpful for patients with the personality disorder. Many traditional psychotherapists find themselves becoming more directive with OCD patients and thereby approach some of the techniques used by behavior therapists. This chapter explores issues that arise in therapy with patients who meet criteria for DSM-IV OCPD. We will outline specific recommendations to maximize the effectiveness of therapeutic interventions and compliance.

COMPULSIVE AND OBSESSIVE-COMPULSIVE PERSONALITY DISORDERS

How Common Are These Personality Disorders in Patients with Obsessive-Compulsive Disorder?

Unfortunately, criteria for personality diagnoses are constantly changing. To help clarify terminology, we will focus for a moment on diagnostic categories as outlined in DSM-III and its modification, DSM-III-R. We will then give some data on the prevalence of these two *separate* disorders among patients with frank OCD. In DSM-III the personality disorder was called *compulsive personality disorder* and a patient was required to have four of five criteria as outlined in Table 27-1 to meet full criteria. In DSM-III-R, the name was changed to *obsessive*-compulsive personality disorder, further confusing the issue with OCD, new diagnostic criteria were added, and now the patients are required to meet five of nine criteria as defined in Table 27-2. There were few substantial changes in DSM-IV and the name remained unchanged (Table 27-3).

A number of years ago, in an effort to determine how often these personality disorders occurred concomitantly with OCD, we evaluated 96 consecutive DSM-III OCD patients in our clinic with the Structured Interview for the Diagnosis of Personality Disorders (SIDP)[1] and found that 50 (52%) of these patients received one or more axis II personality disorder diagnosis.[2] If mixed personality disorder was excluded, 35 patients (36%) met full criteria for one or more of the personality disorders. The assessment instrument and details of this study are more fully discussed in Chapter 4 and only aspects pertinent to the current discussion are covered here.

We found that compulsive personality disorder was diagnosed in six patients (6%), all with onset of OCD prior to age 20. These results replicate two earlier studies[3,4] in finding that compulsive personality disorder is less frequent among OCD patients than previously believed. The prevalence of compulsive personality disorder of from 4% to 6% in OCD outpatients in these studies indicates that compulsive personality disorder, as defined by DSM-III, is not a necessary condition for the development of OCD, and in fact, is not the most common personality disorder in OCD. When patients with significant compulsive features were combined with this personality disorder diagnosis (i.e., including patients with mixed personality disorder with compulsive features), the sample prevalence increased to only 14%. These conclusions are limited to the DSM-III diagnosis of compulsive personality disorder, rather than the traditional psychodynamic concept of obsessional personality. However, changes in the diagnostic criteria in DSM-III-R moved the diagnostic entity of OCPD somewhat closer to the traditional concept;[5] as a result, prevalence of this personality disorder in OCD may be somewhat higher.[1]

The SIDP generates diagnoses for DSM-III axis II disorders, rather than for the DSM-III-R or current DSM-IV. Significant changes were made in the

Table 27-1 DSM-III Criteria for Compulsive Personality Disorder

At least *four* of the following are characteristic of the individual's current and long-term functioning, are not limited to episodes of illness, and cause either significant impairment in social or occupational functioning or subjective distress.

1. Restricted ability to express warm and tender emotions (e.g., the individual is unduly conventional, serious, formal, and stingy).
2. Perfectionism that interferes with the ability to grasp "the big picture" (e.g., preoccupation with trivial details, rules, order, organization, schedules, and lists).
3. Insistence that others submit to his or her way of doing things, and lack of awareness of the feelings elicited by this behavior (e.g., a husband stubbornly insists his wife complete errands for him regardless of her plans).
4. Excessive devotion to work and productivity to the exclusion of pleasure and the value of interpersonal relationships.
5. Indecisiveness: decision making is either avoided, postponed, or protracted, perhaps because individuals cannot get assignments done on time because of ruminating about priorities.

DSM-III-R diagnostic criteria for many of the personality disorders; the greatest changes were in criteria for compulsive personality disorder (OCPD in DSM-III-R and DSM-IV). As noted previously, rather than the DSM-III requirement of four of five criteria, DSM-III-R requires five of nine criteria to meet the diagnosis. New criteria also have been added for overconscientiousness and scrupulosity, lack of generosity, and hoarding of unimportant objects.

Because such changes in criteria may affect the prevalence of this and other personality disorders in the OCD population, we administered an updated version of the SIDP, which was revised to generate DSM-III-R diagnoses (SIDP-R)[5a] to an additional 59 consecutive patients meeting criteria for OCD and found that 15 (25%) met criteria for OCPD, which is significantly higher than the prevalence of 6 of 96 (6%) in our earlier study ($X^2(1) = 11.5$, p < 0.001).[1]

The higher prevalence of OCPD using DSM-III-R criteria may be attributed to at least two factors. First, DSM-III-R requires only 56% (five of nine) of criteria to make the diagnosis, compared with 80% (four of five) required by DSM-III. It is likely that the difference in prevalence between the two versions of DSM-III might have been the result of raising the number of criteria required for this diagnosis.[1]

An alternative explanation for the increased prevalence with DSM-III-R is that the three new criteria that were added move the personality disorder somewhat closer to the traditional psychodynamic entity of obsessional character, by assessing the traits of orderliness and parsimony.[5] As noted earlier, three new criteria were added that partly overlapped these traits.

In any event, it appeared that changes in DSM-III-R personality disorder criteria affected the prevalence of various personality disorders because of

Table 27-2 DSM-III-R Criteria for Obsessive-Compulsive Personality Disorder

A pervasive pattern of perfectionism and inflexibility, beginning by early adulthood and present in a variety of contexts, as indicated by at least *five* of the following:

1. Perfectionism that interferes with task completion (e.g., inability to complete a project because own overly strict standards are not met).
2. Preoccupation with details, rules, lists, order, organization, or schedules to the extent that the major point of the activity is lost.
3. Unreasonable insistence that others submit to exactly his or her way of doing things, or unreasonable reluctance to allow others to do things because of the conviction that they will not do them correctly.
4. Excessive devotion to work and productivity to the exclusion of leisure activities and friendships.
5. Indecisiveness: decision making is either avoided, postponed, or protracted.
6. Overconscientiousness, scrupulousness, and inflexibility about matters of morality, ethics, or values.
7. Restricted expression of affection.
8. Lack of generosity in giving time, money, or gifts when no personal gain is likely to result.
9. Inability to discard worn-out or worthless objects even when they have no sentimental value.

changes in specific criteria and in the number of criteria required to make each diagnosis. The relationship between treatment outcome with pharmacotherapy and behavior therapy and presence of DSM-III-R personality disorders requires further assessment. There have been no adequate studies evaluating OCPD in OCD patients using the current DSM-IV criteria.

Characteristics of Patients with Obsessive-Compulsive Personality Disorder

Patients with this personality disorder may present with a grim and cheerless demeanor to convey an air of austerity and serious-mindedness.[6,7] In such patients, posture and movement reflect their underlying tightness—a tense control of emotions that are kept well in check. They may be viewed by others as industrious and efficient, although lacking in flexibility and spontaneity. Many consider these people to be stubborn, to procrastinate, to appear indecisive, and to be easily upset by the unfamiliar or by deviations from routines to which they have become accustomed.

Content with their "nose to the grindstone," many of these patients work diligently and patiently with activities that require being tidy and meticulous. They are especially concerned with matters of organization and efficiency and tend to be rigid and inflexible regarding rules and procedures. These behaviors often lead others to see them as perfectionistic. They are polite and formal and

Table 27-3   DSM-IV Criteria for Obsessive-Compulsive Personality Disorder

A pervasive pattern of preoccupation with orderliness, perfectionism, and mental and interpersonal control, at the expense of flexibility, openness, and efficiency, beginning by early adulthood and present in a variety of contexts, as indicated by *four* (or more) of the following:

1. Preoccupation with details, rules, lists, order, organization, or schedules to the extent that the major point of the activity is lost.
2. Perfectionism that interferes with task completion (e.g., is unable to complete a project because his or her overly strict standards are not met).
3. Excessive devotion to work and productivity to the exclusion of leisure activities and friendships (not accounted for by obvious economic necessity).
4. Overconscientiousness, scrupulosity, and inflexibility about matters of morality, ethics, or values (not accounted for by cultural or religious identification).
5. Inability to discard worn-out or worthless objects even when they have no sentimental value.
6. Reluctance to delegate tasks or to work with others unless they submit to exactly his or her way of doing things.
7. Adoption of a miserly spending style toward both self and others; money is viewed as something to be hoarded for future catastrophes.
8. Rigidity and stubbornness.

may relate to others in terms of rank or status; they tend to be authoritarian. These patients can be very difficult to manage and certain psychodynamic tactics can be effective in facilitating treatment. Although there are no systematic studies addressing outcome of psychodynamic techniques in improving the quality of life of these patients, abundant anecdotal evidence suggests that certain approaches may help. In patients with both OCD and OCPD, these techniques may enhance compliance with medication trials and behavior therapy. For example, these patients may fear the risk of taking a drug or of exposing themselves to some feared object and may thus avoid treatment that would likely improve their OCD. Systematically encouraging risk taking (Table 27-4) may be an effective adjunct to standard treatments for OCD in such patients. Further exploration of psychodynamic principles and specific treatment recommendations follow.

PSYCHODYNAMIC PRINCIPLES

Psychodynamic therapy is the process in which an individual's behavior is examined to determine those characterologic styles that impair interpersonal relationships, produce symptoms, and interfere with productive and rewarding activity. Behaviors that are not productive or satisfying are labelled neurotic or maladaptive, and the therapist tries to understand the roots of these behaviors and to introduce new ways of adapting. Salzman[8-10] has outlined three premises of

Table 27-4 Characteristics of Obsessional Patients and Therapeutic Strategies

Characteristic Belief or Tendency	Result	Management
Danger is imminent	Exaggerates risks	Encourage risk taking; help assess risks realistically
Gives excessive details	Confuses issues; never gets to the point	Keep treatment plan firmly in mind
Needs to be in control	Resists change	Explore benefits of not controlling; therapist can model less controlling behaviors; therapist and patient partners in therapy
Confuses past with details and qualifications	Unproductive therapy	Focus on "here and now"
Avoids expressions of feelings	Tends to be cognitive and cold	Encourage feelings, whether positive or negative
Persistent doubt	Reluctance to change	Encourage risk taking
Feels superior to therapist	Devaluing and controlling	Therapist and patient partners in therapy
Equates thoughts and impulses with action	Enhances fears	Clarify distinction at every opportunity
Loses sight of normal behavior	Excessive washing and checking	Model and explain "normal" behavior
Excessive insecurity	Fears any action	Reassure repetitively that anxiety is natural
Aggressive or hostile impulses	Fears hurting others	Focus on what is present, rather than underlying impulses
Needs unlimited information before decisions	Procrastinates	Encourage risk taking

psychodynamic psychotherapy that must be mutually accepted by both patient and therapist in any productive relationship. First, behavior is derived from processes that can be defined and traced to motivational or adaptational sources. Some of these sources, however, are outside of one's immediate awareness. Second, distorted maladaptive behavior is caused by anxiety, which transforms goal-directed conduct into activity designed to relieve or eliminate anxiety. These are called *defenses*. Thus, energy that could be channeled into productive and satisfying activities is spent alleviating anxiety.

Freud and later theorists have focused on the defenses of isolation, displacement, reaction formation, and undoing in the obsessional patient.[11] Third, when these defenses are clarified, the resulting insight can be directed toward altering or abandoning the behavior with notable changes in the characterologic structure, productivity, and satisfaction of the individual. All such therapies require verbal interaction and some intellectual capacity, and focus on emotional elements of behavior as well as the relationship between therapist and patient. All involve issues of transference, countertransference, interpretation, and exhortation toward change.[10]

In treating obsessional patients, there can be a role for psychodynamic psychotherapy as an adjunct to behavioral and pharmacologic techniques and, in fact, most behavior therapists are aware of the concepts of unconscious conflicts and drives and are able to use this knowledge to their advantage in helping patients. Therapists must pay attention to the patients' individual personality styles and environments. When obsessional patients are in a therapeutic relationship, issues of aggression, sexuality, and control invariably arise. In addition, such patients have a pervasive and persistent tendency to resist change and to desperately try to be in control of all situations. They tend to be in doubt and ambivalent about almost everything. They may be perfectionistic and feel that any unacceptable thought can produce disaster. When attempting to deal with the obsessional patient's resistance to change, the therapist must be aware that such defenses against change are extremely strong and that they mitigate against exposure to the patient's deficits. Salzman[10] has noted that obsessionals often steadfastly reject any new awareness that would require admissions that there are matters about which they are unaware. Thus they frequently reject an observation as invalid, only to present it later as their own discovery. The therapist may have to tolerate this tactic early in treatment and not confront it aggressively until a strong therapeutic relationship has developed; such a relationship may take considerable time because these patients often have a fear of trust and commitment.

As noted earlier, an issue that arises over and over in the therapy of these patients is the need for control. In fact, symptoms such as doubting and striving for perfection can be viewed as neurotic attempts to control one's internal and external worlds. Patients have the illusion that such mechanisms can make the world safe and secure. For example, the young man who must persistently think of his mother's vagina to keep her safe has the illusion that no harm can come to her as long as he persists in this disturbing thought. Somehow, by his own discomfort, he is able to sacrifice himself and keep a loved one safe and is thus in control. He is therefore opposed to taking any risks; that is, he refuses to try to give up his thoughts for fear of a catastrophic occurrence. Encouraging obsessional patients to take risks is an integral part of any therapy. Salzman[10] noted that obsessional patients spend endless time in distracting avoidances and contentious disagreements, although they are intellectually astute and cognitively capable of clearer analysis. This is likely a mechanism to control the therapist. Another tactic is affective isolation with little acknowledgment of the importance of the therapist in his or her life; this may continue well into the therapy. Patients may be critical of the therapist's inability to alter symptoms, but will resist steadfastly any attempts to do so. Forming a therapeutic relationship may form the bulk of the work in treating the obsessional patient.

Any expression of feeling by the patient should be encouraged, whether positive or negative. The obsessional patient may become even more rigid, controlling, petty, or derogatory instead of the appropriate response of anger toward the therapist who is unavoidably late for an appointment or who raises his fee. Sharing feelings of dislike, distrust, or affection for the therapist is difficult for these patients because of their fear of loss of control. They need to appear rational and calm. Affectionate reactions are tightly controlled and are believed to be undesirable and frightening and in need of tight management. Such control over tender feelings constitutes the essence of the obsessional defense and not infrequently yields hostile reactions from family members and colleagues. Obsessional patients are frequently unable to commit themselves and will explore every aspect of each issue to assure that they are correct and in control. Pervasive doubt is most pronounced in the obsessional patient (who also has OCD) with checking behaviors. For example, they may check the faucet 50 times before going to bed, or open and close the car door a dozen times to be sure it is locked. To be completely safe and certain about everything, patients maintain the illusion that they must never make an error nor admit to any deficiency; thus, they will not risk making definite decisions or committing themselves to a point of view or course of action in case it turns out to be the wrong one.[9] When patients with OCD who are checkers are coerced into not checking, they are surprised that nothing happens. Many obsessionals equate words, impulses, or thoughts with action and feel that somehow particular thoughts may control the behavior of others (Table 27-4). Salzman[10] has labelled this "omnipotence of thought": words can magically undo unacceptable behavior or produce untold malevolence for which obsessional patients assume guilt. To be absolutely precise, clear, and fair to all parties, obsessional patients typically introduce more and more qualifications and explanations to be sure that the issue at hand has been explained to its fullest. Rather than clarifying, this tends to confuse issues even more. Because of this tendency to never get to the point, such patients can be boring to the therapist who is interested in feelings, insight, and change.

COGNITIVE THERAPY

There has been some work on the use of cognitive approaches in patients with obsessive-compulsive symptomatology.[12] Beck[13] described various emotional disorders in terms of their characteristic thought content, primary rules, and other cognitive features. Cognitive therapy is generally directed at correcting faulty premises and beliefs, or altering thinking habits via self-monitoring techniques, discussion, or rehearsal of new thinking habits. Recent work has focused on cognitive approaches to affective illness, but some researchers have applied similar techniques in combination with behavioral therapy to OCD patients.[14,15] Despite lack of success of preliminary studies, some of the principles that derive from this work can be of help to the therapist. One of the basic rules of the obsessive patient is that "danger is imminent," and they therefore tend to exaggerate risks. This behavior suggests that it may be important to reeducate obsessive patients to reappraise situations more realistically.[12] Obsessives also require more information before they risk making a decision; encouragement of risk-taking is a major part of any therapy—behavioral, cognitive, or psychodynamic—and may be helpful to obsessive patients.

More recent and encouraging work involving cognitive therapy is reviewed in Chapter 18.

RORSCHACH FINDINGS AND IMPLICATIONS FOR TREATMENT

As discussed in Chapter 4, there is one study of the use of projective tests in patients with OCD. This will be briefly reviewed here in view of psychotherapy issues that are raised by the data. In a study designed to examine the primary issues and defenses of patients with OCD, Coursey[11] administered the Rorschach inkblot test to 15 patients. He found that although it is rare to have any explicit hostility on the Rorschach, OCD patients had explicitly aggressive responses on 60 of the protocols. If he included mild or symbolically hostile responses, 80 of the patients gave such responses. He noted that these typical responses contrasted markedly with the socially timid, inhibited, and fearful demeanor and behavior of these patients. Except among children, oral-dependent responses such as mouth, food, touching, and oral-aggressive responses are not common; yet among the OCD patients, two thirds gave mouth and food responses and more than one third gave touching and holding responses. In addition, one third of the patients gave unusual genital and anal content for more than 10 responses. Although the OCD patients had been carefully screened to rule out schizophrenia, approximately 20 had some formal thinking impairment of various types. Coursey believed this finding was an indicator that impulsive primitive material is not always repressed and that it is readily and consciously available to at least some of the patients, sometimes forming the basis of the obsessive thoughts. Moreover, this material was not the result of prior psychotherapy experiences, because few patients had had previous therapy, and fewer still had undergone psychoanalytically oriented therapy.

To control and neutralize the primitive material that had erupted into consciousness, these OCD patients displayed a variety of responses. Some expressed the everyday reactions of embarrassment, guilt, and apologies, whereas approximately half used classical defenses such as undoing and denial. These defense mechanisms were usually seen across responses, balancing the impulse with its opposite. For instance, one patient first saw "piercing mean eyes peering at me through the dark"; the next saw "some type of face smiling, a cartoon figure." Interestingly, 20 of the subjects demonstrated denial that failed—first denying any response, then revealing a sexual or hostile one. The most widespread way that these patients controlled their affect was through language, mostly through the choice of emotionally flat, neutral words. Approximately two thirds used this form of cold factual language, rather than emotionally hot words. Coursey[11] concluded that obsessive-compulsive patients are marked by the extent of primitive material invading their consciousness and the neutralizing strategies these patients have developed to manage these impulses. Unlike other neurotic patients in whom the primitive drives never fully reach consciousness except in symbolic or symptomatic forms, and unlike the psychotic for whom primary process is conscious and defenses have completely failed, most of the OCD patients represented a third possibility: primitive impulse material is conscious and the defenses, other than repression and denial, have not failed. Rather, the defenses that work are those that neutralize and contain the primary process material. Thus, the central characteristic of most of these patients is this highly charged impasse, a deadlock between the failure of repression and denial, and the success of the aforementioned neutralizing strategies and other containing defenses such as preoccupation with detail.

Coursey believed his Rorschach data confirmed the observations of Freud and others, in which hostile and sadistic impulses are a central component of this disorder. They also are in accord with a descriptive study by Rachman and DeSilva[16] of the obsessions of patients and normals, which found that 70% of the obsessions in their patients focused on violence and physical aggression, 17% on deviant sexual impulses, another 9% on being "out of control," and 4% on neutral phrases. The descriptive Rorschach material presented by Coursey also suggested that repression and denial are not very effective in preventing primary process material from becoming conscious. So in contradiction to some Freudian theorists, there is no evidence in his material that there are "even more horrible" unconscious underlying impulses. Coursey believes this is strong evidence that the psychotherapeutic process may better focus on what is present than on what might be underlying. This would entail working with the secondary features of the disorder—the anxiety, rituals, and obsessions. In addition, it would be important to help patients manage and accept the heightened impulses they experience.

THERAPEUTIC TECHNIQUES

Some of the difficulties therapists encounter with obsessional patients are outlined in Table 27-4. In traditional psychodynamic psychotherapy, inactivity on the part of the therapist is encouraged, and it is not uncommon for the therapist to listen to the patient for long periods of time without intervening. With the obsessional patient, this method will usually be unproductive. The therapist must, as a general rule, be more active from the beginning of the therapy. It is important, however, not to overwhelm the patient and give him or her the feeling that the therapist is running the therapy. Salzman[10] notes that the patient's detailed communication designed to prevent omission or error must be interrupted to enable the therapist to understand the overall theme and not get caught up in the confusing minutia. Failure to do so caused long and fruitless analyses in the early history of the psychoanalytic treatment of obsessional patients.

For most therapists, interruption will be necessary to remain alert and awake during the therapy sessions. One of the most frequent countertransference reactions in a patient is drowsiness or inability to keep his or her mind on the therapy; this behavior should be an autognostic sign that the patient is not on a productive track. Salzman[10] recommends that the therapist keep a treatment plan firmly in mind. This will allow a framework for deciding which of the patient's random associations or innumerable details are of importance to the task at hand. As an example, the topic under discussion may be the patient's feelings that he or she contributed to the father's death while visiting him in the hospital and the ambivalent relationship with his or her father while he was alive. But the patient may start to discuss the location of the hospital, the food that was served, the level of nursing care, the types of fluids that were being administered, the level that the father's head was tilted, and so on. The therapist can easily forget that the goal at this time is to help the patient to grasp strong opposite feelings of love and anger toward the deceased father.

Salzman[10] has outlined some of the specific goals that are often helpful in the treatment of these patients. First, it is necessary to discover the basis for excessive feelings of insecurity that require absolutes and guarantees before any action is attempted. This requires the examination of each symptom and obsessional tactic to show how these tie into the patient's overriding need to control. Personality traits and rituals in OCD patients are explored in terms of their role in providing the illusory feeling of absolute control. Second, the therapist must demonstrate, by repeated interpretation and encouragement to act, that such guarantees are not necessary but instead interfere with living. This involves motivating the patient to attempt novel and unfamiliar patterns of behavior through active assistance in stimulating new adventures. This can help patients attempt counterphobic activity and overcome conditioned avoidance reactions to unexplored areas of functioning. Third, it is necessary to help the patient accept that anxiety is a natural part of living and a companion to all human endeavors. This means abandoning attempts at perfection and accepting limited goals, using the most creative resources available. Patients must learn to accept their human limitations.

One of the most frequent pitfalls for the therapist is discussing the past with the obsessional patient for long periods of time. Recollections of the patient's past are undoubtedly clouded by doubts that lead to ambivalence. Interpretations of past events are subject to endless bickering, qualifying, and uncertainty.[10] The safest tactic with the obsessional patient is to focus on the present situation and discuss current functioning, relationships, and issues; this is most likely to yield the greatest clarity and conviction, and also is least open to persistent doubt and distortion. Salzman notes that this focus on current issues also maximizes productive exploration of emotions. Although past feelings can be described and experienced calmly, judiciously, and intellectually, present hostilities and frustrations, especially as they involve ongoing relationships, are much more difficult to camouflage because they represent failures or deficiencies and expose many of the patient's feelings. It is important that the obsessional patient learn to recognize and express hostile and affectionate feelings. A tolerant and patient therapist can be of major assistance in this seemingly impossible task. If the patient is keeping appointments, the therapist should assume that the patient is finding therapy helpful, although this is rarely acknowledged, especially early in the relationship. On the one hand, most of these patients suffer from a pervasive lack of self-esteem despite the fact that many are very successful. On the other hand, they often appear condescending and exude contempt for the abilities and sensibilities of others, including the therapist. Salzman[10] notes that secretly these patients feel superior and contemptuous of the therapist and feel they are "on to" all that is going on in the therapy. The obsessional patient will, however, appear to be pursuing the suggested course and will take delight in fooling the therapist and thereby feel in control of the therapy. Therapists must be alert for such tactics and gently confront them when the opportunity presents itself. Obsessional patients resist interpretations that suggest they are not aware of something.

Before patients change in therapy, it is necessary for a firm therapeutic relationship to develop and the patient must experience a desire to change. For example, a woman with severe handwashing compulsions who had been refractory to all therapeutic interventions was referred to a neurosurgeon for evaluation for cingulotomy; she became so frightened at this prospect that she actively engaged in previously ineffective psychodynamic and behavior therapy and improved greatly over the next 3 months. The threat of surgery had brought the seriousness of her situation to the forefront. Any technique that strengthens the patients' awareness of maladaptive patterns will assist them in making changes. Salzman[10] believes that before any moves can be made to change behavior, individuals must have a strong conviction about the need to change and a trust in the understanding derived from collaboration with the therapist. Patients must be encouraged to see how they will benefit, instead of visualizing the disasters that will confront them when they feel helpless and not in total control of everything.

Not all patients will present in the same way, and the effectiveness of the therapist will lie in his or her ability to detect recurring issues and to allow the patient to see them in a new way. It is sometimes helpful for the therapist to define what behaviors are considered normal and to model normal behavior for the patient. Obsessional patients keenly observe the therapist and, if they consider the therapist to be a successful person, will try to copy certain actions. The therapist must be somewhat spontaneous in expressing personal feelings and weaknesses and thus allow the patient to recognize that human fallibility is not a cause for total rejection by others. Whenever possible, it is safest to assume the position that the therapist and the patient together are going to examine pertinent issues rather than the therapist assuming the role of expert who is going to assist a helpless patient. Compulsive symptoms and styles are repeated without deviation, despite the awareness that they are nonproductive and potentially destructive. Thus, much of the therapy must involve a repetitive review of issues that recur over and over. When patients begin to change, anxiety may become very severe, and occasionally low doses of benzodiazepines may facilitate therapy. When anxiety becomes overwhelming, performance is adversely affected; moderate anxiety, however, facilitates performance. The therapist must induce anxiety to produce change but must be mindful of the pain of severe anxiety experienced by the patient. The therapist must maintain anxiety at a level that will facilitate learning rather than impede it. The focus must be on feelings rather than cognitive exchanges and must concentrate on the here and now. Salzman[10] summarizes the essence of the therapeutic process with these patients as follows: "before patients will relinquish their extensive defense system, they must allow themselves to experience and accept failure, some loss of false pride and prestige, and possible humiliation."

SUMMARY

There is no contraindication to simultaneous psychodynamic, cognitive, pharmacologic, and behavioral approaches in the same patient. Cognitive and psychodynamic approaches facilitate active behavior therapy but cannot replace it. The techniques outlined in this chapter optimize the patient's chances for compliance with behavior therapy and medication treatments, which, according to overwhelming scientific data, are most likely to improve symptoms and allow patients to maximize their chances for a normal and satisfying life.

REFERENCES

1. Stangl D, Pfohl B, Zimmerman M, et al: A structured interview for the DSM-III personality disorders, *Arch Gen Psychiatry* 42:591–596, 1985.
2. Baer L, Jenike MA, Ricciardi J, et al: Standardized assessment of personality disorders in obsessive-compulsive disorder, *Arch Gen Psychiatry* 47:826–832, 1990.
3. Joffee RT, Swinson RP, Regan JJ: Personality features of obsessive-compulsive disorder, *Am J Psychiatry* 145:1127–1129, 1988.

4. Steketee G: Personality traits and diagnoses in obsessive-compulsive disorder. Paper presented at the annual meeting of The Association For the Advancement of Behavior Therapy, November 1988.
5. Goldstein WN: Obsessive-compulsive behavior, DSM-III and a psychodynamic classification of psychopathology, *Am J Psychother* 39:346–359, 1985.
5a. Pfohl B: Personal communication, 1989.
6. Millon T: *Disorders of personality–DSM III: Axis II*, New York, 1981, John Wiley & Sons.
7. Shapiro D: *Neurotic styles*, New York, 1965, Basic Books.
8. Salzman L: *The obsessive personality*, New York, 1968, Science House.
9. Salzman L: Psychotherapy of the obsessional, *Psychiatr Ann* 10:491–494, 1980.
10. Salzman L: Psychoanalytic therapy of the obsessional patient, *Curr Psychiatr Ther* 9:53–59, 1983.
11. Coursey RD: The dynamics of obsessive-compulsive disorder. In Insel TR, editor: *New findings in obsessive-compulsive disorder*, Washington, 1984, American Psychiatric Press, pp 104–121.
12. Hamilton JA, Alagna SW: Obsessive-compulsive disorder: Cognitive approaches in context. In Insel TR, editor: *New findings in obsessive-compulsive disorder*, Washington, 1984, American Psychiatric Press, pp 90–102.
13. Beck AJ: *Cognitive therapy and the emotional disorders*, New York, 1976, International University Press.
14. Emmelkamp PMG, van de Helm H, van Zanten B, et al: Contributions of self-instructional training to the effectiveness of exposure in vivo: A comparison with obsessive-compulsive patients, *Behav Res Ther* 18:61–66, 1980.
15. Foa EB, Kozak MJ: Treatment of anxiety disorders: implications for psychopathology. Paper presented at the National Institute of Mental Health Conference on Anxiety and Anxiety Disorders, Tuxedo, September 1983.
16. Rachman S, DeSilva P: Abnormal and normal obsessions, *Behav Res Ther* 16: 233–248, 1978.

28

Discontinuation and Long-Term Treatment of Obsessive-Compulsive Disorder

Michele T. Pato, M.D., Sudeep Chakravorty, M.D.

Much of the work on the pharmacologic treatment of obsessive-compulsive disorder (OCD) has focused on treatment efficacy. Clomipramine (CMI), one of the first agents to prove effective in this once treatment-resistant illness, has been extensively studied and has shown efficacy over placebo and other antidepressants in the treatment of OCD.[1-5] Other serotonin reuptake inhibitors (SRIs) such as fluoxetine,[6-10] fluvoxamine,[11-15] sertraline, and paroxetine also have been shown to be effective, both in acute and maintenance treatment of OCD[16,17] and have all received FDA approval for this indication.

At present, however, there are few guidelines on how long to continue, and when to discontinue, pharmacologic treatment of OCD. One might guess that because these serotonergic agents are antidepressants, and OCD often coexists with depression, similar guidelines as those used in the treatment of depression[18] might apply. However, this does not seem to be the case. Whether this difference is a function of the medications that have been studied or the illness itself remains to be seen.

DISCONTINUING PHARMACOLOGIC TREATMENT

To date there are few systematic trials in discontinuing antiobsessional agents. At the time of this writing, only one small blinded trial of CMI discontinuation in adults has been published (outlined below).[19] Thus most of the data reviewed below come from open clinical trials and anecdotal reports. However, two large blinded trials (one with fluoxetine and the other with sertraline) are presently in progress.

Discontinuation of Clomipramine

There are scattered anecdotal reports in the literature about what happens when CMI is discontinued in OCD patients.[3,20-26] Most of these reports were clinical observations, usually from a study on the efficacy of CMI. In the earliest report,[22] Capstick noted that in a mixed population of patients with obsessional symptoms, "if the drug is withdrawn or reduced too quickly, the patient is able to relate the time of onset of the recurrence of the obsessions, usually 36 to 48 hours after the former dose."

Yaryura-Tobias, et al[26] discontinued CMI blindly for 2 weeks after either 4 or 6 weeks of CMI treatment in a group of 13 patients. They noted that "obsessions and the ability to resist" were significantly worse after only 1 week without CMI. Thoren, et al[25] examined 15 of 16 patients taking CMI at 1 to 4 years and reported that all patients were doing well except for six, who had stopped the CMI and experienced serious relapse "within a few weeks." Eleven of 12 responders were followed up at 5 to 7 years by Asberg, et al.[21] Nine patients remained well with CMI, and two patients were symptom-free without CMI for more than 1 year; however, the authors noted that both these patients had made previous attempts to withdraw from CMI but had experienced a recurrence of symptoms. In a review of the literature on the usefulness of CMI in the treatment of OCD, Ananth[20] commented, "In up to 70% of the patients, withdrawal of the drug produces a recurrence."

More controlled discontinuation trials of CMI have included three in children[3,23,24] and one in adults,[19] both performed at the National Institute of Mental Health (NIMH). In a double-blind placebo versus CMI crossover study in children with OCD[23] the authors noted a "rapid relapse" when patients shifted from the CMI phase to the placebo phase of the study. The 1989 report of children with OCD,[3] used a double-blind crossover between CMI and desipramine and noted that 64% of patients experienced some degree of relapse of obsessive-compulsive symptoms when they switched from CMI to desipramine. The authors further noted that patients received desipramine for only 5 weeks, and they anticipated that with longer drug-free periods even greater relapse would be noted. Finally, in a double-blind crossover trial, Leonard[24] reported that 89% of successfully treated patients on CMI relapsed when switched to desipramine and improved once again when restarted on CMI.

Although anecdotal reports of CMI discontinuation in adult OCD patients indicated recurrence of symptoms, there had been no systematic discontinuation study until our 1988 NIMH study.[19] Although we expected that some patients would have worsening of symptoms, we were surprised to find that almost all patients—94% (17 of 18)—had symptom recurrence.

Our 1988 NIMH study[19] included 21 patients meeting *The Diagnostic and Statistic Manual of Mental Disorder* (DSM-III-R) criteria for OCD (see Table 28-1). Their mean age was 40 ± 10.6 years. Mean age at onset was characteristic of OCD (22.6 ± 13.5 years) as was the fact that approximately half (57%)

Table 28-1 Characteristics of Patients Who Participated in Discontinuation Study*

Gender	Age (yr)	Marital Status	Work Status	Months on CMI	Dose (mg)	CMI Conc (ng/ml)	DCMI Conc (ng/ml)	Washer	Checker	Obsession	Age at Onset (yr)	Duration (yr)	Family History of OCD	History of Depression	Prior Medication	Prior Treatment
M	45	Single	Employed	7	300	84	295	+	+	+	20	25	+	+	Anxiolytic	Psychotherapy
F	40	Single	Employed	4	250	181	289	+	+	+	22	18	0	+	TCA	Psychotherapy
F	26	Single	Employed	14	300	194	636	+	+	+	20	6	+	0	None	Behavior therapy
F	33	Married	Volunteer	12	300	205	578	0	+	+	30	3	0	+	TCA	Psychotherapy
M	42	Married	Employed	7	250	86	323	0	+	+	20	22	0	0	TCA	Psychotherapy
F	39	Married	Employed	10	200	55	207	0	0	+	15	24	0	+	TCA, MAOI	Psychotherapy
M	37	Single	Employed	7	300	847	444	+	+	+	11	26	0	0	TCA, ECT	Psychotherapy
F	35	Single	Unemployed	11	200	114	226	+	+	+	32	3	0	0	TCA	Psychotherapy
F	44	Divorced	Employed	6	200	249	255	+	+	+	30	14	0	+	TCA	Psychotherapy
M	39	Divorced	Employed	7	250	149	218	0	+	+	13	26	0	0	TCA, ECT	Psychotherapy
F	61	Widowed	Volunteer	5	100	66	124	+	+	+	26	35	0	+	TCA	Psychotherapy
M	23	Single	Employed	10	300	208	288	0	+	+	10	13	0	+	Anxiolytic	Psychotherapy
M	30	Single	Employed	14	250	238	655	0	+	+	10	20	0	0	TCA, MAOI, Me	Psychotherapy
M	35	Married	Employed	13	300	151	584	0	+	+	17	18	0	0	None	Psychotherapy
F	32	Married	Unemployed	12	300	577	452	+	+	+	29	3	0	+	TCA	Psychotherapy
F	33	Single	Employed	15	300	148	580	+	+	+	13	20	+	0	TCA, MAOI, Li	Behavior therapy Psychotherapy
F	66	Married	Volunteer	15	150	151	459	0	+	+	63	3	+	+	Anxiolytic	Psychotherapy
F	54	Married	Unemployed	6	100	143	0	+	0	+	50	4	0	+	TCA	None
M	35	Married	Employed	27	100	39	51	0	0	−	22	13	+	+	TCA, MAOI, Li	Psychotherapy
M	46	Divorced	Employed	18	300	100	265	+	+	+	13	33	0	+	None	Psychotherapy
F	46	Married	Unemployed	5	200	89	434	+	+	+	10	36	+	+	TCA, ECT	Psychotherapy
Mean				10.7	235.7	194.0	350.6				22.7	17.4				
SD				5.46	72.7	186.9	189.3				13.5	10.9				

* Data from Pato MT, Zohar-Kadouch R, Zohar J, et al: *Am J Psychiatry* 1988; 145:1521–1525.
CMI, clomipramine; DCMI, desmethylclomipramine; ECT, electroconvulsive therapy; Li, lithium; Me, Mellaril (thioridazine HCl); MAOI, monoamine oxidase inhibitor; TCA, tricyclic antidepressant.

of the patients had had onset before 20 years of age, with all but 3 of the 21 patients having had symptoms before 30 years of age. Duration of OCD symptoms ranged from 3 to 36 years (mean 17.4 ± 10.9 years). Most patients (62%) had a history of depression. Ninety percent of the patients had both obsessions and compulsions and 10% of patients (2) had obsessions only.

Duration of CMI treatment ranged from 5 to 27 months (mean 10.7 ± 5.5 months) (Table 28-1). Patients were divided into three treatment groups: (1) short duration (4 to 8 months, n = 8); (2) middle duration (9 to 12 months, n = 5); and (3) long duration (longer than 12 months, n = 8). Dosage ranged from 100 to 300 mg/day (mean dosage 236 ± 73 mg/day). (These patients were treated prior to the 1990 FDA approval of CMI, which restricted maximum dose to 250 mg because of increased risk of seizure at doses of 300 mg and higher.) Serum CMI and desmethylclomipramine were 194.0 ± 186.9 ng/mL and 350.6 ± 189.3 ng/mL, respectively, prior to discontinuation.

Procedurally, subjects received 2 weeks of CMI in a blinded fashion before they were withdrawn from their entering dosage of CMI over 4 days. Patients then received placebo capsules for a total of 7 weeks; ratings were performed at 1, 4, and 7 weeks of placebo. OCD rating scales included the Yale-Brown Obsessive-Compulsive Scale (Y-BOCS; range 0 to 40), the NIMH Obsessive-Compulsive Scale (range 0 to 56), the NIMH Global Obsessive-Compulsive Scale (range 0 to 15), and the Comprehensive Psychopathological Rating Scale (CPRS) Obsessive-Compulsive Subscale 5 and 8 items, respectively (range 0 to 15 and 0 to 24, respectively). In addition, because anxiety and depressive symptoms often coexist with OCD symptoms, depression and anxiety were assessed using the Hamilton Depression Scale (24 items, range 0 to 78) and the NIMH Global Depression (range 1 to 15) and Anxiety (range 1 to 15) Scales, respectively.

Eighteen of the 21 patients (85.7%) completed the study. Of the three patients who dropped out, two did so because of onset of debilitating depression during the blinded CMI phase of the study, and one patient was withdrawn because of noncompliance with protocol. OCD symptoms returned in 16 of the 18 (88.9%) who completed the study, with significant deterioration on all but the CPRS scales noted by 4 weeks on placebo (Figure 28-1). One patient remained symptom-free at 6 months, and another had recurrence of depression at the end of 7 weeks of placebo, which required treatment with amitriptyline. (This patient also experienced OCD symptom return at week 19 after the discontinuation of CMI and required the therapy to be reinstituted; amitriptyline effectively treated the patient's depression, but OCD symptoms still reemerged at 19 weeks following CMI discontinuation. CMI kept both the depression and OCD symptoms in remission.)

Analysis of variance found no significant effect of CMI treatment duration prior to discontinuation, on subsequent relapse. (Thus, although the patients were divided into groups with short, middle, and long treatment duration, this

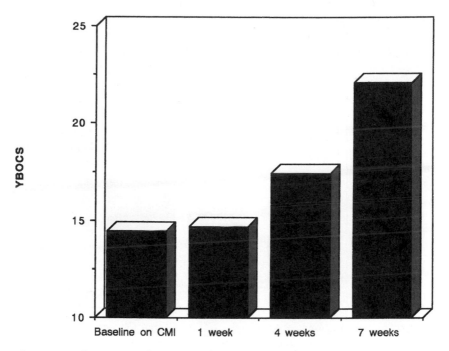

Fig. 28-1 Change in Yale-Brown Obsessive-Compulsive Scale (Y-BOCS) after discontinuation of clomipramine (CMI).

organization seemed to make no difference in recurrence rates.) In addition, no specific pattern of recurrence, other than the almost universal recurrence of symptoms within 4 to 7 weeks, could be discerned. Global ratings for depression, OCD, and anxiety increased two points or more (3.0 to 5.9, 4.9 to 6.9, and 3.7 to 6.1, respectively), and scores on the Y-BOCS and NIMH OCD scale increased by approximately seven points (14.5 to 22.1 and 15.6 to 22.3, respectively).

Eleven of the 18 patients (61.1%) also had significant worsening of depressive symptoms by the end of the study. Only 1 of these 11 (9.1%) experienced no worsening of OCD symptoms during the 7 weeks of placebo. This worsening was noted on both the Hamilton Depression Rating Scale and the NIMH Global Depression Scale, and reached statistical significance at 4 weeks (Figure 28-2). Depressive and OCD symptoms worsened over the same time course.

Following the blinded discontinuation phase of our study,[19] all 16 patients with symptom recurrence chose to have CMI readministered. Open assessment at 8 weeks using the NIMH Global OCD Scale showed that patients had generally returned to their prestudy level of improvement.

This study and earlier anecdotal reports suggest that CMI's antiobsessional effects last only as long as the drug is being administered. It should be noted,

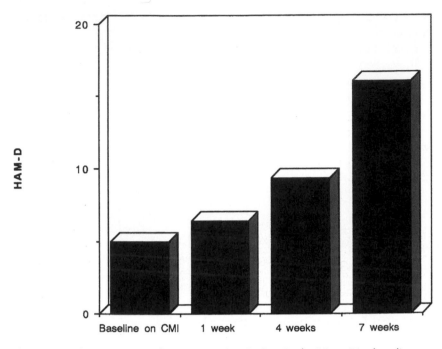

Fig. 28-2 Change in Hamilton Depression Rating Scale (Ham-D) after discontinuation of clomipramine (CMI).

however, that CMI was withdrawn abruptly (over 4 days), and this may have had some effect on the rapid recurrence of symptoms. (Perhaps more gradual withdrawal would lead to less recurrence, although the report below of a maintenance dose study in some of these patients would seem to refute this.[27]) The mean duration of treatment in the 21 patients was 10.7 months, with eight patients having less than 8 months of treatment. It is possible that longer treatment may lead to less recurrence. However, this 10.7-month mean is already higher than the 4 to 5 months recommended before discontinuation of drug therapy in the treatment of depression.[18] Given the high rate of symptom recurrence with withdrawal of medication, one would be prone to recommending continued treatment for all patients. However, occasionally patients remain symptom free without CMI.[19,21,28] In addition, recent data support a role for behavioral therapy for improving the maintenance of long-term symptom remission after acute treatment is discontinued (see following paragraph[29,30]).

Discontinuation Studies with Selective Serotonin Reuptake Inhibitors
Fluoxetine
There are few reports of fluoxetine discontinuation in the literature. Although initially approved for treatment of depression in 1988, fluoxetine has only recently (1994) gained FDA approval for the treatment of OCD. This may

in part contribute to the paucity of data available. An international multicenter trial of fluoxetine discontinuation recently has been completed, but findings are not yet available; so, to date, only the anecdotal reports below can be cited from the literature.

In 1989, Fontaine[7] reported on a trial of 43 patients only 35 of whom agreed to discontinue fluoxetine after 1 year of successful treatment. These 35 patients had been treated for 12 to 20 months with fluoxetine and were abruptly discontinued. At follow-up after 1 year off fluoxetine, only eight (23%) had experienced symptom recurrence. However, symptom recurrence was measured only with a global obsessive-compulsive measure. Further, five patients had a relapse of depression requiring the reinstitution of antidepressants. It is unclear from this report whether an antiobsessional antidepressant was used, so one cannot assess whether these five patients may not have had a relapse in their OCD symptoms as well given more time (as noted in one patient in the Pato, et al study[19]).

In a small open trial,[31] four patients abruptly discontinued 80 mg of fluoxetine after approximately 1 year of treatment and three of the four (75%) had symptom recurrence after 12 weeks off fluoxetine. We postulated that the longer time to relapse, versus the 4 to 7 weeks seen in the CMI study,[19] was the result of longer half-life of fluoxetine. The only patient who did not relapse at 12 weeks also was the only patient who had received behavioral therapy prior to fluoxetine discontinuation.

Orloff, et al[32] reported on the follow-up of a cohort of 85 OCD patients on various antiobsessionals. As a group, 74 (87%) of the patients had greater than 25% response to treatment at least 1 year of follow-up. Remarkably, only four patients had stopped medication (three on fluoxetine and one on CMI), all because of becoming pregnant, and all experienced relapse. Orloff noted that no patients had an adequate course of behavioral therapy prior to discontinuing medication. All four patients restarted medication after delivery and again experienced remission of symptoms. Piacentini[33] and Montgomery[34] have both suggested that fluoxetine is better tolerated than clomipramine and this might contribute to less relapse on discontinuation, but definitive findings await the results of more systematic trials.

Sertraline

At the time of this printing, there is an ongoing multicenter trial of sertraline discontinuation. Although the blind in this study has not yet been broken, patients who dropped out because of relapse during the blinded phase of the trial again showed remission of obsessive-compulsive symptoms when restarted on open-label sertraline.[34a]

Fluvoxamine

There are no systematic, and few anecdotal, data available on the discontinuation of fluvoxamine (and no systematic trial is being planned by Solvay Pharmaceuticals, the manufacturer of fluvoxamine). Mallya[35] noted that seven of nine patients who discontinued fluovoxamine had a recurrence of symptoms within "a few days to weeks." In a recent dosage reduction study by Mundo,[36] five patients were withdrawn from the study because of relapse; two were receiving fluvoxamine when they relapsed and three were receiving clomipramine. However, some of these patients were taking a reduced dose at the time of relapse.

Paroxetine

Few systematic discontinuation data are available for paroxetine, and a review of the existing acute trial data gives no information on discontinuation. One abstract by SmithKline Beecham[37] reports preliminary results of a randomized discontinuation following 12 weeks of acute treatment and 6 weeks of open-label treatment in 104 treatment responders. After a total of 9 months of paroxetine treatment, this sample of patients were blinded and randomly assigned to continue paroxetine (n = 53) or receive placebo (n = 51). Among the placebo group, there was a more rapid return of symptoms, 28.5 days versus 62.9 days, for the group that continued paroxetine blindly. Further, significantly more patients in the placebo group experienced relapse of symptoms, 58.8% (30 of 51), versus those who remained on blinded paroxetine in which only 37.7% (20 of 53) relapsed. Further analysis of these data is not available at this time, including information on patients receiving behavioral treatment.

It is interesting to note that this relapse rate of 58.8% in the placebo group falls between the 89% noted in the Pato[19] single-blind study for clomipramine and the 23% relapse in the open fluoxetine discontinuation by Fontaine.[7] However, this paroxetine study of 104 subjects was larger than either of these cited, involved random assignment, and was double blind, and as such had more rigor. The rate of relapse among the blinded paroxetine group of 37.7% also is worth noting and worthy of further exploration. This represents a high rate of relapse among a group that has been effectively treated and is too high to be attributed to the blinding process alone. However, to date, little information has been published either anecdotally or systematically that would indicate that a loss of efficacy, in up to one third of patients, is typical of any of the antiobsessional agents.

Biologic Correlates of Discontinuation

Although the search for biologic markers in OCD is relatively new, powerful evidence for biologic changes occurring in the brain as a result of treatment is fast accumulating.[38–41] Based on these findings, it seems likely that serotonin is involved in the pathogenesis of OCD. However, lessons from the psychoses and observations in the literature, which state that up to 30% of patients do not respond to selective serotonin reuptake inhibitors (SSRIs),[42,43] suggest that the search for other biologic correlates of the disorder is necessary. Most of the data that presently exist are based on changes resulting from acute treatment. As noted in the following paragraphs, little has been published on (1) whether these changes persist or change with chronic treatment; and (2) what happens when medications are discontinued following treatment.

Imaging Studies

Among the more significant biologic findings in OCD patients are a number of reports citing changes in cerebral perfusion, specifically in the frontal lobe and the caudate nucleus of untreated patients. Molina[44] studied pretreatment, during, and 6 weeks' posttreatment changes in rCBF (regional cerebral blood flow) and measured cerebral perfusion in a previously untreated patient with OCD both qualitatively and semiquantitatively with single photon emission computed tomography before, during, and 6 weeks after treatment with clomi-pramine. The patient's symptoms disappeared when taking medication and relapsed after drug withdrawal. At baseline, there was an increased perfusion ratio in the bilateral orbitofrontal, anterior cingulate, frontotemporal, and right caudate regions. This increased perfusion disappeared during drug therapy. After treatment discontinuation and symptomatic relapse, the same pattern of hyperactivity was found. Semiquantitative measurements after treatment withdrawal showed a return to perfusion values similar to those observed in patients before treatment in subcortical structures. A study of this kind lends biologic credence to clinical reports that discontinuation may lead to symptomatic relapse and that maintenance treatment is indicated in the long-term management of OCD.

Psychopharmacologic Studies

Studies of pharmacologic parameters (e.g., whole blood 5-HT content, plasma 5-HT levels, platelet 5-HT, tritiated imipramine binding, paroxetine binding, platelet benzodiazepine receptors, and sulfotransferases) have been reported with either untreated OCD patients or acutely treated OCD patients. However, there are virtually no studies that have systematically measured these pharmacologic parameters in patients discontinuing treatment or in patients receiving long-term treatment for OCD.

Altemus[45] examined the effect of long-term (mean, 19 months) treatment with clomipramine hydrochloride on cerebrospinal fluid (CSF) levels of several neuropeptides and monoamine metabolites in children and adolescents with OCD. Treatment resulted in significant decreases in CSF levels of corticotropin-releasing hormone and vasopressin and a trend toward a decrease in somatostatin levels. Treatment also significantly increased CSF oxytocin levels. Significant changes in CSF monoamine metabolite levels with treatment included significant decreases in CSF levels of 5-hydroxyindoleacetic acid, CSF homovanillic acid, and 3-methoxy-4-hydroxyphenylglycol and a significant increase in the homovanillic acid/5-hydroxyindoleacetic acid ratio. There is evidence that central administration of corticotropin-releasing hormone, vasopressin, and somatostatin to laboratory animals increases arousal and acquisition of conditioned behaviors. Evidence has accumulated that indicates central administration of oxytocin has opposite behavioral effects, and the authors suggest that these results are consistent with a role for these neuropeptides in the pathophysiologic processes and pharmacologic treatment of OCD.

Maintenance Dosing

As clinical data grow regarding relapse following discontinuation of antiobsessional medications, the next logical question becomes, "If the medication cannot be discontinued, can the dose be decreased to minimize side effects and cost over the course of chronic treatment?" This issue of optimal or maintenance dosing has been approached in two different ways: One is through tapering maximal doses given acutely to see if lower doses bring the same efficacy in the maintenance phase. The second approach to long-term dosing issues has been made through fixed-dose study paradigms in which the question implied is: "Can a patient do well through the acute and maintenance course of treatment receiving a lower than maximum dose?" Because the results from these two types of studies have not agreed, they will be described separately.

Looking first at tapering of doses following maximal dosing during the acute phase of treatment, there have been several anecdotal reports and three more systematic trials to date.[27,36,46] Anecdotally, Solyom[47] commented that six OCD patients who did well with 300 mg CMI during a 6-week trial continued to do well with a smaller dose, with four patients showing further improvement at 1-year follow-up with doses of only 75 to 150 mg. Ananth[20] similarly reported that a maintenance dose of 50 to 75 mg was often adequate to maintain improvement.

In a more systematic open clinical trial of long-term maintenance, we[27] followed 10 patients who participated in the discontinuation study described previously[19] and who were subsequently followed-up after CMI had been reinstituted. Over 17 to 22 months, the dosage of CMI was gradually decreased. Patient reports and clinician impressions were used to establish the dosage below which deterioration was noted. These 10 patients were then given the minimum effective dose of medicine for at least 2 months and were rated twice at this new low dosage, once in an open fashion and once in a double-blind fashion as part of another study. Three measures were used: (1) Y-BOCS; (2) NIMH Obsessive-Compulsive Scale; and (3) NIMH Global Obsessive-Compulsive Scale. These ratings were compared with the same ratings completed at the beginning of the discontinuation study[19] when patients had received a higher dose of medication for a minimum of 5 months. In 7 of the 10 patients, the CMI dose was decreased by 100 mg/day or more, and by 50 mg/day in three of the 10 patients. The mean dose changed from 270 ± 20 mg to 165 ± 19 mg. These changes in CMI dose were accompanied by no significant worsening on the OCD rating scales.

Ravizza, et al[48] studied 130 subjects with OCD for 2 years using an open-label design. These 130 patients had responded to treatment with either clomipramine (150 mg/day), fluoxetine (40 mg/day), or fluvoxamine (300 mg/day) for the prior 6 months and were entered into a maintenance dose study. They were followed in a 2-year, open-label study at either full-dose, half-dose, or discontinuation of previous treatment. Patients were rated with the Y-BOCS and CGI scales at 3-month intervals or whenever symptoms worsened. Maintenance treatments, at both full- and half-dose, were found significantly superior to discontinuation in preventing relapses. No differences in efficacy were found between full- and half-dose treatment. There was also no statistical difference between the three types of medication used—clomipramine, fluoxetine, and fluvoxamine—suggesting that the maintenance efficacy of these three agents might be similar.

In a more recent study, Mundo[36] randomly assigned 30 OCD patients (successfully treated with either clomipramine or fluvoxamine) to three groups: (1) Group 1 was a control group with no change in the dosage of the drug that the patients received; (2) Group 2 included patients whose drug dosage was reduced by 33.3% to 40% compared with baseline; and (3) Group 3 included patients whose dosage was reduced by 60% to 66.6%. The trial was double blind and lasted 102 days. Results indicated no statistical difference between the three dosage groups. Plasma levels of clomipramine and its metabolite decreased significantly as the daily dose was reduced. However, among fluvoxamine patients there was not a correspondence between reduction in daily doses and serum levels. This suggests that unlike clomipramine, fluvoxamine does not have standardized kinetic properties. In fact, in patients remaining at the same dose, serum levels increased over 80 days (see section entitled "Serum Levels").

These results suggest that although patients may not tolerate complete discontinuation of medication, the dosage can be tapered without deterioration in clinical status. In addition, patients found these lower doses easier to tolerate and experienced fewer side effects, including less fatigue, constipation, dry mouth, and impaired sexual functioning.

Fixed-dose studies have generally been structured to allow treatment responders to continue receiving the same dose as in acute treatment, usually about 12 weeks, during 6 to 12 months of follow-up. In addition, patients who are deemed nonresponders in the acute phase are given the option of continuing medication (often at an increased dose for a follow-up period). Perhaps the most systematic study of this kind is that reported by Tollefson.[49] The author studied 274 primary OCD subjects who completed a 13-week, double-blind, placebo-controlled trial of three fixed doses of fluoxetine (20 mg, 40 mg, and 60 mg) with responders (n = 76) continuing the blinded treatment, and acute fixed-dose nonresponders channeled into an open-label trial and receiving the maximally tolerated dose (up to 80 mg/day) for 24 weeks. At the end of that time, most responders had not only maintained the gains of acute treatment, but approximately 50% showed greater than 25% further reduction on Y-BOCS at all three doses combined. Thus, it appears that longer duration of treatment alone improved efficacy for a number of patients. Even more important to the discussion of dosage is the outcome of nonresponders with acute treatment. Nonresponders had dosages titrated to between 20 and 80 mg, and approximately 50% of the patients showed greater than 25% improvement at the end of the extension phase. In both groups, fluoxetine was well tolerated during the 24-week (6 months) continuation periods. Late-emerging side effects (i.e., ones that occurred for the first time or worsened), during the extension phase, of the responders included asthenia (11.4%), rhinitis (10%), flu syndrome (10%), and abnormal dreams (8.6%). There were more late-emerging side effects in the nonresponder extension group as would be expected because their dose of medication was increased. Thus, the side effects were typical of those seen with fluoxetine treatment and consistent with the usual clinical observation that more medication leads to more side effects. Overall there were 20 of 274 patients who dropped out during the extension phase because of adverse events. Thus, continuation treatment with fluoxetine appeared to be well tolerated.

In another fixed-dose study with sertraline, Greist[16] used three dosages (50, 100, and 200 mg) of the drug in a double-blind, placebo-controlled trial of 325 patients from 11 sites who were randomly assigned to 12-week treatment. Three rating scales were used to determine patient outcome. Patients receiving all three doses of sertraline fared better than those receiving placebo. Endpoint analyses also showed significant improvement on all three measures in patients receiving 50 and 200 mg of the drug; patients receiving 100 mg showed improvement on only one measure—the NIMH Global OCD Scale. Those patients who responded at the end of 12 weeks, including placebo responders, were followed for an additional 40 weeks (10 months).[50] Those in the extension phase continued to show treatment efficacy and good toleration of medication.

The paroxetine extension study,[37] published as an abstract, notes that over the 6 months of open-label extension prior to blinding and randomization for discontinuation, mean improvement in Y-BOCS scores continued from a drop of 5.7 points at the end of the 12-week acute trial to 10.2 points at the end of the 6-month, open-label extension. Details are not available on the number of subjects who went to maximal dosing during the 6-month open phase; it is simply noted that flexible dosing between 20 and 60 mg was used. Similar to the fluoxetine extension study,[49] it appears that some patients showed maintained efficacy and even showed further improvement at lower than maximal doses.

Based on the existing data, it appears that a number of patients can maintain continued improvement on less than maximal doses of medication. There is still the question of whether this lower "maintenance dose" should be achieved by tapering down from a higher dose or simply by maintaining a patient at a lower dose throughout treatment. To date, we have no adequate data to predict which patients require higher doses and which patients require lower doses of medication for maximal clinical response. As a clinician, one is left with the notion that more medication may bring more improvement. Thus, if a patient is still experiencing significant symptoms at a less than maximal dose of any antiobsessionals, the physician should discuss with the patient the possibility of increasing the dose, although this increase will likely bring worsening of side effects. On the other hand, it seems likely that maximal dosing is not necessary for long-term treatment,[27,36,46] and it is recommended that after several months of treatment (perhaps 6 months), a patient's dose should be gradually decreased, until symptoms reemerge. As outlined previously, most patients relapse with discontinuation within approximately 4 weeks, except with treatment of fluoxetine which has a much longer half-life than other antiobsessional medications. Thus, a reasonable recommendation might be to allow at least 4 weeks at each dosage decrease before decreasing further.

Serum Levels in Discontinuation and Long-Term Treatment

Data on the relationship between dose, serum level, and therapeutic response have been unable to determine the most effective antiobsessional dose with which to treat OCD, perhaps because the actual mechanism of action of antiobsessional medication in OCD is not well understood. Most data in this area exist for CMI, because the drug has been commercially available in Europe for more than 25 years. Some older studies, mostly performed in acute treatment, support the concept of a therapeutic window for CMI dose.[21,51–53] Assessment of changes in CSF levels of 5-hydroxyindoleacetic acid (5-HIAA), a metabolite of serotonin, has shown that the maximum decrease of 5-HIAA in the CSF occurs at CMI serum levels of 300 ng/mL, with lower and higher levels of serum CMI showing less reduction. Thoren[52] and Traskman[53] reported a positive correlation between CMI serum levels, but not desmethyl-clomipramine serum levels, and improvement of OCD symptoms, but the data are inconclusive.

More recent data continue to provide mixed findings for clomipramine: Mavissakalian, et al[54] found that for 16 of 33 (49%) of OCD patients who responded to treatment with CMI for acute symptoms, plasma levels of CMI, but not desmethyl CMI, correlated significantly with improvement in scores. In addition, a lower ratio of N-desmethylclomipramine/clomipramine was associated with a better antiobsessional response. (This is not surprising, because although the parent compound has serotonergic action, the metabolite, desmethylclomipramine, is a noradrenaline reuptake inhibitor.)

The only study that appears to have measured serum levels in long-term treatment is that by Mundo,[36] in which serum levels were drawn after 6 months or more of treatment during which 10 of 15 patients had a deliberate decrease in the CMI dosages. Despite the predictable decrease in plasma levels of both parent compounds and metabolite in the CMI-treated patients who received one-third and two-thirds dosage reductions, only 1 of 10 patients in the reduction group relapsed. However, one of two patients who did not have CMI dosage reduced also relapsed and was noted to have a drop in serum level despite maintenance at the same dose. Based on this study,[36] it appears that one can lower serum levels in long-term CMI treatment (i.e., > 6 months) and still maintain treatment efficacy.

The data on the more selective serotonin agents regarding serum levels are even scantier and less conclusive, with very few data available on long-term treatment. In a study on acute treatment, after 7 weeks of treatment with fluoxetine, Koran, et al[55] examined the relation between steady-state plasma levels of fluoxetine and norfluoxetine, the sum, and the clinical outcome. (Measuring the parent compound and its metabolite is important because, unlike clomipramine, the active metabolite norfluoxetine also is active serotonergically, so that the antiobsessional effect of fluoxetine is likely affected by serum levels of both parent compound and metabolite.) Using the Y-BOCS, ratings of symptom severity were obtained at baseline and after 13 weeks for 200 adult outpatients with moderately severe OCD treated with fluoxetine at doses of 20 mg/day (n = 68), 40 mg/day (n = 64), or 60 mg/day (n = 68). Mean plasma levels of fluoxetine and norfluoxetine were significantly higher with higher medication doses. However, statistical analyses revealed no significant correlation between plasma level of the parent compound or metabolite, or the sum, in predicting percent change in OCD symptoms. Further, plasma levels of both compounds were not significantly different in responders versus nonresponders, nor was there a gender difference or a suggestion of a therapeutic window. However, because the isomeric forms of norfluoxetine differ in potency, further stereospecific studies might prove useful in differentiating responders and nonresponders based on serum metabolite levels.

In a small discontinuation trial of fluoxetine by Pato,[31] serum levels of both parent compound and metabolite were measured in four patients who had taken fluoxetine at 80 mg for a mean of 52 weeks (SD = 8 weeks). After 4 weeks of abrupt discontinuation, serum fluoxetine had dropped to 9% (from 620 ng/mL to 55 ng/mL) and serum norfluoxetine dropped to 37% (from 496 ng/mL to 184 ng/mL). Despite these dramatic drops in serum levels at 4 weeks, it was not until 12 weeks after abrupt discontinuation that three of the four patients showed significant clinical deterioration.

Sertraline plasma levels were measured acutely[16] in 95 subjects at 50 mg/day (n = 39), at 100 mg/day (n = 25), and at 200 mg/day (n = 31). There was a significant correlation between dose and serum levels but no relationship between serum level and patient response, either at each individual dose or from the pooled group. No long-term treatment data are yet available from this trial.

No data on serum levels in either acute or chronic treatment are available for paroxetine, but there are some data on chronic treatment with fluvoxamine from the Mundo report.[36] Unlike clomipramine levels, which showed a predictable decrease in serum level with a decreased dose, reduction in fluvoxamine dose did not lead to a decrease in fluvoxamine serum levels; rather, most levels remained the same or increased over 80 days of follow-up. This observation may be explained by the fact that fluvoxamine inhibits demethylation, which is the main route of elimination for fluvoxamine itself; hence, the authors indicated that for patients whose medication was not reduced during the study, there was an increase in serum level. Although the importance of this finding is limited by the small sample size of five, one must wonder whether patients receiving fluvoxamine long-term may experience ever-increasing serum levels or wonder when a steady serum level is reached for fluvoxamine.

There are several problems with the use of serum level guides in the long-term treatment of OCD. First, there has been no consistent correlation between serum levels and therapeutic efficacy for any antiobsessional medications. Second, in the case of some agents, particularly fluvoxamine, the medication metabolism is nonlinear and unpredictable, making it difficult to determine the serum level effect of decreasing the dose. Finally, there is marked variability in serum levels of each patient taking the same dosage of medication. Thus, the value of routinely measuring serum levels is questionable except for those patients with severe side effects at low doses, for those patients with no response at high doses, or for use in assessing patient compliance.

DURATION OF TREATMENT

Although CMI does not appear to produce lasting improvement after discontinuation, there are data suggesting that improvements with behavior therapy outlast the actual course of exposure and response prevention[56-58] (see also O'Sullivan[29] for summary and Chapters 17 and 19 in this volume). In both studies by Marks, et al[56,58] (and Mawson,[57] which was an interim follow-up of the same subjects), no treatment group received CMI alone for the entire duration of the study and follow-up. Instead, all patients received some behavioral therapy, making a direct comparison of CMI versus behavioral therapy impossible during prolonged treatment and follow-up. The most powerful conclusion from this study is that patients maintain their improvement at 1- and 2-year follow-up, despite no longer receiving behavioral treatment.[56-58] However, some recurrence of depression and obsessive-compulsive symptoms was reported in some patients at follow-up. In the 1980 study,[56] in which 20 patients received CMI and 20 patients received placebo, Marks concluded that CMI may need to be continued in those patients who had depression along with OCD, because 11 patients in the CMI group and seven in the placebo group had recurrence of depression. The placebo-treated patients who eventually needed antidepressant treatment required it sooner and for a longer duration than the CMI-treated patients. Further data on the state of OCD symptoms were available in 5 of the 11 CMI-treated patients with recurrence of depression.

Reassessment of these five patients showed that the depression recurred to prestudy levels, whereas OCD symptoms in these patients only partially recurred. Thus, patients maintained some of the gains in OCD symptoms despite recurrence of depression. All five patients experienced improvement in both depression and OCD symptoms with reinstitution of CMI treatment. The Marks, et al[58] report is sketchy in reporting recurrence, noting only that the 10 patients who had received CMI and "antiexposure" treatment initially "did badly" at 5-month follow-up after stopping CMI treatment. These results occurred despite patients receiving exposure and response prevention at a later point in the study. Thus, it appears that in some patients, discontinuation of behavioral treatment leads to long-lasting improvement in OCD symptoms, whereas in others, the improvement of OCD symptoms can be maintained only with continued CMI use. Predictors remain unclear as to which patients will need CMI plus behavioral treatment and which patients will experience long-term improvement with behavioral treatment alone.

A more recent review by O'Sullivan[29] on long-term treatment efficacy of behavior therapy supports the findings of the original work by Marks[58]: the majority (79%) of patients continued to do well at follow-up after behavioral therapy for OCD. This report by various authors summarized the findings of nine different behavioral studies totaling 195 subjects, with follow-up periods ranging from 1 to 6 years. To maintain continued remission of obsessive-compulsive symptoms, 14% of patients required booster sessions of behavior therapy, and approximately 33% of patients required pharmacotherapy for depression during follow-up.

Based on these findings, it seems advisable to add behavior therapy to the long-term treatment of OCD. However, although some patients may ultimately be able to have continued symptom improvement with behavior therapy alone, others may need continued pharmacotherapy (either because of OCD or depressive symptom reemergence). Although one would hope that the medication dose could be lower given the addition of behavior therapy, there are no empirical data to date that support this clinical supposition.

Predictors of Long-Term Treatment Response

Predicting treatment response is an important consideration in planning long-term treatment for any psychiatric disorder. Factors such as homogeneity of the disorder, biologic and pharmacologic predictors of response, and psychiatric and medical comorbid conditions may all influence treatment strategies. The reason some patients do not respond to treatment over a given time, whereas others respond rapidly, is a multifaceted problem. Only a few reports have examined predictors in long-term treatment samples: Orloff, et al[32] evaluated the records of 85 patients who had been treated at least 1 year previously (the mean follow-up period was 773 days), with information collected on age of onset of symptoms, time since first evaluation, and scores on several scales measuring symptom severity, including the Y-BOCS. No significant predictors of response were found.

Ravizza[46] studied 53 patients with OCD over a 6-month period, dividing the sample into "responders" and "nonresponders" to treatment with clomipramine or fluoxetine. By the sixth month of treatment, 31 patients (58.5%) were "responders," and among the 22 "nonresponders" (41.5%), there was a significantly earlier age of onset, longer duration of the disorder, higher frequency of compulsions, higher frequency of washing rituals, a more chronic course, more previous hospitalizations, and more concomitant schizotypal personality disorder. Using stepwise regression, poorer response to drug treatment was predicted by: (1) concomitant schizotypal personality disorder; (2) presence of compulsions; and (3) longer illness duration. The authors concluded that there may be distinct types of OCD related to drug treatment response.

SIDE EFFECTS: CONSIDERATIONS IN LONG-TERM TREATMENT

Based on the available data for OCD treatment, the clinician must contend with maintaining many patients on medication for a long time, if not for life. Although many long-term studies report that few patients have a relapse of symptoms even when maintained on the same dose of medication,[18] it is debatable whether this result is true tachyphylaxis, or rather is caused by the waxing-and-waning course of OCD.[20,59–62] Thus, OCD patients warrant regular follow-up and may require adjustment of the medication regimen, depending on the course of illness.

If we are to commit many of our patients to a lifetime of treatment with an antiobsessional medication, it is important to anticipate and make our patients aware of the long-term sequelae of these medications. However, even among the few "long-term" studies in the literature, few long-term detrimental side effects have been noted, other than those that continued after acute treatment. Asberg[21] commented on dental problems resulting from dry mouth effects of CMI treatment and noted that careful oral hygiene can minimize this problem. Other common side effects during CMI treatment include constipation, weight gain, exercise intolerance, mental cloudiness, fatigue, delayed ejaculation, and anorgasmia. Marks[56] warns of more serious side effects, noting that CMI, like other tricyclic antidepressants, can produce cardiac toxicity (arrhythmias and tachycardia), potentiate seizures, induce hypomania, and produce malignant hypertension when given in combination with monoamine oxidase inhibitors. Signs of toxicity should lead the clinician to obtain a serum level and ensure that this level has not risen to the toxic range (usually > 500 ng/mL combined CMI and desmethylclomipramine, though well-tolerated levels can be seen). If the level has risen and side effects are noted, further exploration for a metabolic cause of these elevations is warranted. In addition, as patients age and develop concurrent medical illness, such as cardiac problems, CMI may need to be discontinued and replaced by an SSRI with less cardiac toxicity.

Long-term studies on the safety and tolerability of SSRIs (e.g., fluoxetine, fluvoxamine, sertraline, and paroxetine) in the treatment of OCD are sparse; however, the data available on the use of SSRIs in depression indicate it is likely that SSRIs will become the mainstay of maintenance treatment, given their relatively favorable side-effect profile. The risk of seizures, hypomania, and movement disorders is reported to be less than with tricyclics in general—important considerations in long-term treatment and compliance. Like CMI, SSRIs can cause sexual dysfunction that persists during the course of treatment. The symptoms sometimes can be minimized by decreasing the dose. In other cases, clinicians have recommended brief "drug holidays" (e.g., over a weekend) without a resulting loss of treatment efficacy.[63] This method is not effective with fluoxetine, however, because of the drug's long half-life. Finally, despite reports of weight loss or no weight change in acute treatment, some patients do experience weight gain with long-term use of SSRIs.

Coupland[64] recently studied differences in withdrawal symptoms among 171 patients taking five common antiobsessional agents: (1) clomipramine (n = 13); (2) paroxetine (n = 50); (3) fluvoxamine (n = 43); (4) sertraline (n = 45); and (5) fluoxetine (n = 20). The population studied was not only OCD patients but also included patients with anxiety or mood disorders who had been in treatment for an average of 15 weeks (range, 5 to 28 weeks), although the average duration of clomipramine treatment was longer than that of other SSRIs at 37 weeks (range, 22 to 50 weeks). The most common side effects noted on discontinuation of treatment included dizziness, paresthesia, lethargy, nausea, lowered mood, anxiety, vivid dreams, insomnia, headache, irritability, and movement symptoms. Patients withdrawn from sertraline and fluoxetine experienced virtually none of these symptoms, and this finding was attributed partly to both drugs having active serotonergic metabolites that may, in effect, lengthen the half-life of these agents and make the withdrawal more gradual. Some of these withdrawal symptoms persisted up to 21 days, although symptoms were relieved within 24 hours by restarting the medication.

SUMMARY

Available data indicate that discontinuation of antiobsessional medication in the treatment of OCD leads to recurrence of OCD symptoms in the majority of patients. An exception may be in the case of fluoxetine treatment, in which preliminary studies indicate that a larger number of patients may do well without medication. Some studies also have demonstrated that biologic parameters (e.g., changes in cerebral blood flow with medication treatment) tend to revert to pretreatment levels with discontinuation of treatment. Maintaining clinical improvement after behavior therapy alone or combined with medication appears more promising, although findings remain inconclusive. Results from dosage-lowering studies with clomipramine,[19,36,46] fluvoxamine[36,46] and fluoxetine,[46] and from fixed-dose studies with fluoxetine,[49] sertraline,[50] and paroxetine[37] suggest that lower doses of medication are adequate to maintain clinical efficacy once patients have responded.

The clinician is encouraged to slowly decrease medication dosage even to the point of discontinuation.[64] A trial of medication should be considered, particularly in patients with an adequate course of behavioral therapy or short duration of OCD symptoms. Risk of relapse seems highest in the first 4 to 7 weeks,[19] except in fluoxetine treatment, where it could be 12 weeks or longer before relapse is seen.[31] Although few systematic data are available regarding relapse, there are a number of studies in progress (particularly with sertraline and fluoxetine) that may provide answers about time to relapse, percent of patients who relapse, and patients who are at risk for relapse.

REFERENCES

1. DeVeaugh-Geiss J, Landau P, Katz R: Treatment of obsessive-compulsive disorder with clomipramine, *Psychiatr Ann* 19:97–101, 1989.
2. The Clomipramine Collaborative Study Group: Efficacy of clomipramine in OCD: Results of a multicenter double-blind trial, *Arch Gen Psychiatry* 48:730–738, 1991.
3. Leonard HL, et al: Treatment of obsessive-compulsive disorder with clomipramine and desipramine in children and adolescents. A double-blind crossover comparison, *Arch Gen Psychiatry* 46:1088–1092, 1989.
4. Mavissakalian M, et al: Tricyclic antidepressants in obsessive-compulsive disorder: Antiobsessional or antidepressant agents? II, *Am J Psychiatry* 142:572–576, 1985.
5. Zohar J, Insel TR: Obsessive-compulsive disorder: Psychobiological approaches to diagnosis, treatment, and pathophysiology, *Biol Psychiatry* 22:667–687, 1987.
6. Fontaine R, Chouinard G: Fluoxetine in the treatment of obsessive compulsive disorder, *Prog Neuro-Psychopharmacol Biol Psychiatry* 9:605–608, 1985.
7. Fontaine R, Chouinard G: Fluoxetine in the long-term maintenance treatment of obsessive compulsive disorder, *Psychiatr Ann* 19:88–91, 1989.
8. Jenike MA, et al: Open trial of fluoxetine in obsessive-compulsive disorder (see comments), *Am J Psychiatry* 146:909–911, 1989.
9. Turner SM, et al: Fluoxetine treatment of obsessive-compulsive disorder, *J Clin Psychopharmacol* 5:207–212, 1985.
10. Tollefson GD, et al: A multicenter investigation of fixed-dose fluoxetine in the treatment of obsessive-compulsive disorder (published erratum appears in *Arch Gen Psychiatry* Nov, 51[11]:864, 1994), *Arch Gen Psychiatry* 51:559–567, 1994.
11. Goodman WK, et al: Efficacy of fluvoxamine in obsessive-compulsive disorder. A double-blind comparison with placebo, *Arch Gen Psychiatry* 46:36–44, 1989.
12. Goodman WK, et al: Treatment of obsessive-compulsive disorder with fluvoxamine: A multicentre, double-blind, placebo-controlled trial, *Int Clin Psychopharmacol* 11:21–29, 1996.
13. Koran LM, et al: Fluvoxamine versus clomipramine for obsessive-compulsive disorder: A double-blind comparison, *J Clin Psychopharmacol* 16:121–129, 1996.
14. Perse TL, et al: Fluvoxamine treatment of obsessive-compulsive disorder, *Am J Psychiatry* 144:1543–1548, 1987.

15. Price LH, et al: Treatment of severe obsessive-compulsive disorder with fluvoxamine, *Am J Psychiatry* 144:1059–1061, 1987.
16. Greist J, et al: Double-blind parallel comparison of three dosages of sertraline and placebo in outpatients with obsessive-compulsive disorder, *Arch Gen Psychiatry* 52:289–295, 1995.
17. Wheadon D, Bushnell W, Steiner M: A fixed dose comparison of 20, 40, or 60 mg paroxetine to placebo in the treatment of obsessive-compulsive disorder, American College of Neuro Psychopharmacology Annual Meeting, Hawaii, 1993.
18. Prien RF, Kupfer DJ: Continuation drug therapy for major depressive episodes: How long should it be maintained? *Am J Psychiatry* 143:18–23, 1986.
19. Pato MT, et al: Return of symptoms after discontinuation of clomipramine in patients with obsessive-compulsive disorder, *Am J Psychiatry* 145:1521–1525, 1988.
20. Ananth J: Clomipramine: An antiobsessive drug, *Can J Psychiatry* 31:253–258, 1986.
21. Asberg M, Thoren P, Bertilsson L: Clomipramine treatment of obsessive disorder: Biochemical and clinical aspects, *Psychopharmacol Bull* 18:13–21, 1982.
22. Capstick N: The Grayling well study, *J Int Med Res* 1:392–396, 1973.
23. Flament MF, et al: Clomipramine treatment of childhood obsessive-compulsive disorder. A double-blind controlled study, *Arch Gen Psychiatry* 42:977–983, 1985.
24. Leonard HL, et al: A double-blind desipramine substitution during long-term clomipramine treatment in children and adolescents with obsessive compulsive disorder, *Arch Gen Psychiatry* 48:922–927, 1991.
25. Thoren P, et al: Clomipramine treatment of obsessive-compulsive disorder. I. A controlled clinical trial, *Arch Gen Psychiatry* 37:1281–1285, 1980.
26. Yaryura-Tobias JA, Neziroglu F, Bergman L: Chlorimipramine for obsessive compulsive neurosis: An organic approach, *Curr Ther Res* 20:541–547, 1976.
27. Pato MT, Hill JL, Murphy DL: What is the lowest therapeutically effective clomipramine (CMI) dose in obsessive-compulsive disorder patients? *Psychopharmacol Bull* 26:211–214, 1990.
28. Zohar-Kadouch R, et al: Five-year follow-up of obsessive-compulsive disorder patients. Presented at the American Psychiatric Association, 1989.
29. O'Sullivan G, Marks I: Follow-up studies of behavioral treatment of phobia and obsessive compulsive neurosis, *Psychiatr Ann* 21:368–373, 1991.
30. VanNoppen B, et al: Group and family behavioral treatment for obsessive compulsive disorder. Abstract presented at the American Psychiatric Association, New York, May 1996.
31. Pato MT, Murphy DL, DeVane CL: Sustained plasma concentrations of fluoxetine and/or norfluoxetine four and eight weeks after fluoxetine discontinuation, *J Clin Psychopharmacology* 11:224–225, 1991.
32. Orloff LM, et al: Long-term follow-up of 85 patients with obsessive-compulsive disorder, *Am J Psychiatry* 151:441–442, 1994.
33. Piacentini J, et al: Psychopharmacologic treatment of child and adolescent obsessive compulsive disorder (review), *Psychiatr Clin North Am* 15:87–107, 1992.
34. Montgomery SA, et al: A double-blind, placebo-controlled study of fluoxetine in patients with DSM-III-R obsessive-compulsive disorder. The Lilly European OCD Study Group, *Eur Neuropsychopharmacol* 3:143–152, 1993.

34a. Deleted in proofs.
35. Mallya GK, et al: Short- and long-term treatment of obsessive-compulsive disorder with fluvoxamine, *Ann Clin Psychiatry* 4:77–80, 1992.
36. Mundo E, et al: Long-term pharmacotherapy of obsessive-compulsive disorder: A double-blind controlled study, *J Clin Psychopharmacol* 17(1):4–10, 1997.
37. Steiner M, et al: Long term treatment and prevention of relapse of OCD with paroxetine, 148th American Psychiatric Association Meeting, Miami, 1995.
38. Baxter LR, et al: Caudate glucose metabolic rate changes with both drug and behavior therapy for obsessive-compulsive disorder, *Arch Gen Psychiatry* 49: 681–689, 1992.
39. Rauch SL, et al: Regional cerebral blood flow measured during symptom provocation in obsessive-compulsive disorder using oxygen 15-labeled carbon dioxide and positron emission tomography, *Arch Gen Psychiatry* 51:62–70, 1994.
40. Schwartz JM, et al: Systematic changes in cerebral glucose metabolic rate after successful behavior modification treatment of obsessive-compulsive disorder, *Arch Gen Psychiatry* 53:109–113, 1996.
41. Swedo SE, et al: Cerebral glucose metabolism in childhood-onset obsessive compulsive disorder, *Arch Gen Psychiatry* 46:518–523, 1989.
42. Jenike MA: Pharmacologic treatment of obsessive compulsive disorder, *Psychiatr Clin North Am* 15:895–919, 1992.
43. Rasmussen SA, Eisen JL, Pato MT: Current issues in the pharmacologic management of obsessive-compulsive disorder, *J Clin Psychiatry* 54(6, suppl):4–9, 1993.
44. Molina V, et al: Drug therapy and cerebral perfusion in obsessive-compulsive disorder, *J Nucl Med* 36:2234–2238, 1995.
45. Altemus M, et al: Changes in cerebrospinal fluid neurochemistry during treatment of obsessive-compulsive disorder with clomipramine, *Arch Gen Psychiatry* 51: 794–803, 1994.
46. Ravizza L, et al: Predictors of drug treatment response in obsessive-compulsive disorder, *J Clin Psychiatry* 56:368–373, 1995.
47. Solyom L, Sookman D: A comparison of clomipramine hydrochloride (Anafranil) and behavior therapy in the treatment of obsessive neurosis, *J Int Med Res* 5(suppl 5):49–61, 1977.
48. Ravizza L, et al: Drug treatment of obsessive-compulsive disorder (OCD): Long-term trial with clomipramine and selective serotonin reuptake inhibitors (SSRIs), *Psychopharmacol Bull* 32:167–173, 1996.
49. Tollefson GD, et al: Continuation treatment of OCD: Double-blind and open-label experience with fluoxetine, *J Clin Psychiatry* 55(suppl 10):69–76, 1994b.
50. Greist JH, et al: A 1 year double-blind placebo-controlled fixed dose study of sertraline in the treatment of obsessive-compulsive disorder, *Int Clin Psychopharmacol* 10:57–65, 1995.
51. Stern RS, et al: Clomipramine and exposure for compulsive rituals: II. Plasma levels, side effects and outcome, *Br J Psychiatry* 136:161–166, 1980.
52. Thoren P, et al: Clomipramine treatment of obsessive-compulsive disorder. II. Biochemical aspects, *Arch Gen Psychiatry* 37:1289–1294, 1980.
53. Traskman L, et al: Plasma levels of chlorimipramine and its demethyl metabolite during treatment of depression: Differential biochemical and clinical effects of two

compounds, *Clin Pharmacol Ther* 26:600–610, 1979.

54. Mavissakalian M, et al: The relationship of plasma clomipramine and N-desmethyl-clomipramine to response in obsessive-compulsive disorder, *Psychopharmacol Bull* 26(1):119–122, 1990.
55. Koran LM, et al: Are fluoxetine plasma levels related to outcome in obsessive-compulsive disorder? *Am J Psychiatry* 153:1450–1454, 1996.
56. Marks IM, et al: Clomipramine and exposure for obsessive-compulsive rituals, *Br J Psychiatry* 136:1–25, 1980.
57. Mawson D, Marks IM, Ramm L: Clomipramine and exposure for chronic obsessive-compulsive rituals: III. Two year follow-up and further findings, *Br J Psychiatry* 140:11–18, 1982.
58. Marks IM, et al: Clomipramine, self-exposure and therapist-aided exposure and therapist-aided exposure for obsessive-compulsive rituals, *Br J Psychiatry* 152: 522–534, 1988.
59. Insel TR, Murphy DL: The psychopharmacological treatment of obsessive-compulsive disorder: A review (review), *J Clin Psychopharmacol* 1:304–311, 1981.
60. Rasmussen SA, Tsuang MT: The epidemiology of obsessive compulsive disorder (review), *J Clin Psychiatry* 45:450–457, 1984.
61. Rasmussen SA, Eisen JL: The epidemiology and clinical features of OCD. In Jenike MA, editor: *Psychiatr Clin North Am,* Philadelphia, WB Saunders, 15(4):743–758, December 1992.
62. Eisen JL, Steketee G: Course of illness in obsessive compulsive disorder. In Pato MT, Steketee G, editors: *Annual review of psychiatry: OCD across the life cycle,* vol 16, Washington, 1997, American Psychiatric Association.
63. Rothschild AJ: Selective serotonin reuptake inhibitor induced sexual dysfunction: Efficacy of a drug holiday, *Am J Psychiatry* 152:1514–1516, 1995.
64. March JS, Frances A, Carpenter D, Kahn DA: Expert consensus guideline series on treatment of obsessive-compulsive disorder, *J Clin Psychiatry* 5:4, 1997.

29

Issues in the Assessment and Treatment of Obsessive-Compulsive Disorder in Minority Populations

Steven Friedman, Ph.D., Marjorie Hatch, Ph.D., Cheryl M. Paradis, Psy.D.

This chapter describes our experience in evaluating and treating obsessive-compulsive disorder (OCD) in minority, primarily African-American or Caribbean-American, patients. In this chapter, we refer to our minority patients of African descent as African Americans. However, our patients consist of both U.S.–born and more recent immigrants of color from the Caribbean. We will use multiple case examples to highlight important issues in treating minority patients with OCD, such as help-seeking behavior, misdiagnosis, secrecy, therapist/client ethnicity, the family's role, and adaptations to treatment. Because many clinicians and researchers are likely to be unfamiliar with treating OCD in patients from minority populations, we hope this chapter will highlight a variety of relevant issues.

Demographers have predicted that by the year 2050 more than 50% of the U.S. population will be of Asian, African, or Latin descent. As minority groups continue to grow in number in the United States, the need for mental health service will expand and mental health professionals will be increasingly called upon to provide culturally relevant services.[1] Although published work addressing racial or ethnic issues in mental health has increased in the past two decades, this work has focused on general issues in counseling[2] or on severe forms of psychopathology.[3] Thus, clinicians and researchers may be only minimally familiar with diagnostic and treatment considerations in relation to minority patients with anxiety disorders[4] and with OCD in particular. General issues relevant to various minority groups include poverty, lack of English language skills, levels of low "acculturation," limited access to information and treatment, misdiagnosis, and racism.

PRESENTATION OF OBSESSIVE-COMPULSIVE DISORDER IN MINORITY PATIENTS IN THE UNITED STATES

Although the prevalence of OCD in the United States has been evenly distributed across racial groups,[5,6] African Americans with OCD either do not present for psychiatric treatment in the same proportion as Caucasians do, or they are misdiagnosed. In a survey of major OCD treatment centers, Lewis-Hall[7] found only 30 (2%) African-American patients of a total sample of 1,500 OCD sufferers. In one major medical center with a predominantly African-American clientele, Lewis-Hall found treatment records for only three African Americans with OCD.

Although a detailed analysis of why African Americans have not traditionally sought psychiatric treatment for OCD (as well as for other psychiatric conditions) is beyond the scope of this paper, there are a few points to note. Both culturally influenced help-seeking behavior and mistrust of the psychiatric system on the part of the sufferer, as well as misdiagnosis on the part of mental health professionals, seem to have played a role in this phenomenon.[4]

Help-Seeking Behavior

Neighbors[8,9] argued that African Americans most often consult members of their informal social network, including clergy, in times of emotional distress. More specifically, Friedman and colleagues[10] reevaluated Rassmussen's[11] hypothesis that people with OCD tend to turn to medical specialists such as dermatologists. Examining the rate of OCD in a group of African-American dermatology patients, we found a significantly higher rate of undiagnosed cases in our sample (15%) than would be expected in a general medical population (2% to 3%).

Misdiagnosis

A second clinical issue is that of misdiagnosis in people of color. Paradis and colleagues[13] found evidence of misdiagnosis of anxiety disorders by psychiatric staff at an urban outpatient center with a primarily African-American and Afro-Caribbean clientele. Patients who were initially diagnosed following a clinical interview by outpatient staff were reevaluated by anxiety disorder clinic staff using a structured interview (ADIS-R[14]). None of the original diagnoses of the 100 patients included a diagnosis of an anxiety disorder. Reevaluation resulted in nearly one fourth of these patients being reclassified with either a primary or secondary diagnosis of one or more anxiety disorders. In particular, one case was rediagnosed with a primary diagnosis of OCD.

It is unclear if the dermatologists in the Friedman, et al study[10] or the psychiatric staff in the Paradis, et al study[13] would have had a higher "hit rate" in diagnosing Caucasians. To our knowledge, the differential ability of mental health professionals to correctly diagnose OCD in different ethnic groups has not yet been studied.

Other researchers also have investigated misdiagnosis in minority patients. In his review of the literature, Adebimpe[3] found that African Americans who presented for psychiatric treatment with an affective disorder were more often misdiagnosed with schizophrenia than were Caucasians. A related clinical issue is that of the inappropriate psychiatric hospitalization of minority patients.[15] In clinical practice, OCD sufferers may present in bizarre ways and are sometimes misdiagnosed as having schizophrenia. In an empirical examination of the similar symptomatology between OCD and schizophrenia, Carey and colleagues[16] examined the Minnesota Multiphasic Personality Inventory profiles of a group of 32 OCD patients. The authors found elevations on the schizophrenia scale. This elevation on scale 8 is consistent with the behavioral presentation of OCD in which the patient may present with what appears to be bizzare and senseless behavior and the drive to complete this behavior. Although Carey, et al[16] did not report on the racial background of their sample, it seems likely that such misdiagnosis may be even greater for African Americans than for Caucasians.

One possible explanation for the misdiagnosis of minority patients may have to do with the use of language in people's expression of distress. Many cross-cultural studies have described a great diversity in the language used to describe effects and emotional distress throughout the world.[17,18] Such miscommunication may explain some of the reported misdiagnosis of depression and anxiety in minorities[19] with generally more severe, often psychotic disorders.

PREVIOUS RESEARCH ON OBSESSIVE-COMPULSIVE DISORDER IN AFRICAN AMERICANS

Perhaps the first published paper on OCD in Blacks was a clinical description of five cases in Benin, Africa.[20] The authors reported two patients suffering with checking rituals, one was a doubter, one had washing rituals, and one had mixed washing and religious obsessions. Four of these five patients had a history of affective disorder and two were currently comorbid for minor depression.

The limited number of African Americans with OCD in treatment at university and medical school research clinics has resulted in the failure of this group to be included in research protocols. In extensive review of the literature on anxiety disorders in African Americans, Neal and Turner[4] concluded that, at that time, there was a complete absence of empirical studies dealing specifically with OCD. Hollander and Cohen[21] also published a recent review on OCD in African Americans. Although not presenting any empirical data, they discuss psychopharmacologic treatment considerations and what is known about OCD–related disorders, such as trichotillomania, in this group.

This chapter seeks to add to the information available on OCD in African Americans by discussing the clinical presentation and treatment of a variety of patients. Specifically, we focus on differences in clinical presentation and treatment that we noticed between our African-American and Caucasian patients. A case presentation approach seems especially helpful for clinicians who lack experience with minority populations.

Our clinical experience supports that of others (e.g., Hayes and Toarmino[22]) in concluding that despite the general applicability of treatment principles in the treatment of OCD, understanding the cultural differences between African-American and Caucasian patients can lead to both improved diagnostic reliability and more successful treatment. Finally, although we focus on ethnic group differences as a way to highlight our modified treatment protocol originally developed for Caucasian OCD sufferers, we do not suggest that individual differences within the African-American and other minority communities are unimportant in treatment planning.

The Clinical Population

The Anxiety Disorders Clinic at the Health Sciences Center of the State University of New York at Brooklyn serves a primarily African-American and Caribbean-American clientele. Over the years, the clinic has gained a respected reputation in the community. We have seen a steady increase in the number of African Americans with OCD who present for treatment. The cases detailed in this report are representative of the 13 African Americans and Caribbean Americans with OCD who presented for treatment at our clinic during a 2-year period. Table 29-1 shows demographic data for the entire group. In terms of age, marital status, occupation, and symptom severity, these minority patients did not significantly differ from the Caucasian patients at our clinic. Overall, our patients, both minority and Caucasian, were experiencing severe OCD. Our sample scored an average 24.7 on the Yale-Brown Obsessive-Compulsive Scale (Y-BOCS), which is in the severe range of impairment. The severity of our group is similar to that reported in other studies. Goodman and colleagues[23,24] reported pretreatment mean Y-BOCS scores for two different outpatient groups as 25.3 (± 6) and 26.6 (± 6).

Our clinic's standard treatment for patients with OCD consists primarily of in-session, *in vivo* exposure and response prevention (ERP) as described by Foa and Rowan.[25] The goals include desensitizing the patient to the feared stimulus and demonstrating that anxiety reduction would occur even in the absence of performing rituals. Periodic home visits, therapist-accompanied "field trips," and in-session imaginal exposure also are employed for the same goals.

Our African-American patients were generally seen twice a week for 45- to 90-minute sessions for an average of 37 sessions (range, 8 to 150). The length of treatment in some cases is mainly the result of our clinic policy, which accepts OCD patients for treatment even when there are comorbid psychologic disorders or significant psychosocial problems. A wide range in length of

Table 29-1   Demographic Data for Obsessive-Compulsive Disorder Clients (n = 13)

Ethnic Background
   African American   7
   Afro-Caribbean   5
   African   1

Average Age
   38 years (range = 19 to 69, *SD* = 13.25)

Marital Status
   (n = 9)   Never married   4
             Married   4
             Divorced   1

Occupation
   (n = 12)   Unemployed   5
              Full-time   2
              Homemaker   2
              Student   2
              Retired   1

Average Length of Illness
   14 years (range = 1 to 45 years, *SD* = 14.09)

*Y-BOCS**
   Average Y-BOCS total: 24.7 (out of 40; *SD* = 5.00)
   Average subtotal for obsessions: 10.9 (out of 20, *SD* = 3.09)
   Average subtotal for compulsions: 13.8 (out of 20; *SD* = 5.01)
   Average time spent obsessing: 3–8 hours a day ("severe")
   Average time spent on compulsions: 3–8 hours a day ("severe")

Primary Symptom
   Mixed Washers, Doubters, & Checkers   4
   Washers/Cleaners   5
   Checkers   3
   Trichotillomania   1

Average Number of Treatment Sessions (90 minutes)
   37 (range = 8–150)

Treatment Outcome for Clients who Engaged in CBT (exposure and response prevention) (n = 8)
   Significant improvement   3
   Moderate improvement   3
   No treatment improvement   2

* Yale-Brown Obsessive-Compulsive Scale[23]

treatment is typical for our entire clinic population, regardless of racial or ethnic background or anxiety diagnosis. Notwithstanding, the average length of treatment tends to be longer for our African-American patients, for reasons detailed later in this chapter.

One of the important clinical issues we have struggled with is that although the majority of patients treated for OCD at our clinic receive both behavioral treatment and medication, our African-American patients were more reluctant to agree to a psychiatric consultation for medication. Although medication was recommended by the primary therapist for 60% of the African-American patients, less than half agreed to the medication consultation. The issues in engaging the patients in pharmacologic treatment will be covered in detail.

There are a number of differences in the presentation and process of treatment between our African-American and Caucasian patients related to secretiveness, therapist ethnicity, family tolerance of symptoms, and general knowledge about OCD. We would like to stress that ethnic differences between patient and therapist are not necessarily a problem. Some minority patients, when assigned a Caucasian therapist, initially express concerns that their culture and lifestyle may not be understood, and worry that this will impede rapid amelioration of their presenting problem. But as is demonstrated in the case reports, this obstacle can be overcome with frank discussion of racial differences and concerns early in the treatment process. The constellation of these factors had made it necessary to approach the treatment of our African-American patients in a manner different from the "standard" approach. The following cases are summarized in Table 29-2.

Case 1

A 37-year-old married woman originally from Jamaica was referred from a sex therapy clinic where she had originally presented with a vague complaint of loss of sexual desire. After a number of fruitless sessions, she reported to the sex therapist, "There's something else I should tell you, because I don't think it's right. I wash things a lot."

Once referred to our clinic, the patient was initially unwilling to discuss her symptoms in detail. After several weeks of establishing a trusting relationship with her therapist, she gradually elaborated on her obsessive-compulsive symptoms. Obsessions centered around people and places she believed to have a high concentration of germs, such as homeless people, subways, bathrooms, and kitchens. Compulsions included handwashing (10 times a day for at least 1 minute, often longer) and cleaning, both at home and at the home of the woman for whom she was a home nursing aide. Because the patient's husband worked long hours and her client was blind and bedridden, she was able to carry out her rituals undiscovered. Although strongly encouraged, she refused to discuss her

Table 29-2 Characteristics of Patients in Case Reports

Case	Ethnicity	Gender	Age (yr)	Marital Status	Education	Employment	Primary Symptoms	Sessions (n)	Therapist Gender/ Ethnicity		Y-BOCS Score Pretreatment	Y-BOCS Score Posttreatment
1	Afro-Caribbean	F	37	Married	6th grade	Home attendant	Contamination— dirt/washing	23	F	White	16	8
2	Afro-Caribbean	F	29	Married	H.S. graduate	Unemployed	Primarily obsessional	17	F	White	25	21
3	Afro-Caribbean	F	39	Married	2 years college	Unemployed	Blood, harming, contamination/ washing, checking	14	F	White	30	16
4	African American	F	69	Widowed	8th grade	Unemployed	Dirt/washing	N/A	N/A		32	Refused treatment
5	African American	M	30	Single	H.S. Special Ed.	Unemployed	Contamination washing, checking	12 Dropped out	M	White	31	31
6	Afro-Caribbean	F	33	Married	H.S. graduate	Homemaker	Scrupulosity/ repeating, ordering	35	F	White	27	11
7	African American	F	48	Divorced	Graduate degree	Professional	Safety/checking	78	F	White	14	6

OCD with her husband and would not perform therapy homework when he was at home.

Treatment lasted for 23 sessions and primarily focused on deliberate exposure to germ-laden stimuli during therapist visits to her job, combined with increasing periods of "normal" washing behavior. Normal washing in this case was defined as a 15-second handwash after handling blood or fecal material and before food preparation. Treatment culminated with a flooding exercise in which the patient rubbed her hands on the seat of every toilet at the medical center and then touched personal belongings that she had brought from home. This resulted in the patient's success over the last of her obsessive-compulsive behavior, and she was rated by her therapist as showing "significant improvement." At a 1-year follow-up, the patient reported recurring urges to ritualize, but said that what she learned in treatment kept her from acting on these occasional impulses.

Case 2

A 29-year-old pregnant woman, originally from Jamaica, was referred to our anxiety disorders clinic for the treatment of "panic attacks and generalized anxiety." Despite a lengthy initial evaluation of 3 hours, which included administration of the Anxiety Disorders Interview Schedule-Revised, a structured interview that directly asks about OCD symptoms,[14] the patient did not admit to any obsessive-compulsive symptoms. After six sessions of intervention for her panic attacks, which did result in a decrease in panic and anxiety, she finally confided that she had a 15-year history of "obsessions." Obsessions at the time of treatment involved fears of dying and of going crazy. She was "convinced and thought all day" that she would die in childbirth. When asked to explain why she believed this to be true, the patient related it to her culturally derived belief in voodoo and stated that perhaps someone put a "hex" on her. Only once the real OCD symptoms came to light could proper treatment be initiated.

Case 3

This patient was a 39-year-old unemployed African-American woman living with her two children. She was referred to the clinic by her internist for "the evaluation and treatment of her panic attacks." She had been referred by her internist only after she had refused a variety of medical diagnostic procedures that were necessary to treat her chronic medical illness.

In the initial evaluation, she only admitted to the symptoms of panic and a "fear of blood." When this "fear of blood" was pursued in the second and third sessions, she admitted that she had become "obsessed with thoughts for the past 8 years." She described the initial onset of her symptoms when she would look at dried red-colored spots on the street and wonder whether she had touched the blood and, therefore, became ill and spread illness to her family. She engaged in compulsive activities of cleaning and showering because of her constant fear of contamination.

The evaluation by her internist and her previous treatment experiences with mental health professionals had resulted only in the diagnosis of panic disorder with agoraphobia, missing the OCD. At the same time, the patient had kept her OCD secret from her husband and children, even though she would spend 3 to 5 minutes washing various spots in her house at least 20 times a day using both bleach and cleanser on the spots. She would often wash the children's hands with soap as well. She would check compulsively for red material on her clothes and, in spite of financial problems, throw out clothes that she believed were contaminated. She reported that she yielded to her urges 90% of the time, "Although I know it's crazy." She had only become willing to engage in treatment because her chronic medical condition had worsened and she had needed additional medical evaluation, which she was avoiding because of her obsessions and compulsions.

Case 4

A 69-year-old African-American woman came to the attention of the clinic through the hospital dermatology department, where she had presented with psoriasis on her hands and arms and thickened scabs on her elbows and knees. She and her daughter both described the patient as a "clean person." She reluctantly reported that she washed her hands approximately 100 times a day, washed her clothing in antiseptic solution, and cleaned floors on her hands and knees on a daily basis. This pattern had begun in early adulthood. The patient rejected our offer of psychologic treatment. The patient stated that her activities gave her something to do, a view shared by the family members with whom she lived, who were only mildly distressed by her rituals.

Case 5

This patient was a 30-year-old, single, unemployed African-American man, still living at his parents' home. He was referred to the clinic by his mother because she believed he had "obsessive-compulsive disorder." The patient initially complained only about feeling depressed because "I can't maintain a job." Upon probing and a structured interview, he was able to describe his OCD symptoms. He reported washing throughout the day for approximately 3 minutes after touching objects such as a telephone or coming into contact with people who "looked wrong." His hands were extremely dried and cracked and he would normally handwash his clothes every day. He admitted to additional checking behavior such as moving household objects from place to place, checking the house for intruders, and making sure doors were locked and the stove was off. The patient reported never being able to resist these urges and he imagined that he would "get very nervous if I try to stop." He claimed that he only engaged in this ritualistic behavior in "secrecy" at home and was able to control his behavior outside his home. However, for all intents and purposes, the patient was housebound. We were unable to get his family to attend our clinic for "even a diagnostic consultation," as they appeared to be extremely tolerant of his OCD. This patient, after 12 sessions, dropped out of treatment.

Case 6

A 33-year-old Afro-Caribbean female homemaker, originally from Trinidad, reported suffering from severe repeating rituals since 15 years of age. Hospitalized as a teenager for a "nervous breakdown," she did not tell the treatment staff about her obsessive-compulsive symptoms out of fear that she would be seen as crazy. The patient had never really understood her behavior and had been encouraged to call our clinic for help only because we had successfully helped a member of her church.

Case 7

This patient was a 48-year-old, divorced, African-American woman who worked at a social service agency. She had a 5-year history of increasing obsessions about personal safety and compulsive checking at home. She reported that she severely restricted her social life. She only occasionally attended church services, to avoid revealing her problem. She was especially concerned about concealing her ritualistic behavior from her siblings during occasional family visits. When visiting these siblings, she would wake up 2 to 3 hours before any member of the family so that she could complete her rituals completely unobserved. The patient would experience anxiety in the weeks preceding these visits as she rehearsed how she could perform rituals undetected.

One of the initial treatment issues was her reluctance to agree to home visits at her apartment building for fear that her neighbors would think the Caucasian therapist was a welfare caseworker. These visits were an important component of treatment. After some discussion, she decided to tell her neighbors that the therapist was a supervisor from her job coming by with paperwork. Therapy, initially twice a week, was reduced to once a month over the course of 18 months, as the patient made slow and uneven progress. Progress was slowed by her very gradual revelation of additional symptoms of OCD that she had initially denied during our intake. Treatment concluded when the patient reported 85% to 90% improvement and expressed doubt at achieving any more progress.

TREATMENT ISSUES

Secretiveness

Patients with OCD often show reluctance or hesitance in discussing their OCD symptoms—what Rassmussen and Tuang[26] have called the "secretive and withholding nature of individuals with OCD." It is our clinical impression that African-American patients are even more reluctant than Caucasian patients to discuss details of their obsessive-compulsive symptoms. This is also true of our OCD patients of Caribbean-American descent. This is manifested during the initial evaluation and the treatment phase. An additional observation is that our African-American patients, for the most part, are extremely reluctant to involve family in both the information and treatment phases of therapy. The exact nature of the reasons for this reluctance is unclear, but may be the result of a culturally driven fear of being labeled as "crazy."

In Case 1, the patient's reluctance during diagnostic interviews led to initial misdiagnosis of her problems as being of a primarily sexual nature. In Case 7, the patient's gradual revelation of a greater number of obsessive thoughts and ritualistic behavior kept her in treatment for more than 18 months. Patients in Case 1 and Case 3 both had a history of being inappropriately treated, because their reluctance to disclose symptoms contributed to the clinician's misdiagnosis.

Many of our African-American OCD patients initially believe that taking medication is equated with having a psychotic illness with a chronic and a deteriorating course that will inevitably lead to hospitalization and homelessness. Patients in Cases 1, 2, and 3 described previously had all refused a referral for psychopharmacologic evaluation and treatment. As one of the patients explained to us, "You don't understand. Where I come from only very crazy people take medication." This strongly held cultural belief has led us to spend an increased amount of time educating our minority patients regarding the specific effects of selective serotonergic reuptake inhibitors (SSRIs) on OCD. Clinical experience has shown that African Americans may suffer from more side effects and respond at a lower dose, so we increase the medication very slowly in attaining optimum levels.[25-27]

Family Involvement in Treatment

We made two interesting observations regarding the role of the family in the diagnostic and treatment process. For the most part, our minority patients were extremely reluctant to involve the family in any part of the treatment process. In fact, patients made every effort to keep their symptoms a secret from all family members. In addition, we almost never observed family members being drawn into or asked to participate in compulsive rituals as is typical of many OCD patients (e.g., removing clothes or shoes before entering the house, or the patient insisting family members wash if they "were contaminated").[28] This is illustrated with the patient in Case 3. Despite acknowledging that her family "really suspects something is wrong with me," she refused to acknowledge that she had OCD or explain her odd behavior. She stated that she preferred that her children think she was "just crazy." She steadfastly refused to allow a home visit by her therapist. After several months of treatment, she agreed to participate in a family meeting, but she cancelled that appointment and terminated treatment soon thereafter.

Experiences such as that with the patient in Case 3 have taught us that it is often necessary to broach the idea of family involvement differently for our African-American patients. Successful solutions have included coaching the patient in ways to convey information to family members rather than insisting on a face-to-face meeting, and reconceptualizing to expand our definition of family to include friends and neighbors. In the face of strong resistance, however, we have learned to abandon or postpone this clinical intervention rather than risk premature therapy termination.

The second observation related to the diagnostic and treatment process for our African-American OCD patients was that for those cases in which permission was given and family members were contacted, it was common for these people to be exceptionally tolerant of the patient's OCD–related activities. This was illustrated with the patients in Cases 4 and 5.

This pattern of secrecy also adversely affected our ability to involve family in the treatment. A number of therapists specializing in the treatment of OCD have recommended the inclusion of family members to serve as "cotherapists," to facilitate the completion of homework assignments and encourage compliance with treatment.[29,30] In contrast to our experience with Caucasian patients, this was extremely difficult to achieve with our African-American OCD patients. In Case 7, the severe anxiety the patient experienced before visiting family members for fear they would find out about her OCD is an example of this trend. The patient in Case 3 represents the extreme, in which she ended treatment rather than engage in a family session. Although a significant proportion of our Caucasian patients had convinced family members to engage in ritualistic activities (e.g., shower immediately upon returning home) or to assist the patient in performing rituals, with a few exceptions, our African-American OCD patients did not reflect this pattern.

Understanding Obsessive-Compulsive Disorder

Although it is common for OCD patients to have limited information about the disorder, we found this situation more pronounced for our African-American patients. We have observed that understanding of the disorder was so limited that all patients were secretly convinced they were or would become psychotic. As described earlier, the stigma of being mentally ill appears particularly strong in our Afro-Caribbean patients and appears to contribute strongly to a reluctance to accept evaluations or treatment with appropriate medication.

In fact, in almost every case, our patients expressed a belief that OCD is "a White person's problem." This was given as a reason for not seeking treatment earlier. When questioned, patients in Cases 1 and 3 reported that this belief derived from the fact that the television talk shows and magazine articles about OCD they had seen only featured Caucasian sufferers. Each patient was secretly convinced of being alone among African-American women and believed their OCD was particularly unacceptable in the African-American culture. Early in treatment, the patient in Case 3 believed that having OCD somehow negated her identity as an African American.

In an effort to address our African-American patients' sense of isolation, our clinic has compiled a series of videotapes in which African-American OCD patients discuss their symptoms and treatment. A number of the patients who volunteered to be videotaped also have offered to have their phone numbers given to new patients, to facilitate the creation of a support network. Currently, our new African-American patients who view our videotapes are greatly relieved to know that other African Americans suffer with this disorder. The comfort they derive from this knowledge helps motivate them to work through the difficult exposure and response prevention.

We also have begun to make outreach efforts to the African-American community. We have included information on anxiety disorders and OCD in pamphlets that our university provides as part of the medical school's outreach program for African-American patients in Brooklyn. The Arthur Ashe Institute for Urban Health at our university has promoted prevention and treatment for a variety of illnesses such as hypertension, diabetes, and heart disease, diseases that are particularly prevalent among people of color in urban areas. The institute has welcomed our inclusion of simple and clearly written brochures describing anxiety disorders. The institute has helped distribute this information to churches and to proprietors and clients of beauty salons. Gradually, this effort has led to a number of referrals by clergy and other community health members. In addition, the successful treatment of patients with anxiety disorders continues to spread to other potential clients through word of mouth.

Therapist Ethnicity

The majority of therapists at our clinic are Caucasian. This is certainly not an issue in every case involving ethnic minority patients. However, any patient discomfort with the ethnicity of the therapist is a dimension of the treatment that must be assessed and discussed.

As seen in the treatment of the patient in Case 7, it can be extremely helpful, early in treatment, to raise the issue of ethnicity and prejudice. First, this acknowledgment demonstrates to the patient that the therapist is comfortable discussing potentially sensitive issues. This openness in turn often serves to lessen tension and to promote honesty and trust in the therapist-patient relationship.

We must reiterate that ethnic differences between patient and therapist do not necessarily lead to treatment failure. Some minority patients, when assigned a Caucasian therapist, express concerns that their culture and lifestyle will not be understood, and this factor will impact on treatment of the presenting problem. As demonstrated in the previous case reports, discomfort can be overcome with frank discussion of racial differences and concerns early in the treatment process.

Conclusions

To summarize our key recommendations for clinical practice:

1. As detailed earlier in this book, we strongly recommend the use of a structured interview to help overcome reticence in discussing obsessive-compulsive symptoms. Structured interviews often help normalize the intake process, and directed questions make evasiveness easier to recognize.

2. In terms of family involvement, expect resistance, and broach the topic carefully and flexibly. We have found that suggesting the involvement of a friend or neighbor may meet with less resistance. In the face of strong resistance, however, we have learned to abandon or postpone the idea despite potential therapeutic benefits later in treatment.

3. It is the clinician's responsibility to raise the issue of cultural and ethnic incongruity between therapist and patient. This can both foster a therapeutic alliance and uncover potentially ambivalent feelings the patient may harbor such as, "You can't understand what it's like to be on public assistance."

Relevant topics for future work in the specific area of OCD and minority populations are numerous. In terms of etiology and phenomenology, it is unclear how closely OCD in minority populations mirrors that in the White population. For example, a literature search did not find any papers on Hispanic patients and OCD. More specifically, what is the role of social factors, such as prejudice, in explaining the apparent ethnic differences we observed? In terms of treatment, what are the effects of matching African-American clinicians with African-American patients? What is the effect of educational level and socioeconomic status in the provision of culturally informed treatment? Finally, what are the implications of these and other clinical observations for relapse prevention?

Given that the preponderance of research on OCD has been focused almost exclusively on Caucasian sufferers, a fair question is: does our knowledge apply equally well to African-American and other minority populations? We find no particular reason to assume that important factors in the etiology and maintenance of obsessive-compulsive symptoms differ across cultural groups and, in fact, our observations are that their symptoms are often quite similar. However, we do believe that race and ethnicity are sociocultural factors that influence the way individuals present for treatment, what initial diagnosis they receive, and how the treatment process develops.

SUMMARY

In this chapter we have discussed culturally sensitive approaches for the evaluation and treatment of OCD. A literature search did not show any published data on OCD in other American minority groups. However, we believe that the themes and issues discussed in this chapter are appropriate to minority groups, including Hispanic Americans, Native Americans, and Asian Americans. Ethnic minority groups are overrepresented in lower socioeconomic groups and struggle with the stressors of poverty and immigration. These groups often are less knowledgeable about mental health disorders, and currently there are fewer educational materials and outreach programs targeting these groups. These issues indicate the need for outreach into minority communities to provide education and encouragement for individuals to seek treatment. Emphasis on training clinicians in cultural sensitivity and more clinical research on OCD in minority groups are clearly warranted.

ACKNOWLEDGMENTS

This work was supported, in part, by National Institute of Mental Health Grant #42545 and by funds from the Department of Psychiatry's Practice Plan.

REFERENCES

1. Ponterotto JG, Casas JM: *Handbook of racial/ethnic minority counseling research,* Springfield, 1991, Charles C Thomas.
2. Aponte JF, Rivers RY, Wohl J: *Psychological interventions and cultural diversity,* Needham Heights, 1995, Allyn & Bacon.
3. Adebimpe VR: Overview: White norms and psychiatric diagnosis of Black patients, *Am J Psychiatry* 138:279–285, 1981.
4. Neal AM, Turner SM: Anxiety disorders research with African Americans: Current status, *Psychol Bull* 109:400–410, 1991.
5. Karno M, Golding JM, Sorenson SB, Burnam A: The epidemiology of obsessive-compulsive disorder in five U.S. communities, *Arch Gen Psychiatry* 45:1094–1099, 1988.
6. Robins LN, Hezler JE, Weissmann MM, et al: Lifetime prevalence of specific psychiatric disorders in three sites, *Arch Gen Psychiatry* 41:949–958, 1984.
7. Lewis-Hall F: OCD said to be underdiagnosed in minority populations (quote in report), *Psychiatr News* 5, July 1991.
8. Neighbors HW: The help-seeking behavior of black Americans, *J Natl Med Assoc* 80:1009–1012, 1988.
9. Neighbors HW, Caldwell CH, Thompson E, Jackson JS: Help-seeking behavior and unmet need. In Friedman S, editor: *Anxiety disorders in African Americans,* New York, 1994, Springer, pp 26–39.

10. Friedman S, Hatch ML, Paradis C, et al: Obsessive-compulsive disorder in two black ethnic groups: Incidence in an urban dermatology clinic, *J Anx Dis* 7:343–348, 1993.
11. Rassmussen SA: Obsessive-compulsive disorder in dermatologic practice. *J Am Acad Dermatol* 13:965–967, 1985.
12. Deleted in proofs.
13. Paradis CM, Friedman S, Lazar RM, et al: Panic disorder in an inner-city psychiatric outpatient department: Results of a structured interview, *Hosp Comm Psychiatry* 43:61–64, 1992.
14. DiNardo PA, Barlow DH: The Anxiety Disorders Interview Schedule-revised (ADIS-R), Albany, 1988, Phobia and Anxiety Disorders Clinic, State University of New York at Albany.
15. Friedman S, Paradis C: African-American patients with panic disorder and agoraphobia, *J Anx Dis* 5:35–41, 1991.
16. Carey RJ, Baer L, Jenike MA, et al: MMPI correlates of obsessive-compulsive disorder, *J Clin Psychiatry* 47:371–372, 1986.
17. Guarnaccia PJ: A cross-cultural perspective on anxiety disorders. In Friedman S, editor: *Cultural issues in the treatment of anxiety,* New York, 1997, Guilford.
18. Kirmayer LJ: Culture and anxiety: A clinical and research agenda. In Friedman S, editor: *Cultural issues in the treatment of anxiety,* New York, Guilford Press, in press.
19. Paradis CM, Friedman S, Hatch M: Isolated sleep paralysis in African Americans with panic disorder, *Cult Div Ment Health* 3:69–76, 1997.
20. Bertschy G, Ahyi RG: Obsessive-compulsive disorders in Benin: Five case reports, *Psychopathology* 24:398–401, 1991.
21. Hollander E, Cohen LJ: Obsessive-compulsive disorder. In Friedman S, editor: *Anxiety disorders in African Americans,* New York, 1994, Springer, pp 185–202.
22. Hayes SC, Toarmino D: If behavioral principles are generally applicable, why is it necessary to understand cultural diversity? *Behav Ther* 18:21–23, 1995.
23. Goodman WK, Price LH, Delgado PL, et al: Specificity of serotonin reuptake inhibitors in the treatment of obsessive-compulsive disorder: Comparison of fluvoxamine and desipramine, *Arch Gen Psychiatry* 47:577–585, 1990.
24. Goodman WK, Price LH, Rasmussen SA, et al: The Yale-Brown Obsessive Compulsive Scale: I. Development, use and reliability; II. Validity, *Arch Gen Psychiatry* 46:1006–1016, 1989.
25. Foa E, Rowan V: Behavior therapy of OCD. In Bellack AE, Hersen M, editors: *Handbook of comparative treatments for adult disorders,* New York, 1990, John Wiley and Sons.
26. Rassmussen SA, Tuang MT: The epidemiology of obsessive-compulsive disorder, *J Clin Psychiatry* 45:450–457, 1984.
27. Lesser IM, Smith M, Poland RE, Lin KM: Psychopharmacology and ethnicity. In Friedman S, editor: *Cultural issues in the treatment of anxiety,* New York, 1997, Guilford Press.
28. Calvocoressi L, Lewis B, Harris M, et al: Family accommodation in obsessive-compulsive disorder, *Am J Psychiatry* 152:441–443, 1995.
29. Neziroglu F, Yaryura-Tobias JA: *Over and over again,* Lexington, 1991, DC Heath.
30. Steketee G, White K: *When once is not enough,* Oakland, 1990, New Harbinger.

Part V
Patient and Clinic Management

30

Organization and Operation of an Obsessive-Compulsive Disorder Clinic—Management of the Individual Patient

Michael A. Jenike, M.D., Lee Baer, Ph.D.

Over the past few years, we frequently have been asked how to start and run an obsessive-compulsive disorder (OCD) clinic. The demand for our services has exploded over the past decade. This chapter outlines a few basic principles that we use to organize the clinic and patient care.

ORGANIZATION OF AN OBSESSIVE-COMPULSIVE DISORDER CLINIC

Initial Questions

Prior to setting up an OCD clinic, it is imperative that a few basic questions be addressed. How many patients are expected and how will overflow be managed? Who will do the initial assessments and who will follow through with treatment plans? Will the clinic be primarily directed toward service or research? If directed toward research, where will patients who are not appropriate for protocols be referred, and how will these patients be treated once a study is complete? How will patients be billed and charged? What will come of patients who cannot pay?

The answers to each of these questions will determine to a large extent the types of services that are offered. Because the range of combinations is enormous, we will not address each type of organization, but will instead outline how we handle some of these issues in our OCD Clinic at the Massachusetts General Hospital. Many of our clinic procedures and questionnaires should be applicable to other types of practices. Our initial intake questionnaire is presented in Appendix 5. By having the patient complete this form prior to the initial appointment and bring it to the appointment, we were able to decrease our typical initial evaluation time by approximately 50%.

Preevaluation Screening of Patients

Patients or their physicians usually contact our clinic directly. Initially, we were reluctant to allow patients to be self-referred, but we have found over the past few years that almost all of the patients who report OCD symptoms, in fact, suffer from the disorder; as a result, we get very few inappropriate referrals.

A secretary who is familiar with OCD as well as our clinic procedures and protocols does the initial telephone screening and refers non–OCD patients to our general psychopharmacology clinic for evaluation. The secretary tells each patient that a complete evaluation requires at least 1 hour, and either the patient or insurance company will be billed; this fee may be reduced or abolished based on the patient's ability to pay. Patients without resources are asked to apply to the hospital for free care. Because we are partially supported by grants, we have more flexibility in reducing or waiving fees than do many private clinics.

We request that prior to a clinic appointment, patients obtain a copy of their own psychiatric records or get a letter from any mental health professional who has treated them. The clinic secretary then sends out the following material, some of which is to be completed by the patient and brought to the first appointment:

1. Medical, Psychiatric, and Family Information Questionnaire (see Appendix 5).
2. Maudsley Obsessive Compulsive Inventory (see Appendix 7).
3. Beck Depression Inventory (see Appendix 9).
4. The Yale-Brown Obsessive-Compulsive Scale (Y-BOCS) Symptom Checklist (Appendix 12)
5. The Clinic brochure titled "Information for Patients Attending the Massachusetts General Hospital Obsessive-Compulsive Disorders Treatment and Research Clinic" (Appendix 10). This brochure is updated every few months.
6. Insurance Information form.
7. Directions to our clinic.

The First Appointment

Because our patient flow is heavy, we attempt to gather as much information at the first visit as possible. The initial evaluation includes the following:

1. A 45- to 60-minute interview with a psychiatrist who reviews the previously mentioned questionnaires in detail and attempts to get a complete picture of the patient's symptoms, the level of disability, and the history of the illness. The physician completes the "OCD Clinic Initial Evaluation Information"

Form (Appendix 11). This form is used as a guide for data entry into our computer database and serves as a summary of the patient's symptoms, a master list of problems, and an outline of the proposed treatment plan.

2. For difficult or complicated patients, a research associate (with a bachelor's or master's level degree in psychology or psychiatric nurse) may administer the Structured Interview for the Diagnosis of Personality Disorders (SIDP) to each patient (see Chapter 4); this interview lasts hours. Research associates must be specifically trained in the use of this structured interview and demonstrate adequate interrater reliability. The research associate then spends approximately 30 minutes with an informant (family member or friend) to complete the SIDP.

3. The patient is either referred for a research protocol, open medication treatment, behavior therapy, or to another clinic for treatment.

MANAGEMENT OF THE INDIVIDUAL PATIENT

Many of the previous chapters have provided reviews and recommendations concerning OCD patients in general. This chapter outlines an approach to the individual patient who is referred for evaluation and treatment.

Assessment

To outline a treatment plan for an obsessive-compulsive patient, it is necessary to have a clear idea of exactly what the problem is, what exacerbates and what improves it, how it has evolved over the patient's life, and what other symptoms and difficulties exist concomitantly. Optimally, this history-taking will combine behavioral, psychodynamic, and family principles. The questionnaires that the patients bring with them to the first appointment greatly facilitate information-gathering, and we generally review these with the patient and ask about unclear areas.

A thorough mental status examination is performed and the potential for noncompliance is assessed. A depressed, manic, or psychotic patient will require a special treatment strategy because we have found that behavioral treatments for OCD are often ineffective until associated functional illnesses are well controlled. The issues outlined in Table 30-1 should be addressed in each patient. For patients over 50 years of age, or who appear to have cognitive deficits or attentional difficulties, formal cognitive questions as outlined in the Mini-Mental State Examination[1] in Table 30-1 may help to identify deficits and assist in treatment planning. For example, an elderly patient with memory problems may forget behavioral homework if it is not written down for the patient or if the plan is not communicated to those who live with the patient.[2]

In patients who are not clinically depressed, we have not found an increased prevalence of abnormal dexamethasone suppression tests (DSTs), and we do not routinely perform this test in our patients.[3] We have found the Minnesota Multiphasic Personality Inventory (MMPI) to be helpful in history-gathering

Table 30-1   Mental Status Questions

Mood
  Depression
    Dysphoria
    Sleep
      —decreased or increased
      —early morning awakening
    Interest—loss of interest in daily activities, sex, etc.
    Guilt
    Energy—decreased
    Concentration—difficulty
    Appetite—decreased or increased with weight change
    Psychomotor activity—decreased or increased
    Suicide—thoughts, feelings, or plan
  Mania
    Mood—elevated, expansive, or irritable
    Increase in activity
    More talkative than usual or pressure to keep talking
    Flight of ideas or subjective experience that thoughts are racing
    Inflated self-esteem
    Decreased need for sleep
    Distractibility

Psychosis
  Hallucinations
  Delusions
  Ideas of reference
  Paranoia
  Thought insertion or withdrawal

Cognition: Mini-Mental State Examination

Maximum Score	Patient Score	
		Orientation
5	( )	What is the (year) (season) (date) (day) (month)?
5	( )	Where are we (state) (county) (town) (hospital) (floor)?
		Registration
3	( )	Name 3 objects: 1 second to say each. Then ask the patient all 3 after you have said them. Give 1 point for each correct answer. Then repeat them until he learns all 3. Count trials and record. TRIALS _____
		Attention and Calculation
5	( )	Serial 7's: 1 point for each correct. Stop after 5 answers. Alternately spell "world" backwards.
		Recall
3	( )	Ask for 3 objects repeated above. Give 1 point for each correct answer.

Table 30-1 *(Continued)*

		Language
2	( )	Name a pencil and watch.
1	( )	Repeat the following: "no ifs, ands, or buts."
3	( )	Follow a 3-stage command: "Take a paper in your right hand, fold it in half, and put it on the floor." 1 point for each part done correctly.
1	( )	Read and obey the following: "Close your eyes!"
1	( )	Write a sentence. Must contain subject and verb and be sensible.
		Visual-Motor Integrity
1	( )	Copy design (2 intersecting pentagons). All 10 angles must be present and 2 must intersect.
30	**Patient's Total Score** _____	

in the evaluation of our OCD patients, but we do not use this test to follow outcome or treatment response. The Y-BOCS is more useful, and this scale has well-documented reliability (see Chapter 6).

Evaluating Specific Obsessive-Compulsive Disorder Symptoms

Some of the patient's obsessive-compulsive symptoms and problems will be outlined by the clinic questionnaire (Appendix 5). A more detailed symptom description is provided by the Maudsley Obsessive-Compulsive Inventory (MOCI) (Appendix 7), and a fairly complete list of symptoms is outlined in the Y-BOCS Symptom Checklist (Appendix 12). Hodgson and Rachman[4] have validated the MOCI as a research tool but also report that it is useful in routine clinical practice, because it ensures that most complaints are covered during the initial interview. Further, patients have reported relief after completing this questionnaire; they gain confidence in the therapist's ability to understand obsessional problems, because the questionnaire covers so many of their personal complaints. Hodgson and Rachman found that patients suffering from observable obsessive-compulsive rituals complain of four main types of problems: (1) checking; (2) cleaning; (3) slowness; and (4) doubting. The majority of their subjects had more than one obsessional complaint: 76% of checkers complained of doubting, 58% of slowness, and 55% of cleaning problems; 61% of cleaners complained of doubting, 54% of slowness, and 60% of checking rituals. Of those subjects who complained of slowness, 65% also complained of doubting, 60% of checking, and 50% of cleaning problems.

MOCI items can be separated into four subscales based on type of symptom elicited:

1. Checking items include Numbers 2, 6, 8, 14, 15, 20, 22, 26, and 28.
2. Cleaning items include Numbers 1, 5, 9, 13, 17, 19, 21, 24, 26, and 27.
3. Slowness items include Numbers 2, 4, 8, 16, 23, 25, and 29.
4. Doubting items include Numbers 3, 7, 10, 11, 12, 18, and 30.

Medical Evaluation

In Chapter 11, we have outlined potential medical or neurologic causes of OCD. Textbooks of psychiatry do not address the medical work-up of these patients, and organic etiologies are rarely considered. Because the onset of the disorder is infrequent (< 15%) after 35 years of age, at least a neurologic examination should be performed if symptoms *begin* after this age. If abnormalities are found, an electroencephalogram and computed tomography or magnetic resonance imaging scan are indicated. If the onset of OCD is before 35 years of age, the yield of a medical work-up and neurologic examination is almost nil. In any patient, it is very unlikely that correction of a medical illness will remove the OCD symptoms.[3]

Treatment Plan

Pure Obsessionals or Patients with Disorders Related to Obsessive-Compulsive Disorder

In OCD patients who suffer solely from intrusive thoughts and no rituals and those patients with related disorders such as trichotillomania, monosymptomatic hypochondriasis, body dysmorphic disorder, globus hystericus, obsessive fear of illness such as AIDS, bowel and urinary obsessions, and eating disorders, a trial of antidepressant medication is a reasonable first choice for treatment. A wealth of uncontrolled data indicates that such drugs often produce striking improvement in these patients, even when they do not suffer from clinical depression. In those patients who do not respond, behavior therapy techniques as outlined in Chapters 17, 19, and 20 may be of assistance in reducing or alleviating symptoms.

Patients with Compulsive Rituals

There is controversy concerning the *initial* treatment approach of OCD patients who have overt rituals. Although medications are sometimes of help in treating nondepressed patients with clear-cut rituals, the well-documented success of behavior therapy in such patients leads some investigators to begin most nondepressed and nonpsychotic OCD patients on behavior therapy as soon as possible. The technique of exposure and response prevention (ERP) is the mainstay of behavioral treatment for rituals. Other experts begin antiobsessional medication and wait to begin behavior therapy until the patient responds, at least partially, to medication. These experts believe that behavior therapy will proceed more rapidly and with less suffering in the patient once medication has begun to correct the "underlying biologic problem."

It is likely that the initial approach will depend more on the particular clinician's biases and expertise than on scientific facts. Regardless of initial approach, most researchers agree that the combination of pharmacotherapy and skilled behavioral interventions is necessary for the majority of OCD patients to derive maximal treatment benefit.

In patients with concomitant psychiatric symptoms such as major depression, psychosis, or mania, it is unlikely that behavior therapy for OCD will be helpful until these symptoms are well controlled pharmacologically. In such cases, initial therapy should be drug-oriented and behavior therapy should begin only after other functional illnesses are optimally controlled. In patients who only perform ritualistic behaviors at home, it will be necessary for behavior treatment to take place in the home; in this case, family members must function as surrogate therapists and supervise the ERP therapy. Many patients can be treated with behavior therapy in an office setting, with homework assignments given to the patient at the end of each session.

Patients with Severe Personality Disorder

Recent data suggest that patients with schizotypal personality disorder and possibly other severe personality disorders are largely refractory to the usual therapeutic strategies (see Chapter 4). These patients respond differently both to medications and behavioral techniques. Clearly, before definitive recommendations can be given for these patients, additional research will be required; future outcome studies with OCD patients should analyze data separately for patients meeting the *Diagnostic and Statistical Manual of Mental Disorders* (DSM-IV) criteria for severe personality disorders. Currently, we manage such patients by focusing on reducing stress and conflict in their environments. This is achieved through behavioral family or couples counseling and arranging for day treatment or halfway house placement or other alternative living arrangements away from the stressful environment where obsessive-compulsive symptoms often are exacerbated and reinforced. Once out of a stressful environment, the supportive therapy of these patients, with encouragement in ERP and strong verbal reinforcement of the slightest gains, along with medication is often helpful in producing modest improvements in obsessions and compulsions. Knowing whether these interventions and recommendations will yield long-term improvement requires follow-up research.

REFERENCES

1. Folstein MF, Folstein SE, McHugh PR: Mini-Mental State Examination: A practical method of grading the cognitive state of patients for the clinician, *J Psychiatr Res* 12:189–198, 1975.
2. Jenike MA: *Geriatric psychiatry and psychopharmacology: A clinical approach,* Chicago, 1989, Year Book Medical Publishers.
3. Jenike MA: Obsessive-compulsive disorder, *Comp Psychiatry* 24:99–115, 1983.
4. Hodgson RJ, Rachman S: Obsessional-compulsive complaints, *Behav Res Ther* 15:389–395, 1977.

Part VI

Appendixes

Appendix 1
The Obsessive-Compulsive Foundation, Inc.

James Broatch, Executive Director

Until the mid-1980s, obsessive-compulsive disorder (OCD) was considered to be a rare and hard-to-treat illness. Three events occurred in rapid succession to change this view. First, Ciba-Geigy Pharmaceutical Corporation received approval from the Federal Drug Administration (FDA) to test the efficacy and safety of clomipramine as an antiobsessional medication. The news quickly spread that clomipramine worked, and hope-filled individuals with OCD flocked to participating treatment centers throughout the United States.

The second event occurred in New Haven, Connecticut, at the Yale Neuroscience Research Center. Three women, participating in another experimental antiobsessional medication protocol, improved dramatically with the medication, and vowed that they would spread the word that there was now help and hope for those individuals still suffering in fear and silence. Jenny Amlong, Patricia Perkins, and Gail Taylor formed an OCD self-help support group, and convinced the ABC news magazine "20/20" to broadcast the first television show about OCD. The subsequent thousands of letters and phone calls quickly transformed the self-help group into a fledgling national organization.

Concurrently, Dr. Judith Rapoport, chief of the child psychiatry branch of the National Institute of Mental Health (NIMH) wrote *The Boy Who Couldn't Stop Washing*, a compelling narrative of Rapoport's successful treatment of strange and fascinating sickness of ritual and doubts run wild. The book quickly became a New York Times bestseller and greatly increased public and professional awareness of OCD. Five years after its publication, 1,000 copies were still being sold weekly in the United States.

The Obsessive-Compulsive Foundation (OCF) has become a global advocacy organization whose mission continues to be the expansion of research and treatment of obsessive-compulsive disorder and related spectrum disorders.

Remarkable progress has been achieved in the recognition and treatment of OCD. Five antidepressant medications have received the FDA indication for the treatment of OCD, two of which also have a treatment indication for young children with OCD. In May 1997, Expert Consensus Guidelines for Treatment of Obsessive-Compulsive Disorder were released to help clinicians, medical professionals, individuals with OCD, and their support people determine what is appropriate, state-of-the art treatment.

We have learned that early, appropriate intervention is vital for the successful treatment of OCD; yet, a 1995 survey of OCF members revealed that there was a 17-year gap from when obsessive-compulsive symptoms begin and accurate treatment is received. Estimates vary, but it is currently believed that fewer than 20% of individuals with OCD are in treatment. Although OCD is the fourth most common neurobiologic disorder in adults and children, mental health professionals and primary care physicians do not routinely screen for the existence of OCD, and individuals with OCD rarely self-disclose their obsessive-compulsive symptoms.

One of OCF's foremost priorities is to increase public and professional awareness of OCD as a major public health problem. Our message is simple: OCD annually costs the American public $8 billion. According to a 1990 World Health Organization report, obsessive-compulsive disorders are the tenth leading cause of disability in the world. We need to convince the public that although it is perfectly normal for individuals to have obsessive or compulsive personality traits, full-blown OCD is a very painful, chronic, and disabling disorder that has a devastating impact on the individual with OCD and his or her family. The damage wrought rivals the worst cases of bipolar illness and schizophrenia. Most of OCF's eight affiliates and its 250 mutual help and professionally assisted support group networks are working with local schools to spread the word about OCD and its treatment; they are proving that there is help and hope.

One in every 200 children in elementary schools has OCD. OCF is working to familiarize educators with the common red flags that may signal an OCD–related problem (i.e., frequent requests to be excused to go to the bathroom; the presence of dry, chapped, cracked, and even bleeding hands; continual checking of doors, windows, light switches, electric outlets; checking or rechecking of school assignments to the point that they are submitted late or not at all; endless crossouts, tracing, or reerasing of answers, etc.).

To further increase public awareness, OCF has also established a web site on the Internet. More than 7,000 hits from all over the world are recorded each month. Legislative alerts, ongoing research protocols, announcements of upcoming OCD happenings in the media, listings of OCD support groups, the current edition of OCF's bimonthly newsletter, and other pertinent information is posted and updated as needed. OCF is a lifeline for desperate individuals seeking information on ways to help themselves and their loved ones.

Another priority is to increase the availability of high-quality behavior therapy for individuals with OCD. Although cognitive-behavior therapy is considered to be a first-line intervention for OCD, less than 40% of individuals with OCD have been in cognitive-behavioral therapy. OCF has mounted a three-pronged campaign to increase the availability of high-quality behavior therapy. In conjunction with its Scientific Advisory Board, OCF conducts a 3-day Behavior-Therapy Institute (BTI) for mental health clinicians who are licensed or certified by the state to practice independently. The model combines theory and practice. Participating clinicians administer a standardized assessment packet locally to one of the patients. The resulting data enable BTI faculty to follow-up and design a behavioral treatment plan tailored to each training case. Each participating clinician then implements the customized treatment plan, together with three follow-up phone conversations with a faculty consultant. OCF is conducting regional BTIs. Thus far, clinicians from 16 different states and Canada have participated.

In 1996, OCF raised more than $50,000 in cash and in-kind services for individuals whose finances prevent them from entering behavioral therapy. OCF is currently matching those individuals who are financially eligible with clinicians who have donated a 20-behavior-therapy-session block or have agreed to reduce their fees to participate in the behavior therapy scholarship program.

OCF has begun distribution of a manual and video for forming a behavioral support group for OCD—The GOAL Approach: Giving Obsessive-Compulsives Another Lifestyle. Since 1981, Dr. Jon Grayson, a founding member of our Philadelphia OCF affiliate, has cofacilitated a professionally assisted GOAL group. The biweekly group is divided into three parts. The first part is a general discussion of an OCD–related topic that is selected prior to the meeting. In part two, group members divide into small GOAL groups to devise a behavioral goal with an exposure and response prevention component. If an individual does not accomplish this goal, it is redesigned so that he or she is successful the next time. When the GOAL group concept was introduced at OCF's 1995 and 1996 annual membership meetings, more than 50% of the participating individuals accomplished a behavioral goal prior to the meeting conclusion. For many, it was the first time they were successful in regaining some degree of control over their obsessive-compulsive symptoms. Devising goals in a group setting can be an important motivational factor, because individuals know that they will share their progress at the next group session. During the final part of the meeting, with refreshments and socializing, group members are encouraged to share everything they couldn't during the meeting. We believe all three parts of the meeting are critical. The first part allows a sharing of feelings and ideas of general concern to everyone. Goal planning keeps the meetings focused on what everyone can do to help themselves, and socializing helps bring everyone closer, which is crucial, because members will need to depend on others for support in accomplishing the goals.

Since 1993, OCF has been engaged in fundraising to award annual grants on any aspect of research related to obsessive-compulsive disorders. According to C. Everett Koop, former U. S. Surgeon General, only three cents of every health care dollar is spent on biomedical research. A much greater private and public investment is needed to develop newer medications without side effects that currently discourage an individual's medication compliance. Research into children's pharmacologic treatment, complementary medical interventions, and cognitive-behavior therapy also is needed. In 1996, OCF was only able to fund 5 of the 59 submitted applications.

In less than 11 years, OCF and the obsessive-compulsive community have accomplished a great deal. OCD has achieved widespread recognition and hundreds of thousands of individuals are in treatment and recovery. Marc Summers, a television talk-show host, has publicly self-disclosed that he has OCD and has embarked on an OCF and Solvay Pharmaceuticals and Pharmacia & Upjohn–cosponsored campaign to increase awareness of OCD in children and adolescents. His message is: OCD is real, and treatable, and there is help and hope for the estimated 1,000,000 American children with OCD.

OC Foundation, Inc., 9 Depot Street, P.O. Box 70, Milford, CT 06460-0070, (203) 878-5669, fax: (203) 874-2826, EMAIL: jphs28a@prodigy.com, www OCF home page: http://pages.prodigy.com/alwillen/ocf.html

Appendix 2
Resources for People with Obsessive-Compulsive Disorder and Related Disorders

ORGANIZATIONS

Trichotillomania Learning Center
1215 Mission Street, Suite 2
Santa Cruz, CA 95060
Telephone: 1-408-457-1004
E-mail: trichster@aol.com
Membership: $35 includes information packet and bimonthly newsletter
Internet: e-mail to MAJORDOMO@CS.COLUMBIA.EDU with INFO TTM
in body (no subject) for info on subscribing to a list for trichotillomania.
(Independent of Trichotillomania Learning Center)

Obsessive-Compulsive Disorder Hotline
Telephone: 1-800-639-7462

Obsessive-Compulsive Information Center
Dean Foundation for Health and Education
8000 Excelsior Drive, Suite 302
Madison, WI 53717
Telephone: 1-608-836-8070
    The Obsessive-Compulsive Information Center has the ability to perform computer searches on the latest OCD research and clinical papers. A computer database of more than 4,000 references is updated daily. Computer searches are performed for a nominal fee. There is no charge for quick-reference questions. The Center maintains physician referral and support group lists.

National Institute of Mental Health
c/o Research on Obsessive-Compulsive Disorder
Building 10, Room 3D41
10 Center Drive MSC 1264
Bethesda, MD 20892
Telephone: 1-301-496-3421

Information Resources and Inquiries Branch
Room C-02
5600 Fishers Lane
Rockville, MD 20857
Telephone: 1-301-443-4513

Anxiety Disorders Association of America
6000 Executive Boulevard, Suite 513
Rockville, MD 20852
Telephone: 1-301-231-9350
          1-900-737-3400/24-hour service @ $2.00/minute
    This association makes referrals to professional members and to support groups. Has a catalog of available brochures, books, and audiovisuals. Has an annual meeting wherein professionals and patients meet together.

Obsessive Compulsive Anonymous
P.O. Box 215
New Hyde Park, NY 11040
Telephone: 1-516-741-4901

California Affiliate of the Obsessive-Compulsive Foundation
18653 Ventura Boulevard, Suite 414
Tarzana, CA 91356-4174

National Alliance for Mentally Ill
200 North Globe Road, Suite 1015
Arlington, VA 22203
Telephone: 1-800-950-6264

Freedom From Fear
308 Seaview Avenue
Staten Island, NY 10305
Telephone: 1-718-351-1717

Center for Help for Anxiety/Agoraphobia through New Growth Experience (CHAANGE)

National Headquarters
128 Country Club Drive
Chula Vista, CA 91911
Telephone: 1-619-425-3992

Association for Advancement of Behavior Therapy

Seventh Avenue, Suite 1601
New York, NY 10001-6008
Telephone: 1-212-647-1890

This organization maintains a membership listing of mental health professionals focusing on behavior therapy.

Tourette Syndrome Association, Inc.

42-40 Bell Boulevard
New York, NY 11361-2874
Telephone: 1-718-224-2999

Publications, videotapes, and films are available from this organization at minimal cost. A newsletter is sent to members who pay an annual fee of $35.00.

BOOKS

Baer L: *Getting control: overcoming your obsessions and compulsions.*

Foa E, Wilson R: *Stop obsessing! how to overcome your obsessions and compulsions.*

Neziroglu F, Yaryura-Tobias JA: *Over and over again: understanding obsessive-compulsive disorder.*

Steketee G, White K: *When once is not enough: help for obsessive-compulsives.*

Foster C: *Funny you don't look crazy: Life with obsessive-compulsive disorder.*

Greist JH: *Obsessive-compulsive disorder: a guide,* Madison, 1992, Dean Foundation. This booklet is available through the Obsessive-Compulsive Foundation.

Foster C: *Polly's magic games: a child's view of obsessive-compulsive disorder,* 1994, Dilligaf.

New developments in the biology of mental disorders, Research and Education Association 1995, Section on government funding/research.

Jenike MA, Baer L, Minichiello WE, editors: *Obsessive-compulsive disorders: theory and management,* ed 2, Chicago, 1990, Year Book Medical.

Elfenbein D: *Living with prozac and other selective serotonin reuptake inhibitors,* San Francisco, 1995, Harper. Personal accounts of life on antidepressants.

Jenike MA, Asberg M, editors: *Understanding obsessive-compulsive disorder,*

1990, Stuttgart, Hogrefe & Huber Publishers.

Jenike MA, editor: Obsessional disorders, *Psychiatr Clin North Am* 15(4), December 1992.

Callner J, writer/director: The Touching Tree (videotape), Awareness films. Distributed by the Obsessive-Compulsive Foundation, Milford, Connecticut. A film about a child with OCD.

INTERNET SITES

Obsessive-Compulsive Disorder Newsgroup can be found at alt.support.ocd

OCD-L mailing list on the Internet. To subscribe send e-mail to:
LISTSERV@VM.MARIST.EDU
with blank subject line and in the body of e-mail the command
SUB OCD-L <your real name>
For example: <subject blank> SUB OCD-L John Doe

Prodigy On-Line Bulletin Board Service for Obsessive-Compulsive Disorder
It can be found by: (jump) medical support bb; choose topic "anx/dep/ocd"; look in subject area for subjects beginning with "OCD."

Obsessive-Compulsive Disorder Chat on America Online
Wednesday at 9:00 pm EST
It can be found by keyword: PEN
>chat rooms
health conference room

Internet Relay Chat: IRC
Log onto a server at port 6667.
Type /NICK <name> to register.
Type /JOIN ##OCD to find listserv members.
Type /NAMES ##OCD to get list of current users.
Best times vary. Try noon to 2:00 pm EST and 8:00 to 10:00 pm EST.

World Wide Web Site for Obsessive-Compulsive Disorder
Vast amount of info on OCD including how to get free meds.
http://www.fairlite/ocd/

World Wide Web Site for Psychopharmacology
http://uhs.bsd.uchicago.edu/~bhsiung/tips.html

World Wide Web Site for Medication Support by Drug Companies
http://pharminfo.com

Appendix 3

Obsessive-Compulsive Disorder:
A Guide*

Obsessive Compulsive Information Center,
Dean Foundation for Health, Research and Education

WHAT IS OBSESSIVE-COMPULSIVE DISORDER?

Obsessive-compulsive disorder (OCD) commonly involves both obsessions and compulsions. Occasionally, an afflicted person will have only obsessions or compulsions.

Obsessions are unwanted, intrusive ideas, images, impulses, or worries that run through a person's mind repeatedly. Often the obsessions are senseless, unpleasant, distasteful, or even repugnant, and typically they involve themes of harm. Common obsessions include: (1) repeated impulses to kill a beloved family member; (2) incessant worries about dirt, germs, contamination, infection, and contagion; (3) recurrent thoughts that something has not been done properly even when the individual knows it has; (4) blasphemous thoughts in a religious person; (5) fears of losing something even though it is of little or no importance; (6) feelings that certain things must always be in a certain place, position, or order; (7) worries about the shape or functioning of body parts; or (8) nonsensical sounds, words, numbers, or images. For some, infrequent obsessions cause great anguish, whereas for others, incessant obsessions may be viewed as a mildly annoying "background noise."

Compulsions are strong urges to do something to reduce anxiety or other discomfort from obsessions. Usually certain behaviors (either physical actions or mental thoughts) called rituals are repeated in response to an obsession. Rituals do reduce discomfort or anxiety caused by an obsession. However, relief from rituals is often incomplete and always short-lived, so they must be repeated frequently and soon become a problem in their own right because they are

---

* ©1997 by John H. Greist. Modified with permission from the authors. Inclusion of this booklet is not intended for reproduction. Copies can be purchased from the Dean Foundation Information Centers, 2711 Allen Blvd., Middleton, WI 53562, 608-827-2390.

excessive. Rituals must be performed in a specific manner or even according to self-prescribed "rules." Sometimes, the behavior does not appear related to relieving an obsession, and sufferers are at a loss to explain the overwhelming compulsion they feel to carry out the ritual. Ritualistic behaviors do not provide pleasure but are continued because they reduce tension, discomfort, or anxiety associated with obsessions. Ritualistic behaviors are almost always recognized as excessive or unrealistic, although some children may deny the redundancy of their actions and some older sufferers may have given up resisting their compulsions.

Common cleaning or washing rituals include excessive hand washing, showering, bathing, toothbrushing, or grooming, cleaning household items, and avoiding contaminants. *Checking rituals* often involve doors, locks, and appliances, and assuring that nothing bad has happened. *Repeating behaviors* include putting clothing on, then taking it off, going to and fro through a door, or touching certain objects. *Placing things* in a certain position or order decreases discomfort from obsessions about disorder and dissymmetry. *Hoarding,* so that nothing of value will be lost, and *having to do something exceedingly slowly* to feel that it has been done properly are less common problems but can be very disabling. *Seeking reassurance* that something has or has not happened is a common ritual that involves others, often unwittingly, in a patient's ritualistic behaviors.

Mental rituals deserve special mention. Mental rituals may be mistaken for obsessions because they occur as thoughts rather than external and observable behaviors. Mental rituals are easily distinguished from obsessions. Obsessions *increase* discomfort, anxiety, or rituals and mental rituals *decrease* discomfort, anxiety, or rituals. In technical terms, obsessions are anxiogenic (generating or producing anxiety) whereas rituals are anxiolytic (lysing or breaking down anxiety or other discomfort).

Just as obsessions vary in their frequency and intensity, compulsions may occur only rarely but can consume many hours each day.

Obsessive-compulsive disorder can be a mild problem unnoticed by anyone except the individual involved. It can create varying amounts of difficulty for the sufferer and family members as it waxes and wanes, or it can be of such severity that it consumes the sufferer's attention and energies and involves family members in elaborate rituals to "keep the peace."

Case Histories

One patient described her obsessions and compulsive rituals as follows:

My disorder began around 21 years of age. It has been constantly present in various forms since then. The onset was gradual and I have never been completely free of it. I was a new R.N. (registered nurse) working at a hospital and not very confident. Every so often I would be afraid I contaminated a needle or IV, but I wasn't sure.

I changed jobs 1 year later. I left because I was doubting myself constantly in my nursing tasks. I would aspirate two or three times, afraid I hit a blood vessel when giving an injection. It would take me very long to clean proctoscopes after assisting in the procedure. I would throw things away (at one point a whole tube of KY jelly) because of fear of contamination. I would go from one doctor to another asking many questions regarding germs and air bubbles in syringes and what was safe. At this point, I didn't have the feeling that I was constantly dirty or contaminating things at home—that came later.

I left the clinic and worked for an insurance company in 1976–1977 as a claims adjuster. That was fine until I started to check claims over and over to see if I had coded them right. I felt guilty, and I do to this day, about not working to my fullest and daydreaming a lot of the days away.

At this time, my worst obsessions and compulsions started. I became unsure of whether I was clean enough when I went to the bathroom. I started obsessing and felt I had killed someone. I had trouble doing the wash—not knowing if I put soap in the machine. I had the feeling it was stool (feces) instead. I felt ashamed and guilty having such grotesque thoughts.

Behavior therapy made a big difference. I worked hard to decrease my washing, gradually at first and then more rapidly. At the same time, I stopped avoiding most of the situations that made me worry and want to wash. To my surprise and great relief, my fears decreased rapidly and steadily, and my feelings of being dirty or hurting others became faint thoughts in the back of my mind rather than overwhelming concerns I felt compelled to act on by washing or avoiding.

Another patient describes her problems with hoarding as follows:

For 17 years, I have been afraid I might lose something important. At first, this just led to a quick check to make sure I wasn't leaving something behind. I soon began to doubt that my checking had been thorough enough and intensified my efforts by checking very closely and repeating the process. My concerns about loss first focused on things of obvious value such as jewelry or other important possessions, but I soon began to worry about throwing anything out for fear I might discard something of importance with trash or garbage. This led to difficulty with trash and garbage, and this problem grew to the point that I truly could not throw anything out, including such things as our 3-year-old Christmas tree or the needles that fell from it. When I came for treatment, every room of our house was full to overflowing with junk and garbage because I couldn't discard anything.

After treatment with clomipramine, my fears lessened substantially and I was again able to wear jewelry (before I was afraid I would lose it) and to throw out things from the house (including the Christmas tree!) without excessive worry.

> Behavior therapy was difficult for me because I still believed I needed to be in complete control of things that left my house, but the principles of behavior therapy make sense and, as I have applied them myself, are clearly helpful.

A man illustrates fears of harming others, checking, and avoidance:

> For as many years as I can remember, I have been afraid that I would harm others intentionally, although I have never done so and find the idea of hurting others repugnant. The problem bothers me everywhere although it is least troublesome when I am at home. At work, I am afraid I might put poison in the common coffeepot and not know I had done it, so I don't even walk down the hallway where the coffeepot is located. On the way home from work, I have my wife or children meet me at the bus stop so they can reassure me I haven't harmed any of the children who are playing in their yards as I pass by. When I went to my son's cross-country meet and saw the line indicating the course that was marked with lime, I worried that I had poisoned the powdered sugar donuts I saw at the meet with lime I had picked up.
>
> I have had little benefit from clomipramine and fluvoxamine and had great difficulty following through on the behavior therapy program and still have substantial problems with my obsessions and rituals.

Obsessive-compulsive disorder often begins in childhood. Fully one third of cases have appeared by 15 years of age with the majority of additional cases emerging before 30 years of age. Once present, untreated OCD usually follows a fluctuating course, waxing and waning for the rest of the individual's life. Men and women are equally likely to be affected, but average age of onset is 17 in men and 21 in women. If OCD interferes substantially with life's activities, secondary depression is common. Alcohol and other drugs may be used to the point of abuse in a misguided attempt at self-treatment.

Obsessive-Compulsive Spectrum Disorders

A large number of other disorders share some characteristics with OCD and are sometimes referred to as obsessive-compulsive spectrum disorders. Thus, *hypochondriasis* is typified by obsessions about having a dread disease and rituals of repeatedly asking doctors for reassurance that the disease is not present. *Anorexia nervosa* is characterized by obsessions about being fat despite obvious malnutrition and rituals such as calorie counting, hoarding certain foods, and compulsively exercising to lose weight. Some people are obsessed that their bodies are so misshapen that they are truly ugly (*body dysmorphic disorder*). Others feel compelled to pull out hair (*trichotillomania*— see page 60 regarding a booklet on trichotillomania). Some sufferers of these obsessive-compulsive spectrum disorders respond to treatments effective in OCD–behavior therapy and potent serotonin reuptake inhibitor medications.

COMMONLY ASKED QUESTIONS ABOUT OBSESSIVE-COMPULSIVE DISORDER

How common is obsessive-compulsive disorder? Many sufferers hide their difficulties from friends and coworkers and, sometimes, even family members. They feel alone and are embarrassed about obsessions that are at best silly, often nasty, and sometimes horrific. They recognize that their ritualistic behaviors seem bizarre and worry (unfortunately with some justification) about stigmatization if they disclose their disorder. OCD has been a hidden epidemic. The landmark National Institute of Mental Health Epidemiologic Study of 18,000 Americans interviewed in their homes found that 1.3% reported enough obsessive-compulsive symptoms to meet criteria for the diagnosis in the past month and that 2.5% had suffered the disorder at some point in their lives. The severity of OCD varies. Some cases are so mild that treatment is not sought. Other cases are so severe that the sufferer does nothing but compulsive rituals throughout all waking hours, often late into the night. Now that effective treatments for OCD are becoming available, more sufferers are seeking help, and there is a growing awareness that OCD is more common than previously recognized.

Is obsessive-compulsive disorder inherited? Some families have at least four successive generations with clear cases of OCD. Because family members could have "learned" these behaviors from other family members, the presence of OCD across generations does not prove inheritance. However, successive family members often have different obsessions and compulsions, suggesting that they have not "learned" specific obsessions or compulsions. What appears to be inherited is a capacity to respond to common life experiences with obsessions and compulsions. Specific genetic sites and mechanisms of inheritance of OCD have not been identified.

There are a few studies of inheritance involving identical and fraternal twins that also provide supportive evidence for an inherited component in OCD. However, many individuals suffering from OCD have no family members with any symptoms of OCD.

What causes OCD? There is growing evidence based on several lines of research that OCD involves abnormal metabolism in specific areas of the brain. Further, considerable evidence suggests that abnormalities in functioning of a specific neurotransmitter (chemical messenger) called serotonin may be prominently involved in OCD.

The front part of the brain, which lies just over the eyes (orbital cortex), is involved with social consciousness regarding proper behavior. Underactivity of that part of the brain (whether occurring naturally or as a result of damage from injury, infection, or brain tumor) leads to coarsening of social consciousness and behaviors such as hypersexuality, overeating to the point of massive obesity, and personality changes as, for example, frequent and inappropriate use of profanity and making crude jokes. Overactivity of the same part of the brain appears to result in excessive social concern with meticulousness, fastidiousness, "nitpicking," and, it is believed, symptoms of OCD.

Other brain structures, such as the caudates, filter information coming from the front part of the brain. Some doctors believe that if too many messages regarding worries about how things should be done reach the caudates, they are not filtered properly and spill over into and flood consciousness. Increased metabolism of frontal parts of the brain concerned with order and social propriety and the inability of the caudate structures to properly filter increased messages from these frontal areas may be important components of OCD. Caudate structures also are involved in regular, repetitive behaviors, and abnormalities of the caudates may play a part in rituals.

Both the frontal brain areas and the caudates are richly supplied with serotonin neurons. Operations that interrupt a small number of serotonin neurons and medications that alter functioning of serotonin neurons are helpful to many obsessive-compulsive patients. However, and this is a very important point, although serotonin is an important factor in OCD, that knowledge tells us little about the ultimate causes or triggers of OCD or effective treatments of OCD. Serotonin abnormalities may *result from* rather than be the cause of OCD. Also, changes in serotonin neurotransmission have effects on some of the more than 60 other neurotransmitters and neuromodulators that affect thoughts, feelings, and behaviors. OCD is probably the final expression of many different kinds of abnormalities in the structure and functioning of the brain. This complexity helps us understand why different treatments are helpful and why some sufferers fail to respond to treatments that are effective for others.

What about unconscious conflicts and other causes of OCD? There have been many speculations about factors that may cause OCD. For many years, psychoanalysts held that obsessive-compulsive symptoms were symbolic of and signaled underlying conflicts, often involving aggression, hidden in the unconscious. Despite the elegance of these theories, attempts to change obsessive-compulsive symptoms by uncovering and working through these conflicts have not been effective for most patients. What's more, there is no proof that these theories are even correct.

Currently, some "clinical ecologists" claim that OCD may be related to "allergies," a claim they also make regarding many other mental and physical disorders. To date, there has been no systematic evidence to support this claim.

Specific causes of OCD have been identified infrequently but are impressive when seen. Von Economo's encephalitis, which occurred in epidemic proportions at the end of the First World War, produced compulsive behaviors in some of its victims. This encephalitis (infection of the brain) involved many brain areas, including the caudates. Head injuries that involve the part of the frontal surface (cortex) of the brain overlying the eyes (orbital cortex) can lead to OCD symptoms. Sydenham's chorea (also called St. Vitus dance) results from the body's attempt to throw off a streptococcal infection involving the caudates. This "autoimmune" reaction not only kills the streptococci but also changes the caudates and can result in development of OCD. In one small series of patients with a history of Sydenham's chorea, 14% developed OCD, a rate much greater than that found in the general population.

Individuals who are raised in religions with many ritualistic practices may be more susceptible to developing religious rituals. This raises the possibility that some OCD may be related to learning or other experiences individuals have as they grow and develop. Learning theory provides a good explanation for some aspects of OCD. It suggests that when a person anxious from any cause performs some act, either by intention or accident, that causes the anxiety to decrease, that act is reinforced and repeated. Such acts might be as different as handwashing and making sure the letters on a bar of soap are upright. In time, a whole range of behaviors becomes established in this ritualistic manner, giving rise to OCD. This model does not explain the development of all cases of OCD but fits well with some patients' histories.

There are almost certainly several causes of OCD that are manifested in common symptoms of obsessions and rituals. It seems probable that there is an interaction between genetic predisposition, biochemical factors, and experiences in life that encourage or protect against the development of OCD. Although our knowledge about the causes of OCD is currently fragmentary, it is important not to focus on cause at the expense of what is known about effective treatments. We know a pittance about cause but have a purse full of knowledge about effective treatment.

What other disorders may be confused with OCD? People sometimes wonder if compulsive eating or drinking or gambling or deviant sexual behaviors are forms of OCD. These are not customarily classified as OCD because some pleasure is obtained from these activities and the person would not, ordinarily, wish to stop them except for secondary problems they cause (such as obesity, convictions for driving when intoxicated, gambling debts, and criminal prosecution for sexual deviancy). Nevertheless, a few individuals with these compulsive behaviors may respond to drug and behavioral treatments that are effective for OCD. As our understanding of the spectrum of obsessive-compulsive phenomena improves, some reclassification of these disorders may occur.

Depression may bring on obsessive-compulsive symptoms. Sometimes the content of depressive thinking is typical of OCD (fears about the future), but more often depressive thoughts are focused on the past and appear in the form of self-condemnatory ruminations. This distinction is not absolute, as unrealistic worries about the future also can appear in non–OCD depression.

The distinction between delusions (firmly fixed but false beliefs) in schizophrenia, psychotic depression, or mania and overvalued ideas (strong beliefs that are wrong, which the person grudgingly admits are not true) in OCD is sometimes difficult to make. However, the overall diagnosis of schizophrenia, psychotic depression, or mania is usually straightforward because of other characteristic features such as hallucinations, perplexity, withdrawal, decreased motivation, and hyperactivity.

How do phobias differ from OCD? Both phobic and obsessive-compulsive persons usually avoid feared objects and both kinds of patients retain insight— an awareness that their fears and avoidance behaviors are excessive. But although phobias and OCD have some similar characteristics, there are clear differences between them, and the distinction is usually easy to make.

Phobics are usually most upset about the prospect of actually coming in contact with the thing they fear and do what they can to avoid such contact; obsessive-compulsive patients may be more concerned about the time-consuming rituals such contact will trigger than they are about the contact itself.

Phobic fears are usually more specific than obsessive fears. Even the seemingly general fears of agoraphobics can be summarized as fear of being stuck in some situation from which escape would be difficult or in which they might be alone if they felt frightened. An obsessive-compulsive person fearful of contamination can worry about germs being everywhere and have rituals triggered by many different situations.

Finally, obsessive-compulsive people may express more disgust or discomfort than anxiety when asked to confront their feared objects, although anxiety is frequently apparent too. Phobics usually become or feel noticeably anxious and fearful, seldom expressing disgust at the prospect of contact with their phobic objects or situations.

How do families became involved in compulsive rituals? Sufferers of OCD worry and become anxious or frightened that they will feel tense, anxious, or uncomfortable, or worse, that some calamity may occur unless they take "precautions" to prevent it. These precautions usually occur in the form of compulsive rituals. Sometimes they can relieve their anxiety/tension/discomfort/fears by performing rituals themselves. Sometimes, however, other family members seem to be part of the problem. For example, a father concerned about contamination will worry as his wife and children come home from work, school, or play—who knows where they have been and with what and whom they have come in contact. A wife with OCD may explain to family members that she would "feel better" if they all washed their hands whenever they came into the house.

Contamination obsessions commonly spread to concerns about shoes, because it is easy to imagine what shoes may have come in contact with. The next "request" may be that family members have "inside" and "outside" shoes. If these obsessions spread, it may seem necessary to have "inside" and "outside" clothing; to take showers upon returning home; to exclude nonfamily members because they might carry contamination inside; to "sanitize" food from the market with a cloth soaked in a disinfectant solution; to wash clothing several times to ensure cleanliness; and to clean and order the house in specific ways to reduce the affected member's discomfort. It may seem less troublesome for family members to spend a few minutes or even hours every day or week performing rituals than it is to engage in constant arguments with the obsessive-compulsive family member. Once this process starts, it becomes so habitual that family members often view their participation as "just the way we do things in our family."

When should I seek treatment for OCD? Most of us have occasional thoughts that seem senseless, and many of us also have habits or rituals that we perform infrequently and which interfere little, if at all, with our functioning. These are not the stuff of OCD requiring treatment. In fact, symptoms and signs of such mild severity would not even qualify for a diagnosis of OCD.

When obsessions and rituals reach the level that they interfere substantially with a person's "normal routine, occupational (or academic) functioning, or usual social activities or relationships" or "cause marked distress, are time-consuming (take more than 1 hour a day)," then a diagnosis of OCD is warranted according to criteria in the *Diagnostic and Statistical Manual of Mental Disorders, Fourth Edition* (DSM-IV) (American Psychiatric Association, Wash-ington, DC, 1994). Even after a diagnosis is made, many individuals do not seek treatment because of embarrassment. Deciding when to seek treatment is a personal matter, although family members and the person's physician or therapist can be helpful in making the decision.

How is the severity of obsessions and compulsions evaluated? The severity of obsessions and compulsions may be partly determined by the extent to which an individual tends to avoid certain situations, is slow in completing them, or repeats them. People avoid situations that trigger obsessions, discomfort, or rituals. Slowness may result from repeating rituals or checking to see that something is done "just right." And the hallmark of rituals is the need to repeat them. The Obsessive-Compulsive Checklist (Table A.1) permits an individual to rate these aspects of functioning for activities that are commonly difficult for obsessive-compulsive patients. In general, total scores above 10 raise a question about OCD, and those above 20 indicate it even more strongly. The Yale-Brown Obsessive-Compulsive Scale (Y-BOCS) is another commonly used scale for rating severity of OCD (Table A.2). This 10-item scale has

Table A.1 Obsessive-Compulsive Checklist

People with your kind of problem occasionally have difficulty with some of the following activities. Answer each question by writing the appropriate number in the box next to it.

0 *No problem with activity—takes same time as average person. I do not need to repeat or avoid it.*

1 *Activity takes me twice as long as most people, or I have to repeat it twice, or I tend to avoid it.*

2 *Activity takes me three times as long as most people, or I have to repeat it three or more times, or I usually avoid it.*

Score	Activity	Score	Activity
☐	Taking a bath or shower	☐	Touching door handles
☐	Washing hands and face	☐	Touching own genitals, petting, or sexual intercourse
☐	Care of hair (e.g., washing, combing, brushing)	☐	Throwing things away
☐	Brushing teeth	☐	Visiting a hospital
☐	Dressing and undressing	☐	Turning lights and taps on or off
☐	Using toilet to urinate	☐	Locking or closing doors or windows
☐	Using toilet to defecate		
☐	Touching people or being touched	☐	Using electrical appliances (e.g., heaters)
☐	Handling waste or waste bins	☐	Doing arithmetic or accounts
☐	Washing clothing	☐	Getting to work
☐	Washing dishes	☐	Doing own work
☐	Handling or cooking food	☐	Writing
☐	Cleaning the house	☐	Form filling
☐	Keeping things tidy	☐	Mailing letters
☐	Bed making	☐	Reading
☐	Cleaning shoes	☐	TOTAL

Reproduced from Greist JH, Jefferson JW, Marks IM: *Anxiety and its treatment: help is available,* Washington, DC, 1986, American Psychiatric Press. Used with permission.

five items for obsessions and five for compulsive rituals. Total scores of 16 or above indicate at least moderate severity. Many patients with scores of 10 seek treatment, whereas most individuals with scores below 5 are comfortable enough with their disorder that they do not need treatment. A computer-administered version of the Y-BOCS can be self-administered by dialing an 800 telephone number and is available at no charge from the Dean Foundation. The Obsessive-Compulsive Information Center at the Dean Foundation (see address, page 728) can be contacted for further information about the computer version.

It is important to keep in mind that the Obsessive-Compulsive Checklist and Y-BOCS are only indicators of the possibility of OCD. Even if an individual shows clear obsessive-compulsive symptoms, careful evaluation and diagnosis are necessary to discriminate among the many possible causes of such symptoms. A few obsessive-compulsive symptoms and behaviors that may be severely disabling are not represented in the checklist, and some obsessive-compulsive people do not actively report their distress or tend to minimize its effect. If OCD causes enough distress or dysfunction for a sufferer to seek treatment, then it is probably severe enough to warrant treatment.

YALE-BROWN OBSESSIVE-COMPULSIVE SCALE (Y-BOCS)*

"I am now going to ask several questions about your obsessive thoughts." [Make specific reference to the patient's target obsessions.]

1. TIME OCCUPIED BY OBSESSIVE THOUGHTS
   Q: How much of your time is occupied by obsessive thoughts? [When obsessions occur as brief, intermittent intrusions, it may be difficult to assess time occupied by them in terms of total hours. In such cases, estimate time by determining how frequently they occur. Consider both the number of times the intrusions occur and how many hours of the day are affected. Ask:] How frequently do the obsessive thoughts occur? [Be sure to exclude ruminations and preoccupations that, unlike obsessions, are ego syntonic and rational (but exaggerated).]
      0 = None.
      1 = Mild, less than 1 hr/day or occasional intrusion.
      2 = Moderate, 1 to 3 hrs/day or frequent intrusion.
      3 = Severe, greater than 3 and up to 8 hrs/day or very frequent intrusion.
      4 = Extreme, greater than 8 hrs/day or near constant intrusion.
2. INTERFERENCE DUE TO OBSESSIVE THOUGHTS
   Q: How much do your obsessive thoughts interfere with your social or work (or role) functioning? Is there anything that you don't do because

---

*Used with permission from Wayne K. Goodman, M.D.

of them? [If currently not working, determine how much performance would be affected if patient were employed.]

   0 = None.

   1 = Mild, slight interference with social or occupational activities, but overall performance not impaired.

   2 = Moderate, definite interference with social or occupational performance, but still manageable.

   3 = Severe, causes substantial impairment in social or occupational performance.

   4 = Extreme, incapacitating.

3. DISTRESS ASSOCIATED WITH OBSESSIVE THOUGHTS

   Q: How much distress do your obsessive thoughts cause you? [In most cases, distress is equated with anxiety; however, patients may report that their obsessions are "disturbing" but deny "anxiety." Only rate anxiety that seems triggered by obsessions, not generalized anxiety or anxiety associated with other conditions.]

   0 = None.

   1 = Mild, not too disturbing.

   2 = Moderate, disturbing, but still manageable.

   3 = Severe, very disturbing.

   4 = Extreme, near-constant and disabling distress.

4. RESISTANCE AGAINST OBSESSIONS

   Q: How much of an effort do you make to resist the obsessive thoughts? How often do you try to disregard or turn your attention away from these thoughts as they enter your mind? [Only rate effort made to resist, not success or failure in actually controlling the obsessions. How much the patient resists the obsessions may or may not correlate with his/her ability to control them. Note that this item does not directly measure the severity of the intrusive thoughts; rather it rates a manifestation of health, that is, the effort the patient makes to counteract the obsessions by means other than avoidance or the performance of compulsions. Thus, the more the patient tries to resist, the less impaired is this aspect of his/her functioning. There are "active" and "passive" forms of resistance. Patients in behavioral therapy may be encouraged to counteract their obsessive symptoms by not struggling against them (e.g., "just let the thoughts come"; passive opposition) or by intentionally bringing on the disturbing thoughts. For the purposes of this item, consider use of these behavioral techniques as forms of resistance. If the obsessions are minimal, the patient may not feel the need to resist them. In such cases, a rating of "0" should be given.]

   0 = Makes an effort to always resist, or symptoms so minimal doesn't need to actively resist.

   1 = Tries to resist most of the time.

2 = Makes some effort to resist.

3 = Yields to all obsessions without attempting to control them, but does so with some reluctance.

4 = Completely and willingly yields to all obsessions.

5. DEGREE OF CONTROL OVER OBSESSIVE THOUGHTS

Q: How much control do you have over your obsessive thoughts? How successful are you in stopping or diverting your obsessive thinking? Can you dismiss them? [In contrast to the preceding item on resistance, the ability of the patient to control his obsessions is more closely related to the severity of the intrusive thoughts.]

0 = Complete control.

1 = Much control, usually able to stop or divert obsessions with some effort and concentration.

2 = Moderate control, sometimes able to stop or divert obsessions.

3 = Little control, rarely successful in stopping or dismissing obsessions, can only divert attention with difficulty.

4 = No control, experienced as completely involuntary, rarely able to even momentarily alter obsessive thinking.

"The next several questions are about your compulsive behaviors." [Make specific reference to the patient's target compulsions.]

6. TIME SPENT PERFORMING COMPULSIVE BEHAVIORS

Q: How much time do you spend performing compulsive behaviors? [When rituals involving activities of daily living are chiefly present, ask:] How much longer than most people does it take to complete routine activities because of your rituals? [When compulsions occur as brief, intermittent behaviors, it may be difficult to assess time spent performing them in terms of total hours. In such cases, estimate time by determining how frequently they are performed. Consider both the number of times compulsions are performed and how many hours of the day are affected. Count separate occurrences of compulsive behaviors, not number of repetitions; for example, a patient who goes into the bathroom 20 different times a day to wash his hands 5 times very quickly, performs compulsions 20 times a day, not 5 or 5 x 20 = 100. Ask:] How frequently do you perform compulsions? [In most cases compulsions are observable behaviors (e.g., handwashing), but some compulsions are covert (e.g., silent checking).]

0 = None.

1 = Mild (spends less than 1 hr/day performing compulsions), or occasional performance of compulsive behaviors.

2 = Moderate (spends from 1 to 3 hrs/day performing compulsions), or frequent performance of compulsive behaviors.

3 = Severe (spends more than 3 and up to 8 hrs/day performing compulsions), or very frequent performance of compulsive behaviors.

4 = Extreme (spends more than 8 hrs/day performing compulsions), or near-constant performance of compulsive behaviors (too numerous to count).

7. INTERFERENCE DUE TO COMPULSIVE BEHAVIORS

Q: How much do your compulsive behaviors interfere with your social or work (or role) functioning? Is there anything that you don't do because of the compulsions? [If currently not working, determine how much performance would be affected if patient were employed.]

0 = None.

1 = Mild, slight interference with social or occupational activities, but overall performance not impaired.

2 = Moderate, definite interference with social or occupational performance, but still manageable.

3 = Severe, causes substantial impairment in social or occupational performance.

4 = Extreme, incapacitating.

8. DISTRESS ASSOCIATED WITH COMPULSIVE BEHAVIOR

Q: How would you feel if prevented from performing your compulsion(s)? [Pause] How anxious would you become? [Rate degree of distress patient would experience if performance of the compulsion were suddenly interrupted without reassurance offered. In most, but not all cases, performing compulsions reduces anxiety. If, in the judgment of the interviewer, anxiety is actually reduced by preventing compulsions in the manner described above, then ask:] How anxious do you get while performing compulsions until you are satisfied they are completed?

0 = None.

1 = Mild, only slightly anxious if compulsions prevented, or only slight anxiety during performance of compulsions.

2 = Moderate, reports that anxiety would mount but remain manageable if compulsions prevented, or that anxiety increases but remains manageable during performance of compulsions.

3 = Severe, prominent and very disturbing increase in anxiety if compulsions interrupted, or prominent and very disturbing increase in anxiety during performance of compulsions.

4 = Extreme, incapacitating anxiety from any intervention aimed at modifying activity, or incapacitating anxiety develops during performance of compulsions.

9. RESISTANCE AGAINST COMPULSIONS

Q: How much of an effort do you make to resist the compulsions? [Only rate effort made to resist, not success or failure in actually controlling the compulsions. How much the patient resists the compulsions may or may not correlate with his ability to control them. Note that this item does not directly measure the severity of the compulsions; rather it rates a manifestation of health, that is, the effort the patient makes to counteract the compulsions. Thus, the more the patient tries to resist, the less impaired is this aspect of his functioning. If the compulsions are minimal, the patient may not feel the need to resist them. In such cases, a rating of "0" should be given.]

    0 = Makes an effort to always resist, or symptoms so minimal doesn't need to actively resist.

    1 = Tries to resist most of the time.

    2 = Makes some effort to resist.

    3 = Yields to almost all compulsions without attempting to control them, but does so with some reluctance.

    4 = Completely and willingly yields to all compulsions.

10. DEGREE OF CONTROL OVER COMPULSIVE BEHAVIOR

    Q: How strong is the drive to perform the compulsive behavior? [Pause] How much control do you have over the compulsions? [In contrast to the preceding item on resistance, the ability of the patient to control his compulsions is more closely related to the severity of the compulsions.]

    0 = Complete control.

    1 = Much control, experiences pressure to perform the behavior but usually able to exercise voluntary control over it.

    2 = Moderate control, strong pressure to perform behavior, can control it only with difficulty.

    3 = Little control, very strong drive to perform behavior, must be carried to completion, can only delay with difficulty.

    4 = No control, drive to perform behavior experienced as completely involuntary and overpowering, rarely able to even momentarily delay activity.

TREATMENT OF OBSESSIVE-COMPULSIVE DISORDER

The past 20 years have seen the emergence and evaluation of two effective forms of treatment of OCD. Behavior therapy provides obsessive-compulsive patients with a successful method for decreasing discomfort from obsessions and for reducing or eliminating compulsive rituals. Drug treatment using medications with marked effects on serotonin neurotransmission has also been shown to be effective in decreasing both obsessions and compulsions. The combination of behavior therapy and medications that enhance serotonin neurotransmission is presently the most effective treatment for almost all patients. Although these treatments will be discussed separately for purposes of clarity, it is important to avoid pitting these two complementary approaches against each other.

Table A.2   Yale-Brown Obsessive-Compulsive Scale (Y-BOCS)

Patient's Name _____   Date _____
Patient ID _____   Rater _____

Obsession Rating Scale (circle appropriate score)

	Item	None	Mild	Moderate	Severe	Extreme
1	Time spent on Obsessions	0 hrs/day	0–1 hrs/day	1–3 hrs/day	3–8 hrs/day	>8 hrs/day
	Score	0	1	2	3	4
2	Interference from Obsessions	None	Mild	Manageable	Severe	Incapacitating
	Score	0	1	2	3	4
3	Distress from Obsessions	None	Mild	Moderate	Severe	Disabling
	Score	0	1	2	3	4
4	Resistance to Obsessions	Always resists	Much resistance	Some resistance	Often yields	Completely yields
	Score	0	1	2	3	4
5	Control over Obsessions	Complete control	Much control	Moderate control	Little control	No control
	Score	0	1	2	3	4

Obsession subtotal (add items 1–5) ☐

Table A.2   *Continued*

Compulsion Rating Scale (circle appropriate score)

Item		None	Mild	Moderate	Severe	Extreme
6	Time spent on Compulsions	0 hrs/day	0–1 hrs/day	1–3 hrs/day	3–8 hrs/day	>8 hrs/day
	Score	0	1	2	3	4
7	Interference from Compulsions	None	Mild	Manageable	Severe	Incapacitating
	Score	0	1	2	3	4
8	Distress from Compulsions	None	Mild	Moderate	Severe	Disabling
	Score	0	1	2	3	4
9	Resistance to Compulsions	Always resists	Much resistance	Some resistance	Often yields	Completely yields
	Score	0	1	2	3	4
10	Control over Compulsions	Complete control	Much control	Moderate control	Little control	No control
	Score	0	1	2	3	4

Compulsion subtotal (add items 6–10) ☐

Y-BOCS total (add items 1–10) ☐

TOTAL Y-BOCS SCORE: RANGE OF OCD SEVERITY

0–7 Subclinical	8–15 Mild	16–23 Moderate	24–31 Severe	32–40 Extreme

Adapted with permission from Wayne K. Goodman, M.D.

Behavior Therapy

Behavior therapy or, as it is sometimes called, behavioral psychotherapy, helps patients learn how to quell the discomfort arising from obsessions and to reduce or eliminate compulsive rituals. Behavior therapy is not something done to a patient; it is a structured set of techniques the patient learns to employ whenever anxiety, discomfort, or dysfunction arises because of obsessions or rituals. Because most patients have already thought out the reasons for their obsessions and rituals and have frequently sought advice from friends and family members without improvement, behavior therapy focuses on behaviors and specific steps the patient can take to lessen anxiety.

Basically, patients are asked to find and face the things they fear (exposure) and then to refrain from carrying out compulsive rituals (ritual or response prevention). Exposure and ritual prevention may be carried out gradually or rapidly, much as one might enter a swimming pool filled with cold water by wading in from the shallow end or by diving into the deep end. The total amount of discomfort is probably comparable, and the end result is the same—immersion.

Surprisingly, many patients find that even after years of obsessing, avoiding things they fear, and performing compulsive rituals, very little discomfort occurs when they do intensive and extensive behavior therapy. Instead, obsessions begin to fade and the urge to perform rituals diminishes. Exposure is more effective in decreasing discomfort, anxiety, worry, and obsessions, whereas ritual prevention is more helpful in reducing compulsive rituals.

To illustrate how exposure and ritual prevention are employed, let us assume that a patient has fears of contamination with germs so that he avoids touching doorknobs and public telephones as well as shaking hands, and that he washes his hands more than 40 times each day. The exposure component of behavior therapy would consist of asking him to begin to touch doorknobs and telephones as well as shaking hands. Ritual prevention consists of reducing the number of times he washes his hands. He might choose to begin exposure with objects and people he considers relatively "safe," and to decrease his washing by no more than five times per day (down to a level of 35 handwashings per day). He would monitor his distress, record it in a diary or therapy log, and report results of the specific exposure and ritual prevention treatments to the therapist at his next session. As therapy progresses and he feels ready, he would be asked to touch more "germy" objects and people and to decrease his number of handwashings more and more until a normal level is reached. Ultimately, the patient is asked to "run the same risks" the rest of us do with regard to germs and cleanliness.

Occasionally, it proves helpful for patients to "go beyond normal" in order to "get back to normal." In this variation of behavior therapy, the patient described previously might be asked to touch objects that many of us would have some reluctance to touch, such as the underside of a toilet seat, and then to refrain from washing his hands for an extended period. Although most of us wash after using the toilet, it is striking how many people do not and suffer no ill effects because of their habits. Patients should not be asked to take risks that the therapist would not be willing to accept as well.

Other specific techniques such as "thought stopping" and "semantic satiation" also may be employed to help with OCD. Thought stopping uses some form of negative or aversive stimulation (for example, wearing a rubber band around the wrist and snapping it against the inside of the wrist, which causes pain but is noninjurious) whenever mental rituals occur. Semantic satiation, a form of exposure therapy to thoughts, consists of asking the person to say or write, over and over again, whatever his or her obsession may be. As an illustration of semantic satiation, try saying the word "hundred" a hundred times. You will find that before reaching 100 repetitions, the word loses its meaning. In the same way, formerly distressing obsessions become meaningless and, for some, laughable.

The distinction between thoughts that increase anxiety (anxiogenic) and thoughts that decrease anxiety (anxiolytic) is critical. Exposure is needed for thoughts and objects or situations that increase anxiety, whereas ritual prevention is used for behaviors (rituals) or thoughts (mental rituals) that reduce anxiety. Although obsessions intrude into consciousness and either involve themes of harm or seem silly, mental rituals are voluntary thoughts intended to reduce anxiety from obsessions. Thus, an obsessional thought about harming a child might lead to a mental ritual such as "God would never let me harm a child." This ritual is just as anxiolytic as handwashing is for someone obsessed with fears of germs.

Behavior therapy has few, if any, side effects. Occasionally, patients become somewhat more anxious early in the course of behavior therapy, and sometimes patients report that they dream more actively and, rarely, have nightmares at the start of therapy. Patients with heart disease such as angina pectoris as well as those with stomach ulcers, asthma, and ulcerative colitis may be wise to proceed gradually with behavior therapy, but these problems seldom prevent behavior therapy.

Severe depression interferes with the effectiveness of behavior therapy, and sedative drugs such as alcohol, barbiturates (such as amobarbital, phenobarbital, and secobarbital), meprobamate (Equanil, Miltown), antihistamines (such as diphenhydramine [Benadryl and others] and hydroxyzine [Atarax, Vistaril]), and benzodiazepines (such as alprazolam [Xanax], chlordiazepoxide [Librium], clonazepam [Klonopin], clorazepate [Tranxenel], diazepam [Valium], estazolam [ProSom], flurazepam [Dalmane], halazepam [Paxipam], lorazepam [Ativan], oxazepam [Serax], quazepam [Doral], temazepam [Restoril], and triazolam [Halcion]) may interfere with the effectiveness of behavior therapy through state-dependent learning. State-dependent learning means that what a person learns in one mental state does not carry over well to another mental state. Importantly, antiobsessive compulsive medications such as clomipramine, fluoxetine, fluvoxamine, paroxetine, and sertraline do not interfere with behavior therapy.

Finally, behavior therapy must be carried out according to treatment instructions to be effective. Just as penicillin pills must be taken properly to combat bacterial infections, behavior therapy must be performed according to prescription to alleviate OCD.

Commonly Asked Questions About Behavior Therapy

How successful is behavior therapy?

Depending on which study one reviews, between 60% and 90% of OCD patients benefit from behavior therapy, and they may expect a 50% to 80% reduction in symptoms. However, these results require active patient participation, and approximately 25% of OCD sufferers decline behavioral treatment.

How long does it take before improvement from behavior therapy begins? Sometimes improvement occurs during and after the first session. However, gains may not be recognizable for a few sessions. Some improvement should be apparent within five or six sessions in which real exposure occurred and rituals were resisted, or it is unlikely that substantial gains will occur even with many more sessions. However, once improvement begins, it is likely to increase for many months.

Sometimes there is a lag between improvement in behaviors and trust that the gains are real. These "cognitive" or thinking and "affective" or feeling lags may last up to 4 months and reflect the many years over which obsessions and rituals have become ingrained. Persistent exposure and ritual prevention lead to growing appreciation of progress as real reductions in obsessions and rituals occur.

Because behavior therapy is a treatment patients can apply whenever necessary, the gains realized with behavior therapy are usually maintained for many years and, often, indefinitely.

How can I find out about behavior therapists practicing in my area? Finding a well-trained and experienced behavior therapist is often difficult. Anxiety disorder centers or clinics should have experienced behavior therapists working with them. Departments of psychiatry affiliated with medical schools are also a good place to inquire, as are departments of clinical psychology with graduate training programs. The Obsessive-Compulsive Information Center (address p. 728) maintains a referral list and may know a therapist in your area. The Obsessive-Compulsive Foundation, Inc., 9 Depot Street, Milford, Connecticut 06460 (203-878-5669), the Anxiety Disorders Association of America, 6000 Executive Boulevard, Suite 513, Rockville, Maryland 20852 (301-231-9350), and the Association for Advancement of Behavior Therapy, 305 7th Avenue, New York, New York 10001 (212-647-1890) also have listings of therapists who have indicated special interest in treating OCD and phobias. Some will be experienced and skilled in behavior therapy, whereas others may represent themselves as behavior therapists without proper training, experience, or demonstrated effectiveness. As with all clinicians, reputation in the local community is important, but even when a person's reputation and success with others is established, it is possible that you may not work well together. If this seems to be happening, address the issue directly and, if it cannot be resolved satisfactorily, ask for a second opinion or consultation or referral to another therapist.

It may be possible for you to travel to one of the centers where behavior therapy is available for evaluation and initiation of treatment. Because obsessive-compulsive problems occur outside hospitals, and behavior therapy helps patients confront the things they fear and reduce rituals, hospitalization is seldom necessary. Patients often can stay in a motel, hotel, or with family or friends and attend an outpatient clinic for evaluation and intensive therapy. After a patient has worked with a therapist, some subsequent sessions may be possible by telephone. A few patients may need to be treated in a hospital because of substantial risk of suicide, medical problems requiring treatment, or if intensive behavior therapy is available only on an inpatient basis.

If a therapist is not available nearby and traveling to consult one is not feasible, some patients have been successful in treating themselves with the help of the Self-Help section from the book, *Anxiety and Its Treatment: Help is Available* (see Suggested Readings). This Self-Help section has been used for more than 15 years. Although a higher proportion of obsessive-compulsive patients who receive treatment from well-trained behavior therapists improve and begin to improve somewhat more quickly, some patients who use the Self-Help section achieve the same gains as patients who are treated by therapists. Perhaps this reflects the common experience that to do things on our own, we have to understand fully what we are doing and put the principles we have learned through careful study into practice.

Even those who are receiving treatment from a therapist may benefit from reading this Self-Help section, which provides specific suggestions and may answer questions that commonly arise during the course of treatment.

As an even more abbreviated guide to behavior therapy, the following set of instructions has been adapted from instructions prepared and used in Professor Isaac Marks' Behavior Therapy Treatment Unit at the Institute of Psychiatry, Bethlem-Maudsley Hospital in London. They are printed on the following pages with his gracious permission.

Other patient guides are listed in the section on Suggested Readings.

Behavior Therapy Instructions for Obsessive Compulsive Disorder
AIMS

This treatment aims to help you stop your rituals and confront the triggers of your discomfort, obsessions, and rituals until your discomfort diminishes. It is necessary to accept some discomfort in order to learn how to cope with various situations. The faster you tackle your triggers the sooner you will get better. Your ability to do this will improve with practice.

GENERAL RULES

1. Three-hour homework sessions every day. This can be broken up into three 1-hour sessions. Set aside time for sessions.
2. Try to stop all ritualistic behaviors (e.g., washing, checking, counting, ordering, and repetition). If you don't succeed immediately, reduce them day by day.
3. Your most disturbing problem should be tackled within the first two weeks of therapy.

BEFORE THE SESSION

Only you know what triggers your rituals.

1. Choose your exposure homework tasks as carefully and as clearly as you can. The things you avoid are the guide to the things you must expose yourself to (touching telephones, shaking hands, thinking about sex, saying "unlucky" numbers, etc.).
2. Arrange exposure tasks in order of difficulty.
3. Decide which goals you are going to achieve in each session every day for a full week.
4. Make sure you know exactly what you are to do, e.g., touch ten different doorknobs, then rub hands on your clothes (including pockets) and touch everything in your purse (or wallet). Do not wash for two hours.

COPING WITH FEAR

A certain amount of discomfort or anxiety is normal. If you get very anxious or panicky:

1. Remember that what you are experiencing will pass in time; it won't damage you, and you won't lose control.
2. Don't ritualize.
3. Practice another exposure homework task to keep busy.
4. Wait for the fear to decrease a little.
5. Repeat the task that caused the fear as soon as you can; you have already faced it once and it will be easier the second time.
6. Talk to a friend or a relative if it helps you face the situation and stop the rituals. But do not seek reassurance, which is another ritual.

THREE-HOUR HOMEWORK SESSION

1. Carry out the exposure homework tasks in the way you planned.
2. Make sure that you know and can't avoid the fact that you are in contact with the things you fear (i.e., no hidden rituals).
3. Resist any urges to stop exposure, run away, or ritualize.
4. Doing your homework tasks may increase your anxiety at the time. Wait in the feared situation until your anxiety has come down.

5. Repeat the exposure again and again. In time, your discomfort will decrease.
6. If necessary get a friend to help you (e.g., by modeling contaminating themselves so that you can copy them, and praising you for stopping rituals).
7. It is essential that you not leave the exposure session until your discomfort has come down at least a little.

AFTER THE SESSION

1. Give yourself a treat—you deserve it.
2. If you have not achieved your treatment goal, don't despair. What is most important is that you have made an effort. We all have bad days.
3. Note any problems you had so that you can devise tactics to deal with them.

We would appreciate comments regarding your experience using these behavior therapy instructions. Please write:

Obsessive-Compulsive Information Center
Dean Foundation
2711 Allen Blvd.
Middleton, WI 53562 USA

Are there any other ways to get behavior therapy? One promising approach that's still under development combines a computer program reached by telephone and a workbook that guides the patient through exposure and ritual prevention. Two studies have found that many patients benefitted substantially from the program and like its availability at all times. You can check the status of the program through the Obsessive-Compulsive Information Center.

What about systematic desensitization as a treatment of OCD? The most widely practiced form of systematic desensitization combines muscle relaxation with exposure either in fantasy or in real life (*in vivo*). The theory behind this combination is that relaxation will provide "reciprocal inhibition" for anxiety. However, numerous studies have shown that relaxation adds nothing to the exposure component of systematic desensitization and merely takes time (and presumably money) to achieve. Being relaxed is a generally positive state for most people and there is nothing wrong with seeking relaxation when performing exposure if one wishes, but relaxation is not necessary for effective treatment.

Some therapists also have sought to heighten anxiety (through "flooding" or "implosion") in the belief that this technique would speed up the rate of improvement. Again, the evidence shows that neither reducing nor increasing anxiety affects the rate or amount of improvement—it is exposure that counts.

Some people advise, "If it bothers you, just stay away from it." Isn't that good advice? No! For OCD, avoidance or antiexposure, as it is sometimes called, actually makes the person's obsessions and rituals worse. In fact, in one study, antiexposure was so destructive that it substantially reduced the benefits conveyed by clomipramine (Anafranil), an effective drug treatment for OCD. So, for people with OCD, avoidance is the wrong thing to do.

What should a family member or friend do when an obsessive-compulsive patient seeks reassurance repeatedly to the point of being annoying? Seeking reassurance is a very common compulsive ritual for patients with OCD. After a patient has been reassured that he is not spreading contamination or hasn't hurt someone or needn't repeat another ritual, he will feel better for a brief period. Patients often feel that they can "shift the responsibility" for their worry to the person who has given them reassurance. However, after a short time, the obsessive concern returns full force. Seeking reassurance is a form of avoidance or antiexposure, so it is not surprising that the benefits are short-lived and the long-term results are negative. Obsessive-compulsive patients become reassurance "junkies," seeking their regular "fix" of reassurance. As with other addictions, the "fix" doesn't last long and the addict is soon back for another fix. The cure for this "addiction" is to withdraw the source of addiction, in this case reassurance. This is another example of ritual prevention.

Family members and friends can help obsessive-compulsive patients by withholding reassurance. These patients need to be exposed to the anxiety or discomfort associated with their fears without avoiding it. This exposure usually leads to a reduction in obsessions and compulsive rituals, whereas reassurance perpetuates or even worsens them.

It is important not to be harsh or sarcastic in the process of withholding reassurance. Also, some role-playing rehearsal with family members is often necessary as the habit of giving reassurance is usually well established. It may be helpful to have a neutral statement that can be repeated each time the person seeks reassurance. Phrases such as, "doctor's instructions are I'm not to reassure," are often beneficial. Practicing them aloud with others before the occasion to use them with the patient comes up is often necessary. Obtain the patient's permission and remind the patient that you are not intending to be mean but that you have come to the conclusion, based on understanding and personal experience with the failure of repeated reassurance and information that reassurance is counter productive, that it is best not to reassure.

Does it have to be either behavior therapy or drugs? Patients who have the option of both treatments will often select one or the other. Some prefer the simplicity of taking a medication; others want to avoid medication side effects and worry about possible long-term adverse effects of medications. Some will prefer behavior therapy, but others will not want to invest the time and energy required for behavior therapy or to face things that may raise short-term anxiety to have a long-term gain. Some patients opt to begin with medication in hopes of gaining some initial relief of symptoms before starting behavior therapy. Others want to start with behavior therapy in hopes they will be content with progress they make and, therefore, be able to avoid medications. Finally, patients may begin treatment with behavior therapy and medication simultaneously. For many patients, this combination is the best treatment approach.

There is no single approach that is ideal for every patient. The skillful therapist will carefully assess the obsessive-compulsive patient's problems and attitudes toward treatment and make a recommendation based on that information plus knowledge of the available behavioral and drug treatment resources. Unfortunately, some therapists restrict themselves to one kind of treatment and exclude even consideration of others.

Medication Treatment

From time to time, patients with OCD benefit substantially from treatment with the common tricyclic or the less common monoamine oxidase inhibitor (MAOI) antidepressant drugs (Tables A.3 and A.4). This may occur when the primary problem is depression with obsessions and compulsions occurring secondary to the depression. As depression abates, so do the obsessions and compulsions. However, most currently available antidepressant medications are not predictably effective in alleviating primary obsessive-compulsive symptoms.

By contrast, five medications that enhance serotonin neurotransmission have been shown to reduce obsessive-compulsive symptoms in many patients whether they are depressed or not. These medications are effective antidepressants, but they also have specific antiobsessive-compulsive properties and are valuable treatments for OCD.

Clomipramine (Anafranil) is the most studied of the anti–obsessive-compulsive drugs and the first to be approved by the Food and Drug Administration (FDA) for use in the United States (1990). Many carefully controlled experiments have conclusively proven that clomipramine is a more effective treatment for OCD than either placebo or other tricyclic antidepressants. Approximately 80% of patients improve with average reduction in obsessions and rituals of approximately 50%. In the largest study of clomipramine, 58% of patients rated themselves as much or very much improved, and only 3% of patients treated with placebo (an inactive substance that looked like the clomipramine tablets) gave the same ratings of improvement.

Side effects of clomipramine are similar to those of other tricyclic antidepressants available in the United States, the most common being dry mouth. Other side effects include constipation, tremor, sedation, increased sweating, difficulty urinating, delayed orgasm, weight gain, blurred vision, and some temporary lowering of blood pressure with position change which may lead to lightheadedness or rarely, fainting. When common side effects occur, they usually decrease as patients grow accustomed to the medication, and most patients can take clomipramine without great difficulty. Rarely, as with all

Table A.3 Common Antidepressant Drugs

Generic Name	United States Brand Name	United Kingdom Brand Name	Canadian Brand Name
Selective serotonin reuptake inhibitors (SSRIs)			
fluoxetine	Prozac	Prozac	Prozac
fluvoxamine*	Luvox	Faverin	Luvox
paroxetine	Paxil	Seroxat	Paxil
sertraline	Zoloft	Lustral	Zoloft

*Non*selective serotonin reuptake inhibitor tricyclic antidepressant

clomipramine*	Anafranil	Anafranil	Anafranil

(Clomipramine is a tricyclic antidepressant. It is a more potent serotonin reuptake inhibitor than the other tricyclic antidepressants and the only one predictably effective in OCD.)

Tricyclic antidepressants

Generic Name	United States Brand Name	United Kingdom Brand Name	Canadian Brand Name
amitriptyline	Elavil	Domical	Elavil
		Elavil	Levate
		Lentizol	
		Triptafen	
		Tryptizol	
amoxapine	Asendin	Asendis	Asendin
clomipramine*	Anafranil	Anafranil	Anafranil
desipramine	Norpramin	Pertofran	Norpramin
			Pertofrane
doxepin	Adapin	Sinequan	Sinequan
	Sinequan		
imipramine	Tofranil	Tofranil	Tofranil
nortriptyline	Pamelor	Allegron	Aventyl
		Aventyl	
protriptyline	Vivactil	Concordin	Triptil
trimipramine	Surmontil	Surmontil	Surmontil

Other antidepressants

Generic Name	United States Brand Name	United Kingdom Brand Name	Canadian Brand Name
bupropion	Wellbutrin	Not available	Not available
maprotiline	Ludiomil	Ludiomil	Ludiomil
mirtazapine	Remeron	Not available	Not available
nefazodone	Serzone	Dutonin	Serzone
trazodone	Desyrel	Molipaxin	Desyrel
venlafaxine	Effexor	Efexor	Effexor

Note: Probably no physician uses all of these medications. They are listed because they are all available antidepressants and might be prescribed. Dosage must be individualized in all patients. Older patients usually require lower doses.

Reproduced in revised form from Greist JH, Jefferson JW: *Depression and its treatment,* Washington, DC, 1992, American Psychiatric Press. Reproduced with permission.

* Clomipramine and fluvoxamine have Food and Drug Administration (FDA) approval for only OCD in the United States. Clomipramine is included in this list of antidepressant drugs because it has approval as an antidepressant in more than 70 other countries. Similarly, fluvoxamine is available to treat depression in more than 36 countries.

Table A.4   Monoamine Oxidase Inhibitor Antidepressant Drugs

Generic Name	United States Brand Name	United Kingdom Brand Name	Canadian Brand Name
phenelzine	Nardil	Nardil	Nardil
tranylcypromine	Parnate	Parnate	Parnate

Note: Dosage must be individualized in all patients. Older patients usually require lower doses. Reproduced in revised form from Greist JH, Jefferson JW, Marks IM: *Anxiety and its treatment: help is available*, Washington, DC, 1986, American Psychiatric Press. Reproduced with permission.

antidepressants, patients taking clomipramine can become manic (excessive energy, racing thoughts, decreased sleep, poor judgment) or psychotic (lose contact with reality). Rarely, a seizure might occur, as can happen with any antidepressant.

Fluoxetine (Prozac) became available in the United States in 1988 for treatment of depression. The most common side effects of fluoxetine, a selective serotonin reuptake inhibitor (SSRI) more selective in that property than clomipramine, include nausea, headache, overstimulation, and delayed orgasm. No medication is free of side effects and any medication may prove intolerable to some patients. Three multicenter controlled studies have found fluoxetine clearly effective in OCD, and the FDA gave approval for use of fluoxetine in OCD in March of 1994.

Six controlled studies have shown the effectiveness of fluvoxamine (Luvox), another SSRI, in OCD, and fluvoxamine received FDA approval for treatment of OCD in December 1994. It has been available in other countries as an antidepressant since 1983. Fluvoxamine's side-effect profile is similar to that of fluoxetine.

Paroxetine (Paxil), approved as an antidepressant in 1993, is the third SSRI to receive FDA approval for OCD (May, 1996) based on multicenter controlled trials.

Sertraline (Zoloft) is an SSRI available since 1992 as an antidepressant. It also has been found effective in OCD compared with placebo in multicenter controlled trials and received FDA approval for use in OCD in October 1996.

All of the SSRIs have side-effect profiles similar to that discussed for fluoxetine, although individual patients may respond differently in terms of benefit and side effects from these medications. In general, patients receiving SSRIs experience fewer side effects than patients taking clomipramine, which is a tricyclic compound. All five of these effective compounds are potent serotonin reuptake inhibitors.

Venlafaxine (Effexor) has been reported to be helpful in several individual cases and small case series. The only small controlled trial reported to date had mixed results, and more careful work is needed to establish the proper role of venlafaxine in OCD.

Nefazodone (Serzone) has been reported to be helpful in a handful of patients and will require substantially more research before one would recommend it. Mirtazapine (Remeron) is the newest antidepressant with specific effects on the serotonin system. No studies of mirtazapine's effects in OCD have been reported.

At present, venlafaxine, nefazodone, and mirtazapine are not FDA-approved treatments for OCD.

Beginning Anti–Obsessive-Compulsive Drug Therapy

What will your doctor need to know before prescribing anti–obsessive-compulsive drugs? Some of the information your doctor will need includes:

Your medical history—Do you have other medical conditions? For example, you might be asked about heart disease, liver disease, epilepsy, anemia or other blood diseases, glaucoma, and diabetes. *Any medical condition* you have may be important, so be sure to give the doctor a complete listing.

Any medications you are taking—For example, are you taking medication for your heart or blood pressure, oral contraceptives, blood thinners, antibiotics, or antidepressants? *Any medication* you are taking may be important, so be sure to inform your doctor of *all* medications (including nonprescription drugs). Also, you will be asked if you have ever had any allergic reactions to medication. For example, have you ever had an allergic reaction to an antidepressant?

Your normal diet—Do you drink large amounts of coffee or tea? How much alcohol do you consume? Are you on a special diet of any type? Do you plan to start any special diets in the future?

Your occupation and activities—Do you need to operate dangerous machinery or drive a vehicle? (Sometimes antiobsessive-compulsive drugs cause sedation or impair coordination, but these are usually temporary side effects.)

Of special note to women—Are you pregnant? Is there a possibility of pregnancy while taking anti–obsessive-compulsive drugs? Are you or will you be breastfeeding your baby? (Anti–obsessive-compulsive drugs may be harmful to unborn or breastfed babies, although there is no evidence to date that they are.)

The previous lists of questions are *not* complete but should give some idea of what your doctor will want to know before you begin anti–obsessive-compulsive drug therapy. The *main point* is to inform your doctor about *any* medical conditions, medications, and so forth, even if you are being treated by several doctors. If you are not sure whether certain facts should be brought out, mention them and let your doctor decide how important they are in your treatment. Without such information, a doctor would have difficulty treating you safely and effectively.

Are anti–obsessive-compulsive drugs harmful during pregnancy or breastfeeding? Birth defects have occasionally been found in babies whose mothers were taking anti–obsessive-compulsive drugs during pregnancy. Whether the drugs actually caused these abnormalities is not known. In humans, the risk of birth defects from these drugs appears to be very small; in fact, it is questionable whether the risk is increased at all. If you plan to become pregnant or think you might be, contact your doctor immediately to discuss the risk of birth defects from the particular anti–obsessive-compulsive medication you are taking.

Anti–obsessive-compulsive drugs cross from the mother's blood into the fetus. For this reason, if you are taking an anti-OCD drug during pregnancy, it is important to get your doctor's opinion about temporarily stopping your medication shortly before delivery. As with any drug, the risks and benefits of discontinuing anti-OCD drug therapy before or during pregnancy are best evaluated on an individual basis with your doctor.

It is highly unlikely that there are harmful effects for children whose fathers were taking anti-OCD medications at the time of conception or for children of women who had taken anti-OCD medications prior to but not during pregnancy.

Although anti-OCD drugs are found in breast milk, they don't reach high levels and cause toxicity in the infant. Whether small amounts of an anti-OCD drug can cause other problems in a breastfed baby is not known, but to be on the safe side, breastfeeding is usually discouraged. For some, however, the benefits of breastfeeding may outweigh this potential disadvantage. For more detailed information about a specific anti-OCD drug and its effects on pregnancy and breastfeeding, consult your doctor, pharmacist, or local drug information center.

Are laboratory tests necessary before starting anti–obsessive-compulsive drugs? In the approvals awarded by the FDA for clomipramine, fluoxetine, fluvoxamine, paroxetine, and sertraline for treatment of OCD, there are no specific laboratory or other tests required before they are prescribed. Tests will be ordered as a physician feels they are indicated. For example, patients with a history of heart disease would be likely to have an electrocardiogram (ECG) and blood studies of electrolytes. Those with a history of liver problems would probably have evaluations of liver function, and so on. Many patients receiving these medications will not have tests ordered before they begin treatment.

Investigational or experimental drugs for OCD remain under close scrutiny by the FDA. All patients receiving them in experimental programs are required to have blood and other tests (often a urinalysis, ECG, and physical examination) at regularly scheduled intervals to assess the drug's effect on the body and to ensure that patients participating in experiments with the drugs can do so with acceptable safety. If the FDA approves these drugs for prescription by physicians across the United States, there may or may not be specific requirements for laboratory tests.

How should anti–obsessive-compulsive drugs be taken? Clomipramine (Anafranil) is often initially prescribed in divided doses during the day—usually two or three times daily. Alternatively, it may be taken all at once in the evening so that any side effects are likely to be at their greatest level when the patient is asleep. The dose typically starts at 25 mg and is gradually increased to approximately 100 mg after 2 to 4 weeks and then may be further increased, as necessary, to obtain a good response, to a maximum of 250 mg/day. Controlled trials have shown that, on average, 200 mg/day of clomipramine is as effective in OCD as 250 mg or even 300 mg. Many patients respond at even lower doses. In general, the dosage is gradually increased until beneficial effects are obtained. Later, the dose may again be adjusted with the goal of finding the "minimum effective dose" (i.e., the least amount of drug needed to obtain the desired effect).

Fluoxetine (Prozac) dose should be increased very gradually, and we suggest increments of 20 mg every 3 to 4 weeks, stopping at the lowest dose associated with improvement for at least 10 weeks. The maximum approved dose is 60 mg/day although doctors sometimes prescribe 80 or more mg/day. A subsequent final increase of 20 mg may be tried if improvement is incomplete. Fluvoxamine (Luvox) may be started at 25 or 50 mg/day and then increased by 50 mg every 4 to 7 days as tolerated. The maximum recommended dose is 300 mg/day. Many patients do well on doses of about 150 mg/day. Paroxetine (Paxil) should be started at 20 mg/day and will probably need to be increased to 40 or 60 mg/day to achieve maximum effectiveness, although dosage increase should be delayed at least 1 week to permit the person to adjust to the medication. Sertraline (Zoloft) dose starts at 50 mg and should be increased approximately every month to a maximum of 200 mg. Once improvement begins with any of the potent serotonin reuptake inhibitors, the dose should be maintained at that level until improvement has plateaued. At that point, another increase can be tried to see if further improvement is possible.

Older patients over 60 years of age usually need smaller doses to achieve the same effects. Doses in older patients are often one-half to two-thirds the dose required by younger adults.

Taking anti–obsessive-compulsive drugs regularly as prescribed is important, and people must work out ways to avoid forgetting doses or taking extra doses. Simply put, taking less than the prescribed amount may not be effective and taking more may make a person sick from side effects. A pill holder, divided into days and designed to carry a week's supply of pills, will help avoid these problems.

Many people prefer to take medication with meals, which not only helps them remember to take it but also helps to avoid nausea that may occur if medication is taken on an empty stomach. It is not necessary, however, that anti–obsessive-compulsive drugs be taken with food.

How are antiobsessive-compulsive drugs handled in the body? When taken by mouth, antiobsessive-compulsive drugs are absorbed into the bloodstream and carried to all body tissues, including the brain. Much of the anti–obsessive-compulsive drug is temporarily bound to proteins in the blood from which it is gradually released. It is felt that only the "free" anti–obsessive-compulsive drug (the part not bound to blood proteins) is active and effective in treating OCD.

Anti–obsessive-compulsive drugs are removed from the body by the liver where they are metabolized to byproducts. These byproducts and any remaining unmetabolized drug are excreted into bile or urine. Bile passes out of the body through the intestines.

Since the liver is the major organ of drug metabolism (breakdown) in the body, diseases that damage the liver may affect the level of anti–obsessive-compulsive drug in the body and, therefore, require adjustment of dose. Liver disease, in some instances, may prevent the use of anti–obsessive-compulsive drugs. Other drugs that compete for the same metabolic pathways in the liver also may affect the level of anti–obsessive-compulsive drugs in the body and, therefore, require dosage adjustment.

Small amounts of anti–obsessive-compulsive drugs are excreted unmetabolized in the urine, but kidney disease is seldom a factor in limiting their use. Even when kidney or liver disease is present, many patients can still benefit from anti–obsessive-compulsive medications by taking smaller doses.

Commonly Asked Questions About Anti–Obsessive-Compulsive Drugs

Are anti–obsessive-compulsive drugs addictive? No!

Aren't drugs other than anti–obsessive-compulsive compounds often used to treat OCD? Many other antidepressant (Tables A.3 and A.4), antianxiety (Table A.5), and antipsychotic drugs (such as chlorpromazine [Thorazine], fluphenazine [Prolixin], haloperidol [Haldol], thioridazine [Mellaril], thiothixene [Navane], and trifluoperazine [Stelazine]) have been tried in the treatment of OCD. Although the common antidepressants are occasionally helpful in reducing symptoms of OCD, particularly in patients with substantial depression, they are not as effective as the five more potent serotonin reuptake inhibiting anti–obsessive-compulsive drugs. Antianxiety drugs reduce anxiety in general but seldom reduce specific obsessions or rituals. Antipsychotic medications appear to help only 1% to 5% of patients with OCD (usually those who also have some form of tic disorder), and the risk of tardive dyskinesia, a side effect involving involuntary movements that may be irreversible, makes them a last choice for most physicians treating OCD. The so-called "atypical" antipsychotics, clozapine (Clozaril) and risperidone (Risperdal), have pronounced effects on the serotonin system and can worsen OCD—but not always.

Since clomipramine, fluoxetine, fluvoxamine, paroxetine, and sertraline are now available and have been proved effective in OCD, trials of other antidepressants should not be made unless these compounds have failed (because

Table A.5 Benzodiazepine Antianxiety Drugs

Generic Name	United States Brand Name	United Kingdom Brand Name	Canadian Brand Name
alprazolam	Xanax	Xanax	Xanax
chlordiazepoxide	Librium	A-Poxide	Librium
		Librium	Solium
		Tropium	Tropium
clonazepam	Klonopin	Rivotril	Rivotril
clorazepate	Tranxene	Tranxene	Tranxene
diazepam	Valium	Alupram	Diazemuls
		Atensine	Valium
		Evacalm	Vivol
		Solis	
		Stesolid	
		Tensium	
		Valium	
halazepam	Paxipam	Not available	Not available
lorazepam	Ativan	Ativan	Ativan
oxazepam	Serax	Oxanid	Serax
		Serenid	

Note: Estazolam (ProSom), flurazepam (Dalmane), quazepam (Doral), temazepam (Restoril), and triazolam (Halcion) are also benzodiazepines but are marketed as sleeping pills. Dosage must be individualized in all patients. Older patients usually require lower doses. Reproduced in revised form from Greist JH, Jefferson JW, Marks IM: *Anxiety and its treatment: help is available,* Washington, DC, 1986, American Psychiatric Press. Reproduced with permission.

they are either ineffective or not tolerated). Although antianxiety and antipsychotic drugs also may be tried, the chances of improvement are not as great as with the more specific anti–obsessive-compulsive compounds.

What can be done if an anti–obsessive-compulsive medication doesn't work? *First*, it is important to make certain that both the dose and duration of treatment with any medication are sufficient. With clomipramine, doses up to 250 mg/day should be tried, if tolerated, before concluding that it will not work. For fluoxetine, 60 mg/day may have been slightly more effective than 40 or 20 mg/day. Fluvoxamine should be tried up to 300 mg/day; paroxetine to 60 mg/day; and sertraline to 200 mg/day before concluding that they are ineffective. (Sometimes doctors may prescribe doses above these limits, particularly if patients are having few or no side effects.) Anti–obsessive-compulsive medications need to be given for at least 10 weeks before it can be concluded that they are ineffective. Some patients respond late, but once improvement begins, it often increases for many additional weeks.

Second, switching to another anti–obsessive-compulsive medication may be effective. Although these medications are believed to have similar effects on serotonin neurotransmission, they have different chemical structures, and it has been found that some patients respond to one and not to another.

Third (the second and third steps are interchangeable depending on patient and doctor preference), if an anti–obsessive-compulsive drug has not worked sufficiently after several weeks at the maximum permitted or tolerated dose, several other medications may be added to augment whatever benefits have resulted from the anti–obsessive-compulsive medication. Buspirone, clonazepam, fenfluramine, L-tryptophan (assuming a safe supply is available), lithium, and antipsychotic medications may all prove beneficial in combination with the primary antiobsessive-compulsive compound.

Buspirone (Buspar) has a variety of effects on serotonin neurotransmission. Although one study found buspirone ineffective in OCD, another supported its effectiveness, and two suggested augmenting effects for buspirone when it was added to fluoxetine. Better-designed studies have found less benefit from buspirone augmentation.

Clonazepam (Klonopin) is a benzodiazepine that is approved for use as an anticonvulsant but often is used to treat anxiety disorders. For OCD, clonazepam alone has been shown in a small study to be an effective treatment, although its benefit is probably less than that of clomipramine. Some doctors also believe that clonazepam can be useful as an augmenting agent for potent SSRIs. Benzodiazepines cause physical dependency if taken for long periods and may interfere with behavior therapy at high dosage. As with all medications, the use of clonazepam or other benzodiazepines should be based on a favorable risk/benefit ratio.

Fenfluramine (Pondimin, Redux) is a nonspecific releaser of serotonin that has been shown to augment the effectiveness of clomipramine and fluoxetine in some obsessive-compulsive patients. Fenfluramine has a narrow "therapeutic index" or difference between therapeutic and toxic dose, so gradual and cautious increases in dosing are necessary.

L-tryptophan, an amino acid precursor of serotonin occurring in certain foods and once available over the counter in drug and health food stores, is sometimes given in an attempt to increase the amount of serotonin available for neurotransmission. Controlled trials of its effectiveness have not been conducted, but some patients appear to have benefitted when this medication was combined with other medications. L-tryptophan can be sedating so that its indiscriminate use may be a problem. Tainted supplies of L-tryptophan have been associated with a serious reaction known as eosinophilia-myalgia syndrome. Consequently, until safe supplies of L-tryptophan can be assured, its use in augmentation of other anti–obsessive-compulsive medications, or for any other purpose, cannot be recommended.

Lithium may be combined with other drugs, because it also tends to increase serotonin neurotransmission. Controlled studies of lithium alone or as an augmenting agent in OCD have not found it to be effective. Nevertheless, because it has some effect on serotonin neurotransmission and individual patients occasionally respond, there is still a rationale for its occasional use in combination with anti–obsessive-compulsive drug treatments.

Antipsychotic medications are usually ineffective in OCD and should be avoided because they may cause tardive dyskinesia (see Chapter 22). However, a few patients with OCD, probably less than 5%, may benefit from addition of an antipsychotic medication to an anti–obsessive-compulsive medication. One study found that patients who have tics (tics are involuntary, sudden, rapid, recurrent, nonrhythmic motor movements or vocalizations [sounds]) benefitted from certain antipsychotic medications. Pimozide (Orap) and haloperidol (Haldol) were of some benefit to seven of eight patients (88%) with tic spectrum disorders when added to fluvoxamine (Luvox) or fluvoxamine plus lithium. However, the same antipsychotic medications were helpful to only two of nine patients (22%) without tic spectrum disorders when added to fluvoxamine or fluvoxamine plus lithium. A better-controlled study also confirmed this finding for haloperidol. Substantial short- and long-term side effects can occur with antipsychotics, so their use in OCD should be reserved for these specific indications.

None of the augmentation approaches described previously have been thoroughly evaluated. They must be considered experimental or innovative therapies and should be approached with caution. Nevertheless, some patients are helped by these approaches and may decide, in consultation with their physicians, to try these innovative approaches if more straightforward treatments are ineffective.

Sometimes, combinations of serotonin reuptake inhibitor anti–obsessive-compulsive medications are also tried (e.g., clomipramine plus fluoxetine, fluvoxamine, paroxetine, or sertraline). Blood levels of clomipramine should be measured if it is combined with these other agents because they have been shown to cause substantial increases that could worsen any side effects. One combination that must be avoided is an anti–obsessive-compulsive medication with any monoamine oxidase inhibitor (phenelzine [Nardil] or tranylcypromine [Parnate]), because dangerous interactions (some fatal) have been reported from these combinations. This reaction is characterized by various combinations of fever, muscular rigidity, vital sign fluctuations, agitation, delirium, or coma and is called a serotonin syndrome. Serotonin syndrome may occur (usually more mildly) when buspirone, fenfluramine, L-tryptophan, or lithium is added to anti–obsessive-compulsive drugs.

Obviously, any modification of the treatment regimen should be discussed with the physician before it is made.

Fourth and finally, it is important to remember that medications are only one of the dual cornerstones of effective treatment of OCD, behavior therapy offering a very viable alternative for many patients. Neurosurgery (psychosurgery) is very rarely needed but may prove lifesaving in desperate cases (see Chapter 26).

Are other psychiatric disorders treated with anti–obsessive-compulsive drugs? Clomipramine (Anafranil) is most widely used in other countries to treat depression. Other studies suggest effectiveness in panic disorder and various pain syndromes, including migraine headache. However, the only disorder for which clomipramine has been approved in the United States is OCD.

Fluoxetine (Prozac) is approved as an antidepressant and for OCD and bulimia in the United States. Fluvoxamine (Luvox) is marketed in Europe and Canada as an antidepressant but specific approval for use in the United States is only for OCD. Paroxetine (Paxil) and sertraline (Zoloft) also are approved for both depression and OCD in the United States. Paroxetine and sertraline are also approved for treatment of panic disorder. All of these compounds are being studied as treatments for other disorders, and doctors may use them "off label" in "innovative clinical trials" for these problems.

Isn't behavior therapy the best treatment for OCD? For many patients, behavior therapy (exposure and ritual or response prevention) is highly effective. Behavior therapy avoids the problem of drug side effects and the uncertainty about possible long-term adverse effects.

On the other hand, behavior therapy requires a substantial commitment of time and effort on the patient's part, as well as a willingness to face the things the patient has been avoiding and to endure possible short-term increases in discomfort to gain later long-term reductions. Experienced behavior therapists are unfortunately seldom available and, even with the best behavior therapy, some patients do not benefit.

Medication requires little effort on the patient's part beyond remembering to take it. However, when medication is discontinued, almost all patients relapse rapidly, in striking contrast to patients who learn to treat themselves with behavior therapy and usually maintain their gains for years.

For many patients, a combination of behavior therapy and an anti–obsessive-compulsive drug is the most helpful approach to their problem.

Do anti–obsessive-compulsive drugs have any long-term effects on the nervous system? Only one antiobsessive-compulsive drug (clomipramine [Anafranil]) has been in use for a period long enough (> 30 years) to assess the risk of long-term effects. None has been found to date, which is reassuring. There remains a small possibility that late effects could still develop with clomipramine but the chance of this happening is vanishingly small as the years pass. Newer anti–obsessive-compulsive drugs do not have the advantage of more than 30 years' experience, so some uncertainty will exist for several years regarding the possible development of late side effects from their use. None has been noted to date with fluoxetine (9 years), fluvoxamine (14 years), paroxetine (4 years), or sertraline (5 years).

Do antiobsessive-compulsive drugs affect the heart? In normal doses, anti–obsessive-compulsive drugs cause no problems for patients with normal hearts. Some increase in heart rate may occur with clomipramine, but in general these medications have little effect on blood pressure and heart rhythm. The best protection for the heart and all other organs is use of the lowest possible dose of the drug. Patients with a history of heart disease or who are at risk for heart disease need a careful cardiovascular evaluation, including an electrocardiogram (ECG or heart tracing) before treatment is begun. Patients with underlying heart disease (more common in elderly patients) who are treated with anti–obsessive-compulsive drugs may experience changes in heart rhythm. For patients with known heart disease, one of the SSRIs may be preferred to clomipramine.

Do anti–obsessive-compulsive drugs cause tumors or cancer in humans? There is no evidence that the clinical use of anti–obsessive-compulsive drugs causes tumors or cancer in humans. Extensive animal testing was performed prior to the marketing of these drugs (as with all drugs), and the findings were supportive of their safety in humans.

Are there special effects or special concerns for elderly patients? Older patients are more susceptible to side effects of many drugs, and anti–obsessive-compulsive drugs are no exception. In particular, older patients are more likely to experience confusion, agitation (restlessness or nervousness), or changes in the heart's rhythm or rate (such as unusually slow heart rate). It is important that family members and close associates be aware of this possibility so the patient will receive prompt medical attention if problems appear. Lower doses of anti–obsessive-compulsive drugs are often effective in older patients, whereas higher doses that would be appropriate for younger patients may cause undesirable side effects.

What if I am running out of medication? If you get close to running out of medication, contact your doctor immediately to arrange to obtain more. It is not a good idea to stop anti–obsessive-compulsive drugs abruptly. Instead, a more gradual withdrawal makes it easier for your body to adjust.

How should I store anti–obsessive-compulsive medication? Any anti–obsessive-compulsive drug not needed for the current week's use is best stored in its original prescription container away from sources of heat and moisture and out of contact with direct sunlight. Because anti–obsessive-compulsive medication in large amounts is potentially poisonous, it, as all medication, must be kept out of reach of children. Do not store anti–obsessive-compulsive medication in the bathroom medicine cabinet where heat and moisture may cause it to break down.

What if I forget a dose? Because dosage schedules vary, it is important to ask your doctor what to do if you forget a dose. Until you have done this, a safe rule to follow is:

If you've missed your regular time by 3 hours or less, you should take that dose when you remember it. If it is more than 3 hours after the dose should have been taken, just skip the forgotten dose and resume your anti–obsessive-compulsive medication at the next regularly scheduled time. Your proper blood level will soon be reached again. *Never double up on doses of anti–obsessive-compulsive drugs* to "catch up" on those you have forgotten unless your doctor instructs you to do so. Increased doses may lead to dangerously high blood levels of anti–obsessive-compulsive drugs.

How will I feel when taking anti–obsessive-compulsive drugs? Most people feel like themselves, able to carry on their usual activities, including going to work and driving a car. They experience their normal range of thoughts, feelings, and emotions. If this is not the case, dosage adjustment may be necessary.

What if an anti–obsessive-compulsive drug doesn't work? Unfortunately, like all other treatments, anti–obsessive-compulsive drugs are not effective in all cases. When one drug doesn't work, another drug or augmentation may. Behavior therapy is an alternative treatment that is often effective. Other treatments (see Chapter 22) also are available.

How long do I have to take anti–obsessive-compulsive drugs? The length of therapy varies among individuals. It is determined by the severity of the OCD and how effective and tolerable anti–obsessive-compulsive drugs are for each individual. Although some patients benefit from long-term anti–obsessive-compulsive drug therapy, it is unnecessary for others. The course of treatment for each person should be individually developed with the doctor.

What if I am on a special diet? In general, any diet is acceptable with anti–obsessive-compulsive drugs. For example, balanced vegetarian, low-fat or low-cholesterol, low-sodium, and high- or low-calorie diets are fine.

May I drink alcohol when taking anti–obsessive-compulsive drugs? It is best to ask your doctor for a specific recommendation. Most people may consume alcoholic beverages in small amounts if they wish. However, the ability to drive and to operate hazardous machinery may be dangerously impaired by the combination of alcohol and anti–obsessive-compulsive drugs.

Is it dangerous to take other medications when taking anti–obsessive-compulsive drugs? Most medications may be taken safely with anti–obsessive-compulsive drugs. Some, however, may interact with anti–obsessive-compulsive drugs in such a way as to cause serious side effects. Monoamine oxidase inhibitors (MAOIs) in particular (see Table A.4) should never be combined with anti–obsessive-compulsive drugs (see Chapter 22). Some combinations of anti–obsessive-compulsive drugs may interfere with metabolism of one or another of these drugs and produce unpleasant or even dangerous side effects. It is best to tell *all* doctors treating you that you are taking anti–obsessive-compulsive drugs. Before taking *any* medication (prescription or nonprescription), ask your doctor or pharmacist whether it might interact adversely with your anti–obsessive-compulsive drug.

Examples of some common medications that may be used safely with anti–obsessive-compulsive drugs are aspirin, acetaminophen (a pain reliever such as Tylenol or Datril), ibuprofen (Advil, Medipren, Motrin, Nuprin, and others), antibiotics, and some cough and cold medications (though they may increase drowsiness). Terfenadine (Seldane), astemizole (Hismanal), and cisapride (Propulsid) *should not be taken* with fluvoxamine because of the possibility of a very serious adverse reaction.

Can I use oral contraceptives (birth control pills) when taking an anti–obsessive-compulsive drug? Oral contraceptives are compatible with anti–obsessive-compulsive drugs.

What if I need to see another doctor or have an operation? When seeing other doctors or when undergoing any medical or surgical procedure, always tell those involved that you are taking an anti–obsessive-compulsive drug. This should help ensure that the anti–obsessive-compulsive drug is managed safely and effectively. Do not assume that being on an anti–obsessive-compulsive drug is only important to the doctor who prescribes it for you.

Can I take less anti–obsessive-compulsive medication to reduce side effects and be slightly obsessive-compulsive? Taking an anti–obsessive-compulsive drug at lower doses should reduce side effects but will not usually allow only a "slightly obsessive-compulsive" state. Should symptoms "break through" on a lowered dose of an anti–obsessive-compulsive drug, it is usually possible to regain remission of symptoms by simply increasing the dose to the previously effective level.

What about vitamins and minerals? There is no sound evidence that vitamin or mineral supplements are useful in the treatment of OCD. If a person chooses to take a multivitamin or minerals as diet supplements, no adverse interactions with anti–obsessive-compulsive drugs would be expected.

Can I exercise when taking anti–obsessive-compulsive drugs? By all means! Regular exercise, in moderation, is a healthy activity for people of all ages and has been shown to have antidepressant and antianxiety effects as well. Antiobsessive-compulsive drugs should not interfere with exercise. Although fluid replacement is important during and after exercise, extra salt is seldom needed.

Do anti–obsessive-compulsive drugs cure OCD? No, but they are one effective way to control it. There is currently no cure for OCD, and its causes remain a mystery.

For persons suffering from disabling obsessions and rituals, anti–obsessive-compulsive drugs may be of help in two ways:

1. Gaining remission—anti–obsessive-compulsive drugs can help a person out of a disabling obsessive-compulsive state.

2. Preventing relapses—anti–obsessive-compulsive drugs can help prevent relapses of disabling obsessions and rituals.

The fact that anti–obsessive-compulsive drugs act to *control* rather than *cure* OCD is important. It means that if people stop taking anti–obsessive-compulsive drugs, obsessive-compulsive symptoms and distress are likely to recur.

Controlling rather than curing a disorder with a specific drug is actually a common practice. A well-known example is the use of insulin to control certain forms of diabetes. Here, the insulin does not cure the underlying disease of diabetes, but it does help to control symptoms so that the diabetic patient is able to live a more normal life. If the insulin is stopped, symptoms of the disease reappear. Although insulin helps control many symptoms and prevents many of the damaging effects of the disease, the diabetes itself is still present. Other examples of diseases controlled with medication are high blood pressure, heart failure, and arthritis.

Do anti–obsessive-compulsive drugs help to get a person's life back in order? Although anti–obsessive-compulsive drugs help reduce symptoms of OCD, they are not a "cure-all." Personal problems resulting from prior obsessive-compulsive symptoms may continue to exist. Life problems unrelated to obsessive compulsive disorder will not be helped by anti–obsessive-compulsive drugs. Psychotherapy or other forms of counseling may be helpful in dealing with such difficulties.

How can someone tell if anti–obsessive-compulsive drugs are working properly? Anti–obsessive-compulsive drugs are working properly if they effectively reduce obsessions and compulsive rituals and produce few, if any, side effects.

How long does it take for treatment to be effective? Unfortunately, although side effects begin and usually are at their worst as treatment with medication is started, benefits may not appear for 2 or more weeks. When improvement does occur, it may keep increasing for as long as 5 months before reaching its maximum level. Consequently, patient and doctor must work together to minimize side effects so that the medication may be given sufficient time to work or to establish conclusively that the medication does not work. Continuing a medication for 10 weeks allows sufficient time to determine that it will provide at least some beneficial effects.

What proportion of patients improve with these medications? Different studies have found different improvement rates. Somewhere between 50% and 80% of patients with OCD improved with anti–obsessive-compulsive drugs with average reduction in obsessions and rituals ranging between 30% and 70%. A few patients became virtually symptom-free.

What happens when anti–obsessive-compulsive drugs are stopped? Unfortunately, most patients experience a return toward their previous symptom level when these medications are discontinued. However, some patients maintain improvement they have made, at least for a time. Patients who also have engaged in behavior therapy often maintain their gains when medications are decreased or discontinued.

There is no hard and fast rule one can apply to the issue of whether or when to discontinue medication. Many patients find they can maintain most of the gains they have made through medication with somewhat lower doses than they needed to gain initial relief of symptoms and, at the same time, reduce any side effects that are dose-related. However, below a minimum dose threshold, most patients find that their symptoms worsen and a return to the previously effective dose is necessary.

If someone on anti–obsessive-compulsive drugs has a relapse with increases in obsessions and compulsions, does that mean the anti–obsessive-compulsive drug isn't working? Not necessarily. Ideally, anti–obsessive-compulsive drugs will substantially reduce symptoms of OCD and then maintain improvements for long periods. However, a partial initial response to anti–obsessive-compulsive drugs is common and relapses may occur, even though anti–obsessive-compulsive drugs are continued. Improvement with anti–obsessive-compulsive drugs usually increases as time passes up to a maximum of 5 months. Therefore, it is important to give the drugs a fair trial. If obsessions and compulsions worsen after treatment with anti–obsessive-compulsive drugs has begun, adjustments in dose or addition of other treatments (behavior therapy, other medications, family or individual psychotherapy) may prove helpful.

What feelings accompany anti–obsessive-compulsive drug use for OCD? For most patients, treatment of OCD leads to a less chaotic and more enjoyable life. Some, however, may find that treatment produces confusing feelings. At times, patients find it difficult to accept that they have a chronic medical illness that may require lifelong treatment. Some feel they should be able to use "willpower" to "be like everybody else." Sometimes they feel that being treated will cause others to stigmatize them as being "crazy" or "chronically mentally ill" (and, unfortunately, this is sometimes true). It is often difficult for patients to explain to others that the disorder is a medical condition and not "someone's fault."

Some patients dislike taking medication when they are feeling healthy or find it difficult to take medication because of side effects they experience.

"Giving up" rituals and avoidance that have been the only way to control anxiety and other discomfort is frightening for some patients with OCD, even when the rituals and avoidance have come to dominate their lives.

Discussing these thoughts and feelings with family members, friends, and a doctor is important. As with any illness, successful treatment of OCD consists of more than just taking a pill. Patients are encouraged to learn as much as possible about their illness and its treatment so that they may lead more productive, satisfying lives.

How can I obtain "experimental" medications? At present, the only ways to obtain experimental medications are: through compassionate-use (sometimes called humanitarian) programs that drug companies sometimes have available; by participating in research on the drugs; or by traveling to a country where they are available. In the compassionate-use programs, the drugs must be prescribed by qualified physicians following a protocol of regular assessments for effectiveness and safety (these usually include physical and electrocardiographic examinations as well as tests of the blood and urine).

In the past, when compassionate-use programs were not available, many individuals traveled to Canada or Mexico to obtain clomipramine. A few people traveled to Europe or Canada to obtain fluvoxamine. However, in most situations, it is probably best to use any compassionate-use programs that are available.

Why does it take so long to get new drugs approved for use in the United States after they have been tested and made available in other countries? The Food and Drug Administration (FDA) is responsible for licensing medications in the United States. Only drugs that are both safe and effective receive FDA approval. FDA standards are strict and although they have sometimes delayed introduction of medications that are safe and effective, the FDA's standards also have protected the American public from medicines released elsewhere that were later withdrawn because they were too dangerous.

New drugs are first tested in animals and later in human volunteers free of identifiable illness. The studies by which medicines are tested in humans are very carefully controlled, both to meet high scientific standards and to protect subjects involved in the studies. Final studies with patients usually involve a "placebo-controlled, double-blind design." "Placebo-controlled" means that some patients receive a placebo or inactive substance identical in appearance to the active drug being studied. This helps to determine whether the new drug is better than no drug and offers the subjects in the study who receive placebo the chance of not being harmed by a new drug if it later proves to be dangerous. Placebos are necessary because approximately one third of patients in many studies improve when given placebos, probably because they have faith that whatever a doctor gives them will be helpful. It is interesting that, as a group, patients with OCD have a much lower placebo response rate than patients with other anxiety disorders or depression.

"Double-blind" means that neither the doctor nor the patient knows whether the patient is receiving the new drug or the placebo. This technique tries to eliminate bias that might appear if doctor or patient knew whether the patient was receiving drug or placebo.

Well-controlled studies are costly to perform, both in time and money but, in the end, more effective and safer drugs result from the evaluation process the FDA requires. Although the FDA's system of regulation is not "perfect and all-wise," it is, to paraphrase Winston Churchill's statement about democracy, "the worst form of regulation except for all those other forms which have been tried from time to time."

Other Treatments

Psychotherapy

Psychotherapy or "talk therapy," as it is sometimes called, is widely practiced by psychiatrists, psychologists, social workers, psychiatric nurses, and many others who proclaim themselves "psychotherapists." There are more than 200 specific kinds of psychotherapy. Most of them, however, share nonspecific factors such as a theory regarding what has caused a problem, a belief that the treatment will be helpful, reassurance, positive regard for the patient, empathy, warmth, and information about the problem and its treatment. These common factors are probably more important for improvement than the specific elements that are touted as critical to success by the various schools of psychotherapy.

Every patient needs and deserves support when struggling with obsessions and compulsive rituals. Supportive psychotherapy should be provided in the context of effective medication and behavior therapy and has value in its own right. Supportive psychotherapy emphasizes the patient's strengths; explains, to the extent that accurate information about OCD is available, what the patient can expect from different treatments; empathizes with the distress inevitably associated with OCD; and monitors changes and encourages the patient that improvement is likely. This support must be provided without repeatedly reassuring these individuals that their fears are unfounded, because this reassurance is counterproductive (see Chapters 17–19). Family members and friends also can provide helpful support as long as they understand the role of reassurance rituals in perpetuating OCD.

Unfortunately, the elegant psychoanalytic theories regarding OCD (classically described in Freud's famous case of the "rat man" who was "cured" through a year's analysis) have been helpful to very few, if any, obsessive-compulsive patients. The time and expense involved in psychoanalysis are substantial, and, with little hope for improvement from this approach, it is difficult to justify psychoanalytically based treatments in the face of more efficient and predictably effective treatments. Still, some patients are offered psychoanalytic treatment or variations of that treatment, possibly because of the emphasis given to psychoanalytic theory and practice at the time their therapists were trained.

Cognitive Therapy

This approach seeks to relieve suffering by pointing out incorrect "cognitions" or beliefs patients have. Although theoretically appealing, there has been little controlled research evidence supporting cognitive therapy's effectiveness in the absence of exposure and ritual prevention. One study reported in 1995 did find cognitive techniques aimed at correcting excessive estimation of risks and responsibility to be helpful and will undoubtedly be studied further.

All patients benefit from explorations that correct misconceptions about obsessions and rituals. These corrective cognitions are routinely employed as needed in competent behavior and drug therapies and serve in large part as coping tactics to facilitate these therapies. How to maximize the anti–obsessive-compulsive effects of cognitive techniques remains to be determined.

Most patients with OCD have spent a large amount of time trying to correct their faulty cognitions. Sufferers usually maintain awareness ("insight") that their thinking is abnormal and obsessive. They describe their thoughts as "silly, dumb, stupid, goofy, crazy, irrational, ridiculous, asinine, insane," but are powerless to change their thinking by simply talking with others. Until evidence establishes the effectiveness of cognitive therapy, it would be best to emphasize the other better-established treatments of behavior therapy and anti–obsessive-compulsive drugs instead.

Electroconvulsive Therapy

Electroconvulsive therapy (ECT) has been tried, repeatedly, as a treatment for OCD. Most of the time, ECT is ineffective or, at best, only slightly helpful. ECT usually requires treatment as an inpatient, as well as anesthesia and intravenous muscle relaxants, so that substantial expense is involved. Some temporary memory problems and interference with learning may occur with ECT, although other side effects and complications are uncommon.

When obsessions and compulsions occur in the wake of major depression, ECT may be an effective treatment. In this case, however, ECT is effective in treating the depression that in turn caused the obsessions and compulsions. As the depression is relieved, so are the obsessions and compulsions. Except where major depression is the primary problem and obsessions and rituals are secondary to the depression, ECT is unlikely to be of benefit for obsessions and compulsive rituals.

Antipsychotic Medications

Antipsychotic medications (see Chapter 22) are helpful in alleviating major symptoms of psychosis (loss of contact with reality) such as hallucinations (false perceptions that are heard, seen, tasted, smelled, or felt) and delusions (firmly fixed false beliefs). Hearing voices is the most common hallucination, and beliefs of being spied upon or poisoned or of being an important person (such as the President of the United States) are common delusions.

Because obsessions can be so strange (even bizarre), they are sometimes mistaken as hallucinatory or delusional symptoms of psychosis. When this mistake is made, antipsychotic medications may be prescribed with the best intentions. However, obsessive-compulsive persons only rarely (in no more than 5% of cases, usually those with tics or certain personality disorders) improve when given antipsychotic medication.

Antipsychotic medication can cause a number of annoying short-term side effects (drowsiness, confusion, lethargy, weight gain, lightheadedness, dry mouth, blurred vision, and constipation) and other short-term neurologic side effects (*parkinsonism*, marked by stiffness of the arms and legs, shuffling gate, masklike face, tremor, loss of balance, and difficulty speaking; *acute dystonic reaction*, characterized by fixation of the eyes in one position, twisting movements of the body, muscle spasms of the neck and back and difficulty swallowing; *akathisia*, which usually involves restlessness, pacing, jitteriness, and agitation; and a late-appearing complication called *tardive dyskinesia*, which, unlike the other side effects of antipsychotic medication, may not be reversible and involves various components of lip smacking and puckering, chewing motions, puffing out of the cheeks, and rapid, wormlike movements of the tongue, jaw, face, or arms and legs).

Because antipsychotic medications are seldom helpful for patients with OCD and because they have a number of side effects, a trial of their use in OCD should be reserved for cases that have failed to respond to other potentially more effective treatments.

Neurosurgery (Psychosurgery)

Although psychosurgery (previously called "lobotomy," which means separating a lobe of the brain, or "leucotomy," meaning cutting nerve tracts in the brain) has an extremely bad reputation in the United States, there is a place for the infrequent use of certain specific neurosurgical procedures in the treatment of very severe OCD that is resistant to all other treatments. The bad reputation of earlier brain operations occurred when they were used for disorders for which they were ineffective and when they were crudely done resulting in high rates of surgical complications, including death. Over the past 30 years, neurosurgeons have perfected operations that are done very carefully and safely under strict anatomic control. These operations may produce some temporary side effects but rarely cause any long-term adverse reactions or death. It is proper to rename these operations "neurosurgery," and this revision of this booklet has done so in recognition that surgery is done on neurons and not the psyche and that neurosurgeons do very careful and discrete procedures that differ dramatically from the crude early procedures done largely by oneself-described "psychosurgeon."

Remembering that overactivity of certain parts of the frontal lobes of the brain is believed to be involved in OCD, it is not surprising that the most helpful operations have been made in nerve tracts carrying messages from frontal areas to more central parts of the brain, including the caudates, which are also involved in OCD.

These operations have proven at least somewhat helpful for approximately 80% of the very few patients who have failed to respond to behavior therapy and anti–obsessive-compulsive medications, two treatments usually effective for OCD. Although the operations are very safe in skillful hands, they produce irreversible changes in the brain, and because there is also a risk from anesthesia and muscle relaxants, the operations are rarely used and, happily, are rarely necessary. Nevertheless, neurosurgery can be dramatically effective and has the added benefit of returning many patients to a state of responsiveness to previously ineffective behavioral and anti–obsessive-compulsive drug treatments.

Again, it is important to stress that this neurosurgery is not a routine treatment. It has been recommended for only two of more than 1,000 obsessive-compulsive patients seen by the author. Other therapies had failed these patients, and they had remained severely disabled even after years of treatment. In both of these patients, surgery was helpful.

HOW CAN SOMEONE LEARN ALL THAT IS IMPORTANT ABOUT OBSESSIVE-COMPULSIVE DISORDER AND ITS TREATMENTS?

A booklet of this size cannot provide answers to every question that might be asked about these topics. The material included here was selected because doctors and those suffering from OCD believed it was especially important.

The following suggestions may help you learn more about OCD and its treatment:

- Read this booklet thoroughly, making sure to note any areas where you have questions.
- Ask your doctor these questions and any others you might have.
- Reread the booklet from time to time to refresh your memory. Share it with family members and close friends, and discuss areas that are particularly important to you.
- Refer to the readings suggested on the following pages.
- Self-help groups are forming in different parts of the country to offer sup-

port and information to people with OCD. The Obsessive Compulsive Foun-da-tion, Inc. (9 Depot Street, Milford, Connecticut 06460) (203-878-5669) has a newsletter and can provide information about therapists, clinics, and self-help groups, as well as current research on OCD.

• The Obsessive-Compulsive Information Center (OCIC) provides access to the published literature on OCD, certain obsessive-compulsive spectrum disorders, and their treatments. The OCIC is staffed by medical librarians who provide technical information on any specific topic regarding OCD and its treatments. The OCIC also can provide referrals to therapists, clinics, and self-help groups, as well as the Telephone Assessment Program using the Y-BOCS. Staff also can provide the current status of BT STEPS™, the computer-assisted, telephone-administered, self-help behavior therapy program for OCD. For fur-ther information, please contact the Center (Information Centers, Dean Foun-da-tion, 2711 Allen Boulevard, Middleton, Wisconsin 53562; 608-827-2390, fax 608-827-2399).

SUGGESTED READINGS

The following publications may be helpful in better understanding OCD and related disorders and their treatment. Only those publications marked with an asterisk (*) are available from the Obsessive-Compulsive Information Center. The Center can be contacted for current prices and order forms. The others may be obtained through bookstores and libraries.

Nontechnical

*Greist JH, Jefferson JW, Marks IM: *Anxiety and its treatment: help is available,* Wash-ington, 1986, and New York, 1986, American Psychiatric Press, Warner Books.

Rapoport JL: *The boy who couldn't stop washing: the experience & treatment of obses-sive-compulsive disorder,* New York, 1989. E.P. Dutton, New York Penguin Books.

Schwartz JM: *Brain Lock: Free yourself from obsessive-compulsive behavior,* New York, 1996, HarperCollins.

Baer L: *Getting control: overcoming your obsessions and compulsions,* New York, 1991, Little, Brown and Company, Boston and Penguin Books.

VanNoppen BL, Pato MT, Rasmussen S: *Learning to live with obsessive-compulsive disorder,* ed 3, Milford, CT, 1993, OC Foundation, Inc.

*Marks IM: *Living with fear,* New York, 1978, McGraw-Hill.

de Silva P, Rachman S: *Obsessive-compulsive disorder: the facts,* New York, 1992, Oxford University Press.

*Johnston HF: *Obsessive compulsive disorder in children and adolescents: a guide,* Madison, 1993, Child Psychopharmacology Information Center, University of Wis-consin.

Neziroglu F, Yaryura-Tobias JA: *Over and over again: understanding obsessive-com-pulsive disorder,* rev. ed., New York, 1995, Lexington Books.

Foa EB, Wilson R. *Stop obsessing!: how to overcome your obsessions and compul-sions,* New York, 1991, Bantam Books.

*Anders JL, Jefferson JW: *Trichotillomania: a guide,* Madison, 1994, Obsessive Compulsive Information Center, Dean Foundation.

Steketee G, White K: *When once is not enough: help for obsessive-compulsives,* Oakland, CA, 1990, New Harbinger Publications.

Technical

Phillips KA: *The broken mirror: understanding and treating body dysmorphic disorder,* New York, 1996, Oxford University Press.

Marks IM: *Fears, phobias, and rituals,* New York, 1987, Oxford University Press.

Mavissakalian MR, Prien RF, editors: *Long-term treatments of anxiety disorders,* Washington, 1996, American Psychiatric Press.

Rachman SJ, Hodgson RJ: *Obsessions and compulsions,* Englewood Cliffs, NJ, 1980, Prentice-Hall.

*Greist JH, Jefferson JW: *Obsessive-compulsive disorder casebook,* rev. ed., Washington, 1995, American Psychiatric Press.

Yaryura-Tobias JA, Neziroglu FA: *Obsessive-compulsive disorder spectrum: pathogenesis, diagnosis, and treatment,* Washington, 1997, American Psychiatric Press.

Jenike MA, Baer L, Minichiello WF, editors: *Obsessive compulsive disorders: theory and management.,* ed 2, Chicago, 1990, Year Book Medical.

Hollander E, editor: *Obsessive-compulsive-related disorders,* Washington, 1993, American Psychiatric Press.

Zohar J, Insel T, Rasmussen S, editors: *The psychobiology of obsessive-compulsive disorder,* New York, 1991, Springer Publishing.

Steketee GS: *Treatment of obsessive compulsive disorder,* New York, 1993, Guilford Press.

In addition to *Obsessive Compulsive Disorder: A Guide,* the following publications are available from the Obsessive Compulsive Information Center. The Center can be contacted for current prices and order forms.

Temte JL, Jefferson JW, Greist JH: *Antipsychotic medications and schizophrenia: a guide,* rev. ed., Madison, 1998, Information Centers, Dean Foundation.

Greist JH, Jefferson JW, Marks IM: *Anxiety and its treatment: help is available,* New York, 1986, Warner Books.

Medenwald JR, Greist JH, Jefferson JW: *Carbamazepine and manic depression: a guide,* rev. ed., Madison, 1996, Lithium Information Center, Dean Foundation.

Tunali (Sen) D, Jefferson JW, Greist JH: *Depression and antidepressants: a guide,* rev. ed., Madison, 1997, Information Centers, Dean Foundation.

Greist JH, Jefferson JW: *Depression and its treatment,* rev. ed., New York, 1992, American Psychiatric Press, Washington, and Warner Books.

Jefferson JW, Greist JH: *Divalproex and manic depression: a guide,* Madison, 1996, Lithium Information Center, Dean Foundation, (Formerly Valproate guide).

Dries DC, Barklage NE: *Electroconvulsive therapy: a guide,* rev. ed., Madison, 1996, Lithium Information Center, Dean Foundation.

Greist JH, Greist GL, Jefferson JW: *Fearful flyer's guide,* Madison, 1996, Information Centers, Dean Foundation.

Bohn J, Jefferson JW: *Lithium and manic depression: a guide,* rev. ed., Madison, 1996, Lithium Information Center, Dean Foundation.

Jefferson JW, Greist JH, Ackerman DL, Carroll JA: *Lithium encyclopedia for clinical practice,* ed 2, Washington, 1987, American Psychiatric Press.

Marks IM: *Living with fear,* New York, 1978, McGraw-Hill.

Greist JH, Jefferson JW: *Obsessive-compulsive disorder casebook,* rev. ed., Washington, 1995, American Psychiatric Press.

Johnston HF, Fruehling JJ: *Obsessive-compulsive disorder in children and adolescents: a guide,* Rev. ed., Madison, 1997, Child Psychopharmacology Information Service, University of Wisconsin.

Greist JH, Jefferson JW: *Panic disorder and agoraphobia: a guide,* rev. ed., Madison, 1998, Information Centers, Dean Foundation.

Greist JH, Jefferson JW, Katzelnick DJ: *Social phobia: a guide,* Madison, 1997, Information Centers, Dean Foundation.

Johnston HF, Fruehling JJ: *Attention-deficit hyperactivity disorder in children: a medication guide,* rev. ed., Madison, 1997, Child Psychopharmacology Information Service, University of Wisconsin.

Anders JL, Jefferson JW: *Trichotillomania: a guide,* Rev. ed., Madison, 1998, Obsessive-Compulsive Information Center, Dean Foundation.

Appendix 4
Obsessive-Compulsive Disorder In Children and Adolescents: A Guide*

The University of Wisconsin-Madison, Department of Psychiatry, Child Psychopharmacology Information Service

WHAT IS OBSESSIVE-COMPULSIVE DISORDER?

Obsessive-compulsive disorder is a brain disorder characterized by obsessions and compulsions of such severity that they cause distress or interfere with functioning. In this booklet, the term "obsessive-compulsive disorder" is abbreviated "OCD." The majority of children with OCD experience obsessions or compulsions many times a day. Some common childhood obsessions and associated compulsions are listed in Table A.6. Usually children with OCD have *both* obsessions and compulsions, but some children have only obsessions or only compulsions.

Obsessions

Obsessions are unwanted thoughts or feelings that arise repeatedly in the mind. They are almost always experienced as frightening, disgusting, or otherwise unpleasant. Quite often, children describe obsessions as being very much like worries. Common childhood obsessions include: fears of intruders entering the house, fears of contamination with germs or a toxic substance, and worries about contracting a serious illness. Obsessions are experienced as involuntary. This means that these thoughts come into the child's mind despite attempts to think of something else. Children usually try to resist their obsessions. They may do this by distracting themselves with busywork or by avoiding things that remind them of their obsessions.

Table A.6   Childhood Obsessions and Compulsions*

Obsessions	Compulsions (Rituals)
Fears of harm caused by contamination from toxic substances or germs	Excessive handwashing, showering, cleaning, or avoiding
Worries that a burglar or intruder may enter the house	Repeatedly checking door and window locks
Concerns about contracting a serious illness	Checking temperature, asking others for reassurance, repeated doctor visits
Fears that they, a parent, or loved one, might be injured or killed	Repeated reassurance seeking about safety; excessive concern over storms or bad weather; "clingyness," having difficulty being separated from parents
Vague fears that "something bad may happen" if routine activities are not done "correctly." Fears about not doing things in a predetermined or "usual" manner	Slowness, excessive caution, dressing and undressing repeatedly, repeating actions, reassurance seeking, and others
Fears of something "bad" happening in association with particular numbers	Always doing things in sets (depending on the number), avoiding certain numbers, arranging, mentally counting
Fears that something important will be thrown away or lost	Excessive collecting (often of useless "junk"), hoarding
Fears of being a sinful person	Praying, confessing, seeking reassurance
Beliefs that symmetry or equality prevents bad or harmful things from happening	Arranging, ordering, straightening, or attempting to seek "balance" in other ways

*Note: this list is not all-inclusive; it lists only some of the more common childhood obsessions and compulsions. Obsession and compulsions can take many forms but typically revolve around childhood worries or uncertainties.

Children with OCD usually have a number of obsessions. Some may be focused and specific, such as a fear of catching AIDS from a swimming pool. Others may be vague and difficult for the child to explain. One child described his obsession as, ". . . an uncomfortable feeling that I don't walk through doorways the right way." In general, *the younger the child, the more vague the obsessions.*

Sometimes obsessions change over time for unknown reasons. Some seem to diminish and lose their importance, whereas others grow in significance. For example, a child 9 years of age may be obsessed with having the doors locked, but then gradually has this obsession replaced with an obsession about germs by age 14. These changes are just as baffling to the children as they are to their parents.

Most children older than 8 years of age are aware that their obsessive thinking is abnormal, and they commonly use the word "stupid" or "dumb" to describe the obsessions. Because of this awareness, children are typically embarrassed and uncomfortable talking about the obsessions. They may try to hide or minimize them, and sometimes even deny they exist. Parents can find it quite frustrating when they try to help but their child insists, "It's no big deal!"

Young children are usually much less secretive about their obsessions because they are less socially aware than older children are, and thus not as embarrassed by them. They will often ask their parents endless questions related to their obsessions and make no effort whatsoever to hide their OCD–related discomfort.

Compulsions

Compulsions are deliberate actions that are performed repeatedly. Compulsions are sometimes called rituals, so the two terms are used interchangeably throughout this booklet. They are almost always performed to reduce anxiety associated with an obsession. Some examples of compulsions include repetitive washing, dressing and undressing, and repeatedly checking door and window locks. Children may wash in an attempt to relieve the obsession that they have become contaminated, they may dress and undress to relieve a fear that something bad might happen if they don't dress correctly, or they may check locks because of an obsession about intruders.

Sometimes the connection between obsessions and compulsions is puzzling. This is especially true of younger children. For example, one child compulsively got in and out of bed many times in an effort to relieve an obsession that his mother might become ill. He was unable to explain how his actions could be connected to his mother's health and was very embarrassed to even talk about the topic. As with obsessions, children are often secretive about their compulsions. Children with OCD may spend a lot of time in their bedrooms or bathrooms, often because they are involved in repeated compulsive activities.

Some children have mental rituals. These can be as time-consuming and distressing as other rituals, but because they are performed mentally, they are "invisible" to parents and teachers. Examples of mental rituals include counting, reciting a prayer or a poem repeatedly, and silently repeating a certain word or phrase. Mental rituals can be difficult to distinguish from obsessions because both are entirely "thinking" activities. One key difference is that obsessions are involuntary, whereas mental rituals are performed deliberately.

Although compulsions are typically tied to obsessions, children occasionally have only compulsions. For example, a child treated in our clinic had compulsively collected bits of metal, glass, and shiny rocks. Over time, several large boxes of this material had been accumulated, yet there did not seem to be any associated obsession.

As with obsessions, younger children are much less likely to be secretive about their rituals and may do them in open view of others. This can be an advantage since the frequency of these rituals can be used to assess the severity of the child's OCD. At the same time, it can be a disadvantage, because younger children rarely resist their compulsions and the problem can balloon out of control.

Sometimes compulsive behaviors are seen in disorders other than OCD. For example, some children repeatedly pluck hairs, leading to bald spots. This is called *trichotillomania*. Another example is tic disorder. Children with this problem have frequent tics, which can be simple muscle movements such as eye blinking or shoulder shrugging, or they can be more complex movements that appear quite similar to compulsions, such as gesturing or touching others. Some children have vocal tics (words or phrases). When children have both muscular (often called "motor") and vocal tics, they may have a specific kind of tic disorder called *Tourette's disorder*. Both trichotillomania and Tourette's disorder may be related to OCD. Obsessions and compulsions also can occur along with other psychiatric disorders such as autism, depression, or schizophrenia. Usually, however, obsessions and compulsions play a minor role in these disorders.

Four Case Examples

The following are four actual case histories of OCD. The first three are examples of typical childhood OCD. The last case is complicated and atypical.

Roy T., The Late-Night Lock Checker

Roy was brought to our clinic at 13 years of age because he was often awake until 3 or 4 o'clock in the morning, compulsively checking the door and window locks of his house. Initially, he was reluctant to discuss this problem, but as he began to relax and trust us, he described his difficulties:

"I've been doing this dumb thing since I was 9 years old. After I lie down, I begin to wonder if the doors are locked. I always check them before I go to bed, but then I'm not sure. I lie there in bed thinking to myself forget it, the doors are locked,' but I just can't let it go. So finally, I get up and tiptoe downstairs to check the front and back doors. Usually I check them each three times, just to be absolutely sure. Then I go back to bed. Soon I'm wondering if I might have jiggled the lock loose while I was checking. I know it's really stupid to think this, but at the time I just can't get the thought out of my head. Then I start thinking about all the robberies and murders I have ever heard about. Finally, I'm so scared and disgusted I get up and check them all again. Lately, I've started checking the windows too. I just can't stand it. In the morning I'm so tired I can hardly get to school, and I'm falling asleep in class . . ."

Roy's parents were very surprised to hear that he had been secretly checking the doors since the age of 9. They thought this problem was something that had just come up over the past year. At first they had taken him to a counselor who thought that Roy was insecure because his parents were having marital difficulties. They sought another opinion from our clinic because Roy seemed to be getting worse despite the fact that their marital problems had largely resolved.

Roy was treated with behavior therapy and over several months his checking behaviors had diminished to a manageable level. He still worries a little about burglars and murderers before falling asleep, but he is able to resist getting out of bed and checking.

Ellen P., The Prayerful "Apologizer"

Ellen was 14 years old when she asked her mother for help after watching a television talk show about OCD. Her mother was surprised when Ellen said that she thought she had OCD, because her mother hadn't noticed anything unusual. In fact, she had always thought of Ellen as the "perfect child" who was considerate and thoughtful, and who had always done well in school. In our office Ellen told the following story:

"I thought I was going crazy. I kept having this feeling that I had done something terrible. You know, that I had sinned or something. So, I started saying "Hail Marys" to make up for the sin. But sometimes I didn't say one just right, and that got me thinking I might have sinned, and that meant I had to start over again. Then, I started to feel like I had to say them four times perfectly or I would go to hell. I know it's really stupid, but it really scares me. Now I have this new thing. If I like a boy, it's a sin, and I have to pray or I will go to hell for sure. I tried to explain to Father about it in confession, but he only gave me more "Hail Marys." So, I started to wonder if this was God's way of punishing me or something. Last week I saw this lady on a TV show who sounded just like me. I didn't know what to think, but I told my mom, and she brought me here. I've tried to keep busy and put it out of my head, but it just keeps coming back. I hate it."

Ellen and her mother were given information about OCD and its treatment. Ellen decided she wanted to try behavior therapy. First she was asked to keep a daily journal and write down how often and for how long she was praying. At the next appointment, her behavioral therapist asked her to set aside 1 hour each day when she would try to not do *any* ritual praying. Ellen decided that between 7 and 8 o'clock in the evening would be best. At first it was very hard for Ellen not to pray during this period, but after a week it became fairly easy. For her next assignment her therapist asked her to think about a boy she liked at 7:00 and then refrain from any ritual praying as before. Again, this was initially very difficult but became easier with practice. Ellen continued to do similar exercises in her behavior therapy sessions and at home. After 6 weeks of behavior therapy, she was nearly symptom-free.

Jon K., The Nonstop Handwasher

Jon was 9 years old when he was referred to our clinic by a dermatologist (skin specialist) who had been treating him for a rash on his hands. The dermatologist had told Jon and his mother that the rash was caused by too much hand-washing. His mother tried but was unable to convince Jon to wash less, and when his rash continued to worsen, the dermatologist referred him to us for a psychiatric evaluation.

Jon was downcast and tearful during his first appointment. When his mother tried to talk about the handwashing, he became very angry and told her to "shut up!" Because the interview process was so upsetting, he was excused and his mother provided most of the history. She told the following story:

Jon used to be a very pleasant, happy-go-lucky child. Then, about 6 months ago he started to worry about getting AIDS. His father and I have explained to him in great detail, and on many occasions, that AIDS can only be caught through needles and through sex. Jon understands this, yet he seems to think that AIDS is everywhere. Now he even washes his hands after seeing something about AIDS on the television. As you can see, his hands are raw and chapped. We have tried everything to get him to stop. We've tried bribery, reasoning, and even spankings; nothing works. He has become quite a stubborn and angry child over this.

Because Jon was so irritable and stubborn, we didn't think he should start with behavior therapy. Instead, he was prescribed the anti-OCD medication, fluvoxamine, and after 4 weeks his mood was improved and he was washing his hands much less. Jon then started behavior therapy and made additional gains.

During a portion of Jon's treatment at our clinic, his parents were asked to come in together for a conference to provide them with information about OCD. At that appointment they described their confusion and anger over Jon's behaviors. Once they learned about how OCD had affected Jon, they realized that the harsh punishments they had given him were inappropriate. Both parents had been raised in strict families and had always believed that a no-nonsense approach to child rearing was best. Because this approach had not been helpful in treating their son's OCD, they were initially at a loss about how to cope with his OCD–related behaviors. Consequently, several family sessions were scheduled to help with alternative parenting strategies.

Janet N., Too Slow at Everything

Seventeen-year-old Janet was brought to our clinic because she was becoming progressively slower at nearly everything she was doing. Mornings were especially difficult for her when she was supposed to get ready for school. Janet is mildly mentally retarded and requires special education, which makes it difficult for her to talk about her history and her OCD. During the appointment, Janet was pleasant but seemed quite embarrassed by our questions. She answered most of them by simply saying, "I don't know." Her mother did most of the talking:

Janet has always been a good girl, but I don't know what has gotten into her lately. When she is supposed to get dressed in the morning, I find her staring at the clothes in her drawer. It seems as though she can't decide what to wear. So, now I pick her clothes out for her. But even after I've picked them out, she will sit on the side of the bed and put her socks on and take them off, over and over again. She can't seem to tell me what is wrong other than saying, "They don't feel right." It's the same story with her blouse, pants, everything. I practically have to dress her myself to get her to school on time. In the bathroom she will dawdle all day if I let her. Her teachers say the same thing happens at school. They can't get her to complete any assignments. The special education teacher has no idea what's wrong either.

This case is complex because it is difficult to be certain how much of Janet's slowness is related to OCD rather than to mental retardation. Janet was treated with behavior therapy and anti-OCD medications. The medications were only slightly helpful, and Janet was never able to fully cooperate with the behavior therapy process. She continues to be very slow and she needs a great deal of help in her day-to-day life.

COMMONLY ASKED QUESTIONS ABOUT OBSESSIVE-COMPULSIVE DISORDER IN CHILDREN

How Common is OCD in Children and Adolescents?

Exactly how many children have OCD is unknown. We do know that it is much more common than was once believed. It may be as frequent as 1 out of every 100 children under 20 years of age. It is estimated that about 40% of all the adults who have OCD first began to experience symptoms before 18 years of age. Because of widespread uncertainty about this disorder, as well as attempts by children to hide their OCD, many children are either not diagnosed or are incorrectly diagnosed. This situation is unfortunate, because effective treatments are available.

What is it Like for Children Who Have OCD?

OCD can make day-to-day life very difficult for children and adolescents. They may worry that they are "crazy" because they are aware that their thinking is different from that of their friends and family. Life is often experienced as stressful because OCD symptoms can consume a great deal of time and energy, making it difficult to complete tasks such as homework or household chores. Children with OCD may experience low self-esteem because their inability to control their OCD symptoms has often led to embarrassment and frustration.

Mornings can be especially difficult for children with OCD. Many of these children feel they must do their rituals exactly right or things will not go well during the rest of the day. Yet, at the same time that they are trying to do their rituals very carefully, they are feeling rushed to be on time for school. This combination leads to feeling pressured, stressed, and irritable. Bedtime also can be particularly difficult. Children with OCD may feel they must finish all of their compulsive rituals before they can go to sleep. Yet, they also must finish homework and take care of other chores and responsibilities. Some children stay up late into the night and are exhausted the following day.

Children with OCD sometimes do not feel well physically. This may be due to the general stress of having the disorder, or it may be related to loss of sleep or poor nutrition. Obsessions and compulsions connected to food are common and can lead to sporadic or eccentric eating habits. Because of these, and perhaps other unknown factors, many children with OCD often have many physical complaints such as headache or upset stomach.

Children with OCD usually have periods in which they are extremely angry at their parent(s). Sometimes this is because parents have become unwilling (or are unable) to comply with the child's "unreasonable" demands. For example, children may insist that their clothes be washed multiple times or that they be allowed to shower for hours on end. When parents set limits, the child typically becomes very anxious and angry. This intense anger often seems "out of character" for the child, leaving the parents confused. Sometimes parents will give in to these "temper tantrums," but later will feel powerless and manipulated by their child. It is common for parents to differ between themselves on how these "temper tantrums" should be handled, and this can lead to dissension and inconsistent parenting.

Peer relationships also may be stressful for children with OCD because they often try very hard to conceal their rituals from schoolmates and teachers. When OCD is severe, this becomes impossible, and the child may be teased and ridiculed. Even when OCD is not severe, it may interfere with making friends, because so much time is spent preoccupied with obsessions and compulsions, or because friends react in a negative way to unusual OCD–related behaviors.

What is it Like for the Parents of Children with OCD?

Parents of children with OCD experience a wide range of intense emotions, including bewilderment, guilt, anger, shame, grief, and frustration. Often frustration predominates.

Initially, the behaviors and worries that seem to have overtaken their child often baffle parents, and they usually attempt to reassure their child that the worries are senseless and that the compulsions are unnecessary. These reassurances fail, leaving the parents even more puzzled. In an effort to understand what is happening, parents often ask the child to explain why he or she is acting so irrationally. The child is often unable to understand why these problems are occurring and cannot provide a satisfactory explanation. From the parents' perspective, it can appear that the child is trying deliberately to be stubborn or uncooperative. Over time, family relationships can become strained, and tension is commonplace. Family counseling may be needed to help parents and siblings to reduce their stress and to better understand the behaviors and motivations of a child with OCD. Such counseling can help the family come to an agreement on how OCD is to be viewed and how to respond in a manner consistent with the child's rituals and fears.

In well-meaning attempts to maintain some degree of order and discipline, parents can sometimes find themselves nagging, yelling, or punishing their child, only to feel guilty later. Because obsessions and compulsions can be very compelling, punishment has little effect and only demoralizes both the child and parents.

On the other hand, some parents "bend over backward" trying to help relieve the child's stress and anxiety. They may get caught up in assisting the child with elaborate washing and checking behaviors or other compulsions. This is almost never helpful and can actually add to the family's problems. Going along with rituals may sometimes appear to help reduce anxiety in the short term, but over time, the child usually becomes dissatisfied with the way family members are trying to help. This leads to conflict, resentment, and increasing tension. It is usually best not to give in to the demands of the child, and family members should not conform their own behaviors to fit the child's OCD symptoms. This can be very difficult to avoid, especially with a child who has severe OCD. However, bear in mind that once family members become involved in the child's compulsive rituals, they often need professional help to stop. This is because the child usually becomes upset and angry, and may even become abusive when family members attempt to withdraw from the rituals.

How Does OCD Become Disabling?

OCD disables children primarily when it consumes so much time that they are unable to complete the usual tasks of childhood. Children may have so much difficulty getting dressed in the morning that they do not get to school on time. Once at school, they can become so preoccupied with OCD symptoms that they do not pay attention to the material being taught and fall behind. OCD also can become disabling when it makes the child feel demoralized. Embarrassment over OCD rituals or a loss of self-esteem may cause the child to become unwilling to try new things or engage socially with others. This interrupts the process of normal development and can lead to serious depression.

Are There Other Symptoms Associated with OCD?

Children with OCD are typically quite irritable and moody. They often seem to be chronic worriers and may have difficulty relaxing and enjoying themselves. Children and adolescents with OCD may have many superficial friends and acquaintances but often are unable to form close personal friendships or have a best friend. Children with OCD can be stubborn and demanding, especially around issues related to OCD symptoms. Frequently these children seem inordinately slow in completing seemingly easy tasks, such as getting dressed in the morning or completing household chores. Slowness is sometimes the result of children developing rituals that become intertwined with routine tasks. For example, something as simple as brushing teeth may take hours because the toothpaste must be squeezed out a certain way or each tooth must be brushed in exactly the same manner as every other tooth. Slowness also can occur when children become physically exhausted from OCD symptoms. Finally, in contrast to their stubbornness about certain things, children with OCD also can be frustratingly indecisive about others. A simple decision, such as picking out dessert at a restaurant, can become fraught with obsessional doubts, leading to endless uncertainty and delay.

Can a Child with OCD Have Other Psychiatric Disorders?

Having OCD does not "protect" children from other psychiatric disorders. In addition to OCD, they may have attention–deficit hyperactivity disorder (ADHD), learning disorders, major depressive disorder (MDD), social phobias, or panic disorder, just to name a few. Naturally, when more than one disorder is present, it complicates treatment. A complete discussion of every childhood psychiatric disorder is beyond the scope of this booklet. However, MDD and panic disorder deserve special mention.

Both MDD and panic disorder occur more commonly in adults with OCD than in the general population. This occurrence has not been specifically studied in children, but clinical experience suggests that this relationship also holds true for young people. A diagnosis of MDD is made when a child has become either sad or irritable far beyond what would be considered normal. In addition to problems with mood, children with MDD also may have trouble with sleep, have a poor appetite, or seem unable to have fun or enjoy themselves. When depression occurs in conjunction with OCD, both disorders must be treated. Usually children with MDD are unsuitable for behavior therapy until depression has improved. Fortunately, anti-OCD medications also have antidepressant effects, which often allows both disorders to be treated with the same medication. Children with both disorders also may benefit from counseling therapy for depressive symptoms.

Panic disorder also can complicate the treatment of OCD. Panic disorder is diagnosed when a child suffers from frequent panic attacks. A panic attack is a brief "spell" in which a child becomes extremely frightened for no rational reason. Panic attacks typically last less than 10 minutes, but are nonetheless quite terrifying. Usually physical symptoms are present, including shortness of breath, a pounding heart, trembling, sweating, an upset stomach, or chest pain. Children experiencing a panic attack typically feel as though they might be "going crazy" or dying, and they often look ill and extremely frightened. They quickly learn to avoid anything associated with a previous panic attack. This can result in school avoidance, reluctance to ride in cars or elevators, or avoidance of public places. Children who have both panic disorder and OCD may require more intensive behavior therapy, as well as additional medication. Fortunately, many children find that panic symptoms improve when they take anti-OCD medication, so additional treatment may not be needed.

How Does OCD in Children Differ From OCD in Adults?

In most respects OCD in children is very similar to OCD in adults. Usually both age groups have obsessions and compulsions, and the same treatments are used for each. However, there are some differences, which are discussed in the following paragraphs.

Children with OCD—especially young children—often do not have as much insight into the disorder as do adults. Most adults with OCD recognize that their obsessions are senseless and that their drive to do rituals is irrational and excessive. Children often have some insight, but it is typically limited. They may admit that their OCD symptoms are "dumb" when speaking "in general," but will become insistent that their OCD symptoms are important when confronted with a specific situation. For example, one child always readily agreed that she washed her hands too much. Yet, whenever her parents tried to stop her from doing so, she would insist that this particular washing was very important and that it had nothing to do with OCD.

Children try to involve family members in rituals much more frequently than adults with OCD. They may insist that parents wash their laundry twice (or more), declare their bedroom "off limits," or demand that parents repeatedly check and recheck the accuracy of homework. These demands are often frustrating for parents because children with OCD are seldom grateful for this "extra help." Many times they become angry that their parents won't do more, or because the parents didn't perform their part of the ritual correctly. It is usually best for parents to reduce or eliminate their involvement in the child's rituals. However, this can be very difficult for parents of children with severe OCD. The assistance of a trained behavior therapist or other qualified helper outside the family is often necessary to devise a behavior therapy plan that will help to get parents off the "OCD hook," relieving them of having to perform their part in the child's OCD rituals. The need for this seemingly stern approach is discussed further in the section on behavior therapy. When children with OCD have involved their brothers or sisters in compulsive rituals, these siblings should be included in a behavior therapy plan.

Another way that childhood OCD differs from adult OCD is that the relationship between obsessions and compulsions can be less clear. One child refused to allow her parents to throw out any garbage. Her obsession was a vague fear that something bad might happen, or something important might inadvertently get thrown away. She was unable to explain the connection between "something bad" and the garbage. Another child had to do nearly everything in sets of four or (she felt) her dog would be run over by an automobile. She admitted that there was no connection between doing things in fours and automobiles, yet she was afraid to ignore the obsession.

Why Do Children with OCD Ask So Many Questions?

All children ask repetitive questions at times, but children with OCD take this annoying behavior to extremes because of their compulsive need to be certain. This questioning ritual is called "reassurance seeking." A typical example is as follows:

Child—"What time is my doctor appointment?"
Parent—"Three o'clock."
Child—"Are you sure?"
Parent—"Yes!"
Child—"What if you forgot, or didn't hear it right?"
Parent—"I'm sure I'm right, it's written right here on the calendar."
Child—"Maybe you should call the doctor and check?"
Parent—"I said, I'm sure!"
Child—"But how can you be sure if you don't check?"
Parent—(exasperated) "I am sure it is 3 o'clock, now drop it! . . ." [which the child is unlikely to do until the appointment time arrives!]

This example illustrates several features of reassurance-seeking rituals. It isn't unusual for children to occasionally ask for reassurance, but when reassurance is given to children with OCD, they are not satisfied. It also illustrates how these children can be very persistent about a topic that may be of relatively trivial importance. Lastly, it shows how even the most patient parent can become frustrated in the face of endless questioning. Giving repeated reassurance to children with OCD is unwise because it tends to lead to more questions and actually perpetuates the problem. A better response for the parent to make could be, "The doctor's instructions are that I am not to reassure you." When pestered, another neutral response might be, "The doctor says we all have to take risks." These approaches can help parents or other family members avoid becoming involved in these reassurance-seeking rituals, and place the reason for the refusal upon the doctor's (or behavioral therapist's) shoulders.

What Causes OCD in Children?

The exact cause of OCD remains unclear. It is known that OCD is related to disturbances in brain functioning. These disturbances have not been fully specified, but it seems certain that they involve the brain chemical serotonin. This topic is discussed in greater depth in the companion booklet (see Appendix 3). Recent research has suggested that sometimes childhood OCD may be triggered by certain kinds of infections, such as strep throat. Exactly how or why this happens to some children and not to others is unclear, and this is an area of active research.

Is OCD Inherited?

We know that in many families, OCD follows a pattern of inheritance, suggesting a genetic link. This does not mean that the disorder itself is inherited, but rather that some kind of susceptibility is passed on. People who have this susceptibility may develop OCD or may remain well. Some individuals develop OCD without having any family history of the disorder, strongly suggesting inheritance is not the only factor causing OCD. Other factors such as infections or stresses also may be involved.

There is little doubt that OCD often runs in families. However, it appears that genes are only partially responsible for causing the disorder. If OCD was completely determined by genetics, pairs of identical twins would always either both have the disorder or both not have it. For example, eye color is completely determined by genes and identical twins *always* have the same color eyes. However, in the case of OCD, if one identical twin has it, there is a 13% chance that the other twin will not be affected. This strongly suggests that genetics only partly explains the cause of OCD and that some other factor is also important. At this point, no one really knows what that other factor (or factors) might be, although some have suggested that infection or exposure to an environmental toxin may play a role.

Some experts have speculated that there may be different types of OCD, and that some types are inherited, whereas other types are not. Although the findings are preliminary, there is evidence that OCD that emerges in childhood may be different from OCD that begins in adulthood. Individuals with childhood-onset OCD appear much more likely to have blood relatives who are affected with the disorder than those with adult-onset OCD.

If a parent is affected with OCD, we can roughly estimate how likely it will be that a child also will have the disorder. If one parent has OCD, the likelihood the child will be affected is approximately 2% to 8%. It is important to remember that this statistic is an approximation, and several other factors should be considered when attempting to estimate the risk of an offspring developing OCD. One factor is whether or not the parents themselves have a family history of OCD. For example, if a parent who has OCD also has blood relatives with the disorder, the risk for the child increases somewhat. Conversely, if a parent has OCD but no blood relatives are affected, then the risk decreases. Another factor mentioned earlier is the age at which a parent developed OCD. If the parent's OCD did not start until adulthood, it is less likely that offspring will be affected during childhood. Conversely, if the parent's OCD is the "variety" that starts in childhood, the chances of the child being affected are increased.

Another factor to consider is the family history of other anxiety or tic disorders (such as Tourette's disorder). Having blood relatives with OCD, as well as other anxiety disorders, means that the child not only has an increased risk for OCD but also may have an increased risk of developing a different anxiety disorder or perhaps a tic disorder. In summary, having blood relatives with OCD, anxiety disorders, or tic disorders increases a child's risk of developing any or all of these same disorders.

As the previous information indicates, it is difficult to estimate precisely the chances that a parent will pass OCD on genetically to his or her offspring. This is an area of very active research and new developments appear frequently. Most major medical centers have genetics counselors available. These counselors are highly trained individuals whose jobs dictate that they stay abreast of current literature in this area. They can be an excellent resource for prospective parents who have OCD (or any other disorder with an inherited component). We advise prospective parents to contact a genetics counselor if they would like the most precise estimate possible regarding whether they might transmit a psychiatric disorder such as OCD to their offspring. Additional information on this and other OCD questions related to parenting can be found in the booklet *OCD and Parenting,* which is available from the Obsessive-Compulsive Foundation.

How is OCD Diagnosed in a Child or Adolescent?

Typically, a physician or psychologist makes the diagnosis of OCD after carefully reviewing the child's history and conducting a psychiatric diagnostic interview. Information about the child gathered from family members and teachers is helpful. Usually this diagnostic process is straightforward, but occasionally it may be difficult to diagnose OCD with certainty because symptoms can overlap with those of other disorders. In general, the younger the child, the more difficult the disorder is to diagnose.

At present, there is no specific blood test or other objective medical test used to diagnose OCD. However, this is an area of active research, and there are several promising possibilities being developed. The most interesting research involves positron emission tomography (PET scan) and functional magnetic resonance imaging (fMRI). These technologies allow scientists to identify and measure activity in specific parts of the brain. As medical practice advances, PET and fMRI may someday develop into clinically useful tools for diagnosing OCD.

In summary, diagnosing mental disorders in children is still a highly subjective process. If OCD seems a possibility, the child should be evaluated by a physician or psychologist experienced in the diagnosis and treatment of children with anxiety disorders.

Do All Children Who Have Rituals Suffer From OCD?

Nearly all children go through phases in which certain rituals become prominent. For example, most of us are familiar with the chant "step on a crack, break your mother's back," and have seen children carefully avoiding pavement or sidewalk cracks. In addition, children often have special bedtime rituals, such as having a favorite story read to them. It is only when rituals inter-fere with day-to-day life, or cause significant distress, that a diagnosis of OCD should be considered.

Does OCD Always Require Treatment?

Sometimes the child's OCD is so mild that treatment is unnecessary. We base the decision to treat on two factors:

1. The degree of distress the OCD is causing.
2. How much the OCD is interfering in the child's life.

If a child is not suffering and the OCD is only causing mild interference in the child's life, the inconvenience and expense of treatment may not be justi-fied. In these cases, a "wait-and-see" approach is best, because the problem may not get any worse and could diminish on its own. However, in families with a high prevalence of OCD, adopting a more proactive approach would be pru-dent. In these situations, behavior therapy might serve as a preventive strategy.

Does OCD Occur in Very Young Children?

The youngest child we have diagnosed with OCD was only 18 months old! Instead of playing normally, this young boy spent most of his time anxiously arranging and rearranging his toys. OCD was suspected because his mother and other family members also had OCD. Still, it was not possible to establish the diagnosis with certainty until the child was older and demonstrated more typical OCD symptoms.

Although we know that OCD can occur in very young children, this occur-rence appears to be quite uncommon. In our clinic, we seldom see children with OCD younger than 5 years of age. This may be because the disorder is rare in this age group, or it may be because it is difficult for parents to recog-nize that their young child is having symptoms. Many school-age children with OCD say they remember having OCD symptoms as far back as they can recall and believe they have always had OCD.

What Other Disorders Mimic OCD?

Many disorders, including schizophrenia, autism, eating disorders, and phobic disorders, can produce symptoms similar to those seen in OCD. For example, children with autism often engage in repetitive activities that appear similar to those seen with OCD. It sometimes requires considerable training and experience to unravel the complex symptoms seen in a disturbed child. This is especially true with very young children.

As mentioned earlier, children may have more than one psychiatric disor-der. When two or more diagnoses are present, it is important that each be iden-tified to ensure the child receives appropriate treatment.

Occasionally, a situation is encountered in which an exact diagnosis of OCD cannot be made. This usually occurs when a child has additional developmental difficulties—such as mental retardation—or has a collection of very unusual symptoms. Over time, the typical patterns of specific disorders begin to emerge and the diagnostic confusion can be sorted out. However, this process may take months or even years.

CHILDREN AND ADOLESCENTS WITH OBSESSIVE-COMPULSIVE DISORDER AT SCHOOL

What Should I Tell My Child's Teacher About His or Her OCD?

There is no simple answer to this question. It depends partly on the severity of the child's OCD symptoms. Children who have mild OCD usually do not exhibit any symptoms at school. In this case, it may be best not to inform the teacher because the child might be treated differently or even viewed as "crazy." However, this reaction is the exception and not the rule. Most teachers take a very enlightened view of mental illness and appreciate being informed of their students' challenges. If a child is experiencing OCD symptoms at school, the teacher should almost always be informed, to clear up questions about unusual behaviors and allow the teacher to implement strategies to facilitate the child's learning.

It is helpful to provide the teacher with educational material about OCD (such as this booklet), since prejudice against those who are mentally ill is usually based on ignorance. Almost without exception, teachers who are well informed about a child's OCD are able to teach a child more effectively. If a child is on anti-OCD medications, the teacher and school nurse should always be notified. This information can be extremely valuable if a medical emergency should arise during school attendance, and the parents are not immediately available.

How Can OCD Affect a Child's School Performance?

Sometimes OCD has little or no effect on school performance. As stated earlier, many children with mild to moderate OCD have no symptoms when at school. This has led some parents to wonder whether their child actually has OCD or is intentionally being manipulative or eccentric at home. However, children with OCD commonly say they feel their OCD "building up" when at school, but resist it to prevent embarrassment. When they get home, they "let it all out" and may spend much time with rituals. Although distressing to parents, this indicates that the child views the home environment as safer and less threatening than school.

Children with OCD can become so preoccupied with obsessive thoughts that they do not pay attention to the material being taught. This can give the impression that they have another disorder called attention deficit disorder (ADD). Most children with OCD do not have problems with attention span, but when they are focused on their OCD symptoms, they can appear to be quite inattentive or easily distracted.

At times, OCD symptoms can interfere directly with specific aspects of school performance. For example, some children develop reading or writing rituals. A child may feel that he or she has to read each word a specific number of times or that written material must be done absolutely perfectly. Obviously, this can slow a child's progress greatly. On occasion, obsessions and compulsions can become so time-consuming that children fail to complete homework assignments, and some children develop compulsions around reading or writing that are so upsetting they absolutely refuse to read or write at all.

Do Anti-OCD Medications Affect a Child's Ability to Learn?

Many children with OCD suffer some difficulty with school, and effective treatment of any kind often results in *improved* school performance. However, medication side effects also can lead to problems. Some children experience sedation (sleepiness) when taking anti-OCD medication. Children who are very sleepy obviously do not learn well. Sometimes sleepiness is a temporary side effect, appearing shortly after an anti-OCD medication has been started and slowly diminishing over time as the child adjusts to the medication. If sleepiness persists, the medication dose may need to be adjusted or an alternative medication considered.

Some children experience restlessness or irritability as a side effect of anti-OCD medication. This side effect can result in the child being disruptive in class, although it usually does not interfere with the child's ability to learn. If a teacher suspects that a medication side effect may be causing problems in school, the doctor who prescribed the medication should be notified.

Can Teachers Be Helpful in the Treatment of Children with OCD?

If the child is not having OCD symptoms at school, the teacher may not need to be involved. If there are OCD symptoms causing problems at school, it is usually helpful to have the teacher work with the parent, physician, or behavioral therapist involved in the child's care. Simply understanding more about the disorder and the child's treatment program can be helpful in responding appropriately to OCD–related difficulties. Most often, applying the behavior therapy principles of exposure and response prevention will minimize OCD–related problems at school. These concepts are illustrated in the following paragraphs and are discussed further in the section on behavior therapy.

What Should Be Done About a Child Who Keeps Requesting to Use the Bathroom to Perform Rituals?

This is a common problem that can be very disruptive to the rest of the class. Usually it is best to work with the parent, physician, behavioral therapist, and child to develop a program to address the problem. Often the first step is to accurately assess how many times the child goes to the bathroom and how much time is spent there. It is also helpful to note whether this is a problem only in certain classes or at certain times of the day.

Once this information has been gathered, the next step is to discuss with the child what he or she is doing and feeling that leads to these trips to the bathroom. A specific behavior therapy plan can then be developed by a behavioral therapist with input from the child and teacher. This may consist of limiting bathroom visits to a certain number per hour or limiting the time spent in the bathroom. Often the behavioral therapist will ask both the child and teacher to keep an accurate record of progress. It is helpful to set specific goals and, when the goals are achieved, to ensure that the child receives appropriate rewards and praise.

What Can be Done About Children Who Keep Erasing and Rewriting?

This problem usually occurs when the child has an obsessional fear that something terrible may happen if written homework assignments are not performed perfectly. The result is many rewritten drafts or excessive erasures on the child's papers. The behavioral therapist develops exercises in which the child deliberately writes incorrectly and then refrains from erasing for a prescribed period of time. This time period is gradually lengthened until the child no longer needs to erase at all. These gains are then transferred to the school environment by employing the same behavior therapy techniques. This requires some degree of collaboration between the teacher, behavioral therapist, and child.

It is important for the teacher to be patient while this problem is being addressed, and to recognize that the child's anxiety may increase while resisting the urge to rewrite an assignment. Unfortunately, children are sometimes penalized with bad grades or outright punishment when they fail to complete written assignments. This can lead to power struggles, defiance, or demoralization, none of which is conducive to learning. Some teachers are concerned that overall classroom discipline will suffer if exceptions are made for a child with OCD. But, far-sighted teachers recognize the need to balance short-term discipline with the long-term special needs of students with OCD.

What Can be Done About Children Who Ask an Endless Series of Inappropriate Questions During Class?

This is a common and very disruptive problem. Often children have little insight into this particular OCD symptom. This is not surprising, because children are regularly encouraged to ask questions in class whenever they have doubts about the subject material being taught. As described earlier, the first step is to obtain an accurate record of how often and at what times this problem arises.

Once an accurate assessment of the frequency of inappropriate questioning has been obtained, a behavior therapy approach can be developed. The following is an example of the approach used for a child named Ethan. By his teacher's account, Ethan was initially asking approximately 50 questions per hour (not unusual for OCD). For the first intervention, he was requested to keep a careful count of how many questions he asked each hour and to record his count in a journal. Just by doing this, his rate of question asking was reduced to approximately 30 questions per hour. After several days at this level, Ethan was told that 30 questions per hour was the maximum number he was allowed. If he tried to ask a 31st question, he was simply told, "You have used up all your questions." Because Ethan had become used to asking approximately 30 questions, he wasn't greatly upset by this. He then agreed to have the number of questions he was allowed per hour decreased by 1 each day. When Ethan reached eight questions per hour, which the teacher considered appropriate, no further reductions were made.

It is important for the teacher to handle these problems in a matter-of-fact manner, avoiding harshness or ridicule. This will help prevent the child from becoming demoralized and will reduce the likelihood of testing by classmates. It also is useful to set goals that will result in rewards as the child makes progress.

Do Some Children Use Their OCD as a "Crutch" to Avoid School or Schoolwork?

Children with OCD are first and foremost children. Like all children, they have their moments of laziness or manipulation. Just as children with asthma or a broken bone may use their health problem to get special favors, so may children with OCD use their disorder to get what they want. Much of the time, it is nearly impossible to tell whether an OCD symptom is real or whether it was dreamed up for the convenience of the moment. Because of this, it is best to be as consistent as possible and not try to determine hidden motives. We always encourage parents and teachers to give the child "the benefit of the doubt" but to also be firm, consistent, and supportive. Most children respond quite positively to this approach.

What (If Anything) Should the Teacher Tell the Class About a Pupil's OCD?

First of all, nothing can (or should) be said without the permission of both parent and child. In mild to moderate cases of OCD, the child typically does not have noticeable symptoms at school, and it is best to say nothing. In some severe cases, children with OCD may show obvious symptoms that cause the other children to ask questions. It is sufficient to say something general such as, "Billy has some difficulties and he is working on them." Children who are persistent in questioning should be told that "Billy's difficulties are private."

How Can Teasing be Handled?

Teasing can be demoralizing for any child and is more likely to occur if a child has severe OCD. The only helpful remedy is close supervision and swift intervention when it occurs. It is also very important for teachers to set a good example and always refrain from expressing any ridiculing or demeaning comments toward children. Unfortunately, we have seen instances in which teachers have failed to intervene or, even worse, have laughed when a child was teased. This sends the wrong message to both the child with OCD and the child (or children) doing the teasing. The child with OCD begins to feel that having a mental disorder is shameful. The child doing the teasing is led to believe that it is okay, or even desirable, to torment classmates who are having problems. Teasing children with mental or physical disorders must not be tolerated!

Should Children With OCD be Placed in Special Education Classrooms?

Most special education classrooms are designed for children who are falling behind because of behavior or learning problems, or for children who have behaviors that disrupt the rest of the class. Most children with OCD are neither falling behind nor disruptive. In fact, a substantial number of children with OCD have above-average intelligence! However, a few children with severe OCD have so much difficulty with simple day-to-day activities that they benefit from the additional individual attention provided in a special education classroom. These decisions should be made on a case-by-case basis.

What Should a Teacher Do if He or She Suspects a Child has OCD?

If a child is handwashing excessively, making many erasures on homework, asking an excessive number of questions, or seems extremely slow in the bathroom, teachers may suspect OCD. The first thing to do is contact the parents and have a frank discussion about the behaviors that seem abnormal. If these behaviors are interfering with school performance, or if the child seems significantly distressed, the teacher should recommend a professional consultation.

TREATMENTS FOR OBSESSIVE-COMPULSIVE DISORDER
Behavior Therapy

Behavior therapy is a unique type of psychologic therapy that has been developed primarily for problems with anxiety. It is unique because it involves action. Most psychologic therapies focus on thinking about, talking about, and understanding feelings and thoughts. Although thoughts and feelings are a part of behavior therapy, the main focus is directed at performing (or not performing) certain actions. Because behavior therapy is action-oriented, much less emphasis is placed on insight and understanding. During behavior therapy, the patient performs a series of activities (behaviors), and it is the activities themselves that have the beneficial effect. Although most psychologic therapies rely on insight and understanding for progress, behavior therapy relies heavily on performing a "real-life" activity. The resulting experiential learning produces therapeutic progress.

Experiential learning is an example of the type of learning that takes place when a child learns to ride a bicycle. Just as a child cannot learn to ride a bicycle through imagination or talking or reading about it, neither can a child master OCD–related anxiety through these techniques. Learning to ride a bicycle requires experience and practice. Learning to master OCD requires experience and practice as well.

Commonly Asked Questions About Behavior Therapy

How does behavior therapy work?

The workings of behavior therapy are best illustrated through an example. The two guiding principles of behavior therapy are *exposure* and *response prevention*, which are illustrated in the following case.

Ann was a child who obsessed that she might become contaminated with chemicals and that these chemicals could cause her great harm.

These obsessions plagued her for hours on end and were often triggered by trivial experiences, such as seeing a container of kitchen cleanser, or listening to a radio commercial for ant poison. Because of these obsessions, she felt compelled to shower immediately after any actual or imagined contact with a harmful chemical. These symptoms were severe and interfered greatly in her life. She would shower for several hours, many times each day.

The following behavior therapy exercises were prescribed for Ann. Twice a day, with the help of her mother, Ann sprinkled a small amount of kitchen cleanser (a greatly feared chemical) on her hands. She had agreed to wait 1 full hour before taking a shower. Over a span of weeks, this waiting time was extended to 2 and then 3 hours, and eventually was modified to simply rinsing her hands off 3 hours after the exposure session. The *exposure* consisted of putting cleanser on her hands. The *response prevention* consisted of encouraging her to refrain from showering immediately after the exposure. (Note: Response prevention is sometimes called "ritual prevention.")

These behavior therapy sessions were initially very difficult for Ann. Shortly after putting cleanser on her hands, she experienced high anxiety and a strong urge to take a shower. With help from her mother and her behavioral therapist, she gradually learned to resist these urges and was able to delay showering.

Over several months, these sessions proved helpful because Ann engaged in "experiential learning." She learned by experience that nothing terrible would happen to her after exposure to cleanser. This learning by experience is much more powerful and effective than other kinds of learning activities. Her parents had lectured her on many occasions about the harmless effects of cleanser, an approach that was not at all helpful to Ann and was frustrating for her parents. When she experienced the reality of the harmlessness of the cleanser, and the reality that a shower was unnecessary, her anxiety eventually diminished. These learning experiences enabled Ann to skip many showers that she would otherwise have taken.

This example of how Ann's behavior therapy was conducted is deliberately oversimplified to illustrate the principles of exposure and response prevention.

Typically, behavior therapy is more complex and usually requires the assistance of a trained behavioral therapist. This is especially true in the case of children with OCD because the therapist must take into account the child's developmental age, motivations, and dynamics of the family.

How effective is behavior therapy?

Behavior therapy is often sufficient treatment for many children, or is at least helpful in conjunction with anti-OCD medications (discussed later). The effectiveness of behavior therapy varies from child to child, but it is most beneficial for children who have mild to moderate OCD and who *want* to reduce their symptoms. Motivation is a key factor in behavior therapy success. Children who recognize that the OCD–related behaviors are causing problems are usually interested in behavior therapy and are willing to participate in therapy exercises. Behavior therapy is almost always helpful for motivated children.

Unfortunately, many children with OCD are *not* motivated. Some deny that the OCD is a problem, and others may be so discouraged that they are unwilling to try. Occasionally, a skilled behavioral therapist can inspire an unmotivated child. In our experience, behavior therapy is helpful for most children, highly effective for approximately 20%, and of little value to a small minority of approximately 5%.

How often must behavior therapy be performed?

To be effective, behavior therapy exercises must be performed daily, sometimes several times each day. This does not mean that the child must see the therapist every day. Instead, it means that the child must perform behavior therapy exercises and assignments on a daily basis. This requires that family members be involved in the child's behavior therapy to ensure that behavior therapy assignments are completed consistently. Family involvement usually means identifying a "behavior therapy coach" (usually a parent) who reminds the child when it is time to conduct the therapy and helps the child stay focused on the assigned exercises.

How long does it take before behavior therapy begins to work?

Positive results are usually seen within the first 2 weeks of behavior therapy, although the full benefit often takes months to achieve. Because OCD is a chronic disorder that can persist for years, behavior therapy is an ongoing process. Although initial positive results are seen as early as 2 weeks after beginning therapy, maintaining these gains requires continual work.

Renewed exposure and response prevention therapy also is needed if new obsessions and compulsions emerge. An important goal of behavior therapy is to teach children to recognize developing obsessions and rituals so that they may take action on their own. One child who was a very successful behavior therapy subject described to us how he nipped an obsession in the bud. He had gradually developed an obsession that fast-food hamburgers could be contaminated with lead, and he was starting to avoid eating at fast-food restaurants. Because of his experience with behavior therapy, as soon as he realized that an OCD–related problem was developing, he ran out and ate as many fast-food hamburgers as his stomach could hold. His enthusiasm for behavior therapy led him to conduct his own exposure (eating hamburgers) and response prevention (not avoiding fast-food restaurants).

Why is behavior therapy not always successful?

In approximately 50% of children with OCD, behavior therapy can bring about a satisfactory reduction in symptoms. For the remainder, behavior therapy alone is not enough. Because OCD is almost certainly the result of many different causes, it makes intuitive sense that one type of treatment is unlikely to help all OCD patients. Factors such as the severity of the OCD symptoms, the existence of other psychiatric problems (such as depression), the age of the child, and the involvement of the family in the child's OCD symptoms also can help explain why different children have different responses to the same treatment. In addition, some children are not temperamentally well suited for behavior therapy because of their personality style. Children who are extremely shy, reluctant to take chances, or have a low level of enthusiasm may find that behavior therapy is simply too difficult. When the child is unable or unwilling to complete the behavior therapy assignments consistently, behavior therapy usually fails. The primary challenge of the behavioral therapist is to develop assignments that are both therapeutic and fun.

Occasionally, a child will complete behavior therapy assignments, but still does not seem to improve. This is quite unusual. Again, the vast majority of behavior therapy "failures" are a result of improper or inconsistent completion of the behavior therapy assignments.

My child hates behavior therapy: what can be done?

Because behavior therapy almost always temporarily raises the child's anxiety, it is not surprising that many children don't like it. A few guidelines can make behavior therapy more acceptable to a child with OCD:

1. Nagging and lecturing should be avoided. A schedule for completing behavior therapy assignments should be established and adhered to in a firm but matter-of-fact manner.

2. Part of the behavior therapy time period should include some activity that is genuinely fun for the child and the therapist. For example, a behavior therapy session might start with playing a video game for 10 minutes and then end the same way.

3. The therapist must maintain an attitude of enthusiasm and encouragement, and never force the child to do behavior therapy against his or her will.

4. Behavior therapy progress should be clearly charted on easy-to-understand graphs so that the child is able to see progress as it occurs. Many children can assist in preparing these graphs.

5. A program of rewards and incentives should be designed so that the child will be encouraged and excited about the behavior therapy process. These rewards should be given for *participation* as well as for progress.

It is very easy for children and parents to become embroiled in "power struggles" over behavior therapy. These battles usually prevent progress and lead to unhappiness for everyone involved. Parents and therapist must keep in mind that behavior therapy is, by its very nature, stressful for the child. Because of this stress, behavior therapy must include generous amounts of reward, enthusiasm, affection, and fun.

What if behavior therapy fails?

Many children will not have an adequate response to behavior therapy alone. This is usually an indication to begin a trial of anti-OCD medication. However, it is important not to abandon behavior therapy simply because a medication is being started. Often children who have not responded to behavior therapy alone will begin to respond when an anti-OCD medication is added. When behavior therapy alone fails, it may be helpful to take a behavior therapy "holiday" until the child has begun to respond to a medication, or until the child is older and more mature. Behavior therapy can then be resumed with a better chance for success.

Anti-OCD Medications

Because behavior therapy alone is not always successful, or may not be available, it is fortunate that anti-OCD medications have been developed. Each of these medications is discussed individually (see pages 30–34). However, there are several principles that apply to all of the anti-OCD medications:

• *There is no single "best" anti-OCD medication.* Although all five anti-OCD medications work by affecting the brain chemical serotonin, the response varies from child to child, and there is no way to predict which of the medications will work best for a particular child. Each of the anti-OCD medications was originally developed for use in treating depression. Beginning with clomipramine (Anafranil), it was found that certain antidepressant medications also possessed anti-OCD properties. Not all antidepressant medications have these anti-OCD effects, only those that strongly affect serotonin. Serotonin is a chemical that certain nerve cells in the brain use to communicate. Under the right conditions, certain brain cells (called neurons) release serotonin, which affects communication between neighboring cells. After the serotonin is released and the communication is completed, the serotonin is taken back up into the cell so that it can be reused. Anti-OCD drugs interfere with serotonin being taken up once it has been released. This allows serotonin to spend more time outside of the cell where it continues to affect neighboring cells. Why or how this reduces obsessions and compulsions is unknown.

• Unfortunately, *the therapeutic effects of anti-OCD medication last only as long as the medication is being taken.* When the child stops taking medication, the OCD symptoms almost always gradually return. Although anti-OCD medications are usually effective in controlling symptoms, they are not considered a cure. At this time, there is no known cure for OCD.

• Whenever possible, *medication should be used in conjunction with behavior therapy.* As stated earlier, medication alone is usually not as effective as medication combined with behavior therapy. This is especially true of children who have had OCD for a number of years. Even when anti-OCD medication reduces their symptoms and their anxiety, many of the rituals have become ingrained habits that require behavior therapy to eliminate them.

• *Anti-OCD medications usually work very slowly.* It is not uncommon for the onset of improvement to be delayed as much as 2 months. It is important to keep this in mind, because it is human nature to hope for rapid results. It can be especially difficult to be patient when the child is experiencing side effects and the benefits seem slow in coming. Sometimes, even after taking the drug for months, a child will only improve slightly. Other times, intolerable side effects occur. When medication nonresponse occurs, or problem side effects emerge, it may be helpful to try a different medication or a combination of medications. However, sometimes a child will not improve on any of the anti-OCD medications or medication combinations.

• *All of the anti-OCD medications have the capacity to produce* **behavioral side effects** *in children.* These side effects can include defiance, irritability, excessive energy, or other inappropriate behaviors. Behavioral side effects are more likely to occur in younger children or when higher doses of medication are used. These side effects can be subtle, and at times it can be difficult to tell whether a particular behavior is the result of medication side effects or simply childhood misconduct. However, when a pattern of inappropriate behaviors emerges that seem "out of character" for the child, the possibility of behavioral side effects should be considered. When behavioral side effects do occur, it is usually within the first few weeks of medication treatment, although they can occur at any time. Often, reducing the dose of medication will reduce or eliminate behavioral side effects, although in some instances an alternative medication may be needed.

• *Not all anti-OCD medications have been officially approved for use in children by the U.S. Food and Drug Administration (FDA).* At present, three anti-OCD medications, clomipramine (Anafranil), fluvoxamine (Luvox), and sertraline (Zoloft) have specific FDA approval for use in children, down to age 10, 8, and 6, respectively. It is anticipated that other anti-OCD medications will obtain this approval in the future.

Although some medications do not have specific FDA approval for use in treating childhood OCD—and drug companies are then prohibited from promoting their use in childhood OCD—doctors can still prescribe them to children if they believe it is medically appropriate. Often, doctors prefer to prescribe medications that have a specific FDA approval for use in children.

Following is a brief overview of the currently available anti-OCD medications:

Clomipramine (Anafranil)

Clomipramine was the first anti-OCD medication to become widely available, and it is the medication that has been most studied in children with OCD. As with all the anti-OCD medications, clomipramine exerts strong effects on the brain chemical serotonin. Unlike the other anti-OCD medications, clomipramine exerts effects on other brain chemicals, including norepinephrine, histamine, acetylcholine, and dopamine. Although clomipramine's effects on serotonin appear to be the most important in treating OCD, its effects on other brain chemicals also may be important in reducing symptoms for some children.

Clomipramine is one of three anti-OCD medications with FDA approval for use in children. It has approval for use in children 10 years of age and older. The customary dose range is 25 to 250 mg/day.

What are clomipramine's side effects?

Clomipramine can cause a wide range of side effects—some problematic—although most children taking it only experience a few mild ones. The most common are dry mouth, sleepiness, and constipation.

When children become excessively sleepy when taking clomipramine, waiting may be one simple option because sometimes a child's body will adapt to this side effect. However, if it doesn't, a dose reduction is often helpful.

Dry mouth occurs because clomipramine can reduce the amount of saliva that is produced. Although this sensation can be uncomfortable for a child, it is not medically dangerous. This side effect also seems to diminish by itself over time. Many children feel more comfortable if they chew sugarless gum, which stimulates saliva production. Occasionally dry mouth can be problematic for children who are undergoing orthodontic work (braces). The combination of reduced saliva production and wearing braces can result in an increased rate of tooth decay. If the child has braces and clomipramine therapy is prescribed, the child's dentist should be informed so that he or she can monitor the child more closely for tooth decay and take preventive or corrective steps as needed.

Children also can experience significant constipation when taking clomipramine. Because of this, it is important to monitor the bowel habits of a child taking this drug to prevent serious constipation from developing. This is especially important for younger children who may not complain until several days have gone by without a bowel movement. A high-fiber diet, plenty of fluids, and regular exercise are useful preventive measures. If constipation remains a problem, the child's physician should be alerted, because it may be necessary to prescribe a stool-softening agent.

Another side effect of clomipramine is decreased sweating. For most children this is not a problem. However, caution is advised for those who engage in competitive, endurance-related athletics such as marathon running, basketball, soccer, and bicycle racing. The profuse sweating that occurs in those who participate in these sports is important because it cools the body. Children taking clomipramine may not produce enough sweat to provide this cooling and can thus become dangerously overheated. If endurance-related athletics are an important part of a child's life, one of the other anti-OCD medications may be more appropriate.

Clomipramine also has a small potential to cause irregular heartbeats, especially in children who have preexisting heart problems. Therefore, many physicians obtain an electrocardiogram (ECG) before starting a child on clomipramine. This is a simple and painless test in which the heart's electrical activity is measured. A physician also might order an ECG from time to time during clomipramine treatment, especially if a child is on a higher-than-usual dose, or if a child is experiencing side effects. Because the risk of heart problems is very small in children, some physicians feel that routinely performing ECGs is unnecessary. If you have concerns, you should discuss them with your child's physician.

Fluoxetine (Prozac)

Fluoxetine was the first of a new class of medications (called SSRIs) to become available in the United States. Medications in this class mainly affect the brain chemical serotonin, with negligible effects on other brain chemicals. Because SSRI medications are selective, they tend to have fewer side effects. Of course, doctors and patients alike prefer fewer side effects, and shortly after fluoxetine was introduced, it became the most commonly prescribed antidepressant.

Although research has shown that fluoxetine is an effective anti-OCD drug in adults, it has not been approved by the FDA for childhood OCD. However, some research, as well as clinical experience, indicates that it is also effective for OCD in children.

Fluoxetine is unique among the anti-OCD medications in that it can persist in the bloodstream for a long time—longer than 1 month in some cases. In some situations this property can be an advantage, in others a disadvantage. Some patients, especially adolescents, can be sporadic about taking their medications. This may be because they are forgetful, ambivalent about treatment, or simply cavalier about taking the medication. For these individuals, fluoxetine holds a special advantage because it persists in the bloodstream through those periods of missed doses. On the other hand, a child who has side effects from fluoxetine may have to wait several weeks after stopping the medication before side effects diminish.

For many children fluoxetine has a mild stimulating effect, similar to the sensation produced by drinking several cups of coffee. Because of this, fluoxetine is usually given in the morning to help avoid its stimulating effect leading to insomnia at night.

Fluoxetine is also the only anti-OCD drug available in a liquid preparation. This can sometimes be beneficial for children who cannot swallow pills, and it can be dosed in small amounts for children who are very sensitive to the effects of medication. The customary dose range for fluoxetine is 5 to 60 mg/day.

What are fluoxetine's side effects?

Most children are able to take fluoxetine without experiencing any side effects. Occasionally, children will develop a rash, headache, sleepiness, upset stomach, or difficulty falling asleep. All of these side effects are uncommon and, should they occur, are typically mild. Nonetheless, a doctor should be consulted whenever side effects occur. Like all anti-OCD medications, fluoxetine also may produce objectionable behavioral side effects (see page 29).

Fluvoxamine (Luvox)

Fluvoxamine is another SSRI medication. Like all the other SSRIs, it acts specifically on serotonin and has very limited effects on other brain chemicals. Fluvoxamine has been used for many years as an antidepressant and anti-OCD medication in Europe. It was recently introduced in the United States to treat OCD and has FDA approval for use in treating children with this disorder as young as 8 years of age.

Fluvoxamine does not persist in the bloodstream as long as most anti-OCD medications and is usually prescribed to be taken twice daily. The customary dose range for fluvoxamine is 25 to 250 mg/day.

What are fluvoxamine's side effects?

Most children can take fluvoxamine without experiencing any side effects. Occasionally, some children will experience headache, sleepiness, upset stomach, or difficulty falling asleep. Although not specifically a side effect, fluvoxamine can slow down the rate at which a person's body eliminates caffeine. Many children may experience problems such as jitteriness, excessive sweating, irritability, and insomnia when they are taking fluvoxamine and drink caffeinated beverages. The best solution is to greatly decrease or eliminate caffeine consumption in children taking fluvoxamine. Fluvoxamine also can produce behavioral side effects.

Paroxetine (Paxil)

Paroxetine is yet another SSRI medication that acts very selectively on serotonin, with minimal effects on other brain chemicals. Paroxetine has demonstrated effectiveness for treating OCD in adults. Like fluvoxamine, paroxetine does not persist long in the bloodstream and may require administration twice daily. Studies have not been completed in children, and currently there is little information about the use of paroxetine in those under 18 years of age. Because of this, there are few data to guide proper dosing for childhood OCD. The customary dose range for paroxetine is 10 to 60 mg/day.

What are paroxetine's side effects?

In adults paroxetine's side effects are similar to those of the other SSRI medications. Currently there is little information available about paroxetine's side effects in children, although it is likely that the side effects are similar to those experienced by adults (Table A.7).

Sertraline (Zoloft)

Sertraline is another SSRI medication that was initially introduced for the treatment of depression. Like the other SSRIs, it acts specifically on serotonin and has very limited effects on other brain chemicals. Several studies have been completed that show sertraline to be an effective anti-OCD medication for children. Sertraline has recently received FDA approval for use in children as young as 6 years of age.

Sertraline is usually given once per day, typically in the morning. The customary dose range for sertraline is 50 to 150 mg/day.

What are sertraline's side effects?

Most children can take sertraline without experiencing any side effects. In a few individuals the use of sertraline may lead to overstimulation, sleepiness, tiredness, headaches, or upset stomach. When upset stomach occurs, it is often helpful to take the medication with food. Sertraline also can produce behavioral side effects (see Table A.7).

Commonly Asked Questions About Anti-OCD Medications

Are other side effects possible with anti-OCD medications?

Table A.7 lists the more common side effects of anti-OCD drugs. Although this list may at first appear frightening, it is important to remember that most children experience few, if any, significant side effects. Of course, other side effects can occur, and sometimes these are severe. If you suspect your child is experiencing side effects, contact your physician for further guidance.

Which medication is best?

Research has not shown any one medication to be consistently better than the others. However, some children may respond well to one particular med-

Table A.7 Anti-OCD Medication Side Effects *(Please see explanatory notes below)*

Clomipramine (Anafranil)	Fluoxetine (Prozac)	Fluvoxamine (Luvox)	Paroxetine (Paxil)	Sertraline (Zoloft)
*Dry mouth	*Headache	*Nausea	Sleepiness	*Nausea
*Sleepiness	*Insomnia	*Headache	*Insomnia	*Headache
*Dizziness	*Nausea	Sleepiness	*Weakness	Diarrhea
Weakness	*Diarrhea	*Insomnia	*Nausea	Insomnia
Tremor	Sleepiness	Weakness	Sexual	Dry mouth
*Headache	*Anorexia	*Dry mouth	problems	Sexual problems
Constipation	*Weakness	Nervousness	Dry mouth	Tiredness
Anorexia	Anxiety	Dizziness	Constipation	Dizziness
Upset stomach	*Dizziness	Diarrhea	Dizziness	Tremor
*Abdominal pain	Dry mouth	Constipation	Tremor	Weakness
Insomnia	Sexual	Upset stomach	*Diarrhea	
*Menstrual	problems			
disturbance	Upset stomach			
	Flu syndrome			

Explanatory notes:
1. This table was prepared using *Mosby's Complete Drug Reference,* ed 7, Mosby-Year Book, St. Louis, Missouri, 1997. It lists side effects in descending order of occurrence that had a 10% or higher incidence, as reported in placebo-controlled clinical trials. The data in this table are based on many studies—which were *not* designed to compare the side effects between drugs. Because of this, the table should *not* be used to compare the side effects of one drug with those of another. Only the clomipramine side effect data are exclusive to children and adolescents.
2. Of course, not all children will experience these side effects, and other side effects are possible. Please contact your child's doctor if medication side effects are suspected.
* Adverse effects preceded by an asterisk (*) also had a 10% or higher *placebo* (inactive drug) reporting rate.

ication, and respond poorly, or not at all, to the others. The reasons these medications appear to work inconsistently in different children are unclear. In addition, the occurrence of medication side effects in children varies greatly. One child may have no side effects from a particular medication, and another child may have intolerable ones. In short, there is no one best medication for all children.

If behavior therapy alone is unsatisfactory or unavailable, and medication treatment is contemplated, we recommend beginning with sertraline. Although all of the anti-OCD drugs can be effective, sertraline offers several advantages:

- FDA approval down to 6 years of age.
- Does not interact with caffeine or antiasthma medications (such as theophylline).
- Once-per-day dosing.
- A favorable side-effect profile.

If sertraline treatment is unsatisfactory, therapeutic trials of alternative anti-OCD medications should be considered because—as stated previously—some children may respond to one particular anti-OCD medication.

What if my child does not want to take medication?

Many children are reluctant to take medication, and children with OCD are no exception. The first step in overcoming this is to explore the child's objections. Once the reasons behind your child's concerns are understood, it may be possible to address them satisfactorily.

Quite commonly, children refuse to take medications because they find swallowing pills difficult or unpleasant. This may be because the child gags easily, the drugs have a "funny taste," or the child does not swallow the pill immediately so that it dissolves in the mouth. One effective solution to this problem is to crush the pill (or empty the contents of a capsule) and mix the medicine with a small amount of applesauce or jelly. This mixture can then be given to the child on a spoon, followed by a generous drink of water or milk. Although this approach is mildly inconvenient, it can appease objections to pill swallowing. In addition, fluoxetine is available in a liquid form that most children find acceptable, although this formulation is more expensive than fluoxetine capsules.

Side effects are another reason why children may be reluctant to take medication. Some children find that the anti-OCD medication causes an upset stomach shortly after it is taken. This may be helped by taking the medication with a moderate amount of fluid or with meals. Dividing the dose so the child is taking a smaller amount at several points also may help. If these remedies aren't helpful, it may be necessary to switch to an alternative medication. Some children are reluctant to take medication because of other side effects, such as headache, jitteriness, or sedation. It is important to encourage children to talk about any of the side effects they experience, including ones that are related to sexual functioning.

Sexual side effects are difficult ones for children, adolescents, and parents to discuss. All anti-OCD medications have the potential to produce changes in sexual function. Usually these changes are mild and consist of a modest delay in reaching orgasm. In some cases, more severe sexual problems such as impotence or an inability to reach orgasm occur. Children should be informed of potential sexual side effects and should be given reassurance that these side effects are not harmful, nor medically significant. Sexual side effects are often overlooked, especially in younger children. Most children and adolescents masturbate and may become alarmed if this sexual experience changes. If you suspect that your child is having sexual side effects, you should inform his or her physician, because children are sometimes more comfortable talking to their doctors about these problems than to their parents.

Another reason children with OCD are reluctant to take medications is that the process can become entangled with an OCD ritual. For example, some children with OCD have strong objections to certain numbers. If a child becomes anxious around the number "2," and by coincidence is prescribed a dose of two pills, problems will likely result! Similarly, some children may have obsessions that the medication is contaminated, or they may be involved in rituals such as pill counting, which can be quite time-consuming. These problems are best addressed through behavior therapy in which a focused program can be developed that will enable children to take pills on a consistent basis.

Perhaps the most challenging reason children refuse to take anti-OCD medication is that they are engaged in power struggles with parents. This occurs most commonly with teenagers, although no age group is immune. Sometimes it is helpful to give the child a certain amount of control as a strategy to eliminate power struggles. For example, if the child is allowed to choose the timing of the dose (within a medically sensible range), this may sufficiently reduce conflict. Occasionally some children will respond to rewards for taking their medication, although this strategy can sometimes backfire because, over time, children will often strive to increase the size of the reward. When power struggles seem insurmountable, we usually recommend family therapy.

What should I do if my child skips a dose of medication?

If it is discovered within 3 hours after the dose has been skipped, it may be given late. Beyond 3 hours, it is usually best to resume dosing at the next prescribed time. This is a general recommendation and you may wish to consult your child's physician for more specific guidelines.

How long should my child take anti-OCD medication?

The duration of anti-OCD medication treatment must be individualized for each child. Because OCD symptoms can persist for years, most children need to take medication for a long time. As a general rule, we plan for an initial 6-month treatment period after which a gradual dosage reduction is attempted. If a child's symptoms begin to return, the dosage is readjusted to a level where adequate symptom control is achieved. Because OCD is a disorder that waxes and wanes over time, many children find that their dose of anti-OCD medication must be changed from time to time. Other children make such significant progress with behavior therapy that medication can sometimes be decreased or discontinued altogether.

Can anti-OCD medications affect my child's weight?

Many children will experience weight gain when taking clomipramine. For most children this is of minor consequence, but a few will become significantly overweight. A sensible program of diet and exercise typically manages weight gain. However, if the problem persists, a change to an alternative medication may be necessary.

A few children will *lose* weight when on anti-OCD medication, particularly the SSRI medications fluoxetine, fluvoxamine, paroxetine, and sertraline. This is usually because of appetite suppression or stomach upset. These side effects can sometimes be managed by providing the child with favorite high-calorie foods, having the child take the medication with meals, and always encouraging adequate nutrition. Occasionally, appetite suppression is so severe that a medication change is required.

Are anti-OCD drugs addictive?

These medications do not produce a "high" and, thus, have a very low potential for being abused. This fact should be discussed with the child. We have seen several instances in which children have refused to take their anti-OCD medication after attending school-based anti–drug abuse educational programs. These well-intentioned programs sometimes fail to draw a clear distinction between prescription medications and "street drugs" and can frighten children who are taking medication for OCD.

Can anti-OCD drugs be stopped abruptly, or should the dose be gradually reduced before stopping?

Although these drugs have little abuse potential, it is important to be aware that a child's body does adapt to these medications over time. Because of this adaptation, if an anti-OCD medication is to be discontinued, it is often best to taper the drug and discontinue it gradually. This is especially true of clomipramine, fluvoxamine, paroxetine, and sertraline. If clomipramine has been taken for an extended period of time (greater than 4 months) and is then stopped abruptly, many children will experience flulike symptoms. In the case of fluvoxamine, paroxetine, and sertraline, abrupt withdrawal of the medication can result in the child's feeling dizzy, having an upset stomach, or experiencing other uncomfortable sensations.

Fluoxetine does *not* require a tapered withdrawal because this drug has a very long duration of action and is essentially self-tapering.

Do anti-OCD drugs have any long-term or delayed effects on a child's development?

Probably not, although a definitive answer cannot be given because anti-OCD medications have not been used in children for a long enough period of time to be sure. The only way to detect delayed side effects is by monitoring many children who are taking the drug over an extended period of time. Doctors are most confident about the long-term effects of clomipramine because this medication has been used in adults for many years (in other countries) and no significant long-term harmful effects have yet been reported. There is very little information on the long-term effects of fluoxetine, fluvoxamine, paroxetine, or sertraline on a child's development, although at this point, nothing has emerged that would suggest a problem.

Because uncertainty remains about the use of these medications in children, they should only be given to those who clearly need them and should be continued only if the child is deriving benefit from them. In addition, the dose of medication should be monitored to ensure that a child is receiving no more medication than is necessary to adequately control OCD symptoms.

Do anti-OCD drugs cause cancer?

The vast majority of biochemical studies, both animal and human, indicate that anti-OCD medications do not increase the risk for cancer. As research technologies have become more sophisticated, a few studies have suggested that these medications may slightly increase the risk of certain kinds of tumors and slightly decrease the risk of other kinds of tumors.

Clinical experience suggests that if there is a risk of cancer from these drugs, it is so low that it is essentially insignificant.

Can my child take other medications when taking an anti-OCD drug?

This is usually okay if it is done under the supervision of a physician. Both prescription and nonprescription medications can interact with anti-OCD medications and lead to problems. This is especially true of certain cold remedies and cough medicines, even over-the-counter ones. It is best to avoid the use of these drugs unless you have first consulted with your child's physician. Because of increasing specialization, some children have several physicians involved in their care. It is important to inform all of the physicians about all of the drugs being prescribed to the child. This will help reduce the chances of an adverse drug interaction.

How is the right dose of an anti-OCD drug determined?

The correct dose of anti-OCD medication varies widely from child to child. Typically, the correct dose is achieved over time, through periodic dosage adjustments and the careful monitoring of symptom relief versus the occurrence of medication side effects. Occasionally, your child's physician may recommend obtaining blood levels of the medication to aid in determining the proper dose. The optimum dose also may change from time to time as your child grows. Lastly, because OCD is a disorder that tends to fluctuate over time, the dose of anti-OCD medication may need to be changed to accommodate these fluctuations.

How long does it take for anti-OCD drugs to work?

These drugs typically take a long time to work. In some instances, beneficial effects have not been seen until 2 months after the anti-OCD medication was started. Usually improvement occurs sooner, but it is very important for everyone involved to be patient with anti-OCD medication treatment.

Can my child participate in sports when taking anti-OCD drugs?

Yes. However, as mentioned earlier, some caution is advised for those children taking clomipramine because some children find that they become easily overheated or fatigued while taking it. Children who participate in endurance-related sports can find that clomipramine impairs their performance. Because of these effects, children, coaches, and physical education instructors should be aware that children on clomipramine therapy might need to reduce the intensity or duration of athletic activities. Fluoxetine, fluvoxamine, paroxetine, and sertraline do not appear to have any effect on athletic performance.

What if the anti-OCD drug stops working?

Because OCD is a disorder that typically waxes and wanes in severity over time, it sometimes appears as though the medication has lost its effectiveness. Usually a dosage adjustment will correct this problem. When children are experiencing a worsening of their OCD symptoms, it also may be helpful to consider increasing the emphasis on behavior therapy to help them get through a difficult period.

What about other treatments for OCD?

Other treatments for OCD such as family therapy, play therapy, and counseling therapy remain controversial. There is little evidence to suggest that these other therapeutic approaches are directly beneficial in reducing OCD symptoms. However, it must be remembered that children with OCD experience many of the same problems that commonly face children without the disorder. These include the divorce of their parents, peer pressures, school problems, and the stresses of puberty, to name a few. If a child is experiencing such difficulties, one of these other therapeutic approaches can be helpful.

Periodically, "fad therapies" such as nutritional therapy or megavitamin therapy emerge. These fad therapies are nearly always of little value and are typically promoted by individuals of dubious character and qualifications. If you are contemplating such an alternative therapy for your child, investigate the therapy thoroughly. Discuss it with your child's physician and carefully explore all possible risks, including financial ones. Useful therapies have withstood the test of time and careful research. Fad therapies are usually supported only by personal testimonials. Because parents want to do everything possible to help their child, they are sometimes easy prey for unscrupulous quacks making grand promises for their unproved techniques.

What can be done when a child does not improve with either behavior therapy or medication?

A small percentage of children do not improve with standard medications and behavior therapy. This can be disheartening for the child and the family. In certain instances, it is reasonable to try combinations of medication. Some combinations that have shown promise include: clomipramine plus an SSRI, anti-OCD medication plus an antipsychotic medication such as risperidone (Risperdal), anti-OCD medication along with buspirone (BuSpar), and many others. It is important to be aware that whenever medications are combined, the chances of side effects are increased. This is one of the reasons medication combinations are not used routinely. Most medication combinations have not been systematically studied in either adults or children, leaving their safety and effectiveness suspect. A complete discussion of medication combinations is beyond the scope of this booklet. If combination therapy is being considered, it is best done at a medical center where the physicians are familiar with both OCD and the use of psychiatric medications in children.

COMMONLY ASKED QUESTIONS ABOUT OBSESSIVE-COMPULSIVE DISORDER AND THE FAMILY
How Can a Child's OCD Affect the Family?

The answer is different for every family, but problems related to discipline are common. In many families, it is difficult for parents to agree on how to manage child behavior problems. Because of the special stresses involved in raising a child with OCD, parents are often in sharp disagreement over issues of discipline. One parent may see the other as "too easy" and not firm enough. Conversely, that parent may view his or her spouse as harsh and unsympathetic. The child is usually aware of these differences and often will attempt to get the more sympathetic parent to take his or her side in a conflict. When a parent takes sides with the child against the other parent, the result is usually anger and resentment. This is illustrated in the following dialogue between two parents in a family therapy session. Ann and Bill have an 8-year-old boy, Tim, with severe OCD.

> **Bill**—"You can't keep giving in to Tim. He's already spoiled rotten and you're spoiling him even more."
>
> **Ann**—"If you would take some time to learn about OCD, you would understand that he can't help it. All *you* do is yell at him and lecture."
>
> **Bill**—"Well someone has to make him mind. You know as well as I do that he is fully able to wipe up after one of his 2-hour sessions in the shower. When you're visiting your mother and I tell him to do it, he does it! When you're home and I tell him to clean up after himself, he goes running to his "mommy" and you always give in and clean up after him."
>
> **Ann**—"All you're saying is that he is afraid of you. Do you think that's good?"
>
> **Bill**—"No, it's not good, but if you keep giving in to him he is never going to get over this. You heard what the therapist said—he has to face his fears. He's just using his OCD as an excuse for being lazy. He doesn't even try when you're there to make it easy for him."

Ann—"That's not fair. You think yelling or spanking is the cure for every-thing . . ."

Because this pattern is common, it is important for parents to recognize it early and, if necessary, seek professional help in resolving these issues. Parenting is never easy, but when a child has OCD, the job can seem insurmountable. Many parents have found support groups for parents of children with OCD helpful. The Obsessive-Compulsive Foundation can help you locate a nearby support group. If there isn't one, you may be able to start your own with their help.

Might I Somehow Have Caused my Child to Have OCD?

It is perfectly understandable that some parents may feel guilty and respon sible for their child's psychiatric illness. However, there is absolutely no evidence to suggest that bad parenting causes OCD. Many parents wonder if they have used too much discipline or not enough discipline, if they have been overprotective or underprotective, or if they have made some other error resulting in OCD. Clinical experience has shown that OCD occurs in children from families with every possible parenting style. Parents should be reassured that they have not caused their child's OCD through any error of parenting. Only through genetic endowment might a parent have contributed to a child's OCD, and none of us can control our genes!

Although parenting style does not cause OCD, good parenting techniques can reduce the impact of the disorder on the child and family. Parents who are able to listen to their child in a nonjudgmental fashion and with genuine concern help maintain the child's sense of self-esteem. Setting firm limits on allowable behavior is often difficult, but this gives the child a sense of security that life will not "spin out of control." Focusing on the child's strengths and successes will help the child develop an identity as a "person," rather than as a "sick person." Often OCD magnifies the differences a child's parents have in their philosophies of child rearing. When this occurs, parents should work to resolve their differences to ensure that the child does not receive confusing "mixed messages." Parents must remember that rearing a child with OCD can be confusing, stressful, and frustrating. It is usually helpful to meet and talk with other parents of children with OCD by joining a support group if one is available.

Like most illnesses, OCD tends to worsen during times of stress. Just as children who have asthma or diabetes tend to have more problems when their family is extremely stressed, so do children with OCD tend to experience a worsening of symptoms during difficult times. For example, we commonly see OCD symptoms worsen when families are undergoing a divorce or major financial crisis. Conversely, positive stresses such as play, athletics, and extra-curricular activities often lessen the grip of OCD.

Should We Take Our Child with OCD on the Family Vacation?

Except in severe cases, children with OCD usually function better when away on vacation than they do at home. The reasons for this are complex, but it seems as though many children are able to take a vacation from their OCD! Because of this, we encourage parents to take family vacations away from home. Keep in mind that each child is unique, and a few children will not enjoy the time away from home, but these children are the exception.

Can Parenting Styles or Techniques Influence the Severity of Symptoms in Children Who Have OCD?

We strongly doubt that there is any parenting style that will fully *prevent* OCD symptoms from occurring in a child vulnerable to developing OCD. Similarly, even the worst parenting possible does not seem to *produce* OCD. However, it does appear that if a child develops OCD, parenting techniques *can* influence the degree to which these symptoms affect the child's life. Over the years, we have established a list of "dos and don'ts" that may help to keep a child's OCD symptoms manageable:

- Do create an atmosphere in which the child is comfortable talking about feelings, especially worries.
- Do encourage your child to take reasonable risks.
- Do demonstrate, through example, that anxiety is "no big deal."
- Do work on co-parenting; don't allow the child to "divide and conquer."
- Do adopt a healthy lifestyle, properly balancing social, work, and family life.
- Do help your child to experience the many "unknowns" life has to offer.
- Don't forget that anxiety is often contagious.
- Don't "give in" to demands to provide unnecessary reassurance or cooperate with rituals.
- Don't participate in your child's anxiety.

Although systematic research has not been done on this issue, we believe that the parents' capacity to provide a proper emotional and physical environment can diminish the impact that OCD symptoms will have on a child's life. We also strongly suspect that many compulsions or rituals are often "nipped in the bud" by parents who steadfastly refuse to give in to any excessive or unreasonable demands. Conversely, when parents enable or involve themselves in these rituals, the rituals typically become ingrained, and may grow to become quite problematic, complicated, and miserable for all.

What if Both Parent and Child Have OCD?

This situation actually occurs surprisingly often, although OCD may not be formally diagnosed in both parent and child. For example, the child may have a diagnosis of OCD, whereas the parent may simply have a few OCD-like symptoms, or conversely the parent may have OCD and the child may have only a few OCD traits. There are advantages and disadvantages, which are discussed in the following paragraphs.

The main advantage that occurs when both parent and child have OCD is that usually the parent is much more attuned to the child's difficulties. Parents without OCD often find the symptoms incomprehensible and can have difficulty providing empathy and support for their child. Parents with OCD have a very clear understanding about what the child is experiencing. In most cases, parents with OCD are not only able to empathize and be supportive, but also are better equipped to set limits. They understand both the misery and the fact that the symptoms must be confronted and cannot be allowed to rule the child's life.

Another advantage is that medication response also tends to run in families. This can be very helpful in choosing medication options. For example, if a parent has had a very good response to paroxetine but has experienced many side effects on other medications, we are much more likely to prescribe paroxetine for the child. Although this rule is not absolute, it can be very helpful when optimizing treatment for a child.

One disadvantage that occurs when both parent and child have OCD is obsessions and compulsions interacting in destructive ways. This is illustrated in the following example:

> Both Barbara and her 11-year-old daughter Erin have moderately severe OCD. Over the course of the summer Erin developed an obsession that her vaginal secretions were contaminated and that these secretions could make her (or others) become ill. Because of this, Erin vigorously scrubbed herself after going to the toilet and walked around with her arms folded across her chest because of fear that she would accidentally touch her groin area.
>
> Her mother, Barbara, then began to develop an obsession that Erin had been sexually abused. Although Barbara did not really believe that this had happened, she was plagued with doubts and would repeatedly question Erin about whether anyone had touched her "down there" and would ask to inspect her groin area. These questions raised Erin's anxiety about whether she had contaminated someone, and this caused her to scrub even more. When Barbara inspected Erin's groin area, and saw that she was red and raw (from scrubbing), this would fuel her anxiety about sexual abuse, causing her to question Erin more intensely.
>
> This interaction was very uncomfortable for both Barbara and her daughter. When Barbara brought Erin in for an appointment, a diagnosis of OCD was made and Erin was started on anti-OCD medication. Both mother and daughter were enrolled in a behavior therapy program.
>
> Erin was given a behavior therapy assignment to respond to her mother's questions about sexual abuse by saying, "Well, maybe I have been abused and maybe I haven't!" Erin was absolutely delighted with this assignment although

it was very difficult for her mother. She also was given assignments to gradually reduce the time spent scrubbing her groin area, and her mother was to monitor this with a stopwatch from *outside* the bathroom. Although a complete discussion of the nuances of Erin's and her mother's behavior therapy is beyond the scope of this pamphlet, both she and her mother were enthusiastic behavior therapy participants and made rapid recoveries.

Parent and child OCD can interact in numerous complex ways. When this occurs, medication treatment alone is almost never adequate, and we always advise behavior therapy consultation for the whole family. Often, more traditional family therapy, which focuses on communication patterns, boundaries, family alliances, and so forth, can be an important element of an overall treatment program.

Are There Tests That Can Determine Whether an Unborn Child Might Get OCD?

No, although this is at least *theoretically* possible at some point in the future.

Is OCD Caused by Sexual Abuse?

This question is asked surprisingly often. The prevalence of this question is probably the result of the fact that many children and most adolescents with OCD have sexual obsessions from time to time. Sigmund Freud even proposed a theory that childhood sexual experiences were at the root of OCD. We now know that obsessions are almost always related to something that is inherently anxiety-provoking. This can be disease, injury, natural disaster, or sex. Given the fact that sex is an extremely common topic on television and in popular music, as well as a fundamental part of the child's normal development, it is perfectly understandable that children can develop obsessions that have a sexual theme.

Of course, this does not rule out the possibility that a child with OCD may have been sexually abused or exploited. Unfortunately, sexual abuse of children is all too common in our society, and children with OCD can become victims just like other children. If you are concerned that your child has had a traumatic sexual experience, you should consult your child's physician. Understanding whether a child's sexual obsessions or compulsions are the result of abuse, of OCD, or both, is a difficult task. In situations such as this, consulting with a professional who is experienced with OCD and children should be helpful.

How Can I Ensure That My Child With OCD Will Have Positive Self-Esteem?

This is perhaps the most important question addressed in this booklet. Children with OCD often feel worthless and defeated, and wonder if they are crazy. Education about the nature of OCD is a powerful tool in restoring a child's self-esteem. (Older children should read this booklet.) Children must understand that OCD–related difficulties are not the result of weakness, stupidity, or poor self-discipline. For example, when treating OCD, we often tell young children that they do certain behaviors (such as excessive washing) because of "Oscar the OCD bug." This helps children appreciate that they are still "okay" and that it is simply "Oscar" interfering in their lives.

Self-esteem is closely related to identity. When children believe their OCD symptoms are the result of personal weakness, they soon become demoralized. They may feel that they are fundamentally flawed and lose hope that their lives could be better. This is especially unfortunate because most children with OCD are quite resourceful in minimizing the impact of symptoms on daily life, both socially and academically. We commonly see children who are spending 4 hours per day doing rituals, yet are maintaining passing grades at school and are functioning adequately at home. All too often, parents and professionals emphasize how OCD has been disruptive without acknowledging the child's skill, energy, and spirit in grappling with the disorder. When parents acknowledge this effort, their child's self-esteem improves.

With effective treatment, education, and support from their parents and teachers, most children can maintain or restore their self-esteem. Indeed, children who are able to be successful in school and have friends despite their OCD are justifiably proud of their achievements and thrilled that this troubling disorder did not triumph.

OTHER COMMONLY ASKED QUESTIONS ABOUT CHILDHOOD OBSESSIVE-COMPULSIVE DISORDER
What Are the Early Signs of OCD?

All children are at risk for developing OCD, but children whose parents have OCD are at an increased risk. We advise parents of these "at-risk" children to be watchful of the signs and symptoms of emerging OCD, but to temper their alarm if such symptoms appear. We do so because typically *all* children develop some behaviors suggestive of OCD at differing stages in their maturation. Virtually all children create bedtime or bathing rituals because predictability and routine are calming and comforting. So too, many children develop irrational fears about a confusing world they are trying to "figure out," and may create rituals that help them cope. The childhood chant, "Step on a crack, break your mother's back," is but one example.

It is not unusual for children to become quite fastidious when they first learn about germs—which they obviously cannot see—and they may become afraid to drink out of a glass someone else has touched or to take a bite from another person's cookie. These are all *normal* childhood behaviors and yet are all *possible* signs of impending OCD. To repeat, these behaviors should be monitored, but are not cause for undo concern.

When should a parent's concern be raised? There are three general areas of concern:

1. If these OCD-like behaviors appear to be overly exaggerated when compared with other children the same age
2. If these OCD behaviors have led (or appear to be leading) to unhappiness for the child
3. When these behaviors interfere with the three essential tasks of childhood:
   * To learn knowledge and skills
   * To develop interpersonal and social relationships
   * To have fun

If a child is having difficulty with any of these three tasks, there is reason to be concerned (whether or not OCD–related behaviors are the cause). Any child who is having difficulty learning, seems unable to form satisfying relationships with adults or peers, or frequently expresses unhappiness, is a child in need of help. That is really all there is to it! If a child is having fun, learning at an appropriate rate, and developing quality friendships, a few OCD-like behaviors are of little concern.

If a child is having difficulty achieving the three tasks of childhood, or when OCD-like behaviors grow to problematic proportions, an evaluation by a child psychiatrist or psychologist familiar with OCD is in order.

Will My Child Ever be Cured of OCD?

At present, there is no known cure for OCD. However, behavior and drug treatments are available that are often very effective in reducing or nearly eliminating OCD symptoms. Occasionally, children with mild OCD symptoms seem to "outgrow" the disorder. We do know, however, that this happens rarely and that OCD usually remains throughout childhood and into adulthood. Although it does tend to persist, OCD commonly waxes and wanes in severity and most children find that certain times of the year are more difficult than others.

Although there is no cure (yet) for OCD, only a few children are significantly disabled. With appropriate treatment, most children are able to finish their education, get married, obtain a job, and lead a nearly normal life.

When Should a Child With OCD Be Hospitalized?

It is very rare that a child requires hospitalization for effective treatment OCD symptoms. When hospitalization is being contemplated, the most important question to ask is, "What can be done in the hospital that cannot be accomplished on an outpatient basis?" Occasionally, children with very severe OCD must be hospitalized for their safety, or because their symptoms are too severe to manage at home. For example, this may occur when a child is so obsessed with cleanliness that it is nearly impossible to interrupt the washing rituals. Another example results when a child is so obsessed with food contamination that severe malnutrition results and basic health is in danger. Some children with both OCD and depression become suicidal and require hospitalization to keep them safe. Aside from these extraordinary circumstances, hospitalization for children with OCD is usually not warranted.

How Do I Pick a Doctor for My Child With OCD?

This is a difficult problem, because most physicians are unfamiliar with treating OCD in general and are even less comfortable treating children with OCD. It is usually best to consult with your family doctor or pediatrician for a referral to a qualified child psychiatrist. Other sources of information for referrals are the Obsessive-Compulsive Foundation and the Obsessive-Compulsive Information Center.

How Do I Pick a Behavioral Therapist?

Behavioral therapists who are familiar with treating children who have OCD are rare indeed! The same sources of information given previously may be helpful, and you can also contact the Association for Advancement of Behavior Therapy (page xx).

My Child Refuses to Admit that OCD is a Problem: What Can Be Done?

It is not uncommon for children with OCD to minimize their symptoms or even deny that they have the disorder. This is particularly common during adolescence. It is usually best to avoid arguments or other attempts to persuade the teenager that he or she is suffering from OCD. Instead, focusing on specific problem areas in a collaborative fashion can result in meaningful progress. An example is the approach taken with a 13-year-old boy, Rob.

Rob insisted vehemently that he did not have OCD and said that he took long showers because "I like to be clean!" Rob did not want to participate in behavior therapy, nor would he agree to take medication. When his psychiatrist asked him what could be done to help him, he said, "Get my parents off my back." They worked out a plan in which he agreed to participate in behavior therapy to control his showers in the morning (when the whole family was waiting for their turn). In exchange, his parents agreed to ignore his showering in the afternoon.

This was the beginning of a collaborative relationship that over time unlocked the struggle between Rob and his parents. Eventually, Rob was able to come to terms with his OCD. Adolescence is often a time of struggle. It can be difficult trying to sort through problem behaviors when they may be simply "teenage problems," OCD problems, or a mixture of both. In Rob's case, it was a mixture. In these complex situations professional help can provide an objective viewpoint.

Just How Much Control Does my Child Really Have Over His or Her Behaviors?

This varies enormously from child to child. It is not uncommon for conflict to develop between a child with OCD and parents around this issue. It often appears that a child has control over OCD symptoms and is willfully misbehaving and using OCD as a "crutch" to excuse objectionable behavior. It is helpful to consider two aspects of this dilemma.

First, almost all children have *partial* control over their OCD behaviors. This means that they are sometimes able to delay their rituals, but are almost never able to stop them indefinitely. This is similar to an individual's control over breathing. Everyone can delay breathing for brief periods of time, but no one can stop breathing (voluntarily) for long. It is important that parents not mistake this partial control for complete control.

Secondly, children could use their OCD symptoms as a tool in the struggles that occur in all families. Just as a child might use a cast on a broken arm to obtain special favors from friends, so might a child with OCD use symptoms when it is convenient. As a rule, it is best not to "overanalyze" a child's control over OCD–related behaviors. Instead, try to normalize the situation as much as possible by setting firm yet nonjudgmental limits on behaviors that are unacceptable.

How Can Someone Learn More About OCD in Children and Adolescents?

A booklet of this size cannot provide answers to every question that might be asked about OCD in children. The material included here was selected because patients, doctors, behavioral therapists, parents, and teachers felt it was important. The following suggestions might help you learn more about OCD in children:

- Read this booklet thoroughly, making sure to note any areas where you have questions.
- Ask your doctor these questions, and any others you might have.
- Reread the booklet from time to time to refresh your memory. Share it with family members, friends, and teachers. Discuss areas that apply particularly to your child.
- Refer to the readings suggested on the following pages.
- Self-help groups are available in many areas of the country that offer support and information for adults as well as children. The **Obsessive-Compulsive Foundation, Inc.** publishes a newsletter and provides information about self-help groups, therapists, and clinics as well as current research on OCD. Contact: P.O. Box 70, Milford, Connecticut 06460-0070. Phone: 203-878-5669. Fax: 203-874-2826. Web site: http://pages.prodigy.com/alwillen/ocf.html
- The **Obsessive-Compulsive Information Center** (OCIC) provides access to the published literature on obsessive-compulsive disorder as well as obsessive-compulsive spectrum disorders and their treatments. Medical librarians who provide technical information on OCD and its treatment

staff the Center. Referrals to therapists, clinics, and self-help groups are also provided. Contact: Dean Foundation for Health, Research & Education, 2711 Allen Boulevard, Middleton, Wisconsin 53562. Phone: 608-827-2390. Fax: 608-827-2399. Web site: www.deancare.com/info/info16.htm (or info11.htm)

- The **Child Psychopharmacology Information Service** (CPIS), located at the University of Wisconsin's Department of Psychiatry, provides access to literature on the use of psychiatric medications in children. The CPIS is staffed by a medical librarian and child psychiatrist who provide technical information on any topic regarding the use of psychiatric medication in children. Contact: 6001 Research Park Boulevard #1568, Madison, Wisconsin 53719-1179. Phone: 608-263-6171. Fax: 608-263-0265. Web site: www.psychiatry.wisc.edu

- The **Association for Advancement of Behavior Therapy** provides nationwide referrals to behavioral therapists who treat children with OCD. Contact: 305 7th Ave, 16th Floor, New York, New York 10001-6008. Phone 212-647-1890. E-mail: referrals.aabt.org

SUGGESTED READINGS

The following publications may be helpful in better understanding OCD and related disorders and their treatment. Only publications marked with an asterisk (*) are available from the Obsessive-Compulsive Information Center. The Center can be contacted for current prices and order forms. The others may be obtained through bookstores and libraries.

Nontechnical

*Greist JH, Jefferson JW, Marks IM: *Anxiety and its treatment: help is available,* Washington, 1986, American Psychiatric Press, and New York, 1986, Warner Books.

Rapoport JL: *The boy who couldn't stop washing: the experience and treatment of obsessive-compulsive disorder*, New York, E.P. Dutton, 1989, and New York, 1989, Penguin Books.

Schwartz JM: *Brain lock: free yourself from obsessive-compulsive behavior*, New York, 1996, HarperCollins.

Foster CH: *Funny, you don't look crazy: life with obsessive-compulsive disorder*, Ellsworth, 1995, Dilligaf Publishing.

Baer L: *Getting control: overcoming your obsessions and compulsions*, Boston, 1991, Little, Brown, and New York, 1991, Penguin Books.

Van Noppen BL, Pato MT, Rasmussen S: *Learning to live with obsessive-compulsive disorder*, ed 4, Milford, 1997, OC Foundation.

*Greist JH: *Obsessive compulsive disorder: a guide*, Madison, rev. ed., 1997, Obsessive Compulsive Information Center, Dean Foundation.

Johnston HF, Fruehling JJ: *OCD and parenting*, Milford, 1995, OC Foundation.

Neziroglu F, Yaryura-Tobias JA: *Over and over again: understanding obsessive-compulsive disorder*, rev ed, New York, 1995, Lexington Books.

Foster CH: *Polly's magic games: a child's view of obsessive-compulsive disorder*, Ellsworth, 1995, Dilligaf.

Foa E, Wilson R: *Stop obsessing*, New York, 1991, Bantam Books.

Steketee G, White K: *When once is not enough: help for obsessive-compulsives*, Oakland, 1990, New Harbinger.

Technical

Francis G, Gragg RA: *Childhood obsessive-compulsive disorder*, Thousand Oaks, 1996, Sage Publications.

March J, Mulle K: *How I ran OCD off my land: a cognitive-behavioral treatment program for obsessive compulsive disorder in children and adolescents*, New York, 1998, Guilford Press.

Mavissakalian MR, Prien RF, editors: *Long-term treatments of anxiety disorders*, Washington, 1996, American Psychiatric Press.

Rachman SJ, Hodgson RJ: *Obsessions and compulsions*, Englewood Cliffs, 1980, Prentice-Hall.

*Greist JH, Jefferson JW: *Obsessive-compulsive disorder casebook*, rev. ed, Washington, 1995, American Psychiatric Press.

Rapoport JL: *Obsessive-compulsive disorder in children and adolescents*, Washington, 1989, American Psychiatric Press.

Yaryura-Tobias JA, Neziroglu FA: *Obsessive-compulsive disorder spectrum: pathogenesis, diagnosis and treatment*, Washington, 1997, American Psychiatric Press.

Jenike MA, Baer L, Minichiello WE, editors: *Obsessive-compulsive disorders: theory and management*, ed 2, Chicago, 1990, Year Book Medical.

Zohar J, Insel T, Rasmussen S, editors: *The psychobiology of obsessive-compulsive disorder*, New York, 1991, Springer.

Steketee GS: *Treatment of obsessive-compulsive disorder*, New York, 1993, Guilford Press.

Video

Callner J: *The touching tree*, Milford, 1993, Awareness Films, OC Foundation.

In addition to *Obsessive Compulsive Disorder in Children and Adolescents: A Guide*, the following publications are available from the Dean Foundation Information Centers. The Centers can be contacted for current prices and order forms (see address page 52).

Temte JL, Jefferson JW, Greist JH: *Antipsychotic medications and schizophrenia: a guide,* Madison, 1992, Information Centers, Dean Foundation.

Greist JH, Jefferson JW, Marks IM: *Anxiety and its treatment: help is available,* New York, 1986, Warner Books.

Johnston HF, Fruehling JJ: *Attention-deficit hyperactivity disorder in children: a medication guide,* Madison, 1997, Child Psychopharmacology Information Service, University of Wisconsin.

Medenwald JR, Greist JH, Jefferson JW: *Carbamazepine and manic depression: a guide,* rev. ed., Madison, 1996, Lithium Information Center, Dean Foundation.

Tunali (Sen) D, Jefferson JW, Greist JH: *Depression and antidepressants: a guide,* rev. ed., Madison, 1997, Information Centers, Dean Foundation.

Greist JH, Jefferson JW: *Depression and its treatment,* rev. ed., New York, 1992, Hardback copy, American Psychiatric Press, Washington, DC, and paperback copy, Warner Books.

Jefferson JW, Greist JH. *Divalproex and manic depression: a guide,* Madison, 1996 (Formerly Valproate guide). Lithium Information Center, Dean Foundation.

Dries DC, Barklage NE: *Electroconvulsive therapy: a guide,* rev. ed., Madison, 1996, Lithium Information Center, Dean Foundation.

Greist JH, Greist GL, Jefferson JW: *Fearful flyer's guide,* Madison, 1996, Information Centers, Dean Foundation.

Bohn J, Jefferson JW: *Lithium and manic depression: a guide,* rev. ed., Madison, 1996, Lithium Information Center, Dean Foundation.

Jefferson JW, Greist JH, Ackerman DL, Carroll JA: *Lithium encyclopedia for clinical practice*, ed 2., Washington, 1987, American Psychiatric Press.

Marks IM: *Living with Fear.* New York, 1978, McGraw-Hill.

Greist JH, Jefferson JW: *Obsessive-compulsive disorder casebook,* rev. ed., Washington, 1995, American Psychiatric Press.

Greist JH: *Obsessive-Compulsive disorder: a guide,* rev. ed., Madison, 1997, Obsessive Compulsive Information Center, Dean Foundation.

Greist JH, Jefferson JW: *Panic disorder and agoraphobia: a guide,* rev. ed., Madison, 1997, Information Centers, Dean Foundation.

Greist JH, Jefferson JW, Katzelnick DJ: *Social phobia: a guide,* Madison, 1997, Information Centers, Dean Foundation.

Anders JL, Jefferson JW: *Trichotillomania: a guide,* Madison, 1994, Obsessive Compulsive Information Center, Dean Foundation.

Appendix 5

Obsessive-Compulsive Clinic Questionnaire

MEDICAL, PSYCHIATRIC, AND FAMILY INFORMATION

This questionnaire will be used to gather information from your history and present situation that is important in assisting us to change your problematic behaviors. Your answers will be held in strictest confidence and will not be revealed to anyone without your written consent.

Today's date:_____ Evaluation date:_____

Name: _____ Birthdate: _____

Age: _____ Gender: _____

Height: _____ Weight: _____

Phone numbers:

Work _____ Home _____

Mailing address: _____

_____

Occupation: _____

Person to contact in the event of an emergency (not living with you):

   Name: _____

   Phone number: _____

Who referred you to our clinic? _____

What is your main problem?

What types of obsessive-compulsive behaviors do you have?

At what age did the obsessions or compulsions begin?

Medical History
Allergies
Do you have allergies to any medication?   yes/no

If so, what medication?

If so, what type of reaction did you have?

Medical Illnesses
Have you in the past or do you now have any medical illnesses?   yes/no

What type of illness?

Surgery
Have you ever had surgery?   yes/no

Types and dates of surgery:

Psychiatric History
Hospitalizations
Have you ever been hospitalized for a psychiatric illness?   yes/no

If so, what was the diagnosis and when were you hospitalized?

Outpatient Psychiatric Treatment
Have you been in therapy for a psychiatric condition?   yes/no

If so, where and when?

What type of therapy did you have (e.g., medication, psychodynamic, behavioral, other)?

Medication History
What medications are you presently taking (include medical and psychotropic medications, as well as dosages for all)?

What other medications have you taken in the past (duration and dosage)?

Have you used illegal drugs?   yes/no

If so, what kinds of drugs and when (how much)?

Do you drink alcohol?   yes/no

If so, how much?

Has anyone considered you an alcoholic?

Do you smoke?   yes/no

If so, how much?

Developmental History

Were there any problems with your own birth?

As far as you know, did you walk and talk at roughly the same ages as other children?

Did you have any abnormalities or difficulties in your physical development as you were growing up?

Family History

Has anyone in your family ever been diagnosed with a psychiatric illness? yes/no

Have any of the following family members had psychiatric difficulties (including depression, mania, schizophrenia, drug or alcohol abuse, panic attacks, phobias, Tourette's disorder, other)? Please list diagnosis (if known) and which relative had the disorder.

Children:

Father:

Mother:

Brothers:

Sisters:

Maternal grandparents:

Fraternal grandparents:

Uncles:

Aunts:

Cousins:

Others:

Marital status: Single   Married   Partner   Separated   Divorced

If married or with a partner, how long? _____

Husband/Wife/Partner's age _____

Occupation of husband/wife/partner _____

If separated/divorced:
    Date:_____
    Reason: _____

Children (names/ages):

Others currently living in your household and their relationship to you:

Referral

Have you sought treatment before?   Yes/No

What present compulsive behaviors (e.g., washing, checking, ordering, repeating) or obsessive thoughts do you need help with?

What specific situations or objects trigger your compulsive rituals or obsessions?

What thoughts, images, or impulses trigger your compulsive rituals or obsessions?

How often do the compulsive behaviors occur? Times per day? Times per week?

How often do the obsessive thoughts occur? Times per day? Times per week?

What do you fear will happen if you do not engage in your rituals or obsessions?

How strongly do you believe this? Please circle response below.

0	1	2	3	4	5
Very weak					Very strong

Please estimate the severity of your problem. Circle response below.

1	2	3	4	5
Mildly	Moderately	Very	Extremely	Totally
Upsetting	Upsetting	Severe	Severe	Incapacitating

Is there anything you avoid doing or thinking?

List the benefits you hope to derive from therapy.

Family History

Mother

Name: _____ Age: _____

Occupation: _____ Religion: _____

If deceased, your age at the time of her death? _____

Cause of death: _____

How would others describe your mother?

How would you describe your mother?

What activities did you do with your mother when you were a child?

How did you get along with your mother?

Father
Name: _____ Age: _____
Occupation: _____ Religion: _____
If deceased, your age at the time of his death? _____
Cause of death: _____
How would others describe your father?

How would you describe your father?

What activities did you do with your father when you were a child?

How did you get along with your father?

Brothers and Sisters
Name: Age:

How did/do you get along with him/her/them?

Do (did) your mother or father favor any one?   Yes/No
If so, who and why?

How do (did) your mother and father get along?

Marital History

How well do you and your wife/husband/partner get along? Rate your relationship on a scale from 1 to 5. Circle appropriate response.

1 very poor   2 poor   3 fair   4 good   5 excellent

How often do you and your wife/husband/partner go out socially?
     per week: per month:

How often do you and your wife/husband/partner have intercourse?
     per week: per month:

Who is the dominant member of your relationship?
     You   Your husband/wife/partner

List some of the behaviors of your husband/wife/partner that you find disagreeable.

List some of the behaviors of your husband/wife/partner that you find agreeable.

Educational History

Name of School: _____

Location: _____

Dates: _____

How were your grades? _____

Grammar: _____

Secondary: _____

College: _____

Postgraduate: _____

Highest grade completed: _____

How well did you adjust to school situations?
     Poor   Fair   Well   Excellent

List any significant events relating to school that you think had a bearing on your present problems.

Job History

List the jobs you have held and their dates. Then, note which aspects of each job were the most pleasurable for you (e.g., working with people, type of work, etc.) and which aspects gave you the most anxiety or trouble.

Dates: Job titles: Liked: Disliked:

Ambitions:
    Past:

    Present:

Present hobbies and interests:

List any situations that make you feel calm or relaxed.

Religious History

In what religion were you raised?   Protestant
                                       Catholic
                                       Jewish
                                       Other

Rate the strength of your religious belief. Circle appropriate response.

0	1	2	3	4	5
None					Very strong

Do you presently engage in any religious activity?   Yes/No

If yes, please describe.

Do you think your religious beliefs or practices have played a role in your obsessive-compulsive disorder?   Yes/No

If yes, please describe.

Personality Assessment

List your good points.

List any faults you think you have.

On the other side of this sheet, please add anything not covered in this questionnaire that you feel could help us understand your problem.

Food Intake History

Have you ever been diagnosed as having anorexia or bulimia?   Yes/No

Do you ever eat large amounts of food in a short period of time?   Yes/No

Have you ever made yourself vomit to keep from gaining weight?
   Yes/No

Do you have a fear of gaining weight or becoming fat?   Yes/No

Have you missed your period when not pregnant?   Yes/No/N/A

Do you tend to snack when you are not hungry?   Yes/No

Do you tend to snack almost every day?   Yes/No

When do you snack most often?
   Morning
   Afternoon
   After dinner
   Before bedtime

What snacks would you eat if you were *not worried* about calories?
   a. Salty, crunchy snacks like potato chips, corn chips, crackers
   b. Sweet snacks like candy, cookies, pastries, ice cream

   c. Starchy snacks like crackers, bread, muffins, bagels
   d. Real food like cheese, cold cuts, leftovers
   e. Fruit or vegetables
   f. Cottage cheese, yogurt

If you could choose only one category from this list, what would you choose when you *must* have a snack? _____

If the following snacks had the same number of calories per serving, which types of snack foods would you prefer?
   a. Sweets like pastries or candies or ice cream
   b. Starchy crunchy foods
   c. Soft or chewy starchy foods
   d. Fruit or vegetables
   e. Meal foods like cold chicken, tunafish, cheese, cold cuts, hamburger
   f. Yogurt, cottage cheese, milk

Right before you get your period, do you change your food preferences?
   Yes/No/N/A

If you answered yes, what would you like to eat during those days?
   a. Sweets foods especially chocolate
   b. Salty crunchy foods like potato chips or pretzels
   c. Starchy foods like pasta, potatoes, rice, bread, rolls, pancakes
   d. Salty meal foods like hard cheese or anchovies
   e. Substantial fools like meat, chicken, fish, dairy products

During the dark cold months of the year, do you change your food preferences?
   Yes/No

If you answered yes, what would you like to *eat more* of during those months?
   a. Sweet foods
   b. Starchy foods
   c. Substantial meal foods like meat, fish, chicken, cheese
   d. Fruits and vegetables

Do you ever feel restless, bored, tired, cranky, tense, or distracted before you snack?   Yes/No

Do these feelings get any better after you snack?   Yes/No

Dissociation Experiences

This section consists of questions about experiences that people often have in their daily lives. We are interested in how often you have these experiences. It is important, however, that your answers show how often these experiences happen to you *when you are not under the influence of alcohol or drugs*. To answer the questions, please determine to what degree the experience described in the question applies to you and mark the line with a vertical slash at the appropriate place as shown in the example below.
Example

0% _____100%

1. Some people have the experience of driving a car and suddenly realizing that they don't remember what has happened during all or part of the trip. Mark the line to show what percentage of the time this happens to you.

0% _____100%

2. Some people find that they are listening to someone talk and they suddenly realize that they did not hear part or all of what was just said. Mark the line to show what percentage of the time this happens to you.

0% _____100%

3. Some people have the experience of finding themselves in a place and they have no idea how they got there. Mark the line to show what percentage of the time this happens to you.

0% _____100%

4. Some people have the experience of finding themselves dressed in clothes that they don't remember buying. Mark the line to show what percentage of the time this happens to you.

0% _____100%

5. Some people have the experience of finding new things among their belongs that they do not remember buying. Mark the line to show what percentage of the time this happens to you.

0% _____100%

6. Some people find that they are approached by people whom they do not know who call them by another name or insist that they have met them before. Mark the line to show what percentage of the time this happens to you.

0% _____100%

7. Some people have the experience of feeling as though they are standing next to themselves or watching themselves do something and they actually see themselves as if they were looking at another person. Mark the line to show what percentage of the time this happens to you.

0% _____100%

8. Some people are told that they do not recognize friends or family members. Mark the line to show what percentage of the time this happens to you.
   0%   100%

9. Some people find that they have no memory for some important events in their lives (for example, a wedding or graduation). Mark the line to show what percentage of the time this happens to you.
   0% _____100%

10. Some people have the experience of being accused of lying when they do not think that they have lied. Mark the line to show what percentage of the time this happens to you.
    0% _____100%

11. Some people have the experience of looking in a mirror and not recognizing themselves. Mark the line to show what percentage of the time this happens to you.
    0% _____100%

12. Some people have the experience of feeling that other people, objects, and the world around them are not real. Mark the line to show what percentage of the time this happens to you.
    0% _____100%

13. Some people have the experience of feeling that their body does not seem to belong to them. Mark the line to show what percentage of the time this happens to you.
    0% _____100%

14. Some people have the experience of remembering a past event so vividly that they feel as if they were reliving that event. Mark the line to show what percentage of the time this happens to you.
    0% _____100%

15. Some people have the experience of not being sure if things that they remember happening really did happen or if they just dreamed them. Mark the line to show what percentage of the time this happens to you.
    0% _____100%

16. Some people have the experience of being in a familiar place but finding it strange and unfamiliar. Mark the line to show what percentage of the time this happens to you.
    0% _____100%

17. Some people find that when they are watching television or a movie, they become so absorbed in the story that they are unaware of other events

happening around them. Mark the line to show what percentage of the time this happens to you.

0% _____100%

18. Some people find that they become so involved in a fantasy or daydream that it feels as though it were really happening to them. Mark the line to show what percentage of the time this happens to you.

0% _____100%

19. Some people find that they are able to ignore pain. Mark the line to show what percentage of the time this happens to you.

0% _____100%

20. Some people find that they sometimes sit staring off into space, thinking of nothing and are not aware of the passage of time. Mark the line to show what percentage of the time this happens to you.

0% _____100%

21. Some people find that when they are alone they talk out loud to themselves. Mark the line to show what percentage of the time this happens to you.

0% _____100%

22. Some people find that in one situation they may act so differently compared with another situation that they feel almost as if they were two different people. Mark the line to show what percentage of the time this happens to you.

0% _____100%

23. Some people find that in certain situations they are able to do things with amazing ease and spontaneity that would usually be difficult for them (for example, sports, work, social situations etc.). Mark the line to show what percentage of the time this happens to you.

0% _____100%

24. Some people find that they cannot remember whether they have done something or have just thought about doing that thing (for example, not knowing whether they have just mailed a letter or have only thought about mailing it). Mark the line to show what percentage of the time this happens to you.

0% _____100%

25. Some people find evidence that they have done things that they do not remember doing. Mark the line to show what percentage of the time this happens to you.

0% _____100%

26. Some people find writings, drawings, or notes among their belongings that they must have done, but cannot remember doing. Mark the line to show what percentage of the time this happens to you.

    0% _____100%

27. Some people find that they hear voices inside their head that tell them to do things or comment on things that they are doing. Mark the line to show what percentage of the time this happens to you.

    0% _____100%

28. Some people feel as if they are looking at the world through a fog so that people and objects appear far away or unclear. Mark the line to show what percentage of the time this happens to you.

    0% _____100%

Appendix 6
Obsessive-Compulsive Support Groups

DOMESTIC LIST
Alabama
Birmingham
Phil Shell at (205) 322-1797
Contact: Ralph Dobbs at (205) 786-8288 or (888) 841-8335, then enter 0747, after
tone enter phone number with area code
Open To: Individuals with obsessive-compulsive disorder
Frequency: First and third Thursday at 7:00pm-9:00pm
Location: Brookwood Medical Center, Gallery Complex, Room 545
*MH
Updated 4/97

Huntsville
Contact: Jane Sucic at (205) 881-2295
Open To: Individuals diagnosed with obsessive-compulsive disorders by a physician,
and currently in treatment
Frequency: Second and fourth Monday at 6:00pm
Location: Mayfair Church of Christ
*PA
Updated 2/96

Arizona
Dothan
Contact: Gregory G. Woodham, M.S. at (334) 793-8858
Open To: Individuals with obsessive-compulsive disorder, family, and friends
Frequency: Monday at 6:00pm
Location: Southeast Alabama Medical Center
*MH
Updated 12/97

---

*MH, Mutual Help Groups; *PA, Professionally Assisted Groups

Phoenix
Contact: Steve at (602) 935-7725 or Mental Health Association at (602) 994-4407
Open To: Individuals with obsessive-compulsive disorders, spectrum disorders, and
    family members
Frequency: Thursday 7:00 pm-9:00 pm
Location: Samaritan Behavioral Health Center (Board Room), 7575 E. Earll Dr.,
    Scottsdale, AZ
*MH
Updated 12/97

Tempe
Contact: Shelly at (602) 497-8054, (Church) (602) 838-1446, or (MHA) (602) 994-
    4407
Open To: Children and Adolescents with obsessive-compulsive disorder, and family
    members
Frequency: Fourth Monday at 7:00pm-8:30pm
Location: Bay Spring United Methodist Church, 1365 E. Elliott
*MH
Monthly Newsletter Updated 11/97

Tucson
Contact: Susan Silva-Salgado at (520) 622-5582
Open To: Individuals with obsessive-compulsive disorder, and family members
Frequency: Fourth Wednesday at 7:30pm
Location: Amisa Conference Room, First Floor, 738 N. Fifth Ave.
*MH
Updated 1/96

Tucson
Contact: Randall J. Garland, Ph.D. at (520) 322-9334
Open To: Individuals with obsessive-compulsive disorders, and children
Frequency: Wednesday, once a month at 7:00pm-8:30pm
Location: 5447 E. Fifth St., Suite 210-A
Fee: $10 per group
*PA
Updated 5/97

Tucson
Contact: Randall J. Garland, Ph.D. at (520) 322-9334
Open To: Individuals with trichotillomania
Frequency: Once monthly, typically on Mondays at 6:30pm
Location: 5447 E. Fifth St., Suite 210-A
Fee: $10
*PA
Updated 5/97
Requested that persons wanting to be in group have been previously professionally
    diagnosed or are evaluated by myself prior to entry into either group

Arkansas

Little Rock
Contact: Jackie Weser at (work) (800) 237-3675 or (home) (501) 397-5202
Open To: Individuals with obsessive-compulsive disorder and trichotillomania
Frequency: Third Tuesday at 7:00pm
Location: Hendricks Hall, Room 150
*MH
Updated 11/97

California

Calabasas
Contact: Carla Huffman, M.A., M.F.C.C.
Open To: Young adults (20-30 years of age)
Frequency: Tuesday evening
Cost: $25 per session
*MH
Updated 1/96

El Sobrante
Contact: Irv Bork at (510) 222-3535
Open To: Individuals with obsessive-compulsive disorder, family members,
    and friends
Frequency: Thursday at 7:00pm
*MH
Updated 9/96

Fullerton
Contact: Bob Hohenstein, Ph.D. at (714) 528-9335
Open To: Individuals with obsessive-compulsive disorder, and family members
Frequency: Wednesday at 7:00pm-8:00pm
Location: 3350 E. Birch, Suite 206
Format: Cognitive/Behavioral approach
Fee: $20 per session
*PA
Updated 7/96

Fullerton
Contact: Dr. Fred Ilfeld, M.D. at (916) 488-7795
Open To: Individuals with obsessive-compulsive disorder
Frequency: Wednesday, once a month at 4:30pm
Location: 4300 Auburn Blvd., #205
Format: Support/Behavioral therapy
*PA
Updated 3/96

Garden Grove
Contact: John Henry Foundation at (714) 539-9597
Open To: Individuals with obsessive-compulsive disorder, anxiety, and depression
Frequency: Thursday at 6:00pm-7:30pm
Location: 12812 Garden Grove Blvd., Suite J
*MH
Updated 3/97

Glendale
Contact: Dr. Boone at (310) 375-4855
Open To: Individuals with obsessive-compulsive disorder
Frequency: Monday at 12noon-12:50pm
Location: 116 N. Maryland Ave., #200
*PA
Updated 9/97

Long Beach
Contact: John at (562) 867-2907
Open To: Individuals with obsessive-compulsive disorder
Frequency: Saturday at 4:30pm
Location: Geneva Presbyterian Church, 2625 E. Third St (N.W. Corner Third and Molino)
Format: Twelve-step group
*MH
Updated 3/97

Loomis
Contact: Dan at (916) 427-3935
Open To: Individuals with obsessive-compulsive disorder, and family members
Frequency: First and third Monday at 7:00pm-9:00pm
Location: 5645 Rocklin Rd.
*MH
Updated 10/97

Los Angeles
Contact: Dr. Schwartz or Dr. Gorbis at (310) 392-4044 or (213) 651-1199
Open To: Individuals with obsessive-compulsive disorder
Frequency: Thursday at 4:30pm-6:00pm
Location: UCLA
Format: Cognitive/Behavioral
Fee: Requires Prior Evaluation

Los Angeles
Contact: Karron Maidment at (310) 794-7305
Open To: Family members or individuals involved with someone with obsessive-compulsive disorder
Frequency: Last Thursday of the month at 4:30pm-6:00pm
Format: Support/Educational

Los Angeles
Contact: Karron Maidment at (310) 794-7305
Open To: Individuals with obsessive-compulsive disorder
Frequency: Friday at 3:00pm-4:30pm
Location: UCLA Neuropsychological Research
Format: Research/Treatment
*PA
Updated 5/97

Los Angeles
Contact: Courtney Jacobs, Ph.D. at (310) 358-5984
Open To: Individuals with obsessive-compulsive disorder
Frequency: Monday at 8:00pm-9:30pm
Location: 1100 Glendon Ave., Suite 1601
Fee: $37.50 per month
*PA
Updated 3/97

Los Angeles
Contact: Coast Counseling Center, Janice Held, M.A., M.F.C.C. or Tom Corboy,
    M.A. at (310) 335-5443 or (310) 374-7407
Open To: Individuals with obsessive-compulsive disorder
Frequency: Weekly
*MH
Updated 9/94

Los Angeles
Contact: Edward Glaser at (213) 465-1216
Open To: Individuals with obsessive-compulsive disorder, Tourette's disorder, and
    trichotillomania, and family member
Frequency: Tuesday at 7:00pm-9:00pm
Location: Dialog Copy Shop, 8766 Holloway Dr., West Hollywood (basement)
Format: OCA twelve step
*MH
Updated 5/96

N.W. Los Angeles County
Contact: David Mellinger, M.S.W., L.C.S.W., B.C.D. at (818) 758-1200
Open To: Individuals with obsessive-compulsive disorder who are members of Kaiser
    Permanente
Format: Cognitive/Behavioral therapy
Fee: To be determined
*PA
Updated 9/97

Orange
Contact: Katie Monarch, M.S.W. at (717) 771-8243, extension 8243

Open To: Individuals with obsessive-compulsive disorder
Frequency: Every other Wednesday at 6:00pm-7:00pm
Location: St. Joseph Hospital Community Counselling
Fee: $5 donation
Updated 11/96

Palo Alto
Contact: Scott Granet, L.C.S.W. at (415) 858-2875
Open To: Individuals with obsessive-compulsive disorder and Spectrum disorder
Frequency: Monday at 5:00pm-6:30pm
Location: Palo Alto Medical Clinic
Fee: $30 per session
*MH
Updated 7/96

Petaluma
Contact: June Taylor at (707) 769-7869
Interested in starting a self-help group
Open To: Adults with obsessive-compulsive disorder
Frequency: Weekly for 1 hour
Location: 7 Fourth St., Suite 8
Fee: $25 per session
Format: Parents group
*PA
Updated 3/96

Petaluma
Contact: Darlene at (707) 762-4610
Interested in starting a twelve-step group OCA

Petaluma
Contact: Dawn at (707) 522-9133
Open To: Parents of children and adolescents with obsessive-compulsive disorder
Frequency: Third Monday at 7:00pm-9:00pm
Location: Easter Seal Society office, 5440 State Farm Dr., Rohnert Park
Updated 5/97

Pleasanton
Contact: Don at (510) 828-5184 or Naomi Gaunt at (510) 455-5748
Open To: Individuals with obsessive-compulsive disorder, and family members
Frequency: Wednesday at 7:00pm
Location: 4725 First St., Suite 200
*MH
Updated 3/97

Redlands
Contact: Colleen Woodhouse at (909) 796-3412

Open To: Individuals with obsessive-compulsive disorders, and family members
Frequency: Second and fourth Monday at 7:00pm-9:00pm
Location: Loma Linda University Behavioral Medical Center
*MH
Updated 3/96

Sacramento
Contact: Rachele Junkert at (916) 966-5917
Open To: Individuals with obsessive-compulsive disorder, and family members
Frequency: Second and fourth Monday at 7:00pm
Location: 7700 Folsom Blvd.
*MH
Updated 5/97

San Diego
Contact: Ana Maria Andia, M.D. at (619) 476-2260
Open To: Individuals with obsessive-compulsive disorder, and family members
Frequency: Wednesday at 4:30pm-6:00pm
Format: Psychoeducational and 8-week time limited behavioral therapy group
(Must call psychiatry department to make an appointment)
*PA
Updated 3/97

San Diego
Contact: Jayne at (619) 295-6129
Open To: Individuals with obsessive-compulsive disorder
Frequency: Thursday at 5:30pm-6:45pm, second group Wednesday at 6:30pm
Location: 3851 Rosecrans St., Harbor Room
Format: Twelve-step OCA
Please contact group leader before attending
*MH
Updated 5/97

San Diego
Contact: Guy at (619) 427-7635
Frequency: First Wednesday at 6:30pm-8:00pm
(enter through Walnut entrance and go to top stairs)
Location: 3427 Fourth Ave., Room 214
Format: OCA twelve step
*MH
Updated 3/96

San Diego
Contact: Jim Hatton, Ph.D., M.F.C.C. at (619) 457-8428 or Bonnie for group
    information at (619) 475-8527
Open To: Individuals with trichiotillomania
Frequency: Second Monday at 7:00pm-8:30pm

Location: Mesa Vista Hospital, 7850 Vista Hill Ave.
Second Group
Contact: Jorge at (619) 479-4417
Open To: Individuals with obsessive-compulsive disorder, and family members
Frequency: First and third Friday at 7:00pm-9:00pm
Location: Bayview Hospital, 330 Moss St.
Third Group
Contact: Group leader for information
Open To: Individuals with obsessive-compulsive disorder, and family members
Frequency: Second and fourth Friday
Location: Charter Hospital, 11878 Avenue of Industry
*MH
Updated 5/97

San Francisco
Contact: David at (415) 206-1656 or Adam at (415) 648-8390
Open To: Individuals with obsessive-compulsive disorder, and family members
Frequency: First and third Monday at 7:00pm-9:00pm
Location: UCSF
*MH
Updated 3/96

San Francisco
San Francisco Bay Area OCD Support Group
Contact: Peninsula Network of Mental Health Clients at (415) 591-7688
    (Group coordinator will return call)
Open To: Individuals with obsessive-compulsive disorder
*MH
Updated 3/96

Santa Cruz
Contact: Christina Dubowski at (408) 457-1004
Open To: Individuals with trichotillomania
Frequency: Weekly; quarterly newsletter
Location: Trichotillomania Learning Center
Format: Twelve step
*MH
Updated 3/97

Santa Cruz
Contact: Audrey at (408) 438-1043 or Rhonda at (408) 684-0568
Open To: Individuals with Spectrum disorder, and family members.
Frequency: Thursday at 7:30pm
Updated 3/96

Santa Monica
Contact: David Fogelson, M.D. at (310) 828-5015

Open To: Individuals with obsessive-compulsive disorder
(Referrals from professional required)
Location: 2730 Wilshire Blvd., #325
Fee: $50
*PA
Updated 3/96

Torrance
Contact: James S. Pratty, M.D. at (310) 217-8877
Open To: Individuals with obsessive-compulsive disorder
Location: Azimuth Mental Health Associates, 21081 S. Western Ave., Suite 250
*PA
Updated 3/96

Torrance
Contact: Dr. Rodney Boone at (310) 375-4855
Open To: Individuals with obsessive-compulsive disorder
(Prior to group, individuals must meet with Dr. Boone)
Frequency: Saturday at 10:00am-11:30am
Location: 24445 Hawthorne Blvd., #105
Fee: ?
*PA
Updated 9/97

Torrance
Contact: Dr. Boone at (310) 375-4855
Open To: Individuals with trichotillomania
Frequency: Wednesday at 6:30pm-7:50pm
Location: 24445 Hawthorne Blvd., #105
Fee: ?
*PA
Updated 9/97

Ventura
Contact: Richard Reinhart, Ph.D. at (805) 652-6747
Open To: Individuals with obsessive-compulsive disorder, family, and friends
Frequency: First and third Thursday at 7:30pm-9:00pm
Location: 300 Hillmont Ave.
*MH
Updated 3/97

Westminister
Contact: Mary at (714) 893-3137
Open To: Individuals with obsessive-compulsive disorder and trichotillomania
Frequency: Every other Wednesday at 7:00pm-9:00pm
Location: 8854 Grandville Circle

Colorado

Boulder
Contact: Judy Goldstein at (303) 938-1360
Open To: Individuals with obsessive-compulsive disorder,
   and family members
Location: Boulder Mental
Frequency: First Monday—two groups at 7:00pm-9:00pm: (1) for individuals with
   obsessive-compulsive disorder; (2) for friends and family (Mental health
   professional may attend either group)—and third Wednesday (Informational
   meeting) at 7:00pm-9:00pm
No Fee
*MH
Updated 1/97

Colorado Springs
Contact: Edna Huston at (719) 599-7694
(Interested in starting a support group)
*MH
Updated 1/96

Northglenn
Contact: Ed Sears at (303) 452-2376
Open To: Individuals with obsessive-compulsive disorder and trichotillomania, and
   family members
Frequency: First Saturday at 12:00pm
Location: 622 Melody Circle
*MH
Updated 11/97

Connecticut

Danbury
Contact: Maria Urban at (203) 778-2924
Open To: Individuals with obsessive-compulsive disorder and their
   support people
Frequency: Tuesday at 2:00pm
Location: Exodus, 64 West St.
*MH
Updated 10/97

Danbury
Contact: Bruce Mansbridge, Ph.D. at 790-7001
Frequency: First Monday at 7:00pm-8:30pm informational meeting
Location: First Congregational Chruch of Danbury
Open To: Individuals with obsessive-compulsive disorder, and Spectrum disorder, and
   family and friends
*PA

Enfield
Contact: Joe Rinaldi at (860) 745-5363
Open To: Individuals with obsessive-compulsive disorder, and family and friends
Frequency: Twice a month, first Tuesday of the month at 7:00pm-9:00pm
Location: First meeting at Johnson Wellness Center grounds of Johnson Memorial
    Hospital, Stafford Springs, Connecticut; second meeting at Hartford Courant
    building, Phoenix Ave. at 6:00pm-8:00pm
Updated 11/97

Farmington
Contact: Nancy Fidler, M.S.W. at (860) 679-6700
Open To: Individuals with obsessive-compulsive disorder
Format: Cognitive therapy group
Frequency: Every other week
Fee: ?
*MH
Updated 10/97

Middletown
Contact: Ginger Blume at (860) 346-6020
Open To: Individuals with obsessive-compulsive disorder
Frequency: Monday at 4:00pm-5:30pm
Format: Six-week therapy group
Fee: $50 or $60 (with insurance)
*MH
Updated 10/97

Milford
Contact: Jim Broatch at 878-5669
A teenager interested in starting and co-leading a support group for teenagers with
    obsessive-compulsive disorder. An adult volunteer is also needed to help lead this
    group. For more information please call (203) 623-6109

Milford
Contact: Sheryl Esposito at 877-0563
Open To: Individuals with obsessive-compulsive disorder, family, and friends
Frequency: Every other Thursday at 7:30pm
Location: OCF Headquarters, 9 Depot St., Milford, CT
Please call to confirm dates, times and directions
*MH
Updated 12/97

Orange
Emotions Anonymous
Contact: 795-3351 (anytime before 9:00pm)
Open To: Those willing to become well, emotionally
Frequency: Friday at 7:30pm-9:30pm

Location: Church of the Good Shepard Episcopal (basement),
680 Race Brook Road, Orange, CT 06477
Format: Twelve step
*MH
Updated 10/97
Call before attending group

West Hartford
Contact: Emily Bailey Mental Health Association of Connecticut at (800) 842-1501
    extension 15
Open To: Individuals with obsessive-compulsive disorder
Frequency: First and third Wednesday at 7:00pm-9:00pm
Location: First Congregational Church (lower level family room)
*MH
Updated 11/97

West Hartford
Messie Anonymous
Contact: Tonya at (860) 267-2812
Open To: Individuals who have a desire to be clutter-free, and acquire an organized
    lifestyle
Location: Meetings in Greenwich, Westport, Unionville, and East Hampton
*MH
Updated 7/97

West Hartford
Contact: Terry Parkerson at (860) 247-2606 (DAY) (860) 528-2050 (EVE)
Open To: Individuals with obsessive-compulsive disorder, and family members
Frequency: Saturday at 11:00pm-12:30pm
Location: Unity Church, 730 Farmington Ave., West Hartford, Connecticut 06119
Format: Based on Dr. Jeffrey Schwartz's Book, *Brain Lock*
*MH
Updated 10/97

Delaware

Wilmington
Contact: Kathy Parrish, M.A. at (610) 525-1510
Open To: Adolescents ages 12 to 18 years with obsessive-compulsive disorder
Frequency: Every other Thursday at 6:30pm-7:30pm
Location: Center for Cognitive and Behavioral therapy, 3411 Silverside Rd., Hagley
    building, Suite 102
Fee: $10
Updated: 12/97

Florida

Contact: Janis McClure at (904) 726-0918
OCF of Jacksonville, P.O. Box 16892

(Affiliate in-Formation)

Cocoa Beach
Contact: Faith Brigham at (407) 631-1312
Open To: Individuals with obsessive-compulsive disorder, and family members
Location: St. Mary's Catholic School, teacher's lounge
Format: Twelve step

Del Rey Beach
Contact: Michelle at (305) 341-6830
Open To: Individuals with obsessive-compulsive disorder
Frequency: Every other Thursday at 7:00pm
*PA
Updated 1/96

Gainesville
Contact: Janis McClure at (904) 726-0918
Open To: Individuals with obsessive-compulsive disorder, and support people
Frequency: First and third Monday at 7:00pm
Location: Mandarin Middle School, Room #51, 5100 Hood Rd.
*MH
Updated 10/97

Hollywood
Contact: Bruce M. Hyman, Ph.D. at (954) 987-557-4495
Open To: Individuals with obsessive-compulsive disorder
Frequency: Tuesday afternoons for adolescents; Tuesday evenings for adults
Location: 4350 Sheridan St., Suite 102, Hollywood, Florida 33021
Format: Behavioral therapy group
Must meet with Dr. Hyman prior to admission to group
Fee: ?
*PA
Updated 10/97

Lakeland
Contact: Sylvia Hart at (941) 688-7865
Open To: Individuals with obsessive-compulsive disorder, and family members
Frequency: Friday at 7:00pm
Location: Jeanine Brown Drop-In Center, 2968 Lakeland Highlands Rd.
*MH
Updated 2/96

Largo
Contact: Angela J. Gibson, L.C.S.W. at (813) 586-0636
Open To: Individuals with obsessive-compulsive disorder, and family members
Frequency: Saturday at 11:00am-12:30pm
Location: 10225 Ulmerton Rd., Suite 8B

Fee: $20
*PA
Updated 5/97

Rock Ledge
Contact: Barbara Rhode, M.S. at (813) 586-0636
Open To: Individuals with obsessive-compulsive disorder, and family members
Frequency: Tuesday at 8:00pm
Location: 10225 Ulmerton Rd., Suite 8B
Updated 5/97

Georgia

Atlanta
Contact: Charles Melville, Ph.D. at (404) 266-8881
Open To: Individuals with obsessive-compulsive disorder, and
    family members
Frequency: Second Thursday at 6:30pm-8:00pm
*PA
Updated 4/97

Atlanta
Contact: Delanna Protas at (770) 952-1441
Open To: Individuals with obsessive-compulsive disorder, and family and friends
Frequency: Second Saturday at 11:00am-12:00noon
Location: Contact group leader for location
No fee
*MH
Updated 7/97

Atlanta
Contact: Lisa Terry, L.P.C. at (770) 396-2929, extension 28
Open To: Teens with mental-health disorders
Frequency: Tuesday at 6:30pm-7:30pm
*PA
Updated 3/96

Hawaii

Honolulu
Contact: Ginny at (808) 261-6987
Open To: Professionally diagnosed individuals with obsessive-compulsive disorders
    and family members.
Frequency: Second Saturday at 11:00am-1:00pm
Location: 4470 Aliikoa St.
Contact Ginny for further information
*MH
Updated 5/97

Idaho

Boise
Contact: Charles Bunch, M.C.NCC at (208) 344-5254 or (208) 344-5254; e-mail:
   ckestrel@aol.com
SUPPORT GROUP:
Frequency: Second Tuesday at 7:30pm
Location: 303 Allumbaugh St. (in library)
TEAM:
Frequency: Fourth Wednesday at 6:30pm
No fee
Some insurance coverage required after the second visit
Updated 4/97

Hayden Lake
Contact: Karen Grove at (208) 772-4156
Frequency: Thursday at 7:00pm-8:30pm
Open To: Individuals with obsessive-compulsive disorder, trichotillomania,
   and anxiety
Location: 251 West Miles Ave.
Guest speakers periodically
*MH
Updated 5/97

Illinois

Chicago
Contact: Pam Kohlbeck, M.S. at (847) 604-2502
Open To: Individuals with obsessive-compulsive disorder, and significant others
Frequency: Third Tuesday at 6:00pm-7:30pm
Fee: $5
*PA
Updated 2/97

Chicago
Contact: Angela Di Manno at (773) 973-8243
Open To: Individuals with obsessive-compulsive disorder, and family and friends
Frequency: First and third Tuesday at 7:00pm-8:30pm
Location: Loyola University Campus
*MH
Updated 2/97

Chicago
Contact: Susan Richman at (773) 880-2035
Open To: Individuals with obsessive-compulsive disorder, and family and friends
Frequency: Second and fourth Thursday at 7:30pm-9:00pm
Fee: $5
*MH
Updated 2/97

Chicago
Contact: Sharon Vlasak R.N. M.S. at (773) 413-0997 or Dr. A.J. Allen, M.D. Ph.D at (773) 413-1710
Given by University of Illinois at Chicago Pediatric OCD and TIC disorders clinic staff. A series of informational programs for older children and adolescents with OCD, and for their parents. These programs will be held the first Saturday of each month at 10:00am-12:00noon at the UIC Institute. The first hour will be an interactive didactic program on some aspect of OCD. During the second hour, older children and adolescents will meet in one group and parents in another group to discuss what was learned, and to provide each other with mutual support. A series of six meetings will be repeated every 6 months. The cost of these sessions is $10 per family. The initial series of topics and dates are:
February 1: Introduction, overview of OCD, causes of OCD, and medications
March 1: School issues
April 5: Family issues and stresses—major sources of tension
May 3: Introduction to cognitive/behavioral therapy (including ERP)
June 7: More on cognitive/behavioral therapy (including ERP)
July 12: Family issues and stresses—coping strategies
Updated 2/97

Crystal Lake
Contact: Tim Re at (800) 765-9999
Open To: Individuals with obsessive-compulsive disorder
Frequency: Second and fourth Monday at 7:00pm-8:30pm
Location: Horizons, 970 South McHenry Ave.
Leader has therapy group in Elgin
Updated 2/97

Downers Grove
Contact: Dennis Nakanishi, M.A. at (708) 939-4441
Open To: Individuals with obsessive-compulsive disorder
Frequency: Monday at 6:00pm-7:00pm
Format: Goal-oriented ERP group
Fee: $25 per group

Evanston
Contact: James Dod, Ph.D., Evanston Hospital at (847) 570-2720 or (708) 570-1585 (voice mail)
Format:
(1) Short-term behavioral therapy groups for individuals with obsessive-compulsive disorder;
(2) Individual behavioral therapy;
(3) Home-based exposure treatment (leaving office and going to homes)
Fee: $30 per group session (sliding scale for Evanston residents)
Please contact Dr. Dod for more information
*PA
Updated 2/97

Glenview
Contact: Karol K. at (847) 965-1225
Open To: Individuals with obsessive-compulsive disorder
Frequency: Friday at 7:30pm
Location: Glenview Community Church, 1000 Elm St.
Format: Twelve-step OCA
Updated 5/97

Homewood
Contact: Mark Bornstein, Psy.D. at (708) 461-2333 (pager)
Open To: Individuals with obsessive-compulsive disorder, and family and friends
Frequency: Second and fourth Monday at 7:30pm-8:30pm
Fee: $5 per group
*PA
Updated 2/97

Lisle
Contact: Margaret Wehrenberg, Psy. D at (708) 852-3870
Open To: Individuals with obsessive-compulsive disorder
Frequency: Wednesday at 7:30pm-9:00pm
Location: 5007 Lincoln Ave., Suite #215
Fee: $25 per group
*PA
Updated 2/97

Naperville
Contact: Jane Bodine, M.A. at (630) 416-3146
Four groups formed
(1) Open To: Individuals with obsessive-compulsive disorder and Spectrum disorder,
    and family members
    Frequency: Second and fourth Wednesday at 6:30pm-7:45pm
(2) Open To: Young adults
    Frequency: Wednesday at 3:30pm
(3) Open To: Tric group, support people, children, & adol.
    Frequency: First and Third Wednesday
    Location: 10 West Jefferson
(4) Open To: People currently in treatment
    Frequency: Three to four times a year
Format: Goal-oriented ERP group, 10-week therapy group
Fee: $25
Must contact group leader prior to attending group
Updated 5/97

North Chicago
Contact: John Calamari at (847) 578-3305
Open To: Individuals with obsessive-compulsive disorder, and family and friends
Frequency: First and third Wednesday at 7:00pm-8:30pm

Format: Instruction on cognitive/behavioral principles, including ERP
Fee: $10 (can be waived)
Updated 2/97

Northbrook
Contact: Pam Kohlbeck, M.S. at (847) 604-2502
Open To: Parents of children with obsessive-compulsive disorder
Frequency: Fourth Monday at 7:30pm
Location: Glencoe Public Library
*PA
Updated 2/97

Northfield
Contact: Karen Cassiday, Ph.D. at (847) 577-8809
Open To: Individuals with obsessive-compulsive disorder, and family and friends
Frequency: First and third Monday at 7:30pm-9:00pm
Location: Anxiety and Agoraphobia Treatment Center
Fee: $5 per group

Northfield
Contact: Penny Silverman at (847) 432-0446 if interested in starting
    a group for BDD

Northwest Suburbs
Contact: Kristen at (630) 980-1328 (late afternoon or evening)
Open To: Children and adolescents with obsessive-compulsive disorder
Frequency: Second and fourth Monday at 7:30pm-8:30pm
*MH
Updated 2/97

Springfield
Contact: Janice Phelan at (217) 523-2740
Open To: Individuals with obsessive-compulsive disorders, and family members
Frequency: Last Monday at 5:30pm-7:00pm
Location: Christ Episcopal Church, Jackson St.
*PA/MH
Updated 10/97

Indiana

Fort Wayne
Contact: Robert Collie, Ph.D. at (219) 485-6687
Open To: Individuals with obsessive-compulsive disorder, and family members
Frequency: Monday at 7:30pm-8:30pm
Location: Good Shepard United Methodist Church, Room 37
*PA
Updated 7/97

Indianapolis
(1) Contact: Kerri Bova at (317) 888-6753
    Open To: Individuals with obsessive-compulsive disorder, and family and friends
    Frequency: Monday at 6:30pm
*MH
Updated 11/97
(2) Contact: Vikki Sutton at (765) 963-3210
    Open To: Individuals with trichotillomania, and family and friends
    Frequency: Two Mondays
*MH
Updated 11/97
(3) Contact: Homer at (317) 576-0625
    Open To: Individuals with general anxiety
    Frequency: Fourth Monday at 6:30pm-8:00pm
    Location: 7440 North Shadeland Ave., #202
*PA
Updated 4/97
(4) Contact: Phil Clendenen at (317) 297-0625 or Dr. Hilgendorf at
    (317) 578-4213
    Open To: Individuals with obsessive-compulsive disorder
    Frequency: Monday at 7:30pm-8:00pm
*PA
Updated 4/97

South Bend
Contact: Nancy Sechrest at (219) 299-1483
Open To: Individuals with obsessive-compulsive disorder
Frequency: Thursday at 7:00pm
Updated 4/97

Iowa

Iowa City
Contact: Nancee Blum at (319) 353-6180
Open To: Individuals with obsessive-compulsive disorder; separate group for family
    members
Frequency: Second and fourth Thursday (Second Thursday family group) at
    7:00pm-8:30pm
Location: 1942 JPP, University of Iowa
No Fee
*PA
Updated 5/97

Kansas

Lenexa
Contact: Jane Condra at (816) 763-8174
Open To: Individuals with obsessive-compulsive disorder, and family members

Frequency: Thursday at 7:00pm-9:30pm
Location: CPC College Meadows Hospital, 14425 College Blvd., Conference Room
*MH
Updated 5/97

Wichita
Contact: Rob Zettle, M.D. at (316) 978-3081
Open To: Individuals with obsessive-compulsive disorder
Frequency: First and third Monday at 7:00pm
Location: Charter Hospital of Wichita, Room 23
*MH
Updated 4/97

Kentucky

Lexington
Contact: Deborah A. Krause, Ph.D. at (606) 2710-2881
Open To: Individuals with obsessive-compulsive disorder, and significant others
Frequency: First Thursday at 7:00pm
*PA
Updated 5/97

Louisville
Contact: Dr. Jeff Romer, CMFT at (502) 899-5991
Open To: Individuals with obsessive-compulsive disorder and Spectrum disorder
Frequency: Tuesday at 7:00pm-8:30pm
Location: Lutheran Child and Family Counseling
Need to contact group leader prior to attending group
*PA
Updated 1/96

Louisiana

New Orleans
Contact: Pattie Lemonn at (504) 588-5405
Open To: Individuals with obsessive-compulsive disorder, and family and support
    people
Frequency: Second Tuesday at 6:00pm-8:00pm
*MH
Updated 1/96

Maine

Bangor
Contact: Charles Casey at (207) 794-3501 or (207) 794-3161
Open To: Individuals with obsessive-compulsive disorder, and family members
Frequency: Date to be determined; 7:00pm-9:00pm
Location: Bangor Counseling Center
Contact Charles prior to attending

*MH
Updated 5/97

Berwick
Contact: Sandy Skammels at (603) 692-9851
Open To: Individuals with obsessive-compulsive disorder, and family members
Frequency: Sunday at 4:00pm-5:00pm
Location: Portsmouth Regional Hospital, Pavillion
Updated 11/97

Clinton
Contact: Tina Couturier at (207) 873-0145
Open To: Individuals with trichotillomania, and family and friends
Frequency: Third Friday at 7:00pm-9:00pm
Location: Brown Memorial United Methodist Church
*MH
Updated 1/96

Maryland

Annapolis
Contact: Peg Duvall at (410) 544-5918 or Charlotte Lindsley, M.S.W. at (410) 263-3987
Open To: Individuals with obsessive-compulsive disorder, and support people
Frequency: First Wednesday at 7:00pm-9:00pm
*PA
Updated 10/97

Kensington
Contact: Lorett Gaiser at (301) 929-0156
Available 24 hours a day to talk with individuals with obsessive-compulsive disorder or trichotillomania, and give meeting information
Updated 1/96

Rockville
Contact: Roslyn Lehman LCSW-C at (301) 469-0108, Fax (301) 762-5711
Open To: Family members
Frequency: First Thursday at 2:00pm-4:00pm
Location: 20 Courthouse Square, Suite 217
*MH
Updated 4/97

Wheaton
Contact: David at (301) 495-7806
Open To: Individuals with obsessive-compulsive disorder
Frequency: First and third Tuesday at 7:30pm-9:30pm
Location: 2424 Reedie Dr.

Contact David prior to attending
*MH
Updated 1/96

Massachusetts

Belmont
OCF Greater Boston Affiliate
Contact: Debbie Mcdowell, President at (781) 376-3784

Boston
Obsessive-Compulsive Disorder Institute—Obsessive-Compulsive Anonymous
   Mclean Hospital (617) 376-3653
Contact: Diane Baney, R.N., M.B. at (617) 855-3279
Open To: Individuals with obsessive-compulsive disorder
Frequency: Wednesday at 8:00pm
Location: United Presbyterian Church, 32 Harvard St. (basement)
Format: Partial hospital and intensive residential care
*MH
Updated 11/97

Brookline
Contact: Roberta Brucker, LICSW at (617) 499-7979
Open To: Individuals with obsessive-compulsive disorder, and family members
Frequency: Weekly
Format: 10-week program (1 1/2 hours)
Two therapy groups; must contact leader prior to attending
Updated 1/96

Cambridge
Contact: HPA, P.O. Box 614, Cambridge, MA 02140
Open To: Individuals with trichotillomania
Frequency: Wednesday at 7:15pm-8:45pm
Location: Cambridge Hospital, Macht Building, Room 148, 1493 Cambridge St.,
   Cambridge, MA
Format: Twelve step
*MH
Updated 5/97

Chicopee
Contact: Leslie or Mary at (413) 567-5633
Open To: Individuals with obsessive compulsive disorder, and family and friends
Frequency: First and third Tuesday at 7:00 pm
Location: Charles River Hospital, West 350 Memorial Dr.
*MH
Updated 7/97

Great Barrington
Contact: Brent at (413) 229-2994
Brent is interested in starting a mutual-help support group
Greater Boston Affiliate sponsors four self-help groups: (1) Professionally assisted
    group for individuals with obsessive-compulsive disorder, and family and
    friends; (2) Trichotillomania group; (3) Spectrum disorders group; and (4) Child
    and Adolescents group. For further information, please call the helpline at
    (617) 376-3784

Ludlow
Contact: Patricia Ricci at (413) 583-6750
Open To: Family members
Frequency: Wednesday evenings
Updated 1/96

N. Cambridge
Contact: Joris Jones or David Ligon at (617) 458-0925 (beeper) or (617) 864-9902
    (He will return your call)
Open To: Individuals with obsessive-compulsive disorder, and family and friends
Frequency: Third Wednesday at 7:00pm-9:00pm
Location: Rear Mefitz Gerald School, 70 Rindge Ave.
*MH
Updated 1/96

Salem
Contact: Christina at (617) 231-9053
Open To: Individuals with obsessive-compulsive disorder, and family members
Frequency: Wednesday at 7:00pm-8:00pm
Location: Shaughnessy-Kaplan Rehabilitation Hospital
Format: Twelve-step OCA
*MH
Updated 11/95

Stoughton
Contact: Phill at (508) 583-3205
Open To: Individuals with obsessive-compulsive disorder, currently in treatment
Frequency: Monday at 7:00pm-9:00pm
*MH
Updated 5/97

Worcester
Contact: Ann at (508) 799-6784
Open To: Individuals with obsessive-compulsive disorder,
    and family members
Frequency: Every other Tuesday at 7:30pm-8:30pm
Location: Hahnemann Hospital, 281 Lincoln St. (use rear entrance), Fourth Floor,
    Classroom #2

Format: Twelve-step OCA
*MH
Updated 1/96

Worcester
Contact: William Ferrarone at (508) 792-8785
Open To: Individuals with obsessive-compulsive disorder
Frequency: Friday at 3:00pm-4:30pm (follow-up group meets monthly)
Location: Psychiatric Outpatient Service Medical Center, 15 Belmont, Lincoln
    Square Pavillion
Must contact group leader for evaluation and diagnosis
Updated 1/96

Michigan

OCD Foundation of Michigan
Ms. Robert P. Slade, President
P.O. Box 510412
Livonia, MI 48151
(313) 438-3293

Ann Arbor
Contact: Mary Jo at (313) 761-9167
Frequency: Fourth Wednesday at 6:00pm-8:00pm
Location: Washtenaw County Mental Hospital, 2140 Ellsworth
*MH
Updated 8/97

Battle Creek
Contact: Gerda at (616) 965-4529
Frequency: Third Tuesday at 7:00pm-9:00pm
Location: St. Peter's Lutheran Church, 1079 Riverside
*MH
Updated 8/97

Dearborn
Contact: Wally Green at (313) 563-5200
Open To: Individuals with obsessive-compulsive disorder
Frequency: First and third Thursday at 7:00pm-9:00pm
Location: First United Methodist Church, Garrison and Mason Sts.
*MH
Updated 8/97

Escanaba
Contact: Val at (906) 474-9369
Open To: Public
Frequency: Third Monday at 7:00pm-9:00pm

Location: Delta Community Mental Health Building, 2820 College Ave.
Updated: 8/97

Farmington Hills
Contact: Greg at (313) 438-3293
Open To: Adolescents and their supporters
Frequency: Third Wednesday at 7:00pm-9:00pm
Location: Davis Counseling Center Park on the Green Center, 37923 West 12 Mile
    Rd., Building A (between Haggerty and Halstead)
*MH
Updated 8/97

Farmington Hills
T.H.E.O. = Trichotillomania Helping Each Other
P.O. Box 871083
Canton, MI 48187
Contact: Bobbie at (313) 522-8907
Open To: Individuals with Trichotillomania
Frequency: First and third Sunday at 1:00pm-4:00pm
Location: Botsford Hospital, 28050 Grand River
*MH
Updated 8/97

Flint
Contact: David at (248) 694-4845
Open To: Individuals with obsessive-compulsive disorder,
    and family members
Frequency: Second Wednesday at 7:00pm-9:00pm
Location: Perry Center, 11920 South Saginaw St., Grand Blanc
Updated 8/97

Grand Blanc
Contact: Ellen Craine at (810) 695-0055
Open To: Parents of children and adolescents with obsessive-compulsive
    disorder
Frequency: Tuesday, once a month at 6:00pm-7:30pm
Location: 8341 Office Park Dr.
Fee: Most insurance accepted
*PA
Updated 8/97

Lake Orion
Contact: Susan at (248) 628-8029
Open To: Individuals with obsessive-compulsive disorder
Frequency: Saturday at 10:00am
Location: "Keep Them Coming Back" Club, 33 Broadway St.
Updated 10/97

Lansing
Contact: Jon at (517) 485-6653
Open To: Individuals with obsessive-compulsive disorder, and family members
Frequency: First and third Thursday at 7:00pm-9:00pm
Location: Delta Presbyterian Church, 6100 West Michigan Ave
*MH
Updated 8/97

Lansing
Contact: Sandi at (517) 484-8205 or El at (517) 351-7362
Open To: Individuals with Trichotillomania
Frequency: Second Sunday at 2:00pm-4:00pm
*MH
Updated 8/97

Monroe
Contact: Doug at (313) 390 6484
Frequency: First and third Tuesday at 6:00pm-8:00pm
Location: Monroe Community Mental Health, 1001 Raisonville Rd.
*MH
Updated 9/97

Plymouth
Contact: Lois Turpel at (313) 522-3022
Open To: Individuals with obsessive-compulsive disorder, and family members
Frequency: Second and fourth Thursday at 7:00pm
Location: First Baptist Church, 45000 North Territorial Rd.
*MH
Updated 8/97

Royal Oak
Contact: Bob Cato at (248) 542-5909
Open To: Individuals with obsessive-compulsive disorder, and family members
Location: St. John Episcopal Church, 115 South Woodward
Frequency: First and third Tuesday at 7:00pm-9:00pm
*MH
Updated 8/97

Saginaw
Contact: Barb Bacon at (517) 777-6042
Open To: Individuals with obsessive-compulsive disorder, and family members
Frequency: Tuesday at 7:30pm-8:30pm
Location: Healthsource-Dining, Room B, 3340 Hospital Rd. (rear entrance)
Updated 8/97

West Bloomfield
Contact: Ellen Craine, I.D. C.S.W., A.C.S.W. at (810) 539-3850

Open To: (1) Children and adolescents with obsessive-compulsive disorder
(2) Parents and family members with a child with obsessive-compulsive disorder
Frequency: (1) Monday and Wednesday at 4:00pm-5:30pm; (2) Monday and Thursday at 6:00pm-7:30pm
Format: Education/Professionally facilitated support
Fee: $40 per session
*PA
Updated 4/97

Windsor, Ontario
Contact: YMCA at (519) 256-7330
Frequency: Second and fourth Thursday at 7:00pm-9:00pm
Updated 8/97

Minnesota

Chanhassen
Contact: Sharon Lohmann at (612) 646-5615
Open To: Parents and children with obsessive-compulsive disorder
Frequency: Third Saturday at 1:00pm
*MH
Updated 7/97

Duluth
Contact: Mental Health Association Office at (218) 726-0793
Open To: Individuals with obsessive-compulsive disorder, and family members
Frequency: Third Thursday at 7:00pm-8:30pm
Location: 502 East Second St.

Hopkins
Contact: Justus Burggraff at (612) 724-0931, or call Minnesota affiliate for further information
Open To: Individuals with obsessive-compulsive disorder, and family and friends
Frequency: Monday 7pm-8:30pm
Location: Eisenhower Community Center, 1001 Highway #7
Fee: Donation
*MH
Updated 7/97

Minneapolis/St. Paul
Contact: Sharon Lohmann, President, OCF St. Paul Affiliate at (612) 646-5615 or (612) 646-5616
Open To: Individuals with obsessive-compulsive disorder, and family and friends
Frequency: Second and fourth Saturday 11:00am-1:00pm
Location: Please contact leader for meeting place
Updated 7/97

St. Louis Park
Contact: Sharon Lohmann at (612) 646-5615 or (612) 825-0963

Open To: Individuals with obsessive-compulsive disorder, and family members
Frequency: First, third, and fifth Saturday at 11:00am-1:00pm
No Fee
*MH
Updated 7/97

St. Paul
Contact: Gail Meyer, R.N., M.S.N., C.S. at (612) 649-1105 or (612) 649-0050, EXT #3
Location: Pioneer Clinic, 2550 University Ave., West
Format:
(1) Support Group for individuals with obsessive-compulsive disorder (must be Pioneer Clinic patients)
(2) Monthly support group for individuals with Trichotillomania
(3) 10-session treatment group for individuals with Trichotillomania
(4) 1-week intensive treatment group program for individuals with Trichotillomania (program will occur in April, June, and August)
*PA
Updated 5/97

Missouri

Kansas City
Contact: Jane Condra at (913) 469-1100
Open To: Individuals with obsessive-compulsive disorder, and family members
Frequency: Thursday at 7:00pm
Location: College Meadows Hospital, CPC, Pink Unit, Room #A
*MH
Updated 1/96

St. Louis Metropolitan Area
OCD Support group
Contact: Edna or Bernie at (314) 842-7228
Open To: Individuals with obsessive-compulsive disorder, and family and friends
Frequency: Third Saturday at 10:00am
Location: St. John's Mercy Medical Center, 615 South New Ballas Rd.
Format: Professional speaker, individual group
Updated 4/97

St. Louis
Contact: George M. at (314) 394-2662
Open To: Individuals with obsessive-compulsive disorder
Frequency: Saturday at 10:00am (except third Saturday)
Location: Missouri Baptist Hospital, Nursing School Building, Room 108
Format: OCA
Updated 11/96

St Louis
Barnes Hospital
Contact: Elliot Nelson, M.D. at (314) 362-2465

Frequency: Second and Third Wednesday at 7:00pm-8:15pm
Location: Barnes Hospital, 15th floor
*PA
Updated 1/96

Montana

Bozeman
Contact: Sharon Mohr at (406) 587-5718 or Bozeman Help Center at
    (406) 586-3333
Open To: Individuals with obsessive-compulsive disorder and Spectrum disorder, and
    support people
Frequency: Thursday at 7:00pm
Please call coordinator; time and place are subject to change
*MH
Updated 5/97

Nebraska

Hastings
Contact: Nabil Faltas, M.D. at (402) 463-7711
Open To: Individuals with obsessive-compulsive disorder
(an initial screening interview is necessary)
*MH
Updated 5/96

Lincoln
Contact: Pat Diesler at (402) 483-3480
Open To: Individuals with obsessive-compulsive disorder and Trichotillomania, and
    family members
Frequency: First Wednesday at 7:00pm-8:00pm
Location: Bryan Memorial Hospital, 1600 South 48th St.
*MH
Updated 2/96

Omaha
Contact: Dan Hegarty at (402) 496-0242 or (402) 390-6093
Open To: Individuals with obsessive-compulsive disorder, and family and
    support people
Frequency: Third Thursday at 7:00pm-9:00pm
Location: Pathways Center, Building #7701, Suite 319
*MH
Updated 2/96

Omaha
Contact: Creighton-Nebraska Department of Psychiatry, Child and Adolescent Divi-
    sion
3528 Dodge

Omaha, NE 68131
Open To: Parents of children with obsessive-compulsive disorder;
    children's group
Frequency: First and third Monday at 4:15pm-5:15pm
Updated 10/97

Nevada

Contact: Jeff at (702) 642-8775
Open To: Individuals with obsessive-compulsive disorder
Frequency: Monthly
Location: Varies
Fee: None
The Tourette O.C.D. Society of Southern Nevada, Inc. (T-OCD SOSN)
*MH
Updated 1/96

Las Vegas
Contact: Nancy Quinones at (702) 252-4596 or A.D.D. Clinic at (702) 796-1919
Open To: Individuals with obsessive-compulsive disorder, Tourette's disorder, and
    Trichotillomania, and support people
Frequency: First Monday at 7:00pm-9:00pm
*PA
Updated 8/97

New Jersey

Cliffside Park
Contact: James Pinto at (201) 941-8143
Open To: Individuals with obsessive-compulsive disorder
Frequency: Thursday at 6:00pm-7:00pm
Location: The Oasis, 619-A Palisade Ave.
Updated 5/97

Dover
Contact: Michelle Shine at (201) 347-7508 or Helene at (201) 335-6185
Open To: Individuals with obsessive-compulsive disorder, and family members
Frequency: Wednesday at 7:30pm
*MH
Updated 1/96

Haddonfield
Contact: John at (609) 429-1571
Open To: Individuals with BDD
Frequency: Second Thursday at 7:00pm-8:30pm
Location: Institute of Pennsylvania, 111 North 49th St., Philadelphia, Kirkbride
    Building, Room 5
Updated 5/96

Lakewood
Contact: Nancy Spader at (908) 295-8883
Open To: Individuals with obsessive-compulsive disorder, and family members
Frequency: Second Tuesday at 7:00pm
Location: Axelrad Building, Route 9
*MH
Updated 1/96

Montclair
Contact: New Jersey Self-Help Clearinghouse at (800) 367-6274 or (973) 625-9565
*MH

Montclaire
Contact: Nancy Maller at (201) 472-8215
Open To: Individuals with obsessive-compulsive disorder, and family members
Frequency: First and third Thursday at 8:00pm-10:00pm
Location: Mountainside Hospital, 300 Bay Ave., Room 6191
*MH
Updated 1/96

Newton
Contact: OCD Support Group at (201) 619-1207
Open To: Individuals who suffer from obsessive-compulsive disorder, and family and
    friends
Frequency: First and third Thursday at 8:00pm-9:00pm
Location: Newton Memorial Hospital, Center for Mental Health, Conference Room
    239, 175 High St.
*MH

Oradell
Contact: Nina Simon, A.C.S.W. at (201) 265-4793
Frequency: To be determined
Location: 377 Loretta Dr.
Fee: $25 per person/per family
Format: OCD family group and behavioral/cognitive group
*PA
Updated 5/97

Parsippany
Contact: Helene at (201) 335-6185
Open To: Individuals with obsessive-compulsive disorder
Frequency: Wednesday at 7:30pm-9:30pm
*MH
Updated 4/95

Pennington
Contact: Linda Flower, A.C.S.W. at (609) 737-0233

Open To: Individuals with Trichotillomania
Frequency: Monthly therapy group
Fee: $35 for 1 1/2 hours
*PA
Updated 1/96

Piscataway
Contact: Dr. Michael Petronko at (908) 445-5384
Open To: Individuals with obsessive-compulsive disorder
Frequency: First and third Wednesday at 7:00pm-8:30pm
Location: Rutgers University, 807 Hoes Lane
Fee: $1 donation per session
*PA
Updated 1/96

Princeton
Contact: Dr. Allen at (609) 921-3555 ext. 21 or (908) 905-3777
Open To: Individuals with obsessive-compulsive disorder, and family and friends
Frequency: Second and fourth Thursday at 7:00pm
Location: 256 Bunn Dr., Suite #6
*MH
Updated 1/96

Randolph
Contact: Christopher Lynch, Ph.D. at (201) 366-9444
Open To: Individuals with obsessive-compulsive disorder
Frequency: Tuesday at 7:00pm-8:00pm
Updated 3/96

Randolph
Contact: Karen at (908) 269-9044 or (908) 315-1912 (pager)
Open To: Individuals with obsessive-compulsive disorder, and family and friends
Frequency: Friday at 7:30pm-9:00pm
Location: Community Medical Center Auditorium "C"
*MH
Updated 4/97

Somerdale
Contact: Ruth at (609) 627-2971 (available for phone help)
Updated 1/96

Somerville
Contact: Joseph A. Donnellan, M.D. at (908) 725-5595
Open To: Individuals with obsessive-compulsive disorder, and family members
Frequency: Third Thursday at 7:30pm-9:00pm
Location: Somerset Medical Center, Fuld Auditorium
Fee: None

*PA
Updated 1/96

Sussex County
Contact: Wade or Joan at (201) 619-1207
Open To: Individuals with obsessive-compulsive disorder, and family members
Frequency: First and third Thursday at 8:00pm-9:00pm
Location: Newtom Memorial Hospital, Conference Room 239, Second Floor
*MH
Updated 1/96

New Mexico

Albuquerque
Contact: Kathleen McLellan at (505) 299-0266
Open To: Individuals with obsessive-compulsive disorder,
    and family members
Frequency: Third Thursday at 7:30pm-9:00pm
Location: Charter Heights Psychiatric Hospital, 5901 Zuni Southeast
*PA
Updated 5/97

New Hampshire

Portsmouth
Contact: Kim at (603) 778-2906
Open To: Individuals with obsessive-compulsive disorder
Frequency: Second and fourth Sunday at 7:00pm-8:30pm
Location: The Pavillion Hospital, P.H.P. Room 343, Borthwick Ave.
*MH
Updated 9/96

Portsmouth
Contact: Tom Luby at (603) 683-7991
Open To: Individuals with obsessive-compulsive disorder, and support people
Frequency: Sunday at 7:00pm-8:30pm
Also has a group in Lebanon, NH
*MH
Updated 10/97

New York

Brooklyn
Contact: Ron at (718) 624-5716
Open To: Individuals with obsessive-compulsive disorder, and family members
Frequency: Thursday at 7:00pm-8:30pm
Location: Father Demphsey Center
Format: Twelve-step OCA
Updated 10/96

Buffalo
Contact: Jerry Horowitz at (716) 881-2186
Open To: Individuals with obsessive-compulsive disorder, and family and friends
Frequency: First and third Tuesday at 7:00pm-9:00pm
Location: Bry-Lin Hospital
*MH
Updated 2/96

Buffalo
Contact: Patti at (716) 885-1106
Open To: Individuals with obsessive-compulsive disorder
Frequency: First and third Friday at 7:30pm
Location: 1272 Delaware Ave.
Format: OCA group
Updated 2/96

Buffalo
Contact: Susan Arnold Gunn at (716) 859-2703
Open To: Individuals with obsessive-compulsive disorder
Frequency: Tuesday at 7:00pm
Location: Buffalo General Hospital, Auditorium
*PA
Updated 4/97

Comack
Contact: Warren at (516) 681-7861
Open To: Individuals with obsessive-compulsive disorder, and family members
Frequency: Monday at 7:00pm-9:00pm
Location: 155 Indian Head Rd. (enter through rear building entrance)
*MH
Updated 1/96

Commack
Contact: Warren at (516) 681-7861
Open To: Individuals with obsessive-compulsive disorder, and
    family and friends
Frequency: Monday at 7:00pm-8:45pm
Location: 155 Indian Head Rd. (at Mental Health Association, Catholic Charities
    building)
*MH
Updated 5/97

Farmingdale
Contact: Linda at (516) 249-8175 or (516) 741-4901
Open To: Individuals with obsessive-compulsive disorder, and family members
Frequency: Monday at 8:00pm
Location: Brunswick Medical Center, Brunswick Hall

Format: Twelve-step therapy
Updated 1/96

Glen Oaks
Contact: Emily Klass, Ph.D. at (718) 470-3500
Open To: Parents of children with obsessive-compulsive disorder
Therapist must call first
Updated 1/92

Great Neck
Contact: Institute for Biological/Behavioral Therapy and Research at (516) 487-7116
Open To: Individuals with obsessive-compulsive disorder
Frequency: Last Friday of month at 7:30pm-9:00pm
Location: 935 Northern Blvd., Suite 102
Updated 2/96

Herkimer
Contact: Helen Hansen at (315) 866-0300, ext. 373
Open To: Individuals with obsessive-compulsive disorder
Frequency: Second and fourth Thursday at 6:30pm-8:00pm
Location: Herkimer Community College, Room 244
*MH
Updated 9/97

Hicksville
Contact: Donna at (516) 681-5091
Open To: Individuals with obsessive-compulsive disorder
Frequency: ??
Location: Parkway Community Church
Format: OCA
*MH
Updated 5/97

Huntington
Contact: Fred Penzel, Ph.D. at (516) 351-1729
C/O Western Suffolk Psychiatric Services, OCD Support and Information Group
Open To: Individuals with obsessive-compulsive disorder, and family and friends
Frequency: Friday at 7:30pm-9:00pm
Location: 755 New York Ave., Suite 200
*PA
Updated 1/96

Huntington
Contact: Christine Cannella, Ph.D. at (516) 351-1729 or (516) 424-5408
Open To: Family members of Individuals with obsessive-compulsive disorder
Frequency: Thursday at 7:30pm-9:00pm
Location: Western Suffolk Psychiatric Services

Huntington
Contact: Robert Araujo at (516) 351-1828
C/O W.S.P.S.
Open To: (1) Families of individuals with obsessive-compulsive disorder;
    (2) children of parents with obsessive-compulsive disorder and children with
    obsessive-compulsive disorder
Location: 790 New York Ave.
*PA

Huntington
Obsessive-Compulsive Post-Recovery Group
Contact: Erin at (516) 661-2718
Open To: Individuals with obsessive-compulsive disorder
    who have been in Tx
Frequency: Every other Tuesday at 7:00pm
Location: 755 New York Ave., Suite 200
*MH
Updated 2/96

Manhasset
Obsessive Compulsive Anonymous
Contact: Roy at (516) 741-4901
Location: Manhasset Congregational Church, 1845 Northern Blvd.
Format: Twelve-step program
*MH

New York City
Contact: Dr. Josephson, Ph.D. at (212) 288-2777
Dr. Josephson is interested in starting a GOAL
(Giving Obsessive-Compulsives Another Lifestyle) support group
*PA
Updated 1/96

New York City
Contact: Howard at (212) 229-1043
Frequency: (1) Monday at 6:15pm;
(2) Wednesday at 7:00pm
Location: (1) Payne Whitney, Room 129 (2) Gracie Square Hospital,
    423 East 7th St.
Format: Twelve-step OCA
*MH
Updated 2/96

New York City
Contact: Shelby Howatt, C.S.W. or Naomi Sarna, C.S.W. at (212) 865-1331
Open To: Women with Trichotillomania
Frequency: Wednesday and Thursday at 6:30pm-8:00pm

Format: Professionally Assisted group therapy
Fee: $25 per session
*PA
Updated 1/96

New York City
Contact: Naomi Sarna, C.S.W. at (212) 802-9496
Open To: Individuals with Trichotillomania
Frequency: Monthly at 1:00pm-4:00pm
Location: Washington Square United Methodist Church, 135 West 4th St.
Format: TLC group
Fee: None
Updated 1/96

New York City
Contact: Dr. Phillipson at (212) 686-8778
Institute for Behavior Clinic
Open To: Individuals with obsessive-compulsive disorder
Frequency: Tuesday at 6:45pm or Friday at 6:15pm
Format: Behavioral therapy
Fee: $25 per session
*PA
Updated 1/96

New York City
Contact: Shelly Goldberg, C.A.C. at (718) 852-2390
Interested in starting a structured therapy group for individuals who self-injure
*MH

New York City
Contact: Elizabeth Brondolo, Ph.D. at (212) 942-8532
Open To: Individuals diagnosed with obsessive-compulsive disorder (must meet with
    Dr. Brondolo prior to attending group)
Frequency: Every other Monday at 6:00pm-7:00pm
Format: Behavioral therapy group
Fee: $40
*PA
Updated 2/96

New York City
Contact: Stacie at (212) 696-8692
Open To: (1) Hoarders (packrats);
(2) Individuals with obsessive-compulsive disorder, and family members
Frequency: Tuesday at 7:00pm-8:45pm
Location: Payne Whitney Psychiatric Institute, Room #126
Fee: (2) $6 for support group meeting
Updated 2/96

New York City
Contact: Norman Levy at (212) 684-FAMI
Open To: Individuals with obsessive-compulsive disorder
Frequency: Third Thursday at 6:00pm
Location: 432 Park Ave., South, Suite 710
*MH
Updated 3/97

New York City
Contact: Joa Silvestre, C.S.W. at (212) 543-5627 or Mark Hollander, Ph.D.
    at (718) 935-7681
Open To: Individuals with obsessive-compulsive disorder who want to develop and
    practice social skills in the area of employment, relationships, and recreational
    activities
Frequency: Wednesday (20 sessions)
Updated 9/97

New York City
Contact: Marlene Cooper, Ph.D. at (212) 877-8017
Open To: Family members of individuals with obsessive-compulsive disorder
Fee: Monthly
*PA
Updated 1/97

Peekskill
Contact: Robin Goldsand at (914) 739-4029
Open To: Individuals with obsessive-compulsive disorder
Frequency: Every other Tuesday at 7:00pm
Location: 401 Claremont Ave.
Fee: $20
Format: Cognitive therapy group
*MH
Updated 10/97

Peekskill
Contact: Dr. Cantos at (516) 467-5070
Open To: Individuals with obsessive-compulsive disorder who have gone through or
    are in the process of behavioral Tx
Frequency: Last Thursday of month at 8:00pm-9:30pm
*PA
Updated 10/97

Pomona Rockland City
Contact: Self-Help Clearinghouse at (914) 639-9431
Open To: Individuals with obsessive-compulsive disorder
Frequency: Monday at 7:30pm
Location: Pomona Health Center, Room #112

*MH
Updated 1/96

Poughkeepsie
Contact: Krista at (914) 473-2500 or Chris Vertullo (email) at **CHRIS.VERTULLO
@MARIST.EDU**
LCATI Vassar Hospital, Cafeteria, First floor, Conference Room
Open To: Individuals with obsessive-compulsive disorder, and family and friends
Frequency: Second and fourth Tuesday at 7:00pm-9:00pm
*MH
Updated 9/97

Queens
Contact: Albert at (718) 441-7718
Open To: Individuals with obsessive-compulsive disorder
Frequency: Tuesday at 8:00pm
Location: St. John's University
Format: Twelve-step OCA
Updated 2/96

Rego Park
Contact: Albert at (718) 441-7718
Open To: Individuals with obsessive-compulsive disorder
Frequency: Saturday at 1:00pm-2:30pm
Location: Resurrection Ascension Church
Format: Twelve-step OCA
Updated 2/96

Rocklin
Contact: Dan Lloyd at (916) 427-3935
Open To: Individuals with obsessive-compulsive disorder
Frequency: First and third Monday at 7:00pm-9:00pm
Location: 5645 Rocklin Rd.
*MH
Updated 11/96

Ronkonkoma
Contact: Andrew at (516) 232-7429 or (516) 654-9331
Open To: Individuals with obsessive-compulsive disorder
Frequency: Monday at 8:00 pm
Location: Pace Center, 3555 Veterans Memorial Highway
Format: OCA
*MH
Updated 9/97

Schnectady
Contact: Barbara O'Connor at (518) 372-6198

Open To: Individuals with obsessive-compulsive disorder, and family members
Frequency: First Friday at 7:30pm-9:30pm
Location: Ellis Hospital, Conference Room #A6
*MH
Updated 4/97

Staten Island
Contact: Jeanine or Theresa at (718) 351-1717
Open To: Individuals with obsessive-compulsive disorder, and family members
Frequency: Second Monday at 7:30pm
Location: 308 Seaview Ave.
*MH
Updated 1/96

Syracuse
Contact: Joanne Kuneman or Carol Bass at (315) 451-6340
Open To: Individuals with obsessive-compulsive disorder,
    and family members
Frequency: Tuesday 7:30pm-9:30pm
Location: Lyncourt Wesleyan Church
*MH

Utica
Contact: Kathy at (315) 735-2370
Open To: Individuals with obsessive-compulsive disorder, and family members
Frequency: Tuesday at 6:30pm-8:00pm
Location: Mohawk Valley Community College, Room 218, College Center
*MH
Updated 9/97

Utica
Contact: Susan Connell or Scott at (315) 768-8947 or (315) 768-7031
Open To: Individuals with obsessive-compulsive disorder, and
    family members
Frequency: Monday at 6:30pm-8:00pm
Location: St. Elizabeth Hospital School of Nursing, 2215 Genesee St.
*MH
Updated 9/97

Vestal
Contact: Tim Peters at (607) 785-4621
Open To: Individuals with obsessive-compulsive disorder,
    and family members
Frequency: Thursday at 7:30pm
Location: Vestal Library
*MH
Updated 8/95

Westchester
Contact: Meryl at (914) 478-4212
Open To: Parents of children and adolescents with obsessive-compulsive disorder
Frequency: Monthly
*MH
Updated 4/97

Westchester
Contact: Charity Paul at (212) 242-7893
Open To: Individuals with obsessive-compulsive disorder and Spectrum-related disorders
Frequency: Monday or Thursday at 7:00pm-9:00pm
Location: 74 Perry St.
Fee: Sliding scale
*MH
Updated 8/97

Westchester County
Contact: Institute for Biological/Behavioral Psychiatry at (616) 487-7116
A family member of an individual with obsessive-compulsive disorder is interested
    in starting a support group for adults with obsessive-compulsive disorder in
    Westchester County, NY. If interested, call and leave your name and phone
    number. Someone will contact you
*MH
Updated 5/97

White Plains
Contact: Lisa or Sharon at (800) 345-0199
Open To: Individuals with obsessive-compulsive disorder, and family and friends
Frequency: Tuesday at 6:30pm-8:00pm
Location: 5 Waller Ave., Suite 302
Fee: $75
*PA
Updated 1/96

White Plains
Contact: Dr. Alvin Yapalater at (800) 345-0199
Open To: Individuals with obsessive-compulsive disorder, and family members
Frequency: Tuesday at 6:30pm-8:00pm
Fee: Sliding scale
*PA
Updated 8/95

White Plains
Contact: The Center for Holistic Therapy at (212) 961-1378
Open To: Individuals with obsessive-compulsive disorder
Frequency: Monthly
Updated 2/96

North Carolina

Burlington-Central Piedmont
Contact: Lisa at (910) 227-3893 (before noon)
Open To: Individuals with obsessive-compulsive disorder, and family members
Frequency: Second and fourth Wednesday at 7:00pm
Location: First United Methodist Church of Elon College, 1630 Westbrook Ave.
Updated 5/97

Charlotte
Contact: Cecil King at (704) 367-0005
Open To: Individuals with obsessive-compulsive disorder
Frequency: Wednesday at 7:00pm
Location: 1903 Charlotte Dr.
Updated 5/97

Greensboro
Contact: Robert Milan at (910) 378-1200
Open To: (1)(2) Individuals with obsessive-compulsive disorder; (3) Individuals with
    Trichotillomania
Frequency: (1)(2) Every other Thursday; (3) Every Friday and every other Wednes-
    day
Location: 200 East Bessemer Ave.
Format: Support, education, cognitive/behavior therapy
Fee: Sliding scale
*PA
Updated 5/97

Wilmington
Contact: Chris Savard, Ph.D. at (910) 763-1888
Open To: Individuals with obsessive-compulsive disorder and Spectrum disorder
Frequency: First and third Thursday at 7:00pm-8:30pm
Location: First Baptist, 1939 Independence Blvd.
Fee: None
*MH/PA
Updated 12/97

Winston-Salem
Contact: Mary Beck at (910) 722-7760
Open To: Individuals with obsessive-compulsive disorder, and family support people
Frequency: Tuesday at 7:30pm-9:00pm
Location: New Philadelphia Moravian Church, Country Club Rd.
Updated 2/96

Ohio

Cincinnati
Contact: Tami at (513) 662-3830

Open To: Individuals with obsessive-compulsive disorder, and support people
Frequency: Monday at 7:00pm
Location: Holy Name Church, Basement, 2448 Auburn Ave.
*MH
Updated 5/97

Cincinnati
Contact: Susan R. Eppley, Ed.P. at (513) 861-9797
Open To: Individuals with obsessive-compulsive disorder, and their significant others
Location: 2330 Victory Parkway
Fee: $45
Format: Behavioral/Cognitive therapy
*PA
Updated 1/96

Cleveland
Contact: Dennis Klinkiewicz at (216) 883-4801, Andrea at (216) 656-3653, or Tim at
    (216) 747-3944
Open To: Individuals with obsessive-compulsive disorder
Frequency: Monday at 7:00pm
Location: The Independence Ohio Public Library
Format: Twelve step
*MH
Updated 1/96

Cleveland
Contact: Mary Ann Miley at (216) 442-1739
Open To: Individuals with obsessive-compulsive disorder, and family and friends
Frequency: Second and fourth Thursday at 7:00pm
Location: Merida Hillcrest Hospital
*MH
Updated 5/96

Cleveland
Contact: Joyce Williams at (614) 366-2885
Open To: Individuals with obsessive-compulsive disorder, and support people
Frequency: Wednesday at 6:30pm-8:00pm
Location: Mental Health Association, Nessimer Dr., Newark, OH
Format: Combined obsessive-compulsive disorder and eating disorders
Fee: None
Updated 9/96

Cleveland
Contact: The Benhaven Program, Gene Benedetto at (216) 526-0468
Open To: Individuals with obsessive-compulsive disorder, and anxiety disorders
Frequency: Tuesday at 7:00pm
Location: Brecksville Commons Building 4, 8221 Brecksville Rd.

Fee: None
*PA
Updated 5/97

Columbus
Contact: Larry R. at (614) 444-8806 or OCA Hotline at (614) 470-0935
Open To: Individuals with obsessive-compulsive disorder, and family and friends
Frequency: Wednesday at 8:00pm
Location: 95 West Fifth Ave.
Format: OCA, OC-ANON
Updated 2/96

Cuyahoga County
Contact: Bob at (216)252-1065
Open To: Friends and family members of individuals with obsessive-compulsive disorder
*MH
Updated 1/96

Dayton
Contact: Susan Kaspi, Ph.D. at (513)220-2554 (TWTh)
Open To: Individuals with obsessive-compulsive disorders, and family and friends
Frequency: First and third Monday at 7:00pm-9:00pm
Location: Miami Valley Hospital
*PA
Updated 1/96

Marion
Contact: Amy Baldauf at (614) 387-1577
Interested in starting a support group
Updated 1/96

Parma
Contact: Mrs. Zorko at (216) 582-1310 or (216) 591-8684 (pager)
Open To: Individuals with obsessive-compulsive disorder, and family members
Frequency: Tuesday at 7:00pm-8:30pm
Location: Parma Hospital, 7007 Powers Blvd. (orientation classroom)
Call Hospital for directions at 888-1800
Updated 2/96

Toledo
Contact: Nancy at (419) 882-1602, Sally at (419) 475-6963, or Lola at
    (419) 352-6476
Open To: Individuals with obsessive-compulsive disorder, and family and friends
Frequency: Second and fourth Wednesday at 7:00pm-9:00pm
Location: Harbor Behavioral Healthcare, 4334 Secor Rd.
*MH
Updated 5/97

Oklahoma

Edmond
Contact: Joe Hale, L.P.C., Christian Growth Resources at (405) 478-8101
Open To: Individuals with obsessive-compulsive disorder
Frequency: Tuesday at 7:30pm-9:00pm
Location: 2801 East Memorial Rd. #101
Fee: $40-$50
*MH
Updated 8/97

Lawton
Contact: Stacy Winkelman at (405) 357-1457
Open To: Individuals with obsessive-compulsive disorder
*MH
Updated 1/97

Oregon

Grant Pass/Medford
Contact: Kai Bray, c/o OCF
Open To: Individuals with obsessive-compulsive disorder, and support people
*MH
Updated 10/97

Portland
Contact: Dr. James Hancey, M.D. at (503) 494-6173
Open To: Individuals with obsessive-compulsive disorder and Trichotillomania, and
    family members
Frequency: First and third Thursday at 7:00pm-8:30pm
Location: Oregon Health Science University
Individual must meet with Dr. Hancey prior to attending group
*PA
Updated 2/96

Pennsylvania

OC Foundation Philadelphia Affiliate
Contact: Marie Sirolli, V.P. at (215) 499-6425

Allentown
Contact: Marilyn Barkan at (610) 821-8929
Open To: Individuals with obsessive-compulsive disorder,
    and family members
Frequency: First and third Tuesday, at 6:30pm-7:30pm
Location: St. James Evangelical Church, 11th and Tilghman St.
Format: Twelve-step OCA
Updated 10/97

Clearfield
Contact: Ian Osborn, M.D. at (814) 765-5337
Open To: Individuals with obsessive-compulsive disorder
Frequency: First and third Monday at 2:30pm-4:00pm
Location: Clearfield-Jefferson Community Mental Health Center
Fee: None
*PA
Updated 5/97

Erie
Contact: Kimberly Morrow at (814) 838-9155
Open To: Children and adults with obsessive-compulsive disorder
Frequency: First and third Thursday at 6:30pm-7:30pm
Location: 183 West 14th St., Union Station
*PA
Updated 5/97

Indiana
Contact: Jean Clark at 465-5576 or Beverly Lindsey at 459-9558
Open To: Individuals with obsessive-compulsive disorder, and family and friends
Frequency: Thursday at 7:00pm-8:00pm
Location: Indiana City Guidance Center, 699 Philadelphia St., Suite 201
Format: Dr. Ray Hornyak will talk on the role of support groups in the treatment of
    obsessive-compulsive disorder
*MII/PA
Updated 11/97

Johnstown
Contact: Ed at (814) 536-3038
Open To: Individuals with obsessive-compulsive disorder, and
    family members
Frequency: Second Wednesday at 7:00pm-9:00pm
Location: Cornemaugh Memorial Hospital, Education Building, Room 117
*PA
Updated 10/97

Lancaster
Contact: Christina Slick at (717) 397-7461
Open To: Individuals with obsessive-compulsive disorder, and family members
Frequency: Second and fourth Wednesday at 7:00pm
Location: MHA of Lancaster City, 630 Janet Ave., Community Service Building,
    Blair Room
*MH/PA
Updated 5/97

Malvern
Contact: Connie Krasucki, R.N. at (610) 644-9749

Interested in starting a obsessive-compulsive disorder support group
Updated 2/96

Malvern
Contact: Connie Krasucki at (610) 644-9749
Open To: Individuals with obsessive-compulsive disorder
Frequency: Every other Wednesday at 7:00pm-8:30pm
Format: OCA group
Updated 10/97

Monroe County
Contact: Carol L. Denny at (717) 424-8725
Open To: Individuals with obsessive-compulsive disorder
Location: Laurel Manor Nursing Home, Living Room
Frequency: Second Tuesday
*MH
Updated 10/96

New Castle
Contact: Beverly Morosky at (412) 652-6019 or Roger Smith at (412) 658-3578
Would like to start a support group; please contact if interested
Updated 2/96

Philadelphia
Contact: Dr. Harvey Doppelt at (610) 446-8555
Open To: Family members of individuals with obsessive-compulsive disorder
Fee: $10
*PA
Updated 5/95

Pittsburgh
Contact: Joan Kaylor, M.S., Ed., at (412) 942-5448
Open To: Individuals with obsessive-compulsive disorder, and family members
Frequency: Saturday at 2:00pm-3:00pm
Location: Bethel Park
Fee: None
Updated 5/97

Rosemont
Contact: Jon Grayson Ph.D.
1062 Lancaster Ave., Suite 9, Rosemont, PA 19010
(610) 667-6490
Open To: Individuals with obsessive-compulsive disorder
Frequency: Wednesday at 8:00pm
Location: Rosemont Counseling Associates, 1062 Lancaster Ave., Suite 9, Rosemont, PA
*PA
Updated 1/96

Rosemont
Contact: Sally Allen, Ph.D. at (610) 525-1510
Open To: (1) Individuals with Trichotillomania; (2) family members
Frequency: Every other Wednesday at (1) 6:45pm-8:00pm;
    (2) 8:00pm-9:30pm
Location: Rosemont Counseling Center, Suite 9
Fee: None
*MH/PA
Updated 11/97

Rosemont
Contact: Diane Lee at (610) 525-1510
Open To: Children and adolescents with obsessive-compulsive disorder
Frequency: Every other Thursday at 7:00pm 8:00pm
Location: Rosemont Counseling Center, Suite 9
Fee: None
Updated 1/96

Rosemont
Contact: Kathy Parrish, M.A. at (610) 525-1510
Open To: Adolescents 12 to 18 years of age
Frequency: Every other Wednesday at 6:30pm-7:30pm
Location: Rosemont Counseling Associates
Fee: None
Updated 7/97

Scranton
Contact: Beverly Day at (717) 562-4044
Open To: Individuals with obsessive-compulsive disorder, and support people
Frequency: First Saturday at 2:00pm
Location: The Mental Health Association, 846 Jefferson Ave.
*MH
Updated 1/96

University Park
Contact: Ian Osborn, M.D. (CAPS Center) at (814) 863-0395
Open To: Individuals with obsessive-compulsive disorder
Frequency: Thursday at 4:00pm
Location: Ritenour Health Center, Pennsylvania State University, University Park, PA
    16803
Fee: None
*MH/PA
Updated 5/97

West Reading
Contact: Berks County Mental Health Association at (610) 376-3905 or Rusty at
    (610) 372-3080

Open To: Individuals with obsessive-compulsive disorder, and family and friends
Frequency: Wednesday at 7:30pm-9:00pm
Location: First Church of the Brethren, 2200 Bern Rd.
*MH
Updated 1/96

Wilkes-Barre
Contact: Ruth at (717) 675-5867
Open To: Individuals with obsessive-compulsive disorder, and family and friends
Frequency: Third Wednesday at 7:00pm
Location: Human Services Building, 111 North Pennsylvania Blvd., Wilkes-Barre
*MH
Updated 11/97

York
Contact: Julie Rhoades at (717) 845-6417 or Mental Health Association at
    (717) 843-6973
Open To: Individuals with obsessive-compulsive disorder, and family and friends
Frequency: Fourth Monday at 7:30pm-9:00pm
Location: Luther Memorial Evangelical Lutheran Church,
1907 Hollywood (Next to York Suburban High School)
Fee: None
*MH
Updated 5/97

Rhode Island

OCF Rhode Island Affiliate
Contact: Catherine Snell, President at (401) 635-8888
Open To: Individuals with obsessive-compulsive disorder
Frequency: First Tuesday at 7:00pm
Location: Ray Conference Center, Butler Hospital
Fee: $2 per person
*MH
Updated 10/96

South Carolina

Columbia
Contact: Kay York, M.S.W. at (803) 252-0914 or (803) 799-2406
Open To: Individuals with obsessive-compulsive disorder, and family and friends
Frequency: Third Tuesday at 6:45pm
Location: Family Connections Office
*PA
Updated 1/96

Greenville
Contact: Albert C. Bennett, M.A. at (864) 232-6216
Open To: Individuals with obsessive-compulsive disorder, and family members

Frequency: Fourth Thursday at 6:30pm-8:00pm
Fee: $10 for individuals; $15 per family
*PA
Updated 5/97

Hartsville
Contact: Jane Crowley at (803) 332-2823, Nick Menendez at (803) 383-3780,
    Lynn Jordan at (803) 332-1386, or Judy Johnson at (803) 332-3005
Open To: Individuals with obsessive-compulsive disorder, and family members
Frequency: Second Monday at 7:00pm-9:00pm
Location: St. Luke Methodist Church, 302 Dunlap Dr.
*MH
Updated 5/97

South Dakota
Rapid City
Contact: Ron Schuller at (605) 341-1261
Interested in starting a support group

Tennessee
Memphis
Contact: Hadley Hury, Executive Director at (901) 323-0633
Open To: Individuals with obsessive-compulsive disorder, and family and friends
Frequency: Every other Saturday at 10:00am-11:30am
Location: Mental Health Association of Mid-South, 2400 Poplar Ave., Suite #410
*PA
Updated 1/96

Texas
OC Foundation Texas, Inc.
Contact: Ms. Donna Friedrichs, President
P.O. Box 110
Friendswood, TX 77546
(281) 992-1555
EMAIL: WING1PRAY@AOL.COM

Arlington
Contact: Kathleen Norris, M.A. at (817) 461-5454
Open To: Individuals with obsessive-compulsive disorder
Frequency: Monday at 5:45pm
Location: 1521 North Cooper St., Suite 480
*PA
Updated 2/96

Austin
Contact: Andrew Howard at (512) 305-4548
Open To: Individuals with obsessive-compulsive disorder, and family members

Frequency: Tuesday at 7:00pm-9:00pm
Location: Please call leader for location
Updated 2/96

Dallas
Contact: OCD Association-DFW at (214) 278-0318

Fort Worth
Contact: Bette Bolles at (817) 336-1112
Interested in starting a support group for individuals with obsessive-compulsive
    disorder and family members
Updated 2/96

Houston
OC Foundation of Texas, Inc.
Contact: Donna Friedrich, President at (713) 482-2147
Open To: Individuals with obsessive-compulsive disorder, and family and friends
Frequency: Second and fourth Thursday at 7:30pm-9:30pm
Location: Memorial Southwest Hospital, 7600 Beechnut, Level C (1) Room E;
    (2) Room C
*MH
Updated 10/97

San Antonio
Contact: Rick at (210) 816-2019
Phone Support Only
Updated 9/96

San Antonio
Contact: Penny Cooperider at (210) 614-9595 or Jean McRae at (210) 614-9597
Open To: Individuals with obsessive-compulsive disorder who have been evaluated
    by Dr. Nathan
Frequency: Tuesday at 4:00pm-5:30pm
Location: 2829 Babcock Rd., Suite #640
Fee: $65
*PA
Updated 1/96

INTERNATIONAL LIST

Australia

Mutual Help Groups
Attn: Barbro Gill-Larsson
Chairman
Queensland: Friendship House
Rikstoreningen Ananke

20 Balfour St., Box 7003
New Farm, Qld. 4005 S-172 07 Sundbyberg Sweden
Tel. (07) 358-4224, (08)628-3030 tel&fax# E-MAIL-ANANKE3@ODATA.SE
    HTTP://WWW.ODATA.SE/HOTEL/ANANKE/ANANKE.HTML
Updated 5/97

North Sydney
Anxiety Disorders Foundation of Australia
P.O. Box 6198
Shopping World
NSW 2060
(016) 282 897
Fax (02) 9716 0416 (F)

Wallsend
South Australia: Room 55, Epworth Building
Tel. (09) 385-7081\
Frequency: Weekly
Western Australia: Co-ordinator

Brazil

Protoc
Rus Dr. Ouslio
Pires de Caupo S/NE
Instituto de Psipuistio
30 A SALA 4025
5403-010
Phone: 55-11-2809198
Fax: 55-11-2800842
E-MAIL: MIGUELEX@USP.BR

Canada

Coquitlam, British Columbia
Contact: Truman Spring at (604) 522-8593 or Fax at (604) 522-8501
Open To: Parents of children with obsessive-compulsive disorder and individuals with
    obsessive-compulsive disorder
Location: 2773 Barnet Highway
Frequency: Once a month at 7:00pm-9:00pm
*PA
Updated 11/97

Etobicoke
Contact: Tom at (905) 472-0494
Open To: Individuals with obsessive-compulsive disorder
Frequency: Second and last Wednesday at 7:30pm
Location: Our Lady of Sorrows School, 32 Montgomery Rd.

*MH
Updated 10/97

London
Contact: Jim Wallis at (519) 644-2368
Open To: Individuals with obsessive-compulsive disorder, and family members
Frequency: First Tuesday at 7:00pm-9:00pm
Location: 648 Huron St.
*MH
Updated 5/97

Winnepeg, Manitoba
Contact: Calvin at (204) 947-4514 (voicemail)
Open To: Individuals with obsessive-compulsive disorder and anxiety disorder
Frequency: Wednesday at 6:00pm-7:30pm
Location: Health Action Center, 425 Elgin Ave., Second Floor
OCAD/The Obsessive-Compulsive and Anxiety Disorders and Akin Matters Association
*MH
Updated 1/96

Winnipeg, Manitoba
OC Information and Support Center
C/O Manitoba Clearinghouse
Contact: Marie at (204)772-6979 or Fax at (204) 786-0860
Frequency: Second and fourth Tuesday at 7:00pm-9:00pm
Location: 825 Sherbrook St.
*MH
Updated 9/97

North Bay
Contact: Larry at (705) 497-9460
Open To: Individuals with obsessive-compulsive disorder
Frequency: Thursday at 7:00pm
Location: 163 First Ave. East
*MH
Updated 10/97

Sydney, Nova Scotia
Contact: Fred Chezenko at (902)733-3018
Open To: Individuals with obsessive-compulsive disorder, and
    family members
Frequency: Once a month at 7:00pm-9:00pm
Location: McConnel Library
*MH
Updated 5/97

Newmarket, Ontario
Contact: Marianne Small at (905)836-4777 or EMAIL:
    GSMALL@SYMPATICO.CA
(Website–HTTP://WWW3.SYMPATICO.CA/gsmall/nmktocd/)
Open To: Individuals with obsessive-compulsive disorder, and significant others
Frequency: First and third Monday at 7:30pm
*MH
Updated 12/97

Ontario
Contact: Obsessive-Compulsive Disorder Network (OCCDN)
P.O. Box 151
Markham, Ontario L3P 3J7
(905) 472-0494
Open To: Individuals with obsessive-compulsive disorder
*MH
Updated 10/97

Ontario
Contact: Denise at 462-4807
Open To: Individuals with obsessive-compulsive disorder
Frequency: Wednesday at 6:30pm (except two weeks during Christmas)
Location: Grey Nuns Hospital, The Level 0 Auditorium, 1100 Youville Dr. West
*MH
Updated 10/97

Ottawa, Ontario
Contact: Rolland Boisvenu at (613)722-3607
Frequency: Second Wednesday at 7:30pm-10:00pm
Location: The Hintonburg Community Center, Champlain Room, Wellington St.
*MH
Updated 11/97

Pickering, Ontario
Contact: Free From Fear or The Anxiety Disorders Network at (905) 831-3877; 1848
    Liverpool Rd., Suite 199, Pickering, Ontario L1V 6M3 Canada
*MH
Updated 10/97

Toronto, Ontario
Contact: Jan Stewart at (416) 364-0222
Open To: Parents of children with obsessive-compulsive disorder
Location: Hospital for Sick Children
*PA
Updated 10/97

Unionville, Ontario
Contact: Diane at (905) 472-0494; EMAIL: OOCDM@INTERHOP.NET
Open To: Individuals with obsessive-compulsive disorder
Frequency: First and third Thursday at 7:30pm
Location: St. Justine Lamarter Church, 3898 Highway 7
*MH
Updated 10/97

Windsor, Ontario
Contact: Family YMCA, P.A.T.H. PROGRAM at (519) 258-9622 ext. 57 or 58
Open To: Individuals with obsessive-compulsive disorder, and family and friends
Frequency: Second and fourth Thursday at 7:00pm-9:00pm
Location: 511 Pelissier
*MH
Updated 1/96

Montreal, Quebec
Contact: Stephanie Aylwin, Ami Quebec at (514) 486-1448
Open To: Individuals with obsessive-compulsive disorder, and family and friends
Frequency: Two groups a month
Location: AMI QUEBEC
Format: Psychoeducational
*MH
Updated 10/97

Kitchener, Waterloo
Contact: Astride at (519) 746-9644 or EMAIL: ABSILIS@SCIBORG.
    WATERLOO.CA
Open To: Individuals with obsessive-compulsive disorder, and family members
Frequency: Second and fourth Wednesday at 7:00pm
Location: Adult Recreation Centre, 185 King St. South
*MH
Updated 10/97

France

Contact: Marc Lalvee
Association Francaise Des Toc
Et Du Syndrome Gilles De La Tourette
24, Rue Leon Gambetta 59790 Ronchin
Newsletter, Referrals OCD & TS SPECIALISTS
Updated 6/93

India

Maharashtra State
Thane (West)400601-B/103-Cent.
Contact: Dr. Anand Nadkarni at the Institute for Psychological Handicapped

Format: Behavioral therapy group; "Perfect Group"; and 6-week Educational/Behavioral therapy group

Italy

Paolo L. Morselli, M.D. at (39) 02-65-3994 or Fax (39) 02-65-4716
IDEA
Via Statuto 8
20121 Milano

Puerto Rico

NAMI III OF PR
P.O. BOX 902
2569 VIEJO SAN JUAN
P.R. 00902
(787) 745-1760
(787) 743-8475
EMAIL: PRAMI5185@AOL.COM
Contact: Silvia Arias
Sao Paolo, Brazil
(5511) 280.9198
(5511) 280.0842 (F)
Astoc
Associado de Portadores de
Sindrome de Tourette, Tiques e Trastornos
Obsessivo Compulsivo
Contact: Maria C. De Luca
Pereira, Presidente
Rua Dr. Ovidio Pires De
Campos, S/N SALA 4025

Scotland

Contact: Jamie Booth
1277 Dumbarton Rd.
Glasgow, Scotland G1R 9VY
Ms. Booth is starting a group for individuals with obsessive-compulsive disorder
Updated 7/97

South Africa

Houghton
Contact: Janet Serebro, Chairperson
OCD Association of South Africa
P.O. Box 87127
Houghton, 2041
(011) 887-3678
(Fax) (011) 786-6617
O.C.D.S.G.

P.O. Box 4195
Christ church
366-0560
Open to: Individuals with obsessive-compulsive disorder
Frequency: Wednesday at 7:30pm
Updated 5/97

Sweden

Ananke Foundation
Mistelgatan 7
722 25 Vasteras
SWEDEN
EMAIL:KENNETHE@FRYX.VASTERAS.SE
Contact: Kenneth Erickson at 46-21-183132 or Fax 46-21-411305

United Kingdom

England
Durham Health Centre Chester
Contact: Kathleen Savory at 091-3891765
Open To: Individuals with anxiety-related problems
Frequency: Tuesday

England
First Steps to Freedom
22 Randall Rd.
Kenilworth, Warwickshire CV8 1JY
Contact: Helpline Telephone Numbers at Warwick Line: (0926) 851608
    Darbyshire: (0332) 760982
This Charity aims to help phobics, anxiety sufferers, sufferers from obsessive-
    compulsive disorders, and their carers, as well as those who wish to come off of
    tranquillizers

England
Contact: Terri Conley
Wallsend Self Help Group
P.O. Box 5
Wallsend
Tyne & Wear
NE28 6DZ
ENGLAND
Open to: Patients with obsessive-compulsive disorder and Tourette's disorder

England/Bath
Contact: Celia Bonham Christie at (0225) 314129
Advisor: Prof. I.M. Marks, M.D.
Open To: Individuals with phobia or obsessive-compulsive disorder

Frequency: Thursday at 6:30pm
Location: Royal National Hospital for Rheumatic Diseases (The Main Upper Boro Walls)
Format: Structured self-help group using living with fear

England/Worcester Park Surrey
Contact: Sue Scerri at 081-337-2362
Open To: Individuals with obsessive-compulsive disorder, and support people
Frequency: Monday at 8:00pm-10:00pm
Location: A Centre in Mitcham Surrey
Fee: 30 per session
Updated 10/91

England/London
Contact: Laura Olivieri
Administrator/Editor
P.O. Box 6097
London W2 1W2
England
Open To: Individuals with obsessive-compulsive disorder, and family members
Updated 5/96

New South Wales: Mental Health Info. 62 Victoria Rd Gladsville, NSW 2111.
Tel. (07) 816-5688
Victoria: Mental Health Centre
1 Cookson St.,
Ccamberwell, Vic. 3124
Tel (03) 813-3736
Contact: Terri Conley at (091) 262-9678
33 Pirie St.
Adelaide, SA 5000
Tel. (08) 231-1588 or
(08) 362-6772

South Wales
Contact: D.M. Bonney at (0446) (722941)
Open To: Individuals with obsessive-compulsive disorder with a referral by a Mental Health Professional, and family members
Frequency: Tuesday at 7:00pm-8:30pm
New Members Admitted First Tuesday of each month
Location: The Elms Centre, Four Elms St., Cardiff S.,
Glamorgan, South Wales, UK
*MH
Updated 11/97

Appendix 7
Maudsley Obsessive-Compulsive Inventory

The Maudsley obsessive-compulsive inventory (MOCI) is a useful instrument to give at or prior to initial evaluation to identify various types of obsessive-compulsive disorder symptoms. We usually only use this for initial history-gathering and use Y-BOCS initially and at subsequent visits to follow treatment response to medication or behavior therapy.

MAUDSLEY OBSESSIVE-COMPULSIVE INVENTORY

Please answer each question by circling "true" or "false." There are no right or wrong answers and no trick questions. Work quickly and do not think about the exact meaning of the question.

1. I avoid using public telephones because of possible contamination.
   True   False
2. I frequently get nasty thoughts and have difficulty in getting rid of them.
   True   False
3. I am more concerned than most people about honesty.
   True   False
4. I am often late because I can't seem to get through everything on time.
   True   False
5. I don't worry unduly about contamination if I touch an animal.
   True   False
6. I frequently have to check things (e.g., gas or water taps, doors) several times.
   True   False
7. I have a very strict conscience.
   True   False
8. I find that almost every day I am upset by unpleasant thoughts that come into my mind against my will.
   True   False
9. I do not worry unduly if I accidentally bump into somebody.
   True   False

10. I usually have serious doubts about the simple everyday things I do.

| True | False |

11. Neither of my parents was very strict during my childhood.

| True | False |

12. I tend to get behind in my work because I repeat things over and over again.

| True | False |

13. I use only an average amount of soap.

| True | False |

14. Some numbers are extremely unlucky.

| True | False |

15. I do not check letters over and over again before mailing them.

| True | False |

16. I do not take a long time to dress in the morning.

| True | False |

17. I am not excessively concerned about cleanliness.

| True | False |

18. One of my major problems is that I pay too much attention to detail.

| True | False |

19. I can use well-kept toilets without any hesitation.

| True | False |

20. My major problem is repeated checking.

| True | False |

21. I am not unduly concerned about germs and diseases.

| True | False |

22. I do not tend to check things more than once.

| True | False |

23. I do not stick to a very strict routine when doing ordinary things.

| True | False |

24. My hands do not feel dirty after touching money.

| True | False |

25. I do not usually count when doing a routine task.

| True | False |

26. I take rather a long time to complete my washing in the morning.

| True | False |

27. I do not use a great deal of antiseptics.

| True | False |

28. I spend a lot of time every day checking things over and over again.

| True | False |

29. Hanging and folding my clothes at night does not take up a lot of time.

| True | False |

30. Even when I do something very carefully, I often feel that it is not quite right.

| True | False |

Appendix 8

Yale-Brown Obsessive-Compulsive Scale

The Yale-Brown Obsessive-Compulsive Scale (Y-BOCS) is useful for quantifying level of obsessive-compulsive disorder symptoms and for following response to treatment. It is not a diagnostic tool. It is also important to ask patients about avoidance, because they may have low level of symptoms but may be avoiding everything that sets off their symptoms.

1. Time occupied by obsessive thoughts

0 = None

1 = Mild (less than 1 hour/day), or occasional intrusion (occur no more than eight times a day).

2 = Moderate (1 to 3 hours/day), or frequent intrusion (occur more than eight times a day, but most hours of the day are free of obsessions).

3 = Severe (greater than 3 and up to 8 hours/day), or very frequent intrusion (occur more than eight times a day and occur during most hours of the day).

4 = Extreme (greater than 8 hours/day), or near-constant intrusion (too numerous to count and an hour rarely passes without several obsessions occurring).

2. Interference caused by obsessive thoughts

0 = None
1 = Mild, slight interference with social or occupational activities, but overall performance not impaired.
2 = Moderate, definite interference with social or occupational performance, but still manageable.
3 = Severe, causes substantial impairment in social or occupational performance.
4 = Extreme, incapacitating.

3. Distress associated with obsessive thoughts

0 = None
1 = Mild, infrequent, and not too disturbing.
2 = Moderate, frequent, and disturbing, but still manageable.
3 = Severe, very frequent, and very disturbing.
4 = Extreme, near-constant, and disabling distress.

4. Resistance against obsessive thoughts

0 = Makes an effort to always resist, or symptoms so minimal doesn't need to actively resist.
1 = Tries to resist most of the time.
2 = Makes some effort to resist.
3 = Yields to all obsessions without attempting to control them, but does so with some reluctance.
4 = Completely and willingly yields to all obsessions.

5. Control over obsessive thoughts

0 = Complete control.
1 = Much control, usually able to stop or divert obsessions with some effort and concentration.
2 = Moderate control, sometimes able to stop or divert obsessions.
3 = Little control, rarely successful in stopping obsessions, can only divert attention with difficulty.

4 = No control, experienced as completely involuntary, rarely able to even momentarily divert thinking.

6. Time spent performing compulsions

0 = None

1 = Mild (less than 1 hour/day performing compulsions), or occasional performance of compulsive behaviors (no more than eight times a day).

2 = Moderate (1 to 3 hours/day performing compulsions), or frequent performance of compulsive behaviors (more than eight times a day, but most hours are free of compulsive behaviors).

3 = Severe (spends more than 3 and up to 8 hours/day performing compulsions), or very frequent performance of compulsive behaviors (occur more than eight times a day and compulsions performed during most hours of the day).

4 = Extreme (spends more than 8 hours/day performing compulsions), or near-constant performance of compulsive behaviors (too numerous to count and an hour rarely passes without several compulsions being performed).

7. Interference caused by compulsive behaviors

0 = None

1 = Mild, slight interference with social or occupational activities but overall performance not impaired.

2 = Moderate, definite interference with social or occupational performance, but still manageable.

3 = Severe, causes substantial

impairment in social or occupational performance.

4 = Extreme, incapacitating.

8. Distress associated with compulsive behaviors

0 = None

1 = Mild, only slightly anxious if compulsions prevented, or only slight anxiety during performance of compulsions.

2 = Moderate, reports that anxiety would mount but remain manageable if compulsions were prevented, or that anxiety increases but remains manageable during performance of compulsions.

3 = Severe, prominent and very disturbing anxiety if compulsions interrupted, or prominent and very disturbing anxiety when performing compulsions.

4 = Extreme, incapacitating anxiety from any intervention aimed at modifying activity, or incapacitating anxiety develops during performance of compulsions.

9. Resistance against compulsions

0 = Makes an effort to always resist, or symptoms so minimal doesn't need to actively resist.

1 = Tries to resist most of the time.

2 = Makes some effort to resist.

3 = Yields to all compulsions without attempting to control them, but does so with some reluctance.

4 = Completely and willingly yields to all compulsions.

10. Degree of control over compulsive behaviors

0 = Complete control.

1 = Much control, experiences pressure to perform the behavior, but usually able to voluntarily control it.

2 = Moderate control, strong pres-

sure to perform behavior, must
be carried to completion, can
only delay with difficulty.
3 = Little control, very strong
drive to perform behavior,
must be carried to completion,
can only delay with difficulty.
4 = No control, drive to perform
behavior experienced as completely involuntary and over-
powering, rarely able to even
momentarily delay activity.

Appendix 9

Beck Depression Inventory

Instructions: Use as a screening tool for all patients. Give to patient to fill out. Tell them to put down most fitting response for each letter.

A. (Sadness)
   0. I do not feel sad
   1. I feel sad
   2. I am sad all the time and I can't snap out of it
   3. I am so sad or unhappy that I can't stand it
B. (Pessimism)
   0. I do not feel particularly discouraged about the future
   1. I feel discouraged about the future
   2. I feel I have nothing to look forward to
   3. I feel that the future is hopeless and that things cannot improve
C. (Sense of failure)
   0. I do not feel like a failure
   1. I feel I have failed more than the average person
   2. As I look back on my life, all I can see is a lot of failures
   3. I feel I am a complete failure as a person
D. (Dissatisfaction)
   0. I get as much satisfaction out of things as I used to
   1. I don't enjoy things the way I used to
   2. I don't get any real satisfaction out of anything anymore
   3. I am dissatisfied or bored with everything
E. (Guilt)
   0. I don't feel particularly guilty
   1. I feel guilty a good part of the time
   2. I feel quite guilty most of the time
   3. I feel guilty all of the time

F. (Sense of punishment)

    0. I don't feel I am being punished

    1. I feel I may be punished

    2. I expect to be punished

    3. I feel I am being punished

G. (Self-dislike)

    0. I don't feel disappointed in myself

    1. I am disappointed in myself

    2. I am disgusted with myself

    3. I hate myself

H. (Self-accusations)

    0. I don't feel I am any worse than anybody else

    1. I am critical of myself for my weaknesses or mistakes

    2. I blame myself all the time for my faults

    3. I blame myself for everything bad that happens

I. (Self-harm)

    0. I don't have any thoughts of killing myself

    1. I have thoughts of killing myself but I would not carry them out

    2. I would like to kill myself

    3. I would kill myself if I had the chance

J. (Crying spells)

    0. I don't cry any more than usual

    1. I cry more now than I used to

    2. I cry all the time now

    3. I used to be able to cry but now I can't even cry, although I want to

K. (Irritability)

    0. I am no more irritated now than I ever am

    1. I get annoyed or irritated more easily than I used to

    2. I feel irritated all the time now

    3. I don't get irritated at all by the things that used to irritate me

L. (Social withdrawal)

    0. I have not lost interest in other people

    1. I am less interested in other people than I used to be

    2. I have lost most of my interest in other people

    3. I have lost all of my interest in other people

M. (Indecisiveness)

    0. I make decisions about as well as I ever could

    1. I put off making decisions more than I used to

    2. I have greater difficulty in making decisions than before

    3. I can't make decisions at all any more

N. (Self-image change)

    0. I don't feel I look any worse than I used to

    1. I am worried that I am looking old or unattractive

   2. I feel there are permanent changes in my appearance that make me look unattractive
   3. I believe that I look ugly
O. (Work difficulty)
   0. I can work about as well as before
   1. It takes extra effort to get started at doing something
   2. I have to push myself very hard to do anything
   3. I can't do any work at all
P. (Sleep disturbance)
   0. I can sleep as well as usual
   1. I don't sleep as well as I used to
   2. I wake up 1 to 2 hours earlier than usual and find it hard to get back to sleep
   3. I wake up several hours earlier than I used to and cannot bet back to sleep
Q. (Fatigability)
   0. I don't get any more tired than usual
   1. I get tired more easily than I used to
   2. I get tired from doing almost anything
   3. I am too tired to do anything
R. (Anorexia)
   0. My appetite is no worse than usual
   1. My appetite is not as good as it used to be
   2. My appetite is much worse now
   3. I have no appetite at all any more
S. (Weight loss)
   0. I haven't lost much weight, if any, lately
   1. I have lost more than 5 pounds
   2. I have lost more than 10 pounds
   3. I have lost more than 15 pounds
   I am purposely trying to lose weight by eating less: Yes   No
T. (Somatic preoccupation)
   0. I am no more worried about my health than usual
   1. I am worried about physical problems such as aches and pains, upset stomach, or constipation
   2. I am very worried about physical problems and it's hard to think of much else
   3. I am so worried about my physical problems, I cannot think about anything else
U. (Loss of libido)
   0. I have not noticed any recent change in my interest in sex
   1. I am less interested in sex than I used to be
   2. I am much less interested in sex now
   3. I have lost interest in sex completely

Appendix 10
Obsessive-Compulsive Disorder Clinic Brochure

Dear Patient, Family Member, or Clinician:

Thank you for inquiring about our clinic. You have no doubt contacted us because you, your patient, or someone close to you suffers from obsessive-compulsive disorder (OCD) or a related disorder such as trichotillomania, Tourette's disorder, or body dysmorphic disorder (BDD). As you may already know, these disorders are believed to be neurologic disorders that are reinforced by certain behaviors and aggravated by stressors in our lives. They often exist in conjunction with other problems such as depression and anxiety.

We are a clinical research and treatment unit for OCD and related disorders. The doctors on our staff are also teachers at Harvard Medical School. Our psychiatrists, psychologists, and clinical research associates are among the most experienced clinicians in the world.

In addition to open treatment, we have a number of special clinical research programs for which patients may qualify. These programs have some valuable benefits, which often include free treatment in the form of medication and other therapies.

We have a policy of reviewing each individual case even before the patient is scheduled for an evaluation. This review gives the clinic doctors an idea about the possible direction of care for each prospective patient. Although a fee is charged for the complete initial evaluation, there is no charge for the confidential telephone intake interview or the preliminary case review by the clinicians.

In the past, we have been an important part of the research that led to the Food and Drug Administration approval of clomipramine (Anafranil), sertraline (Zoloft), fluvoxamine (Luvox), paroxetine (Paxil), and fluoxetine (Prozac). Our clinical psychologists, who are among the most experienced behavior therapists, have made contributions to the behavioral treatment of these disorders.

In an effort to unravel the causes of these disorders, we also are performing neuroimaging studies of the brain by means of positron emission tomography and magnetic resonance imaging scans. We are developing communications systems by which patients will not only be able to tell us how they are doing symptomatically on a given day, but also will be able to partake of behavioral treatment by telephone without leaving their homes. These are just a few of our current research studies.

We hope you will assist us as we continue to break new ground into discovering the causes and establishing more effective treatments. If you qualify for some of our free research programs, your participation will not only help us find out how best to treat your disorder, but also will help us learn how to treat future patients more effectively. In this way, you will be adding to the personal contributions of the thousands of patients who have allowed us, and centers like ours across the country, to discover the currently used effective treatments. In some of the research studies done here, professionals from the OCD clinic review information from charts. Reports of these research studies never identify an individual patient by name. The people who review the charts are bound by the same confidentiality obligations as the clinician who is evaluating or treating you.

Our primary goal is to help you overcome your disorder. To that end, we enthusiastically look forward to working with you. If you have any questions about our clinic that you would like to discuss before you come in for an evaluation, do not hesitate to call or write us. We also recommend contacting the Obsessive-Compulsive Foundation at 9 Depot Street, P.O. Box 70, Milford, Connecticut 06460-0700 or by phone at 203-878-5669 for further information about OCD and related disorders. They also can be reached by electronic mail: jphs28@prodigy.com. There is also a local Obsessive-Compulsive Foundation affiliate that has a help line, which can be reached by calling 617-376-3784.

Sincerely,

OCD Clinic Staff

Appendix 11

Obsessive-Compulsive Disorder Clinic Initial Evaluation Form

OCD CLINIC INITIAL EVALUATION INFORMATION

Patient name: _____ Evaluation date: _____

Type of obsessive-compulsive disorder: Checking _____
                                           Washing_____
                                           Obsessions_____
                                           Bowel obsessional_____
                                           Urine obsessional _____
                                           Face picking _____
                                           Slowness _____
                                           Others _____
                                           _____

Mental status: Appearance:

                                        Depression:

                                        Psychosis:

                                        Cognition:

                                        Anxiety:

Current medications:

Seizure history:

Insurance:

Diagnosis: Axis I: _____

_____

Axis II: _____

_____

Axis III: _____

_____

Other impressions:

Recommendations:

Test Scores

Y-BOCS: 1 __, 2 __, 3 __, 4 __, 5 __, 6 __, 7 __, 8 __, 9 __, 10 __, Total ____

MAUDSLEY: _____

BECK: _____

CAT scan: _____

EEG: _____

NMR: _____

PET: _____

SIDP: _____

SIDP minus 1: _____

Appendix 12
Yale-Brown Obsessive-Compulsive Scale Symptom Checklist

The Yale-Brown Obsessive-Compulsive Scale Symptom Checklist is useful for systematically identifying obsessive-compulsive disorder symptoms

YALE-BROWN OBSESSIVE-COMPULSIVE SCALE SYMPTOM CHECKLIST

Circle only those symptoms that have bothered you during the past week or that have ever bothered you in the past.

Aggressive Obsessions

Past week	Ever	Fear I might harm myself
Past week	Ever	Fear I might harm other people
Past week	Ever	Violent or horrific images in my mind
Past week	Ever	Fear blurting out obscenities or insults
Past week	Ever	Fear doing something else embarrassing
Past week	Ever	Fear I will act on an unwanted impulse (like stabbing a friend)
Past week	Ever	Fear I will steal things
Past week	Ever	Fear I will harm others because of not being careful enough
Past week	Ever	Fear I will be responsible for something else terrible happening (e.g., fire, burglary)
Past week	Ever	Other:

Contamination Obsessions

Past week	Ever	Concerns or disgust with bodily waste or secretions (e.g., urine, feces, saliva)

Past week	Ever	Concern with dirt or germs
Past week	Ever	Excessive concern with environmental contaminants (e.g., asbestos, radiation, toxic waste)
Past week	Ever	Excessive concern with household items (e.g., cleansers, solvents)
Past week	Ever	Excessive concern with animals (e.g., insects)
Past week	Ever	Bothered by sticky substances or residues
Past week	Ever	Concern that I will get ill
Past week	Ever	Concern that I will get others ill
Past week	Ever	Other:

Sexual Obsessions

Past week	Ever	Forbidden or perverse sexual thoughts, images, or impulses
Past week	Ever	Content involves children or incest
Past week	Ever	Content involves homosexuality
Past week	Ever	Sexual behavior toward others
Past week	Ever	Other:

Hoarding/Saving Obsessions

| Past week | Ever |

Religious Obsessions (Scrupulosity)

Past week	Ever	Concerned with sacrilege and blasphemy
Past week	Ever	Excess concern with right/wrong or morality
Past week	Ever	Other:

Obsession with Need for Symmetry or Exactness

| Past week | Ever |

Miscellaneous Obsessions

Past week	Ever	Need to know or remember
Past week	Ever	Fear of saying certain things
Past week	Ever	Fear of not saying just the right thing
Past week	Ever	Fear of losing things
Past week	Ever	Intrusive (neutral) images
Past week	Ever	Intrusive nonsense sounds, words, or music
Past week	Ever	Bothered by certain sounds/noises
Past week	Ever	Lucky/unlucky numbers
Past week	Ever	Colors with special significance
Past week	Ever	Superstitious fears
Past week	Ever	Other:

Somatic Obsessions

| Past week | Ever | Concern with illness or disease |

Past week	Ever	Excessive concern with a body part or aspect of appearance (e.g., dysmorphophobia)
Past week	Ever	Other:

Cleaning/Washing Compulsions

Past week	Ever	Excessive or ritualized handwashing
Past week	Ever	Excessive or ritualized showering, bathing, toothbrushing, grooming, or toilet routine
Past week	Ever	Excessive cleaning of household items or other inanimate objects
Past week	Ever	Other measures to prevent or remove contact with contaminants
Past week	Ever	Other:

Checking Compulsions

Past week	Ever	Checking that I did not/will not harm others
Past week	Ever	Checking that I did not/will not harm self
Past week	Ever	Checking that nothing terrible did/will happen
Past week	Ever	Checking that I did not make a terrible mistake
Past week	Ever	Checking tied to somatic obsessions
Past week	Ever	Other:

Repeating Rituals

Past week	Ever	Rereading or rewriting
Past week	Ever	Need to repeat routine activities (e.g., in/out door, up/down from chair)
Past week	Ever	Other:

Counting Compulsions

Past week	Ever

Ordering/Arranging Compulsions

Past week	Ever

Hoarding/Collecting Compulsions

Past week	Ever

Miscellaneous Compulsions

Past week	Ever	Mental rituals (other than checking/counting)
Past week	Ever	Need to tell, ask, or confess things
Past week	Ever	Need to touch, tap, or rub
Past week	Ever	Measures (not checking) to prevent: harm to self; harm to others; terrible consequences

Past week	Ever	Ritualized eating behaviors
Past week	Ever	Superstitious behaviors
Past week	Ever	Pulling hair out
Past week	Ever	Other self-damaging or self-mutilating behaviors
Past week	Ever	Other

Index

869